QM Medical Libraries

24 1006931 4

ST BARTHOLOMEW'S AND THE ROYAL   C   N
'OOL OF MEDICINE AN
IBRA

GENETICS
in Obstetrics
and Gynecology

THIRD EDITION

GENETICS
in Obstetrics
and Gynecology

Joe Leigh Simpson, MD
Ernst W. Bertner Chairman and Professor
Department of Obstetrics and Gynecology
Professor, Department of Molecular and
    Human Genetics
Baylor College of Medicine
Houston, Texas

Sherman Elias, MD
G. William Arends Chair and
Phillip C. and Beverly Goldstick Professor
Head, Department of Obstetrics and Gynecology
Professor, Department of Molecular Genetics
University of Illinois at Chicago
Chicago, Illinois

SAUNDERS
An Imprint of Elsevier Science

SAUNDERS
An Imprint of Elsevier Science

The Curtis Center
Independence Square West
Philadelphia, Pennsylvania 19106

GENETICS IN OBSTETRICS AND GYNECOLOGY   ISBN 0–7216–4164–4
Copyright © 2003, Elsevier Science (USA)

All rights reserved. No part of this publication may be reproduced, stored in a retrieval system, or transmitted, in any form or by any means, electronic, mechanical, photocopying, recording, or otherwise without written permission of the publisher.

Notice

Obstetrics is an ever-changing field. Standard safety precautions must be followed, but as new research and clinical experience broaden our knowledge, changes in treatment and drug therapy may become necessary or appropriate. Readers are advised to check the product information currently provided by the manufacturer of each drug to be administered to verify the recommended dose, the method and duration of administration, and contraindications. It is the responsibility of the treating physician, relying on experience and knowledge of the patient, to determine dosages and the best treatment for each individual patient. Neither the Publisher nor the authors assume any liability for any injury and/or damage to persons or property arising from this publication.

THE PUBLISHER

First Edition 1982. Second Edition 1992.

SBRLSMD

CLASS MARK	QZ50 SIM
CIRC TYPE	ORD
SUPPLIER	CISL 161263 £62.99
READING LIST	
OLD ED CHECK	

EXPO/MVY

Printed in the United States of America

Last digit is the print number: 9 8 7 6 5 4 3 2 1

▼

We dedicate this book to our sons

Reid Steven Simpson and Scott Alan Simpson

Benjamin Artman Elias and Kevin Meyer Elias

Preface ▼

•

The three editions of *Genetics in Obstetrics and Gynecology* have appeared at approximately 10-year intervals: 1982, 1992, 2003. Although honesty dictates that these hiatuses did not really reflect the authors' foresight, in retrospect such intervals seem salutary. The intervals covered prior to each edition could be imagined as representing the different epochs of integrating genetics into clinical obstetrics and gynecology. In the Preface to this first edition, it thus sufficed merely to state that advances in genetics had truly impacted the practice of obstetrics and gynecology and could be expected to continue. This reflected the first edition being published, only half a decade after the clinical acceptance of genetic amniocentesis (1976). Relatively few gynecologic disorders were even suspected of heritable tendencies, and whether this was even due to genes was arguable to some. The chromosomal basis of spontaneous abortions was appreciated, but in general, few clinicians thought genetic testing could facilitate diagnosis or provide information on causation. Save for advanced maternal age, genetic screening was mostly preconceptional. By the second edition in 1992, genetic etiology and genetic counseling had been firmly accepted, indeed codified in the curriculum of obstetrics and gynecology training. Many diagnostic standards had been set, genetic screening was routine for selected Mendelian and cytogenetic disorders and all pregnant women were routinely offered either invasive or noninvasive screening for chromosomal abnormalities. First trimester prenatal genetic diagnosis by chorionic villus sampling had been shown to be safe and efficacious; preimplantation genetic diagnosis had recently been accomplished. More portentous, molecular technology (e.g., polymerase chain reaction, PCR) allowing for future advances had been developed barely half a decade earlier, yet already the first clinical fruits were recognized. The sex-determining region Y (SRY) had been identified as the long elusive testicular-determining factor, and genes causing a few Mendelian disorders (e.g., cystic fibrosis) had first been laboriously localized by positional cloning and then sequenced in their entirety. However, molecular tools were still inchoate and high throughput analysis just a hope. The impact of genetics and molecular biology on gynecologic disorders may still have seemed distant to many.

A decade since this last edition, the time of this third edition finds both the general public and physicians alike anxious to pick the fruits of the modern molecular era. The problem is now less evoking genetic vision or justifying once fanciful hypotheses than controlling the media hype and the public's unrealistic near-term expectations. Still, the "laboratory to bedside" interval has never been shorter. Noninvasive prenatal genetic diagnosis has continued to become more sensitive and specific; preimplantation genetic diagnosis is no longer simply boutique medicine, but an integral part of contemporary prenatal genetic diagnosis. Not only can fetal cells in maternal blood be recovered and analyzed, but cell-free fetal DNA offers additional diagnostic promise. Many common gynecologic disorders and a host of the disorders of sex differentiation are well on the way to molecular elucidation. Cancer is universally accepted as a genetic disease, even while the specific genes and mutagens affecting these genes continue to be sought. Increasingly, specific genes are identified whose disturbance leads to a specific clinical disorder. Leiomyomas often involve perturbations of the gene HMGI-C (high mobility group protein IC) or (in Reed syndrome) the Krebs cycle gene fumarate hydrolase (FH). One form of transverse vaginal septum is caused by a mutation in a chaperonin gene (MKKS), which probably acts by directing protein folding. Incomplete müllerian fusion when part of the hand-foot-genital (HGF) syndrome is caused by mutation of the developmental (homeobox) gene HOXA13. The relevance of genetics to clinical obstetrics and gynecology has long since evolved from speculation to explanation, diagnostic application and, in the foreseeable future, doubtless therapy.

These and other advances make this a propitious time for the new third edition of *Genetics in Obstetrics and Gynecology*, not just to reflect on past accomplishments but to prepare us for those that ineluctably will follow. Quickly. The 2001 success in sequencing the human genome is the obvious touchstone. Yet while the number of human genes is now known to be 30,000–40,000, we have evidence of function for only about 5,000. These discrepant numbers hint just where we stand in the evolution of molecular medicine. Given experience of the past decade, however, the velocity of knowledge acquisition will be rapid and the trajectory of its clinical application steep. Imagine the altered landscape of medicine once the remaining 80–90% of genes are elucidated and their gene products (medicine) available!

Despite the authors' exuberance for genetics now being more widely shared, the purpose of *Genetics in Obstetrics and Gynecology* remains the same. As both geneticists and obstetricians-gynecologists, we seek to provide a practical volume on genetics that relates to the clinical practice of obstetrics/gynecology and women's health care. We assume no prior knowledge of genetics, even while realizing younger physicians are increasingly well versed. Our goal remains to provide the practicing physician – in particular the obstetrician-gynecologist – with sufficient material in a single volume to handle most genetic problems that arise in one's practice. Of course, this text is not at all intended to encompass the much greater body of knowledge that is needed by those fewer obstetrician/gynecologists for whom genetics is their primary discipline.

Each chapter has been thoroughly revised, and the entire book written exclusively by the two of us. We have expanded almost all chapters to accommodate the many recent advances. In order to maintain a reasonable book length, we have chosen not to cover teratogenic agents in this edition. Other texts cover this topic in depth. Neither this nor previous editions seek to discuss techniques or criteria for ultrasonographic diagnosis of fetal anomalies. Works by many of our obstetrical colleagues handsomely provide this information. Genetically as well, some readers may wish to consult more general volumes for broader genetic principles or, conversely, more focused coverage of a specific field of human genetics. This especially applies to pediatric disorders and adult onset genetic disorders that are not predominately gynecologic in nature.

We gratefully acknowledge the many professional colleagues who have served as mentors or awarded us so many rich opportunities. In particular, the two of us worked in the 1970s and 1980s with Drs. Albert Gerbie and Henry L. Nadler while at Northwestern University. Dr. Gerbie was a pioneer in development of genetic amniocentesis and Dr. Nadler in amniotic fluid analysis for prenatal diagnosis of genetic disorders. Together they seamlessly melded obstetrics and genetics, a visionary and defining concept at the time. We were privileged to be part of this exciting beginning for reproductive genetics. Other colleagues have been sentinel in our academic development: James L. German (Cornell Medical College) as an incomparable mentor to one of us (JLS); Fritz Fuchs (Cornell Medical College), John T. Queenan (then of University of Louisville), Roy T. Parker (Duke University) as Chairmen during our years of training; John J. Sciarra (Northwestern University) and Robert L. Summitt (University of Tennessee, Memphis) as leaders who generously created space and provided resources to facilitate our endeavors.

We acknowledge the superb clerical assistance of our staff at Baylor College of Medicine (Belinda Felder, Lan Baumann). In particular, Ms. Felder deserves a flotilla of kudos for her clerical coordination and editorial oversight. She prepared the entire text and references, and held sway over the myriad of details that are necessary in a volume of this type. We also acknowledge the editorial assistance and support of Elsevier Science by Ms. Judith Fletcher, Executive Publisher, and the production staff at Bermedica Production, Ltd. (Ms. Berta Steiner).

Joe Leigh Simpson, M.D., Houston, Texas
Sherman Elias, M.D., Chicago, Illinois

CHAPTER 1

Chromosomal Abnormalities

Chromosomal abnormalities are a major cause of congenital anomalies, reproductive loss, and gynecologic disorders. Both numerical and structural changes exist, the latter in particular having the secondary effect of distributing mendelian genes. In this chapter we discuss the principles underlying chromosomal abnormalities as well as methods to identify and analyze abnormalities.

Chromosomal Identification

A characteristic number of chromosomes exists in each species. In humans, there are 46 chromosomes in all nuclei except germ cells: 22 pairs of autosomes (no. 1.2) and one pair of sex chromosomes (XX in females, XY in males). Figure 1–1 shows a cell arrested in mitosis (metaphase).

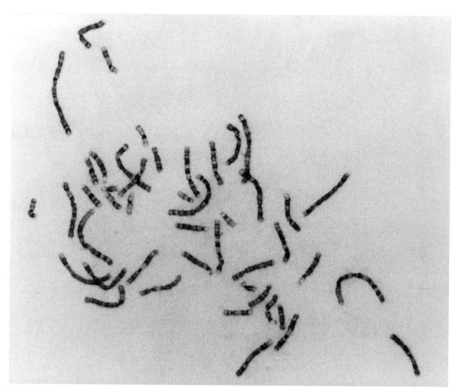

FIGURE 1–1 • Metaphase derived from a normal female (46,XX, G-banding technique). (From Simpson JL, Tharapel AT: Principles of human cytogenetics. *In* Philipp E, Setchell M (eds): Scientific Foundations of Obstetrics and Gynaecology, 4th ed. London: Butterworth-Heinemann, 1991.)

Figure 1–2 shows chromosomes aligned by pairs (karyotype). Chromosomes are numbered according to size and centromere position. The centromere divides the chromosome into a short arm (p) and a long arm (q). The relative centromeric position permits chromosomes to be classified morphologically as *metacentric* (p and q equal in length), *submetacentric* (q slightly greater than p), *acrocentric* (q much greater than p, the centromere nearly terminal), or *telocentric* (the centromere terminal) (Fig. 1–3).

Banding techniques permit identification of specific chromosomes or parts of chromosomes, as illustrated in Figures 1–1 and 1–3. The first banding technique involved staining chromosomes with quinacrine, followed by fluorescent microscopy (Q-banding). Many other methods later became available, with the general category of G-banding techniques (see Figs. 1–1 and 1–2) most widely used. Some banding techniques identify telomeric regions and others identify centromeric regions. Some identify only certain chromosomes.

Cytogenetic Nomenclature

An official chromosomal nomenclature exists (ISCN:1985; ISCN:1995). According to this nomenclature, the chromosomal complement is designated in the following manner:

1. The total number of chromosomes (e.g., 46 or 47).
2. A comma.
3. The sex chromosomal complement (XY in normal males; XX in normal females).
4. The specific abnormality, if any.

A normal male chromosomal complement is thus designated 46,XY (Table 1–1). A complement containing an abnormal number of chromosomes is designated by listing the total number of chromosomes and the appropriate sex chromosomal complement. For example, 45,X is the complement most commonly associated with Turner syndrome. A complement containing additional or missing autosomes is signified by

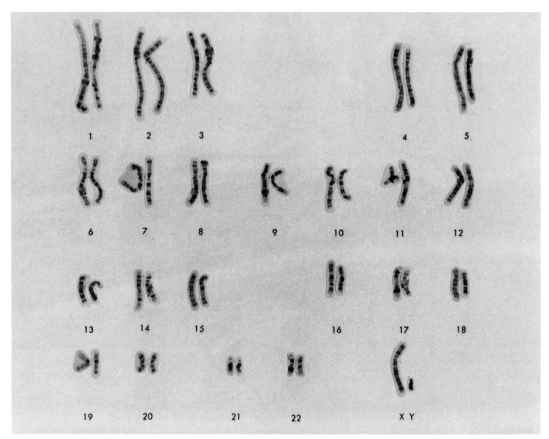

FIGURE 1–2 • Metaphase derived from a normal male (46,XY) G-banding techniques. (From Simpson JL, Tharapel AT: Principles of human cytogenetics. *In* Philipp E, Setchell M (eds): Scientific Foundations of Obstetrics and Gynecology, 4th ed. London: Butterworth-Heinemann, 1991.)

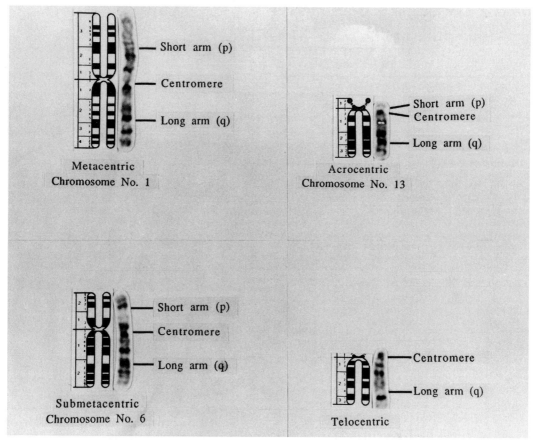

FIGURE 1–3 • Parts of chromosome bands illustrating actual and schematic chromosomes having different arm ratios. Bands are numbered from centromere to telomere, beginning with 1.0. The short arm is abbreviated p and the long arm is abbreviated q. (From Simpson JL, Tharapel AT: Principles of human cytogenetics. *In* Philipp E, Setchell M (eds): Scientific Foundations of Obstetrics and Gynaecology, 4th ed. London: Butterworth-Heinemann, 1991.)

▼ **Table 1–1.** EXAMPLES OF CORRECT
• NOMENCLATURE FOR CHROMOSOMAL
COMPLEMENTS, PARIS CONFERENCE (1971)
AND SUPPLEMENT (1975)

Official Designation	Description
46,XY	Normal male karyotype
46,XX	Normal female karyotype
45,X	Monosomy X
47,XXX	Polysomy X
47,XY, +21	Trisomy 21
46,XX, 1q+	Increase in length of the long arm of No. 1
46,X,del(X)(p21) or 46,X,del(X)(qter→p21:)	Terminal deletion of the short arm of X distal to band 21
46,X,i(Xq) or 46,X,i(X)(qter→qter)	Isochromosome of the long arm of X
46,X,r(Y)	Ring Y chromosome
46,X,t(X;3)(q21;q31)	Balanced translocation between band 21 of the long arm of X and band 31 of the long arm of No. 3
45,X/46,XX or mos 45,X/46,XX	45,X/46,XX mosaicism

+ or – followed by the specific chromosome responsible. A male with trisomy 21 (Down syndrome) is designated 47,XY,+21; a female with monosomy 21 is designated 45,XX,–21. Placing + or – signs after a symbol indicates an increase in the length of chromosome (e.g., 46,XX,+8q+). Complements containing structurally abnormal chromosomes require the symbol for the aberration present as well as the number of the aberrant chromosome(s).

Table 1–2 lists symbols used to designate parts of chromosomes and certain rearrangements. Chromosome bands are designated as shown in Figure 1–3. A band is designated by listing sequentially the chromosome, the arm (p or q), the region, and finally the specific band. Bands are numbered consecutively from the centromere distally. Standardized methods to designate translocations and other rearrangements are reviewed elsewhere in greater detail (ISCN, Basel, 1985).

▼ **Table 1–2.** SYMBOLS USED TO DESIGNATE
• CHROMOSOMAL STRUCTURE,
RECOMMENDED FIRST BY THE PARIS
CONFERENCE (1971) AND ITS SUPPLEMENT
(1975)

Centromeres	cen
Short arm	p
Long arm	q
Isochromosome	i
Deletion	del
Translocation	t
Reciprocal translocation	rcp
Mosaicism	mos
Chimerism	chi
Ring	r
Dicentric	dic
Duplication	dup
Inversion	inv
Break without reunion (e.g., terminal deletion)	:
Break and join	::
From ... to ...	→

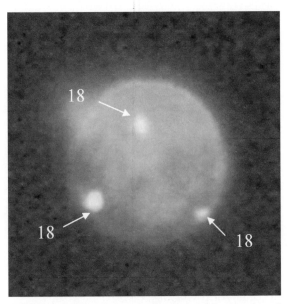

FIGURE 1–4 • FISH fluorescent in situ hybridization of a cell showing signals for the three No. 18 chromosomes. (Preparation of Dr. Farideh Bischoff, Baylor College of Medicine, Houston, Texas.) *See Color Plate*

In 1995, updated nomenclature provided instructions for higher resolution banding, bands increasingly having the need to be subdivided (ISCN, Mitelman, 1995). A decimal is placed after the original band designation, followed by the number assigned to each new subband, e.g., 1q11.1. Further subdivisions follow sequences such as 1q11.11, 1q11.12, 1q11.13. Systems exist to communicate results of in situ hybridization (ISH), with or without the concomitant complete chromosomal complement (see Table 1–2).

Conventional Chromosomal Analysis

Chromosomal analyses are usually performed on peripheral blood (lymphocytes) or fibroblasts cultured from skin, gonads, chorionic villi (mesenchyme), or amniotic fluid cells. Very rapidly dividing cells (e.g., bone marrow, chorionic villi, trophoblasts, fetal cord blood, cord blood, or cancer cells) may sometimes be analyzed without culturing. Rapid techniques have also been developed to yield metaphases from neonatal cord blood or percutaneous umbilical cord blood. However, this is now largely supplemented by fluorescent *in situ* hybridization (FISH) analysis using chromosome-specific probes (Fig. 1–4). Results can produce results within hours. A special advantage is that FISH can be performed on nondividing (interphase) cells, (see later on), whereas metaphase preparations requires dividing cells. Use of different fluores and combina-

tions of fluores permits the assessment of several different chromosomes in a single nucleus. FISH is limited by providing information only on the chromosomes or chromosome regions tested. This may suffice if a specific disorder (e.g., trisomy 21 or 18) must be excluded; however, the information obtained is obviously more limited than in complete chromosomal analysis. On the other hand, in fetal cell analysis (see Chapter 17) and preimplantation genetic diagnosis (see Chapter 16), FISH is virtually the only cytogenetic technique applicable.

If cells are to be cultured to yield dividing cells, nutrient media are used, to which fetal calf serum, perhaps antibiotics, and perhaps growth factors are added. A period of growth specific for a given tissue exists: overnight for bone marrow, cord blood, and chorionic villi trophoblasts; 48 to 72 hours for peripheral blood; and 7 to 14 days for chorionic villi mesenchyme or amniotic fluid cells. Preparation of cells for chromosomal analysis usually requires the sequential addition of (1) colchicine or desoxymethylcolchicine, (2) a hypotonic solution that causes cells to swell, (3) an acetic acid–methanol fixative, and (4) a dye to enhance chromosome visibility. In the past, metaphases were photographed, photographic prints developed, and individual chromosomes cut out and aligned. Automated systems can now produce karyotypes directly from metaphases.

Irrespective of the method, karyotypes portray realigned chromosomes rather than the original metaphase. Analysis generally constitutes counting 20 to 25 cells and karyotyping perhaps two to five. Not all cells remain intact. Some are damaged ("broken") artifactually in preparation and show spurious hypodiploid counts. Hyperdiploid counts are less likely to be spurious. Unless a consistent pattern of chromosome loss or gain is observed, no clinical significance is ascribed. This seemingly tedious point is clinically relevant to obstetricians because approximately 2% of chorionic villi or amniotic fluid specimens contain one or more spurious cells.

Sometimes two or more cell lines exist in a single person. The cytologic basis of this phenomenon (mosaicism) is discussed later, but it is relevant to note here that the likelihood of detecting mosaicism depends not only on the frequency of the minority cell line but also on the number of cells analyzed. In turn, this frequency reflects not only the stage of embryogenesis at which mosaicism originates but also whether any of the cell lines has a selective disadvantage or advantage. The number of cells necessary to exclude a minority cell population with a given level of confidence depends on the statistical power desired to exclude a minority cell. For example, analysis of 50 cells excludes (P <0.05) a minority line of 10% or more. More cells would be required to exclude a minority line of 5%. Mosaicism is naturally more likely to be detected if multiple tissues and many cells are studied, but routine analysis of more than one tissue is not practical. If mosaicism is suspected (e.g., gonadal dysgenesis), it may be advisable to analyze 50 or more cells from each of several tissues. In straightforward prenatal cytogenetic diagnosis in pregnant woman over the age of 34 years, it usually suffices to analyze 20 to 25 cells from a single tissue (amniotic fluid or chorionic villi). If the initial analysis raises suspicion (e.g., two non-model cells with the same complement), additional cells should be analyzed.

Routine cytogenetic analysis usually reveals about 450 to 500 bands per haploid set of chromosomes. Using high-resolution chromosome analysis, it is often possible to obtain resolution of about 1000 bands. At this level each band consists of approximately 3000 to 4000 kilobases (kb) of DNA (3,000,000 to 4,000,000), an amount capable of translating perhaps 30 to 40 genes. Deletions, duplications, and rearrangements involving considerable amounts of DNA can thus pass undetected even with high-resolution chromosome analysis.

Organization of DNA Within The Nucleus

The human diploid (2n = 46) nucleus contains approximately 3×10^9 base pairs of DNA. Three thousand base pairs occupy 1 m; thus, 1×10^6 m is the total length of DNA per nucleus. Since nucleus is only 10 μm in diameter, obviously a mechanism must exist for packaging DNA. Integral to DNA packaging are histone proteins, present virtually unchanged throughout the animal kingdom. There are several types of histones: H1, H2A, H2B, H3, H4. Two units each of all histones except H1 form a core structure called a nucleosome, a cylinder about 8 × 11 nm in size. Around each nucleosome is wound, in two turns (Fig. 1–5A), approximately 140 base pairs of DNA. Another 60 base pairs bridge adjacent nucleosomes, assisted by histone H1. Overall, five nucleosomes exist per 1000 base pairs of DNA. The average gene consists of many individual nucleosomes and their linker DNA segments. For this reason, the structure of the gene has been likened to beads on a string.

At the next level of packaging, beads become arranged into cylindrical form (solenoid) (Fig. 1–5B). These progressively supercoiled packages eventually aggregate into a chromatin fiber and finally into a visible chromosomal band (Fig. 1–6).

Unique Sequence Versus Repetitive DNA

The DNA (repetitive and unique sequences) that actually codes for proteins is called *unique sequence* DNA. Usually only a single copy of the nucleotide sequence codes for a given protein (e.g., enzyme), although some genes are present in duplicate (e.g., α-globin on chromosome 16). DNA characterized by other types of sequences also exist, and in fact constitute by far the majority of human DNA. The nucleotide sequence in most DNA is *repetitious*, that is, too repetitious to code for structures as complex as proteins. An example of a nucleotide sequence consisting of no repetitious sequences would be ATATATAT or (AT_n). The function of highly repetitive sequences is not known, but dispersement of DNA of this type among unique DNA sequences suggests a role in DNA packaging (see earlier). Nucleotide sequences are sometimes only *moderately repetitive*. Such sequences are capable of coding for simple compounds like histones or

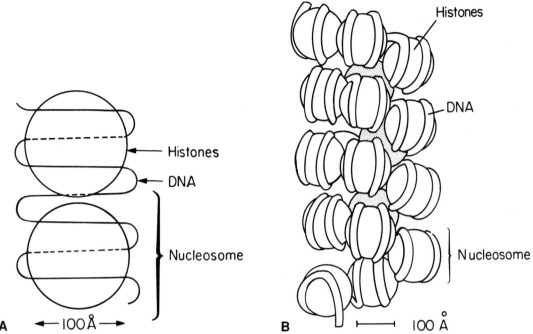

FIGURE 1–5 • *A*, DNA coiling around the histone core. The core is composed of two molecules each of histones H2A, H2B, H3, H4. The DNA and its histone core constitute a nucleosome. *B*, Nucleosomes are then progressively supercoiled and compacted, eventually aggregating into a chromatin factor. (Prepared by Simpson JL: Genetics. Basic Science Monograph in Obstetrics and Gynaecology. Washington, DC: Council on Resident Education in Obstetrics and Gynecology, 1986.)

ribosomes. The various types of DNA are integrated throughout the genome. Unique sequences within a single gene are separated from one another by noncoding sequences, the latter called intervening sequences or *introns*. Coding sequences are *exons*. A given protein is thus characterized by discontinuous unique sequence DNA, interrupted by sequences of DNA that do not code for amino acids. Repetitive sequences are doubtless of functional (spatial) importance in their own right, but serve invaluable diagnostic roles by existence of polymorphic markers, used for linkage analysis. This is applicable for gene localization and diagnosis when the presence or absence of a mutant gene must be assessed but the precise molecular perturbation is not known. The polymorphisms used are most often dinucleotide or trinucleotide repeats AT_n, where (n) could be 5, 7, 9, or other with nearly equal frequencies. Chapter 2 discusses this topic in greater detail.

Mechanism of Chromosomal Banding

The aggregation of different types of DNA—unique sequence, moderately repetitious, highly repetitious—in a given chromosomal region is reflected by chromosomal banding. Positive G- and Q-bands predominantly represent moderately or highly repetitious DNA, particularly AT-rich sequences. Positive C-bands represent highly repetitious DNA. By contrast, positive R-bands and negative G- or Q-bands are more likely to represent relative aggregates of unique sequence DNA (i.e., DNA coding for proteins). Not surprisingly, perturbations in positive R-band regions (negative G- or Q-bands) carry greater clinical consequences than aberrations involving repetitious DNA.

Molecular Cytogenetics: Fluorescent In Situ Hybridization (FISH), Chromosome Painting, Comparative Genome Hybridization (CGH)

As already alluded to, exciting advances have resulted from merging molecular techniques with traditional cytogenetics. The basic principle is first identifying a DNA sequence specific for a given chromosome and then rendering the

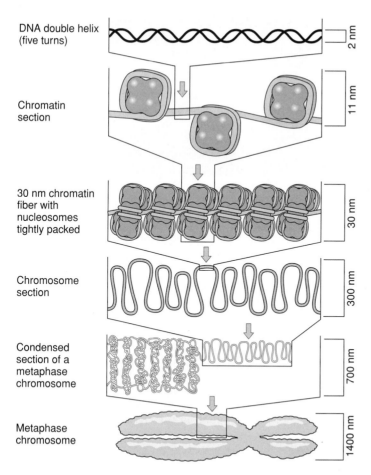

DNA double helix (five turns) — 2 nm

Chromatin section — 11 nm

30 nm chromatin fiber with nucleosomes tightly packed — 30 nm

Chromosome section — 300 nm

Condensed section of a metaphase chromosome — 700 nm

Metaphase chromosome — 1400 nm

FIGURE 1–6 • Relationship between DNA double helix, nucleosomes, and metaphase chromosome. (From Passarge E: Color Atlas of Genetics. New York: Thieme Medical Publishers, Inc., 1995.)

sequence fluorescent for cytologic identification. With in situ hybridization (ISH) or fluorescent *in situ* hybridization (FISH), a single-stranded DNA probe will hybridize to its complementary DNA sequence if the latter is present (see Fig. 1–4). The DNA probe may be labeled directly with a fluorochrome or labeled indirectly. If labeled indirectly, another compound (e.g., biotin) is attached to the probe, and it is this compound that is capable of conjugating with a fluorochrome. If the probe is directly labeled, the fluore intercalates into the DNA. In either case, FISH can be used to derive information from interphase cells (e.g., uncultured amniotic fluid cells).

Chromosome-specific probes can be used to determine chromosomal status of interphase nuclei. Using different fluores allows simultaneous analysis of more than one chromosome in a given interphase cell. At least three is routine and five is readily possible (Iitsuka et al., 2001). Moreover, more than five different chromosomes can be assessed at any given time. Rehybridization is especially applicable for preimplantation genetic diagnosis to exclude aneuploidy.

▼ **Table 1–3.** NOMENCLATURE FOR IN SITU
• HYBRIDIZATION (ISH)

FISH	Fluorescent In Situ Hybridization
ISH	In situ hybridization; when used without a prefix, applies to chromosomes (usually metaphase or prometaphase) of dividing cells
nuc ISH	Nuclear interphase ISH
−	Absent from a specific chromosome
+	Present in a specific chromosome
++	Duplication of a specific chromosome
x	Multiplication sign; precedes the number of signals seen
.	Period; separates cytogenetic observations from results of ISH
;	Semicolon; separates probes on different derivative chromosomes

An official nomenclature exists for FISH (ISCN, 1995). In Table 1–3, symbols for a variety of complicated circumstances are provided (e.g., split or separated signals). However, the general rules remain simple. Absence of a signal for a specific chromosome is indicated by −, presence of a signal by +, and duplication by

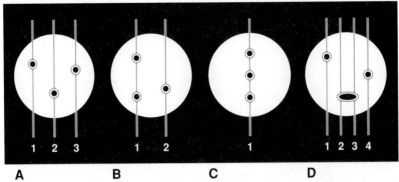

FIGURE 1–7 • Diagram showing geometric vicissitudes of FISH analysis. If two or more cells overlie one another, only a single signal will be evident. The number of signals will appear as fewer than the number of chromosomes. In plane a all three signals are visible. In planes b and c one would score only 2 or 1 signal, respectively. If a chromosome is dividing (d), it may be scored more than once. (Preparation of Dr. Farideh Bischoff, Baylor College of Medicine, Houston, Texas.)

++. If multiple signals are present, a multiplication sign (x) precedes the number of signals seen. Nuclear or interphase *in situ* hybridization is designated nuc ish. Moreover, adherence to rigid criteria is necessary in screening cells. For example, focusing on more than one plane is necessary to detect all signals and avoid misinterpretation (Fig. 1–7). Care must be taken not to record dividing chromatids (split domain) as two different signals (chromosomes). Strict adherence to definitions is crucial.

Mixing varying proportions of the limited number of primary fluorescent colors (fluores) can produce enough distinct colors to allow identification of all 22 autosomes and the sex chromosomes (X,Y). This is termed spectral karyotyping (SKY) (Fig. 1–8). The fluorochromes used can be nonisotopic. This technique is especially useful for identifying rearrangements not easily recognizable on high resolution karyotypes. The principle is that an unexpected color on a given chromosome would indicate a previously unsus-

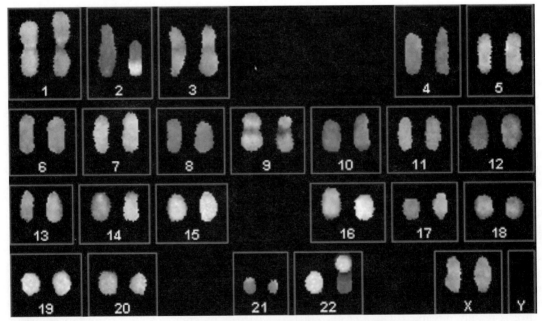

FIGURE 1.8 • Spectral karyotyping (SKY). The power of spectral karyotyping is demonstrated by the identification of a rearrangement between chromosomes 2 and 22. Note that a portion of chromosome 2 has exchanged places with a portion of chromosome 22. Each chromosome is characterized by its own color, a kaleidoscope that is not appreciated in this black and white illustration. (From Jorde LB, Carey JC, Bamshad MJ, et al.: Medical Genetics, 2nd ed. St. Louis: Mosby, 2000. Courtesy of Dr. Art Brothman, University of Utah Health Sciences Center.) *See Color Plate*

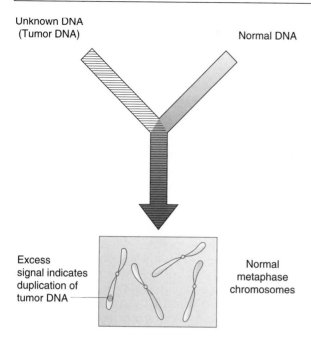

Unknown DNA
(Tumor DNA)

Normal DNA

Excess
signal indicates
duplication of
tumor DNA

Normal
metaphase
chromosomes

FIGURE 1–9 • Comparative genomic hybridization (CGH). In an experiment, green-labeled test DNA (from an unknown sample) and red-labeled reference DNA (from normal cells) would both hybridized to normal metaphase chromosomes. (Mere green is indicated by horizontal lines, red by light stippling.) The ratio of green to red signals on the hybridized metaphase chromosomes indicates the location of duplications (excess green) or deletions (excess red) in the tumor chromosomes. (From Jorde LB, Carey JC, Bamshad MJ, et al.: Medical Genetics, 2nd ed. St. Louis: Mosby, 2000.)

pected excess of DNA. Cancer cytogeneticists find spectral karyotyping especially useful.

The availability of sequence-specific DNA probes that can be amplified by PCR and tagged with fluorochrome reporter molecules has bridged the gap between microscope and molecule. Probes can be constructed enabling hybridization of specific chromosomal regions or even of a single gene. In chromosomal painting composite probes can be coupled with suppressive hybridization to allow selected whole chromosomes or chromosomal segments to be "painted" and uniquely visualized. This technique can be more easily subtle rearrangements or deletions exist.

A variant of this technique is comparative genome hybridization (CGH). A metaphase or interphase nucleus from a normal individual is labeled with a fluore of one color (e.g., red in Figure 1–9). DNA from an unknown specimen labeled with a different fluore (e.g., green in Figure 1–9) is then added. If the DNA content is equal in reference and unknown, the result is uniformly yellow (red plus green). If the unknown has more DNA than the reference (e.g., trisomic), an area of green highlight will exist; if deletion exists, the highlight will be red.

X Chromatin and X Inactivation

One of the two X chromosomes in normal females is the last chromosome in the comple-

ment to complete DNA synthesis, presumably reflecting the tighter condensation during interphase of this X compared with the other X chromosome. The late-replicating X is termed the heterochromatic X. During interphase it forms a planoconvex body, termed X-chromatin (Fig. 1–10). Synonymous terms include sex chromatin or Barr body. In diploid cells the number of X-chromatin masses equals the number of X-chromatin masses minus one. Information about sex chromosomes can obviously be deduced by analyzing interphase nuclei.

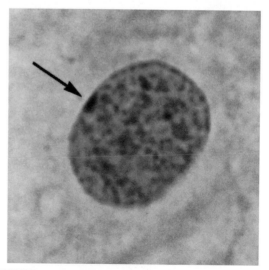

FIGURE 1–10 • X-chromatin (arrow). (From Simpson JL: Disorders of Sexual Differentiation: Etiology and Clinical Delineation. New York: Academic Press, 1976.)

Much but not all of the heterochromatic X chromosome in humans is genetically inactive, a relationship first elucidated by Lyons (1961) (Lyon hypothesis). X inactivation occurs at least by the time of implantation, if not before. The X chromosome (maternal or paternal) inactivated in a given cell is random, provided both X chromosomes are normal (Fig. 1–11). After a given X becomes inactivated, however, all descendants of that cell maintain the identical pattern. Because X inactivation occurs only after the embryo contains hundreds of cells, normal females have two populations of cells. In one population the maternal X is active; in the other the paternal X is active. It is theoretically possible that in every single cell the same X (maternal or paternal) would be independently chosen for inactivation; however, the statistical likelihood of such an event approaches zero. If 100 cells exist when X inactivation is initiated, the probability of the maternal X's always being inactivated approaches zero ($1/2^{100}$).

In humans, some loci on the heterochromatic (inactive) X remain active, especially those on the distal short arm. Ovarian maintenance determinants located on both the X short arm and the X long arm (see Chapter 10) are important exceptions, but many other noninactivated genes have ostensibly nothing to do with reproduction. To date, 275 of the 1500–3000 X loci outside the pseudoautosomal region (Yp-Xp) have been assessed to determine whether they are inactivated. Of these 275, 43 escape inactivation, all but 3 on Xp.

X inactivation does not occur in germ cells. Over 40 years ago, electrophoretic studies of oocytes from females heterozygous for glucose-6-phosphate dehydrogenase (G-6-PD) showed a G-6-PD-A band, a G-6-PD-B band, and the dimer indicating active synthesis of both G-6-PD-A and G-6-PD-B (Gartler et al., 1972). Thus, both X chromosomes were active in oocytes, potentially explaining the deleterious effect of a 45,X complement in which only a single X existed. Finally, in certain extraembryonic tissues, X inactivation is *not* random. In the placenta the paternal X is always active.

X inactivation depends upon a gene located on Xq13, the gene product of which is XIST. The inactive X shows peripheral location within the cell (see Fig. 1–10), nuclease insensitivity, and hypermethylated CpG islands and nonacetylated histones. A novel chromatin protein called Barr-d1 (Barr body deficient) proved deficient in the inactive X and X-chromatin mass (Barr body). The protein is related to histone H2A (Chadwick et al., 2000). The inactive X is coated with more XIST RNA than the active X. Although X inactivation and methylation are integrally related, methylation is not necessarily the primary event.

Y Chromosome

The Y is a submetacentric chromosome slightly longer than chromosomes 21 and 22. The distal two thirds of the Y long arm (Yq) are brilliantly fluorescent (positive Q-bands); this region is also

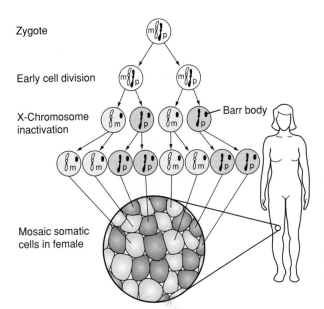

FIGURE 1–11 • X-inactivation. The maternal (m) and paternal (p) X chromosomes are both active in the zygote and in early embryonic cells. X inactivation then takes place, resulting in cells having either an active paternal X or an active maternal X. Females are thus X-chromosome mosaics, as shown in the tissue sample at the bottom of the figure. (From Jorde LB, Carey JC, Bamshad MJ, et al.: Medical Genetics, 2nd ed. St. Louis: Mosby, 2000.)

Zygote

Early cell division

X-Chromosome inactivation

Barr body

Mosaic somatic cells in female

C-band positive. The Y varies in length from person to person, variant Y chromosomes being either unusually long or unusually short. Varying fluorescent portions of Xp are responsible for this polymorphism. The lengths of Yp and non-fluorescent Yq are relatively constant in a given family, whereas the length of the fluorescent portion of the Yq varies in direct proportion to the total length of the Y. The fluorescent region can be absent in otherwise normal people; thus, this region must not be crucial for normal testicular and somatic development. Existence of the fluorescent region permitted Y-containing cells to be identified during interphase long before chromosome-specific probes became available (Fig. 1–12). Nonfluorescent Yp contains the gene (*SRY*) directing male sex differentiation, whereas genes pivotal to spermatogenesis (*DAZ*) are located on nonfluorescent Yq (see Chapter 10).

The number of Y chromosomes is equal to the amount of Y chromatin per interphase cell. A caveat is that regions of autosomal fluorescence may be mistaken for Y chromatin; thus, sex determination should now be made on the basis of complete cytogenetic analysis or chromosome-specific DNA probes rather than on the basis of Y-chromatin analysis alone. Much older literature is derived from use of Y-chromatin. Y-specific DNA probes have now supplanted Y-chromatin analysis. Y- probes utilize unique sequence (e.g., SRY-specific DNA sequences or alphoidcentromeric repeats that are chromosome-specific).

X- or Y-specific probes can also complement metaphase analysis. A good example is using X- or Y-probes to determine the origin of a minute sex chromosomal marker (X or Y fragment) found in chorionic villi or amniotic fluid cells.

Cell Division

Mitosis

Mitosis is the process by which daughter cells receive identical copies of their parental cells' genome. Several distinct stages of mitosis exists, even though each occupies only a small portion of the cell cycle.

Cell Cycle

Periods of the cell cycle are designated gap 1 (G1), synthesis (S), gap 2 (G2), and division or mitosis (D) (Fig. 1–13). G1 is usually the longest part of the cycle. During this period, nucleotides, amino acids, proteins, and other substances are accumulated in preparation for DNA replication. DNA synthesis occurs during S, at the end of which the DNA content is doubled. Before S, each chromosome consists of a single chromatid. After S, each chromosome consists of two sister chromatids connected at their single centromere. After completion of DNA synthesis, a relatively short resting period (G2) lasts until mitosis.

Although it is continuous and lacking well-demarcated points, mitosis is in turn traditionally divided into four stages: prophase, metaphase, anaphase, and telophase (Fig. 1–14).

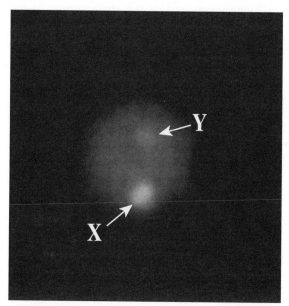

FIGURE 1–12 • FISH showing signals for X and Y chromosomes. (Preparation of Dr. Farideh Bischoff, Baylor College of Medicine, Houston, Texas.) *See Color Plate.*

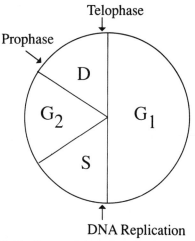

FIGURE 1–13 • Stages of the cell cycles. G_1, gap 1; S, synthesis; G_2, gap 2; D, division. (From Simpson JL: Disorders of Sexual Differentiation: Etiology and Clinical Delineation. New York: Academic Press, 1976.)

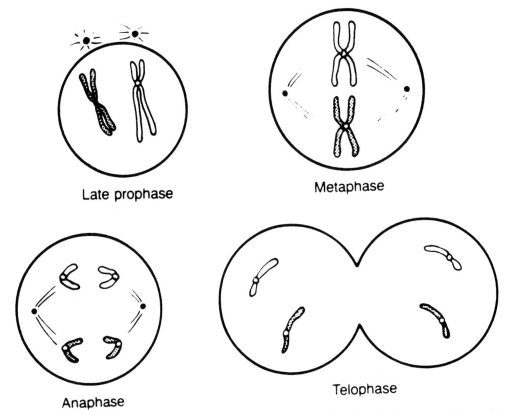

FIGURE 1–14 • Stages of mitosis. Two chromosomes are represented, not homologous. After DNA synthesis, each chromosome consists of two sister chromatids. After centromeric division in the longitudinal plane, each chromatid passes to different cells. (From Simpson JL: Disorders of Sexual Differentiation: Etiology and Clinical Delineation. New York: Academic Press, 1976.)

Prophase

At the onset of prophase, chromosomes are elongated. On light microscopic examination, each chromosome appears to consist of only a single unit. Actually DNA replication has already occurred; each chromosome consists of two sister chromatids. Thereafter, chromosomes become shorter, more compact, and stain more darkly. Toward the end of prophase, a structure called the centriole divides into two daughter centrioles. Each new centriole migrates to opposite poles.

Metaphase

Metaphase begins when the nuclear membrane disappears and the mitotic spindle forms between centrioles. The mitotic spindle consists of protein fibers that attach to the centromeres, allowing the chromosomes to become oriented prior to cell division. During metaphase it becomes apparent on light microscopy that chromosomes consist of paired sister chromatids, joined at the single centromere and arranged on the spindle roughly equidistant between centrioles (equatorial

region). After division of the centromere along the longitudinal axis of the chromosome, sister chromatids pass to opposite poles (see Fig. 1–14). Chromosomes are usually analyzed at metaphase because this stage can be arrested by colchicine, an agent that disrupts the spindle.

Anaphase

During anaphase, chromosomes, each consisting of a single chromatid, move to opposite poles.

Telophase

Telophase begins when the chromatids reach opposite poles. The mitotic spindle disappears and two nuclear membranes form. After division of the cytoplasm (cytokinesis), two complete cells are formed. Each is now in G1 of the subsequent cell cycle.

Meiosis

The diploid complement (2n = 46) of chromosomes is derived from both paternal and maternal sources. Each parent contributes a haploid (n = 23) number of chromosome (n = 23) to the zygote; thus, a process must exist by which chromosomes in gametes (oocytes and spermatozoa) can be reduced to the haploid (n = 23) number of chromosomes. Otherwise, offspring would have twice the number of chromosomes as their parents. This process of chromosomal reduction is *meiosis*. Through recombination (see later on) meiosis also provides the opportunity for a mechanism to generate genetic variability, serving as the basis for natural selection.

Meiosis has two divisions: I and II. During meiosis I the chromosome number is reduced from 2n to n; during meiosis II each haploid germ cell divides its two chromatids between daughter cells (Fig. 1–15). Four haploid cells can thus be formed from a single diploid germ cell. In males all four products persist as functional spermatozoa; in females only one ovum persists, the remaining products becoming nonfunctional polar bodies (1st or 2nd).

Meiosis I. Meiosis I has four stages: prophase, metaphase, anaphase, and telophase. These stages are analogous to the four stages of mitosis, but meiotic prophase is longer and more complex. Several subdivisions of meiosis I are recognized: leptotene, zygotene, pachytene, and diplotene. In *leptotene*, chromosomes are long, slender, and darkly staining. Although it consists of two sister chromatids, each chromosome appears to be only a single unit. During zygotene, homologous chromosomes pair with each other, a process known as *synapsis*. Synapsis occurs at homologous sites, that is, between allelic forms of DNA. Autosomes undergo side-by-side synapsis, but the human X and Y chromosomes undergo end-to-end synapsis between their short arms. At *pachytene*, the two sister chromatids of a given chromosome first become distinguishable. A pair of homologous chromosomes can be visualized as a group of four chromatids, a configuration known as a *tetrad* (Fig. 1–16).

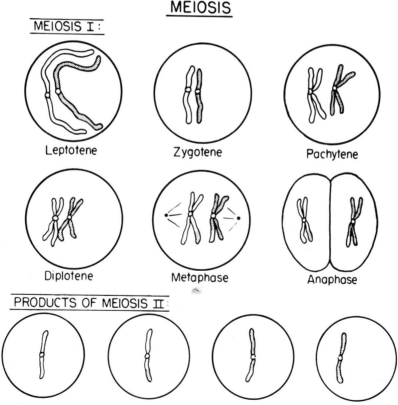

FIGURE 1–15 • Stages of meiosis I and gametes after meiosis II. The behavior of one pair of autosomes is shown. Although each chromosome consists of two sister chromatids, it appears as a single unit initially. At zygotene, homologous chromosomes pair with each other along their longitudinal planes by a process known as synapsis. Synapsis occurs between the alleles at a single locus. At some sites, chromosomal material is exchanged between nonsister chromatids. During diplotene, chromosomes begin to separate. If crossing-over occurs, no two of the four chromatids of a given chromosome pair are genetically identical, as illustrated by the four different gametes at meiosis II. (From Simpson JL: Disorders of Sexual Differentiation: Etiology and Clinical Delineation. New York: Academic Press, 1976.)

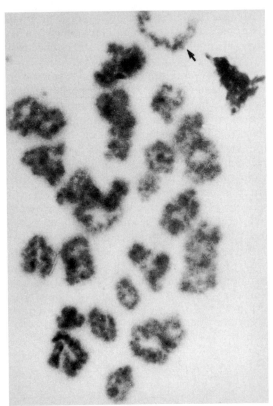

FIGURE 1–16 • Testicular germ cell in meiosis. Chiasmata (sites of crossing-over) are evident. The X and Y chromosomes are designated by the arrow. (Courtesy of RSK Chaganti and J. German, The New York Blood Center.)

Nonsister chromatids of homologous chromosomes can exchange genetic material during synapsis. Sites of exchange are *chiasmata*, and the process of genetic exchange is *recombination*. During *diplotene*, chromosomes shorten and chiasmata appear to move toward the telomeres *(terminalization)*. This process facilitates orderly separation *(disjunction)* of homologous chromosomes. Chiasmata serve two key teleologic functions. First, chiasmata prevent homologous chromosomes from separating prematurely, a process that could lead to nondisjunction and, hence, trisomy. Second, in doing so exchanges of genes between homologous chromosomes occur, providing a source for genetic variability. This is the cytologic basis for natural selection.

Onset of meiotic *metaphase* is heralded by disappearance of the nuclear membrane and equatorial orientation of chromosomes on the spindle. Homologous chromosomes repulse one another and move toward opposite poles during *anaphase*. Centromeres do not divide in meiosis I. Telophase may or may not occur in meiosis I; its occurrence is species-specific.

Meiosis II. In meiosis I the chromosome number is reduced, whereas in meiosis II additional gametes are produced. Meiosis II is thus analogous to mitosis in that centromeres divide. An interphase G1 may or may not occur between meiosis I and II, but in either case little or no DNA synthesis is required in meiosis II. Meiosis II lacks the well-defined prophase characteristic of meiosis I; instead, chromosomes pass directly into metaphase. Metaphase, anaphase, and telophase are similar in both meiosis II and mitosis.

After completing meiosis II, the single originally diploid cell is now divided into four haploid cells. In spermatogenesis the final product is four sperm; in oogenesis the final product is one oocyte and several (two or three) nonfunctioning polar bodies (Fig. 1–17). If recombination has occurred, no two haploid cells will be genetically identical (see Fig. 1–15). In fact, a recombinational event usually occurs at least once if not more per chromosome. In humans, recombination occurs twice as frequently in females as in males. Taking recombination into account is a key principle underlying linkage analysis, either for prenatal genetic diagnosis or for testing candidate genes to determine relevance to a given mendelian or polygenic disorder.

Numerical Chromosomal Abnormalities: Definitions and Cytologic Origin

Trisomy and Polysomy

If a haploid gamete or diploid cell lacks the expected number of chromosomes (n or $2n$), *aneuploidy* exists. If an additional chromosome is present ($2n + 1$), *trisomy* exists. The term *polysomy* is frequently applied if the additional chromosome is a sex chromosome (e.g., 47,XXY). Irrespective of the consequence of meiotic nondisjunction, the resulting zygote has an identical chromosomal constitution in all cells. This contrasts with the effect of nondisjunction during mitosis, which results in two or more cell lines (mosaicism). Rarely, trisomy arises through normal meiotic segregation in a trisomic parent, who should produce equal numbers of n and n + 1 gametes. This is called secondary trisomy.

Autosomal trisomy usually arises following meiotic nondisjunction. The formal possibilities include nondisjunction originating following failure of homologous chromosomes to disjoin in meiosis I, sister chromatids failing to disjoin in meiosis II, or nondisjunction during mitosis.

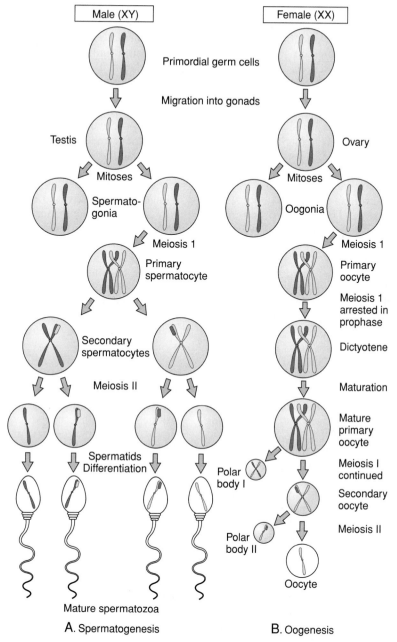

FIGURE 1–17 • *A*, Spermatogenesis and *B*, oogenesis. (From Passarge E: Color Atlas of Genetics. New York: Thieme Medical Publishers, Inc., 1995.)

Irrespective of this process, trisomies usually involve maternal meiotic errors, but there are chromosome-to-chromosome variations (Nicolaidis and Petersen, 1998). Errors in maternal meiosis I have long been accepted as predominantly accounting for trisomies 13, 15, 16, and 21. Virtually all cases of trisomy 16 are caused by maternal meiosis I errors. Trisomy 18 has been considered exceptional in that two thirds of maternal meiosis errors seem to arise at meiosis II.

Recent cytogenetic findings have reinterpreted the origin and significance of trisomy once thought to arise at meiosis II. The idea that cytologic errors causing trisomy could originate at meiosis II was initially considered plausible on the basis of pericentromeric markers being homozygous in the two chromosomes contributed by the parent in whom the nondisjunctional event arose. In contrast, heterozygosity for the markers was considered to indicate meiosis I origin. It is now known that errors in meiosis I and meiosis II differ predominantly on the site of exchange. In many cases of aneuploidy, absence of recombination is observed in meiosis I, but when exchanges are observed in "known" meiosis I errors (i.e., heterozygous markers), they are more likely to involve telomeric regions. Errors once deduced as "meiosis II" on the basis of homozygous markers involve exchanges occurring in proximal regions of the chromosomal arm (Lamb et al., 1996; Yoon et al., 1996). Thus neither telomeric nor proximal exchanges confer the same degree of cytologic stability against nondisjunction as intermediately located exchanges (midarm). The current consensus among cytogeneticists is that almost all aneuploidy arises in meiosis I. So-called meiosis II cases are now considered to reflect cytologic errors originating in meiosis I and continuing in meiosis II. These conclusions are highly relevant clinically. Because meiosis II is not complete until fertilization, nondisjunction at meiosis II was considered more likely to result from periconceptional perturbations. As long as errors arising at meiosis II had to be explained, the hypothesis of aging gametes remained highly attractive. Given current conclusions that virtually all aneuploides arise at meiosis I, periconceptional phenomena such as fertilization involving aging gametes (Simpson et al., 1988) no longer need to be invoked to explain maternal meiosis II errors.

Paternal nondisjunction is uncommon in autosomes, but 10% of trisomy 21 cases arises in paternal meiosis I or II. Trisomy 2 (abortuses) not infrequently arises in paternal meiosis. Mitotic nondisjunction (with subsequent loss of the monosomic line) may arise, and mitotic nondisjunction predominates in trisomy 8, usually in mosaic form.

Approximately 50 to 60% of all 47,XXY cases arise in maternal meiosis (47,X^m,X^mY) (Thomas et al., 2000, 2001); 40% arise in paternal meiosis (47,X^m,X^pY). The fact that approximately equal maternal and paternal contributions exist contrasts with autosomal trisomy, in which by far the most common cytologic origin involves maternal meiosis (90 to 95%). In 47,X^m,X^mY the distribution of maternal errors is 48% meiosis I, 29% meiosis II, 16% mitosis, and 7% unknown (Thomas et al., 2000).

In 47,XXY frequency of recombination in maternal cases can be assessed by determining whether the number of exchanges (recombinants) between the two Xs is that expected for the two homologous Xs. In male and female origin cases, the frequency of exchange between X and Y in the pseudoautosomal region (PAR) is disturbed. Maternal meiosis cases ($X^m$$X^m$Y) constituted

54% of cases studied by Hassold (1980), and in these there were 37 cases in which no recombination occurred (expected number = 6). In 28 cases, one recombinant was observed versus the expected 60. In the 46% of cases arising from paternal meiosis I, recombination between paternal X and paternal Y was observed far less than expected, with two thirds of X^m X^p Y^p cases failing to show exchanges (Thomas et al., 2000). Studying sperm, exchanges are far less common in XY disomic sperm than in normal X sperm. Consistent with the above, paternal age effect is only slightly increased in X^m X^pY, whereas maternal age effect is increased in X^m X^mY.

In poly-X Klinefelter syndrome (XXXY; XXXXY), the additional sex chromosomes generally arise from a single parent, usually the mother (Hassold et al., 1990). Successive meiotic or sequential meiotic and mitotic errors are presumed to be the cytologic mechanism.

Almost all 47,XXX cases arise in maternal meiosis (MacDonald et al., 1994), and 47,XYY obviously arises in paternal meiosis.

Monosomy

Monosomy ($2n - 1$) arises by mechanisms similar to those resulting in trisomy. Indeed, meiotic nondisjunction leading to a disomic gamete should produce a complementary gamete lacking that chromosome. However, monosomy may also result from a chromosome that lags behind and fails to pass to daughter cells (*anaphase lag*).

Polyploidy

In *polyploidy* more than two haploid sets of chromosomes exist. Polyploidy is detected frequently among human abortuses but rarely among neonates. The most common form of polyploidy is triploidy ($3n = 69$). Triploidy may consist of either two maternal or two paternal haploid complements. In humans, dispermy is the most common mechanism responsible for polyploidy. Triploidy accounts for 25% of chromosomally abnormal first-trimester losses or 10 to 15% of all abortuses.

Mosaicism

Mosaicism arises if nondisjunction occurs after syngamy. The number of cell lives depends on when the initial event occurs. If it occurs at the first cell division (Fig. 1–18), only two cell lines are possible. If nondisjunction occurs at a later cell division, two or more cell lines could persist. The ultimate chromosomal complement depends on selection and survival.

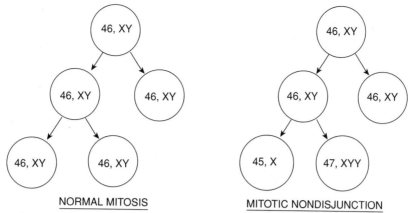

FIGURE 1-18 • Diagrammatic representation of the products of normal mitosis and mitosis characterized by nondis-junction of a Y chromosome. If all daughter cells survived, the complement would be 45,X/46,XY/47,XYY. (From Simpson JL: Disorders of Sexual Differentiation: Etiology and Clinical Delineation. New York: Academic Press, 1976.)

Biologic Basis of Numerical Chromosomal Abnormalities (Aneuploidy)

Decreased Chromosome Exchanges

Autosomal trisomies usually result from nondis-junction, arising at maternal meiosis I. The underlying basis of nondisjunction is less clear, but two related observations are germane. First, autosomal trisomies increase with increasing maternal age (Table 1-4). Second, nondisjunction increases as recombination between homologous chromosomes decreases. The assumption is that a maternal age-dependent effect reflects intrinsic ovarian aging as manifested through decreased recombination (Sherman et al., 1994). In mice, older females show fewer ovarian chiasmata than younger mice, and an inverse relationship exists between chiasmata formation and nondisjunction (Henderson and Edwards, 1968). The corollary is that younger women are more likely to produce an oocyte that has undergone recombination. This long-cited "production-line hypothesis" assumes that the better oocytes are ovulated pref-erentially (Henderson and Edwards, 1968). That is, the dominant follicle in young women is more likely to be derived from a normal oocyte than is the dominant follicle in older women.

Reproductive Aging Rather Than Chronologic Aging

A variant of this idea is that not chronologic aging per se but ovarian (reproductive) aging is the key factor. This was first proposed by Brook and coworkers (1984), who noted that unilateral oophorectomy in mice not only advanced the cessation of reproduction but also was associ-

▼ Table 1-4. MATERNAL AGE AND CHROMOSOMAL ABNORMALITIES (LIVEBIRTHS)

Maternal Age	Risk of Down Syndrome at Birth	Risk of any Chromosome Abnormality at Birth*
20	1/1,667	1/526
21	1/1,667	1/526
22	1/1,429	1/500
23	1/1,429	1/500
24	1/1,250	1/476
25	1/1,250	1/476
26	1/1,176	1/476
27	1/1,111	1/455
28	1/1,053	1/435
29	1/1,000	1/417
30	1/952	1/384
31	1/909	1/385
32	1/769	1/322
33	1/625	1/317
34	1/500	1/260
35	1/385	1/204
36	1/294	1/164
37	1/227	1/130
38	1/175	1/103
39	1/137	1/82
40	1/106	1/65
41	1/82	1/51
42	1/64	1/40
43	1/50	1/32
44	1/38	1/25
45	1/30	1/20
46	1/23	1/15
47	1/18	1/12
48	1/14	1/10
49	1/11	1/7

*47,XXX excluded for ages 20 to 32 years (data not available). Data from Hook (1981).

ated with increased trisomic offspring. If this were true in humans, women having trisomic offspring should have menopause at an earlier age than the general population.

Following the initial observation of Brook and coworkers (1984) in mice, our group (Phillips et al., 1995) pursued the hypothesis that maternal reproductive age (distance in time from approaching menopause) rather than chronologic age is associated with nondisjunction. We found no difference in age at menopause between women ≥ 30 years old at delivery of a child with trisomy 21 (i.e., age-related nondisjunction) and controls. However, in a population-based, case-controlled study, women who did not have a reduced ovarian mass were significantly less likely to have delivered a child with Down syndrome than women who had surgical removal of all or part of an ovary or congenital absence of one ovary (odds ratio 0.61; 95% confidence interval 1.18–446.3) (Freeman et al., 2000).

The study of Kline and associates (2000) differs from others in that ascertainment was by trisomic abortuses, whereas in others ascertainment was by trisomy 21 liveborns. They concluded that women with trisomic abortuses (n = 111) experienced menopause 0.9 years earlier than women with nontrisomy abortuses (n = 157) or nontrisomic liveborn (n = 221).

Overall, the hypothesis is intriguing but considerably more data are needed before arriving at a definitive conclusion.

Accumulated Exogenous Factors

Alternative hypotheses have been raised and rejected. One possibility is that increased aneuploidy accompanied by with increased maternal age merely reflects cumulative accumulation of exogenous factors. This seems unlikely, if for no other reason than mathematically. It seems implausible that toxins could result in the observed exponential increase in aneuploidy. In the fourth decade the maternal age effect increases exponentially, whereas cumulative exposures to toxins should be additive with increased age.

Over the years, a host of hypotheses have revolved around the idea that women who have certain clinical features are predisposed to aneuploid gametes. Maternal antithyroid antibodies have long been proposed as a cause for nondisjunction (Petersen et al., 2000), and other markers have been proposed more recently (e.g., presenilin). Often initial excitement is followed by failure of others to confirm, as exemplified by observations concerning folate polymorphism and trisomy 21. Initial reports suggesting a *MTHFR* 677C→T mutation in mothers of Down syndrome cases (James et al., 1999; Hobbs et al., 2000) were later not confirmed (Hassold et al., 2001).

Relaxed Selection

A discounted hypothesis is that the maternal age effect reflects the mother's being unable to reject trisomic fetuses (relaxed selection) (Hook, 1981). Observations against this idea include lack of a maternal age effect in translocation Down syndrome and presence of an effect in trisomy 21 abortions.

Aging Gametes

Ideally, fertilization involves fresh sperm (recent coitus) exposed to an oocyte ovulation. Fertilization can also involve gametes aged *in vivo* or *in vitro*. Sperm can persist for days before an oocyte is available to fertilize them, and the oocyte may await sperm for 1 or more days. Fertilization could involve a moribund oocyte. Gametes aged *in vivo* are a contribution to nondisjunction in nonhuman mammals, and circumstantial data suggest that a role also exists for this phenomenon in humans (Simpson et al., 1988). However, cohort and case-control studies by our group involving populations that practice periodic abstinence have provided no evidence that aging gametes are a substantive cause of human trisomy (Castilla et al., 1995; Simpson et al., 1997, 2002). Failure to find an association between aging gametes and aneuploidy is consistent with recent data indicating that almost all maternal meiotic errors arise in meiosis I, even if some do not become manifest until meiosis II (see previously) (Yoon et al., 1996). If aging gametes contribute to human aneuploidy, the attributable risk is very small.

Genes Predisposing to Aneuploidy

Genetic predisposition toward aneuploidy clearly exists. After one liveborn aneuploid child, the likelihood of a second trisomic offspring is increased. The idea that a trisomic abortus confers an increased risk for having a liveborn trisomic child is accepted but less rigorously proved. If the first abortus is trisomic, the second is highly likely (70%) to be trisomic (Hassold, 1980; Warburton et al., 1987). If the first abortus is chromosomally normal, the second is likely (80%) to be so as well. The same chromosome is not necessarily involved in successive pregnancies (e.g., trisomy 21 might occur in one pregnancy and trisomy 13 in the next). The manner by which the postulated mutant genes might predispose to aneuploidy is unclear, but plausible hypotheses exist: abnormal centromeric proteins, suppression of recombination, cell cycle check point perturbations. Of relevance is that a predisposition exists toward certain women's having chromosomally "chaotic" embryos, i.e., embryos in which every cell is abnormal but without a consistent cytogenetic abnormality (Delhanty et al., 1997). This topic is explored in detail in Chapter 16, given its obvious relevance to preimplantation genetic diagnosis. Clinically, it is prudent to offer antenatal cytogenetic studies to couples having either trisomic abortuses or liveborns, regardless of their age (see Chapter 5).

Paternal Age

Paternal meiotic errors account for few cases of autosomal trisomy; their contribution ranges from essentially zero (trisomy 16) to perhaps half for trisomy 2 or 47,XXY. Advanced *paternal* age does not predispose to aneuploidy to any meaningful extent. Some studies using FISH (chromosome-specific probes) on ejaculated sperm reveal a slight but statistically significant increase in aneuploid sperm with advanced paternal age (age 55) (Griffin et al., 1995; Martin et al., 1995; Kinakin et al., 1997; McInnes et al., 1998; Guttenbach et al., 2000; Bosch et al., 2001). The magnitude of the increase was arithmetic, not exponential, and thus much lower than observed in women. Whether this connotes an increase in liveborn aneuploidy is even more arguable, although Shi and Martin (2001) reported increased sperm aneuploidy in men who require intracytoplasmic sperm injection (ICSI), a population in which offspring have increased sex chromosomal abnormalities. Certainly those autosomal trisomies (No. 2) known to show a paternal contribution do not seem to show an obvious paternal age effect.

Transmission of Numerical Chromosomal Abnormalities

Autosomal Trisomy

In a trisomic cell, the three homologous chromosomes usually relate spatially in a trivalent configuration at meiotic pachytene. At any given point along their chromosome length, only two of the three chromosomes can pair; however, at another point, two different chromosomes may be paired. Alternatively, the three chromosomes can align themselves as one bivalent and one univalent. This configuration is more likely if the

smaller chromosomes are involved. In either configuration, two chromosomes should pass to one pole at anaphase, with a single chromosome passing to the opposite pole. The final result would be equal numbers of $n+1$ and n gametes.

Although direct human data are limited, several general principles derived from plant and animal studies are noteworthy. *First,* fewer than expected (50%) $2n + 1$ progeny, especially liveborns, are universally recovered.

Autosomal trisomy usually leads either to death or to such severe anomalies that affected individuals fail to reproduce. Those with trisomy 13 or 18 invariably have germ cell failure (Cunniff et al., 1991; Simpson, 1998) (see Chapter 10). Women with trisomy 21 have become pregnant and could transmit a 24, X, +21 gamete (secondary trisomy); males with trisomy 21 are sterile. Among pregnant females with trisomy 21, approximately one third of liveborn offspring have trisomy 21 (Van De Velde et al., 1973). This risk is substantial, although it is less than theoretically expected (50%) and doubtless reflects the spurious elevation of reporting or ascertainment bias.

Potential explanations for empirical risks being lower than theoretical risks include elimination of the additional chromosome during meiosis, reduced viability of $n + 1$ gametes, and reduced viability of $2n + 1$ embryos. The chromosomes most likely to be eliminated are the smaller ones, presumably because their short length minimizes the opportunity for chiasmata formation. Univalents form, and they may behave irregularly, producing various secondary rearrangements. In addition, interchromosomal effects exist. Trisomies for other chromosomes occur with increased frequency. Presumably generalized interference with disjunction arises, or univalents are induced in other chromosomes. Of note, females transmit the additional chromosome more often than males. Differences between transmission rates by sex presumably reflect the higher chiasmata frequency in females than in males.

Sex Chromosome Polysomy

47,XXX. Females with a 47,XXX complement should theoretically yield 46,XX, 46,XY, 47,XXX, and 47,XXY zygotes in equal numbers. However, aneuploid offspring appear to arise only rarely. The theoretical discussion already provided for autosomal trisomy is likely to be applicable here as well. Early reports claiming increased spontaneous abortions in 47,XXX women (which could have a chromosomal basis) probably simply reflect selection biases. Spurious conclusions would be drawn if analyses were restricted to 47,XXX women ascertained only after repetitive abortions (Dewhurst, 1978; Simpson, 1981); 47,XXX women not experiencing abortions would never be ascertained. Nonetheless, antenatal cytogenetic studies should be discussed with pregnant 47,XXX patients.

47,XYY. 47,XYY men should theoretically produce 46,XX, 46,XY, 47,XYY, and 47,XXY offspring in equal numbers. Again, very few chromosomally abnormal offspring seem to occur, despite the high incidence of occurence (1:800 liveborn males) of 47,XYY. Reports exist of 47,XYY fathers having 47,XYY sons (Sundequist and Hellstrom, 1969), but far more often offspring show chromosomally normal offspring (Stoll et al., 1979) if in fact they are fertile. Reports of increased abortions and nonchromosomal abnormalities in 47,XYY offspring are generally considered reflective of biases of ascertainment (Grass et al., 1984). These observations are consistent with animal data suggesting that primary spermatocytes in XYY mice are usually X or Y but not XY or YY (Evans et al., 1978). Thus, the rarity of aneuploidy probably reflects aneuploid gametes not found. Shi and Martin (2000) found few disomic sperm using FISH in studying 30,078 sperm from a 47,XYY male. They found 0.07% 24,YY and 0.44% 24,XY. The frequency of 24,XX was 0.05% and of 24,+21, 0.21%. The risk of gonosomal aneuploidy was only 1%, far less than the theoretical 50%.

47,XXY. With ICSI, men with Klinefelter syndrome can now sire their own offspring. This statement holds even if gonadotropins are elevated and even if the ejaculate is azoospermic. (Sperm can be obtained by testicular biopsy.) In this context, the possibility of transmitting sex chromosomal abnormalities to offspring becomes real.

Relevant data are first available from the XXY mouse. In these animals XY disomy is found more frequently than in XY control mice; still, frequency is less than the theoretically expected 50%. Mroz and associates (1998) showed the frequency of XY sperm to be 1.7% in XXY versus 0.2% in XY mice; frequency of other abnormalities (non-X, non-Y) was .54% versus .05%. The authors concluded that the only germ cells in the XXY Klinefelter mouse capable of completing meiosis were XY, having originated either by mosaicism or by trisomic rescue. In another study of two 41,XXY mice, 80% of embryos would have been predicted to be XY and only 11% XXY (Bronson et al., 1995). Both mice were X^mX^pY.

Theoretical expectations dictate that 50% of sperm and, hence, embryos of XXY men should be hyperhaploid (disomic). As in the mouse, however, the frequency of sex chromosomal polysomy is much less. Based on FISH studies, the frequency of sex chromosomal disomy in sperm is about 0.2% in fertile XY males, 1% in infertile XY males, and 3 to 4% in XXY males (Moosani et al., 1995; Guttenbach et al., 1997; Aran et al., 1999; Okada et al., 1999). No liveborn offspring of XXY fathers sired through ICSI have had sex chromosomal abnormalities. Ron-El and coworkers (2000) collected 14 liveborns reported as of August 2000, and more extensive data from Brussels have been provided by Staessen (2002). Using preimplantation genetic diagnosis (see Chapter 16), a total of 31 couples with KS fathers have undergone 41 cycles, all involving ICSI and preimplantation genetic diagnosis (PGD). In 24 cycles a total of 39 embryos were transferred, yielding 5 fetuses with heart rates. Among all preimplantation embryos, only 59.6% were chromosomally normal. Comparing PGD in these 24 XXY cycles to 78 PGD cases performed for X-linked recessive traits revealed lower fertilization rates (54.6% versus 79.8%), increased chromosomally abnormal embryos (40.4% versus 22.9%), and increased gonosomal abnormalities (30.0% versus 15.2%) in the former group. In 15 PGD embryos recovered outside Brussels, nine were chromosomally abnormal (Tournaye, 1997; Reubinoff, 1998; Bielanska, 2000; Ron-El, 2000); five of these nine were "chaotic," showing different chromosomal abnormalities in different cells of the same embryo (Delhanty et al., 1997).

Overall, there are fewer than expected XY disomic sperm and embryos. This could indicate strong selection against disomic sperm or, perhaps more likely, only XY germ cells being capable of leading to a pregnancy. The latter possibility would help explain the relatively good liveborn outcome. Nonetheless, the high rate of chromosomal abnormalities in preimplantation genetic embryos remains a concern. Monitoring by prenatal genetic diagnosis is recommended.

Distinct from any risk owing to offspring of 47,XXY, about 1% of all ICSI-assisted pregnancies show sex chromosomal aneuploidy (Bonduelle et al., 1998). As discussed in Chapters 12 and 16, this need not necessarily be the result of transmission from a 47,XXY cell line.

Monosomy X

Autosomal monosomy is lethal; thus, the issue of transmission is moot. By contrast, monosomy (45,X) is usually, but not always, lethal. Surviving individuals universally display gonadal and often somatic abnormalities. Although it is rare, fertility in such offspring is rare but reported. In a 1990 review, Kaneko and coworkers (1990) collected 13 nonmosaic cases and 50 mosaic cases who had achieved pregnancy.

In plants, a monosomic chromosome must by definition remain as a univalent at meiotic prophase. This univalent initially lies separately on the equatorial plate, after which three major possibilities can occur. (1) The univalent may lag and become lost, yielding two n-1 products in meiosis I. (2) The univalent may pass undivided to one pole to yield n and n-1 products in meiosis I. (3) The univalent may undergo abnormal transverse centromeric division to yield two or more telocentric chromosomes. If it fails to divide during meiosis I (option 2, above) the univalent may still divide normally at meiosis II to yield two sister chromatids, each contributing to complementary daughter cells having n chromosomes. Alternatively, both chromatids may pass undivided to a single cell or undergo abnormal transverse division at the centromere to yield an isochromosome. If the univalent divides prematurely during meiosis I, the two products may be able to separate normally at meiosis II, especially if telocentric chromosomes or isochromosomes form in the interim. Trisomies and monosomies for chromosomes other than those involved in univalent formation may also arise, presumably as result of indirect meiotic disturbances that induce univalent formation.

Given the above, it is not surprising that far fewer than 50% of progeny of monosomic plants are monosomic. The complexities of segregation evident in plant univalents should caution against simplistic approaches to the rare fertile 45,X human.

Unadjusted tabulations of pregnancies in 45,X or 45,X/46,XX patients superficially would lead one to believe clinical spontaneous abortion rates of approximately 30% (Dewhurst, 1978; Simpson, 1981; Kaneko et al., 1990). Abnormalities in liveborn offspring of 45,X mothers would further appear to be increased. One 45,X mother had an abortion in which chorionic villi were said to show 45,X (Kaneko et al., 1990); no other 45,X offspring had sex chromosomal abnormalities. A few 45,X/46,XX or 45,X/46,XX/47,XXX mothers have had 45,X or mosaic offspring, but these occur in a minority of cases. Trisomy 21 and noncytogenetic conditions (e.g., anatomic defects) have also been recorded.

Actually, the most likely conclusion is that the preceding results merely reflect biases of reporting and ascertainment. Chromosomal studies in the mother were often initiated only *after* an abnormal child was identified. Since pregnant mothers with a 45,X cell line have normal ovarian function and usually have few somatic anomalies, they would not have been subjected to cytogenetic studies if their offspring had not been abnormal. If analysis is restricted to cases ascertained because of maternal infertility, there is clearly no increase in anomalies and abortions in offspring. Similarly, if analysis is restricted to offspring born *after* ascertainment (truncate analysis), there is clearly no increased risk (Dewhurst, 1978; Simpson, 1981).

Given the above caveats, a maternal 45,X line may or may not predispose to abnormal progeny. Both the theoretical considerations reviewed earlier and interchromosomal effects provide reason to suspect that chromosomal abnormalities will be uncommon among liveborn progeny, but it still seems prudent to discuss antenatal diagnosis.

Frequency and Spectrum of Chromosomal Abnormalities

The frequency of chromosomal abnormalities in liveborns is 1 per 160 (Table 1–5). A few clinical generalizations concerning phenotype associated with chromosomal disorders will be offered. This is intended for the obstetrician who may encounter such abnormalities during prenatal studies or in the delivery room. Geneticists and others wishing detailed descriptions and management recommendations should consult standard genetic texts. In this section we merely briefly review the salient clinical and cytogenetic features characteristics of the most common autosomal abnormalities. Sex chromosomal abnormalities are discussed in detail in Chapters 10 and 12.

Autosomal Trisomy

Trisomy 21. Trisomy 21 (Down syndrome, mongolism) is the most frequent autosomal chromosomal syndrome, occurring in 1 of every 800 liveborn infants (see Table 1–5). Its relationship to advanced maternal age is well known. Characteristic craniofacial features include brachycephaly, oblique palpebral fissures, epicanthal folds, broad nasal bridge, a protruding tongue, and small, low-set ears with an overlapping helix and a prominent antihelix (Fig. 1–19). The mean birth weight in Down syndrome—2900 g—is decreased but not as much as in some other autosomal syndromes. At birth, these

▼ **Table 1–5.** CHROMOSOMAL ABNORMALITIES
• IN LIVEBORN INFANTS

Type of Abnormality	Incidence
Numerical aberrations	
Sex chromosomes	
47,XYY	1/1,000 MB
47,XXY	1/1,000 MB
Other (males)	1/1,350 MB
47,X	1/10,000 FB
47,XXX	1/1,000 FB
Other (females)	1/2,700 FB
Autosomes	
Trisomies	
13-15 (D Group)	1/20,000 LB
16-18 (E Group)	1/8,000 LB
21-22 (G Group)	1/800 LB
Other	1/50,000 LB
Structural aberrations	
Balanced	
Robertsonian	
t(Dq;Dq)	1/1,500 LB
t(Dq;Gq)	1/5,000 LB
Reciprocal translocations and insertional inversions	1/7,000 LB
Unbalanced	
Robertsonian	1/14,000 LB
Reciprocal translocations and insertional inversions	1/8,000 LB
Inversions	1/50,000 LB
Deletions	1/10,000 LB
Supernumeraries	1/5,000 LB
Others	1/8,000 LB
Total	1/160 LB

MB, male birth; FB, female birth; LB, liveborn birth.

infants are usually hypotonic. Other features include iridial Brushfield spots, broad short fingers (brachymesophalangia), clinodactyly (incurving deflections resulting from an abnormality of the middle phalanx), a single flexion crease on the fifth digit, and an unusually wide space between the first two toes. Contrary to widespread opinion, a single palmar crease (simian line) is not pathognomonic, being present in only 30% of individuals with trisomy 21 and in 5% of normal individuals. Relatively common internal anomalies include cardiac lesions and duodenal atresia. Cardiac anomalies and increased susceptibility to both respiratory infections and leukemia contribute to a reduced life expectancy. However, the mean survival is still into the fifth decade, and many affected individuals survive to older ages.

Patients with Down syndrome who survive beyond infancy invariably exhibit mental retardation. However, the degree of retardation is generally not as severe as that produced by many other chromosomal aberrations. Mean IQ ranges from

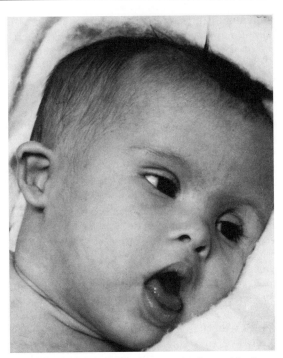

FIGURE 1–19 • Photograph of an infant with Down syndrome.

approximately 25 to 70. 46/47, +21 Mosaicism should be suspected if Down syndrome cases show IQs in the 70 to 80 range. Females are fertile. Although relatively few trisomic mothers have reproduced, about 30% of their offspring are also trisomic. Except for possibly exceptional cases, affected males are not fertile.

Several different cytogenetic mechanisms may be associated with Down syndrome, but the actual cause is triplication of a small portion of the No. 21 chromosome, namely, band q22. This triplication may be caused either by the presence of an entire additional No. 21 or by addition of only band q22. Of all cases of Down syndrome, 95% have primary trisomy (47 instead of the normal 46 chromosomes). These cases show the well-known relationship to maternal age.

By contrast, translocations show no definite relationship to parental age and may be either sporadic or familial. The translocation most commonly associated with Down syndrome involves chromosomes 14 and 21. With translocation Down syndrome [t(14q;21q)], one parent may have the same translocation chromosome, that is, 45,t(14q;21q). For parents with a translocation, the recurrent risk for a child with an unbalanced chromosome complement far exceeds the risk for recurrence of nondisjunction (1%). Empirical risks are approximately 10% for offspring of female translocation heterozygotes and 2% for offspring of male translocation heterozygotes.

Other structural rearrangements resulting in Down syndrome include t(15q;21q), t(21q;22q) and translocations involving No. 21 and chromosomes other than a member of group D (Nos. 13 to 15) or G (Nos. 21 to 22). In t(21q;21q), no normal gametes can be formed. Thus, only trisomic or monosomic zygotes are produced, the latter presumably appearing as preclinical embryonic losses. Parents with the other translocation have a low empirical risk of having offspring with Down syndrome.

Trisomy 13. Trisomy 13 occurs in about 1 per 20,000 live births. Intrauterine and postnatal growth retardation are pronounced, and developmental retardation is severe. Nearly 50% of affected children die in the first month, and relatively few survive past 3 years of age. Characteristic anomalies include holoprosencephaly, eye anomalies (microphthalmia, anophthalmia, or coloboma), cleft lip and palate, polydactyly, cardiac defects, and low birth weight (Fig. 1–20). Other relatively common features include cutaneous scalp effects, hemangiomas on the face or neck, low-set ears with an abnormal helix, and rocker-bottom feet (convex soles and protruding heels).

Trisomy 13 is usually associated with nondisjunction (primary) trisomy (47, + 13). As in trisomy 21, a maternal age effect exists. Translocations are responsible for less than 20% of cases, invariably associated with two group D (Nos. 13 to 15) chromosomes joining at their centromeric regions (robertsonian translocation). If neither parent has such a rearrangement, the risk for subsequent progeny is not increased. If either parent has a balanced 13q; 14q translocation, the recurrence risk for an affected offspring is increased but only by 1 to 2%. Homologous 13q;13q parental translocation carries the same dire prognosis as 21q;21q translocation.

Trisomy 18. Trisomy 18 occurs in 1 per 8000 live births. Among liveborn infants, females are affected more often than males (3:1). Among stillborns and abortuses, however, the sex distribution is more equal.

Facial anomalies characteristic of trisomy 18 include microcephaly, prominent occiput, low-set and pointed "fawn-like" ears, and micrognathia. Skeletal anomalies include overlapping fingers (V over IV, II over 111), short sternum, shield chest, narrow pelvis, limited thigh abduction or congenital hip dislocation, rocker-bottom feet with protrusion of the calcaneum, and a short dorsiflexed hallux ("hammer toe") (Fig. 1–21). Cardiac and renal anomalies are common.

Mean birth weight (2240 g) is below average. The mean survival time for these infants is only a few months. Those surviving show pronounced developmental and growth retardation. Fetal movement is feasible, and approximately 50% develop fetal distress during labor. Trisomy 18 is often detected among stillborn infants not clinically suspected of being trisomic. Approximately 80% of trisomy 18 cases are caused by primary nondisjunction (47,XX, + 18 or 47,XY, + 18). In such cases, the recurrence risk is about 1%.

Other Autosomal Abnormalities (Trisomies and Polyploidies)

Trisomies for several other autosomes have been observed in liveborns, but such pregnancies terminate in abortuses much more often. Trisomies for chromosomes 8, 9, 14, and 16 probably exist in mosaic form, even if this is not always demonstrable. All trisomies show mental retardation, various somatic anomalies, and intrauterine growth retardation. The extent of retardation and the spectrum of anomalies vary. Trisomy 8 mosaicism has a recognizable phenotype: prominent forehead, upturned nose, everted lower lip, micrognathia, low-set ears, high arched palate, cleft palate, and especially osteoarticular abnormalities.

Triploidy and, less often, tetraploidy occur. Again, multiple anomalies occur in these usually lethal conditions.

Cytogenetically recognizable deletions or duplications of portions of autosomes occur. Table 1–6 summarizes the most common. All are characterized by mental retardation and somatic

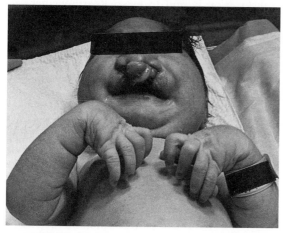

FIGURE 1–20 • Photograph of an infant with trisomy 13.

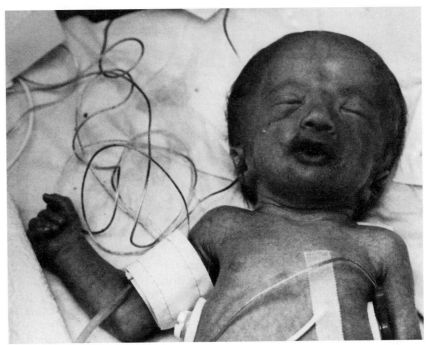

FIGURE 1–21 • Photograph of trisomy 18.

anomalies. Specific features are associated with specific chromosomes. Table 1–7 summarizes so-called microdeletion syndromes. These disorders result from a deletion of a small chromosomal region. They may be difficult to detect by conventional cytogenetics but can be recognized through the use of locus-specific DNA probes applied to metaphases.

Structural Chromosomal Abnormalities: Definitions and Origins

Not all visually evident chromosomal aberrations confer phenotypical abnormalities. Minor structural variation, called *polymorphism*, exists without phenotype effect. Occurring in 1 to 5% of the normal population, examples include prominent satellites on acrocentric chromosomes, variation in the length of the Y long arm, and varying amounts of heterochromatin in centromeric regions (e.g., No. 9). These "variants" are transmitted in dominant fashion. Before molecular technology, chromosomal variants were exploited for tracking chromosomal segregation. Now DNA polymorphic variants are utilized.

Polymorphism should be contrasted with major structural alterations, which by definition are associated with phenotypical abnormalities. Here it can be assumed that many genes are

duplicated or deficient. Phenotypical abnormalities can also result if the position of a gene with respect to its neighbors is altered (*position effect*).

Chromosomal *deletion* involves loss of one portion of one chromosome, either terminal or interstitial. Deficiencies usually result from breakage and loss of an acentric fragment. Deficiencies may also arise following crossing-over within a pericentric inversion loop, as will be discussed later on. Autosomal deficiency usually leads to embryonic death or malformation, but deficiency in a sex chromosome is not necessarily so deleterious.

If, following chromosome breakage, material is exchanged between two or more chromosomes, a *translocation* is said to exist. Rearrangement of chromosomal material need not be deleterious provided genes are neither lost nor gained. If an individual with a translocation is phenotypically normal, it can be assumed that no genetic material is lost. The translocation is thus said to be *balanced*. If a translocation shows deficiency or duplication of genetic material, the rearrangement is said to be *unbalanced*. If a de novo translocation exists, and the individual is phenotypically abnormal, an unbalanced rearrangement can be assumed. If a fetus or offspring shows the same translocation as a normal parent, the translocation can also be assumed to be balanced and the fetus normal. When a de novo translocation is detected in chorionic villi or amniotic fluid cells, however, it is hazardous to assume normalcy even if the translocation seems balanced. A subtle

▼ **Table 1-6.** COMMON DELETIONS AND THEIR CLINICAL MANIFESTATIONS

Deletion	Clinical Abnormalities
4p-	Wolf-Hirschhorn syndrome. The main features are a typical "Greek helmet" facies with ocular hypertelorism, prominent glabella, and frontal bossing; microcephaly, dolichocephaly, hypoplasia of the eye socket, ptosis, strabismus, nystagmus, bilateral epicanthic folds, cleft lip and palate, beaked nose with prominent bridge, hypospadias, cardiac malformations, and mental retardation.
5p-	Cri du chat syndrome. The main features are hypotonia, short stature, characteristic cry, microcephaly with protruding metopic suture, moonlike face, hypertelorism, bilateral epicanthic folds, high arched palate, wide and flat nasal bridge, and mental retardation.
9p-	The main features are craniofacial dysmorphology with trigonocephaly, slanted palpebral fissures, discrete exophthalmos, arched eyebrows, flat and wide nasal bridge, short neck with pterygium colli, genital anomalies, long fingers and toes, cardiac malformations, and mental retardation.
13q-	The main features are low birth weight, failure to thrive, and severe mental retardation. Facial features include microcephaly, flat wide nasal bridge, hypertelorism, ptosis, and micrognathia. Ocular malformations are common. The hands have hypoplastic or absent thumbs and syndactyly.
18p-	A few patients (15%) are severely affected and have cephalic and ocular malformations, cleft lip and palate, and varying degrees of mental retardation. Most (80%) have only minor malformations and mild mental retardation.
18q-	The main features are hypotonia with "froglike" position with the legs flexed, externally rotated, and in hyperabduction. The face is characteristic with depressed midface and apparent protrusion of the mandible, deep-set-eyes, short upper lip, everted lower lip ("carplike" mouth); antihelix of the ears is very prominent; varying degrees of mental retardation and belligerent personality.
21q-	The main features are hypertonia, microcephaly, downward-slanting palpebral fissures, high palate, prominent nasal bridge, large low-set ears, micrognathia, and varying degrees of mental retardation. Skeletal malformations may be present.

From Hall JG: Chromosomal clinical abnormalities. *In* Behrman RE, Kliegman RM, Jensen MB (eds): Nelson Textbook of Pediatrics, 16th ed. Philadelphia: WB Saunders, 2001.

▼ **Table 1-7.** MICRODELETIONS AND THEIR CLINICAL MANIFESTATIONS

Deletion	Syndrome	Clinical Malformations
7q23	Williams	Round face with full cheeks and lips, stellate pattern in iris, strabismus, supravalvular aortic stenosis and other cardiac malformations, varying degrees of mental retardation, and a very friendly personality.
8q24.1	Langer-Giedion or tricho-rhino-phalangeal, type II	Sparse hair, multiple cone-shaped epiphyses, multiple cartilaginous exostoses, bulbous nasal tip, thickened alar cartilage, upturned nares, prominent philtrum, large protruding ears, and mild mental retardation.
11p13	WAGR	Hypernephroma (Wilms tumor), aniridia, male genital hypoplasia of varying degrees, gonadoblastoma, long face, upward slanting palpebral fissures, ptosis, beaked nose, low-set poorly formed auricles, and mental retardation.
13q11-13	Prader-Willi	Severe hypotonia at birth, obesity, short stature (responsive to growth hormone), small hands and feet, hypogonadism, and mental retardation.
13q11-13	Angelman	Hypotonia, fair hair, midface hypoplasia, prognathism, seizures, jerky ataxic movements, uncontrollable bouts of laughter, and severe mental retardation.
16p13	Rubinstein-Taybi	Microcephaly, ptosis, beaked nose with low-lying philtrum, broad thumbs and large toes, and mental retardation.
17p11.2	Smith-Magenis	Brachycephaly, midfacial hypoplasia, prognathism, myopia, cleft palate, short stature, behavioral problems, and mental retardation.
17p13.3	Miller-Dieker	Microcephaly, lissencepahly, pachygyria, narrow forehead, hypoplastic male external genitals, growth retardation, seizures, and profound mental retardation.
20p12	Alagille syndrome	Bile duct paucity with cholestasis, heart defects, particularly pulmonary artery stenosis, ocular abnormalities (posterior embryotoxin), skeletal defects such as butterfly vertebrae, long nose with broad midnose.
22q11	DiGeorge-velocardiofacial CATCH 22	Hypoplasia or agenesis of the thymus and parathyroid glands, hypoplasia or auricle and external auditory canal, conotruncal cardiac anomalies, cleft palate, short stature, behavioral problems.

From Hall JG: Chromosomal clinical abnormalities. *In* Behrman RE, Kliegman RM, Jensen MB (eds): Nelson Textbook of Pediatrics, 16th ed. Philadelphia: WB Saunders, 2001.

rearrangement may not be appreciated, accounting for the 10 to 15% empirical risks of phenotypical abnormality (Warburton et al., 1997).

Translocations may be either reciprocal or robertsonian. In *reciprocal* translocations, breaks and rearrangement involve two or more chromo-

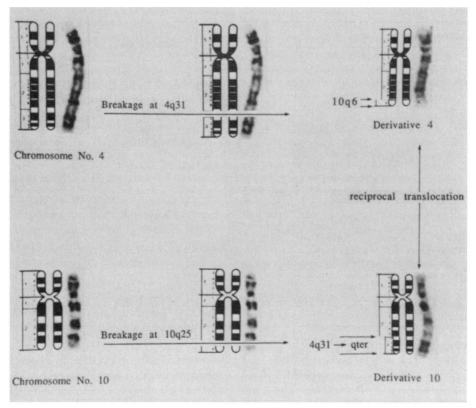

FIGURE 1–22 • A reciprocal translocation between chromosomes 4 and 10. Origin of derivative chromosomes is shown. (From Simpson JL, Tharapel AT: Principles of human cytogenetics. *In* Philipp E, Setchell M (eds): Scientific Foundations of Obstetrics and Gynaecology, 4th ed. London: Butterworth-Heinemann, 1991.)

somes but do not involve centromeres (Fig. 1–22). Translocation heterozygotes have 46 chromosomes, but the homologous chromosomes of two pairs differ in morphology and composition (Fig. 1–23). In *robertsonian* translocations, acrocentric chromosomes (Nos. 13, 14, 15, 21, and 22) fuse at their centromeres. Robertsonian heterozygotes thus have only 45 chromosomes (centromeres). The short arm of acrocentric chromosomes contains genes for ribosomal RNA, but these genes are coded by more than one chromosome. Because no single acrocentric short arm is essential, heterozygotes are phenotypically normal.

An *inversion* (Fig. 1–24) is an intrachromosomal rearrangement in which the sequence of genes in the inverted segment is reversed. Such a rearrangement is usually caused by two chromosomal breaks, followed by reversal and reinsertion of the chromosomal segment produced by the breaks. Two types of inversions exist. Those in which the inverted region includes the centromere are *pericentric*; those in which the inverted region does not encompass the centromere are *paracentric*. Heterozygotes for either inversion may be normal provided genes are not lost, gained, or altered as result of the breaks leading to the inversion.

Isochromosomes are chromosomes with identical arms. This aberration arises if the centromere divides in horizontal rather than longitudinal fashion (Fig. 1–25). One product is acentric, lost at the next cell division. The other product is telocentric, capable of replicating at the next S period to form a metacentric chromosome. The isochromosome thus formed is completely duplicated for one arm and completely deficient for the other arm. Isochromosome for the X long arm (i(Xq)) is the most common structural abnormality associated with gonadal dysgenesis.

A *dicentric* chromosome has two centromeres. Its formation most often begins with an isochromatid break in G2 (Fig. 1–26). Regardless of initial formation, the presence of two centromeres (dicentric) confers mitotic instability because centromeres may migrate to opposite poles during mitotic anaphase. The dicentric chromosome stretches until breaking, followed by either loss of chromosomal material or secondary rearrangements (breakage—fusion—bridge cycle).

A *ring chromosome* arises following a break in both the long arm and the short arm (Fig. 1–27). Chromosomal regions contiguous with the cen-

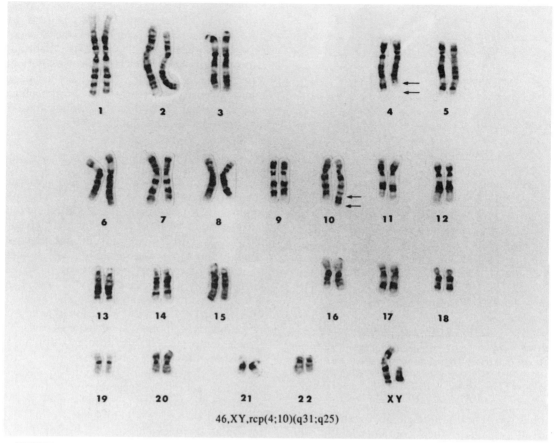

FIGURE 1–23 • Karyotype of a female with a balanced reciprocal translocation between chromosomes 4 and 10. (From Simpson JL, Tharapel AT: Principles of human cytogenetics. *In* Philipp E, Setchell M (eds): Scientific Foundations of Obstetrics and Gynaecology, 4th ed. London: Butterworth-Heinemann, 1991.)

tromeres fuse; acentric telomeric regions of each arm are lost, thus resulting in deficiency. Like dicentrics, ring chromosomes are inherently unstable.

Duplications may originate by various mechanisms. Often duplications for certain loci are accompanied by deficiencies for other loci. This is the usual situation when duplication arises following meiotic segregation in a parent having a chromosomal translocation.

Causes of Structural Chromosomal Abnormalities

Chromosomal breaks responsible for structural chromosomal abnormalities may be caused by irradiation, chemicals, or viruses. Breakage may also arise spontaneously or as result of mutant genes. Chromosomal breaks are also part of the background biologic "noise," arising ubiquitously and being repaired continuously. Chromosomal

breakage may thus be observed in ostensibly normal individuals or their cultured cells.

Agents that break chromosomes are termed *clastogens*. In vitro studies identified immummerable agents as clastogens, but whether exposure in vivo to these agents confers increased risks for abnormal liveborns or abortuses is less certain. Usually couples exposed before or during pregnancy can be reassured concerning the consequences of exposure to clastogens.

Transmitting Structural Chromosomal Abnormalities

Deletions and Duplications

Deletions or duplications affecting large chromosomal regions may produce such severe phenotypical abnormalities that reproduction is precluded. However, individuals with deletions or duplications who are capable of reproduction

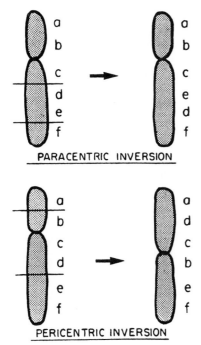

FIGURE 1–24 • Origin of paracentric (top) and pericentric (bottom) inversions. (From Simpson JL: Disorders of Sexual Differentiation: Etiology and Clinical Delineation. New York: Academic Press, 1976.)

should theoretically produce 50% gametes with the abnormality. When compared with other chromosomal abnormalities, the empirical risk could be much less. The question most often arises in individuals with 46,X, del(Xp) or 46,X, del(Xq), distal deletions of which are frequently associated with reproduction (Chapter 10).

Dicentric and Ring Chromosomes

Dicentric and ring chromosomes are mitotically unstable. The two centromeres in a dicentric can pass to opposite poles, causing the chromosome to break and leading to its loss or secondary rearrangement (see Fig. 1–26). During each mitotic cycle ring chromosomes must open in order to replicate (see Fig. 1–27). Offspring of parents with dicentric or ring chromosomes may inherit the same dicentric or ring as their parent, inherit a secondarily rearranged chromosome, or inherit neither and thus be monosomic. No empirical data are available.

Robertsonian Translocations

Robertsonian translocations involve acrocentric chromosomes—13–15 and 21–22. The most important robertsonian translocation involves chromosomes 14 and 21. Two to three percent of individuals with Down syndrome are affected as result of this translocation [t(14q 21q)]. In theory one third of liveborn offspring of t(14q 21q) translocation heterozygotes should have Down syndrome; however, empirical data reveal that only about 10% of viable offspring of female carriers and only about 2% of male carriers have Down syndrome. This sex differentiation has not been shown for other robertsonian translocation involving chromosome 21, e.g., t(15q 21q), but this may merely reflect relatively few cases studied. Liveborn normal offspring have an equal likelihood of having a completely normal chromosomal complement (2n = 46) or being a translocation carrier (2n = 45) like one of their parents. Deficiency of expected versus observed outcomes with respect to abnormal products could be accounted for by (a) preferential segregation of unbalanced products into polar bodies; (b) decreased fertilizability of unbalanced ova or sperm; (c) increased loss of unbalanced zygotes or early embryos; or (d) unrecognized loss of unbalanced fetuses later in gestation.

In t(21;22), female heterozygotes are at relatively high risk (10 to 15%) for Down syndrome

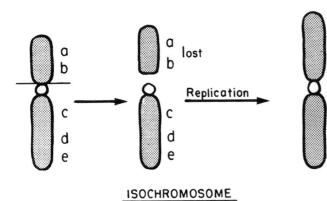

FIGURE 1–25 • Diagrammatic representation of the origin of an isochromosome. (From Simpson JL: Disorders of Sexual Differentiation: Etiology and Clinical Delineation. New York: Academic Press, 1976.)

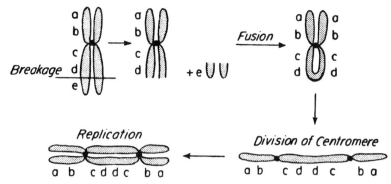

FIGURE 1–26 • Formation of a dicentric chromosome, which usually occurs after an isochromatid break. (From Simpson JL: Disorders of Sexual Differentiation: Etiology and Clinical Delineation. New York: Academic Press, 1976.)

offspring. Risks to carrier males appear similar. Abnormal liveborn infants have also been observed for most other robertsonian translocations. In t(13;14), fewer than 1% of offspring have trisomy 13. These empirical data are not surprising given that liveborn trisomy 14 and trisomy 15 are extraordinarily rare. If survival occurs, infants are usually mosaic. Nonetheless, individuals with all robertsonian translocations should be counseled concerning antenatal chromosomal studies. A recent concern has been whether robertsonian translocations are associated with uniparental disomy (Chapter 2), even if balanced. However, this appears not to be a major clinical concern. Berend and colleagues (2000) found UPD in only 2 of 48 nonhomologous translocations. Both involved chromosome No. 14 in a t(14q15q).

If a robertsonian translocation involves homologous chromosomes, the prognosis is bleak. All liveborns of individuals with translocations involving the two No. 13 chromosomes [t(13q13q)] or the two No. 21 chromosomes [t(21q21q)] should be abnormal (trisomy 13 or trisomy 21); all other conceptions also should terminate in spontaneous abortions because the complement is lethal. Homologous translocations involving Nos. 14, 15, and 22 would virtually always result in abortions, given the absence of liveborns with these trisomies. Females with homologous translocations should be counseled concerning sterilization or assisted reproduction with donor oocytes. Using sperm donors should be discussed for homologous male heterozygotes. Exceptionally, "correction" has been reported by expulsion of a normal 21 to yield a 45, -21,-21, +t(21q21q) complement (trisomic rescue). If this occurs, uniparental disomy may exist and could be a concern (see Chapter 2). Indeed Berend et al. (2000) found UPD in 4 of 6 homologous neuromegawatts to be isochromosomes. Again, chromosome 14 is of greatest concern (McGowan et al., 2002).

Reciprocal Translocation

Theoretical. During meiosis I, the two translocation chromosomes involve a reciprocal translocation and the two structurally normal chromosomes may segregate in several possible ways (Fig. 1–28). Gametes would be balanced if both translocation chromosomes pass to one

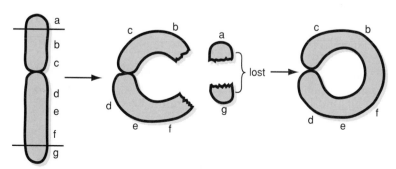

FIGURE 1–27 • Formation of a ring chromosome. (From Simpson JL: Disorders of Sexual Differentiation: Etiology and Clinical Delineation. New York: Academic Press, 1976.)

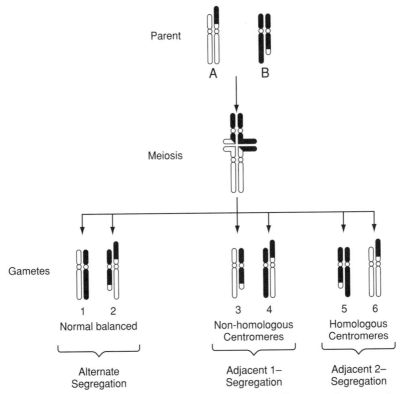

FIGURE 1–28 • Meiotic segregation in a reciprocal translocation (top). Alignment of two translocation chromosomes and two normal chromosomes at pachytene (bottom). Segregation is said to be alternate if centromeres of normal chromosomes segregate, opposed and N2 passing to the opposite pole by centromeres of two translocation chromosomes. Adjacent 1 segregation occurs if nonhomologous centromeres segregate together. Homologous centromeres segregate in adjacent 2 segregation. (Redrawn from Hsu LYF: Chromosomal disorders. *In* Reece EA, Hobbins JC (eds): Medicine of the Fetus and Mother, 2nd ed. Philadelphia: Lippincott, 1999.)

gamete and both normal chromosomes pass to the other gamete (alternate segregation). Gametes would be unbalanced if other types of segregations occur. If nonhomologous centromeres pass to the same gamete, adjacent segregation I is said to occur. If homologous centromeres pass to the same gamete, adjacent segregation II occurs. In either adjacent I or adjacent II segregation, abnormal segregants result in abortions or anomalous liveborns (Phillips et al., 1991). Factors favoring alternate segregation (and, hence, balanced gametes) include chromosomes of equal size, metacentric chromosomes, translocations involving interchanges of approximately equal length, and chiasmata formation involving terminal rather than interstitial segments. Carefully considering the relative likelihood of alternate adjacent I and adjacent II segregation is highly relevant in preimplantation genetics (see Chapter 16). Sometimes segregation favors unbalanced gametes such that very few (e.g., 10 to 20%) of embryos are normal.

Sometimes three chromosomes segregate into one gamete, whereas the other gamete receives only one. In fact, 3:1 segregation is more likely than 2:2 segregation in certain translocations, notably t(11q:22q). Factors favoring 3:1 segregation include disparities in lengths between involved chromosomes, acrocentric chromosomes, and short interstitial segments.

Occasionally two chromosomes are involved in a balanced translocation, and one additional normal chromosome is present. If both arms (short and long) of the additional chromosome are derived from nonhomologous chromosomes, tertiary trisomy is said to exist. In tertiary trisomy the remaining 46 chromosomes are all morphologically normal.

Empirical. Translocations involving all chromosomes have been described, and ideally empirical data should be available for each translocation. However, usually empirical data exist only for general categories. Generalizing, reciprocal translocations carry an empirical risk of about 10 to 15% for abnormal offspring. Counseling would ideally take into account mode of ascertainment. If a reciprocal translocation is ascertained through a balanced (normal) proband (e.g., during a survey of normal individuals), the risk of having a liveborn child with chromosomal duplication or deficiency is extremely low. This low risk probably reflects meiotic or embryonic selection against unbalanced products. If, by contrast, a reciprocal translocation is ascertained through an abnormal (unbalanced) proband (e.g., abnormal liveborn offspring proved to have chromosomal imbalance), the risks of having an abnormal liveborn are much higher. In these latter families unbalanced products are presumably viable.

Females with reciprocal translocations carry risks of unbalanced fetuses of approximately 10%; risks for offspring of carrier males are similar (Boué et al., 1984; Daniel et al., 1988; Gardner et al., 1989). Although substantial, these risks are less than the 50% or higher theoretical risks, assuming random segregation and no crossing-over. (The risk can be derived by recalling that the two products of alternate segregation yield normal gametes, whereas both adjacent segregation I and adjacent segregation II crossing-over products yield only abnormal gametes. At least half the theoretically possible products are abnormal, although the exact proportion depends upon assumptions made concerning whether all three types of segregations are equally likely.) Liveborn offspring who are phenotypically normal are equally likely to show either completely normal chromosomes (46,XY or 46,XX) or the two balanced translocation chromosomes present in the parent. Risks are higher with complex rearrangements involving more than two chromosomes or in situations predisposing to 3:1 segregation (Daniel et al., 1986).

Of considerable clinical importance is whether a translocation ascertained through repetitive abortions confers a risk for abnormal liveborns equal to that conferred if ascertainment occurs through an abnormal liveborn. When ascertainment occurs through repetitive abortions, risks appear to be lower (Daniel et al., 1986).

Pericentric Inversions

Abnormal reproductive outcome among offspring of individuals with either pericentric or paracentric inversions is the result of normal meiotic phenomena. However, the underlying cytologic mechanisms are complex.

Recall that genes seek to pair with their alleles on homologous chromosomes; pairing, in turn, is accompanied by exchanges (crossing-over) of genetic material. This phenomenon is visualized as chiasmata. For each pair of homologous chromosomes to be oriented properly for cell division, at least one chiasma is necessary per tetrad. (A tetrad consists of two homologous chromosomes, each subdivided into two chromatids connected by a centromere; therefore, a tetrad is composed of four 'strands'.) In order for chromosomes with an inversion to pair, a loop is formed (Fig. 1–29). Crossing-over may or may not occur within an inversion loop, but it is likely to do so if the loop encompasses a relatively long length of the chromosome. A single cross-over at any site within a pericentric loop yields four types of gametes: two of the four have the parental sequences (one normal, one inverted); the other two have combinations of genes present in neither parent (recombinants). In each of the latter, crossing-over results in duplication for those genes distal to one break

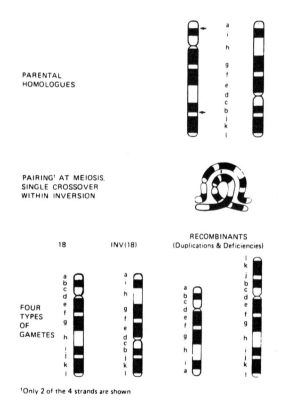

PARENTAL HOMOLOGUES

PAIRING[1] AT MEIOSIS, SINGLE CROSSOVER WITHIN INVERSION

18   INV(18)   RECOMBINANTS (Duplications & Deficiencies)

FOUR TYPES OF GAMETES

[1]Only 2 of the 4 strands are shown

FIGURE 1–29 • Recombination in an inv (18) heterozygote. Pericentric inversion for No. 18. Crossing over at meiosis I would be expected to produce the four types of gametes shown. Two of these would be genetically unbalanced. The chromosomal region outside the inverted segment appears as duplications or deficiencies in the two types of unbalanced gametes. Thus, the smaller the inversion, the greater the genetic imbalance in recombinant gametes and the more severe the expected phenotypical effect. Only two of the four strands are shown. (From Martin AO, Simpson JL, Deddish DB, et al.: Clinical implications of the chromosomal inversions: A pericentric inversion is no. 18 segregating in a family ascertained through an abnormal proband. Am J Perinatol 1:81, 1983.)

point and deficiency for other genes. Actually the four gametes described above result only if an uneven (e.g., 1, 3, 5) number of cross-overs occurs. Even numbers of cross-overs (e.g., 2, 4, 6) do not produce unbalanced gametes.

It is the chromosomal region outside the inverted segment that constitutes the duplicated or deficient regions in unbalanced gametes. As result, a paradox exists when crossing over occurs within the inverted segment. The smaller the inversion, the greater the genetic imbalance in recombinant gametes and, hence, the more deleterious the phenotype. That is, when crossing-over involves inversions characterized by only a small portion of the total chromosomal length, large duplications and deficiencies result. These imbalances may be so great that lethality occurs, the clinical consequences thus being almost nil. Inversions of intermediate length, namely, those involving 30 to 60% of total chromosomal length, are most likely to produce duplications and deficiencies compatible with survival.

Given the above, it is not surprising that counseling regarding risks of pericentric inversions requires empirical data. Data are limited, but a few guidelines may be derived from theoretical principles and from clinical information. Empirical risks are lower than the theoretical risks; thus, it becomes crucial to use empirical risks when counseling patients carrying an inversion. As for translocations, the method by which an inversion is ascertained influences risk to offspring. Pericentric inversions ascertained through an anomalous (presumably recombinant) proband have a higher likelihood of recurrence in that family. Pooled empirical data indicate that a female inversion heterozygote has approximately a 10% risk for an abnormal liveborn; a male inversion heterozygote has a 5% risk. Data derived from prenatal genetic diagnosis registries indicate that female carriers have about an 8% risk, whereas male carriers have only a 2% risk (Boué et al., 1984; Daniel et al., 1988; Gardner et al., 1989). The fact that empirical risks are higher for female carriers is consistent with recombination frequencies being higher in females than males (Sutherland et al., 1976).

Inversions ascertained among couples who have experienced repetitive spontaneous abortions carry a lower risk for anomalous liveborns or second trimester fetuses. Presumably, recombinants are lethal in most of those families.

Pericentric inversions ascertained through phenotypically normal probands (e.g., surveys) are much less likely to result in abnormal liveborns than those ascertained as a result of abnormal clinical consequences. The risk may not even be increased, and antenatal cytogenetic studies may or may not be indicated on statistical grounds. Recombinants are presumably lethal in certain kindreds.

Paracentric Inversions

A single cross-over within a paracentric inversion results in both dicentric and acentric chromatids. Both chromatids are characterized by duplications and deficiencies. Acentric fragments cannot persist beyond subsequent cell divisions because a centromere is required for orderly chromosomal disjunction. The fate of a dicentric chromosome varies, subject to vicissitudes of breakage-fusion-bridge cycles. A dicentric gamete could interfere with reproductive fitness, but more data are required in order to determine the magnitude of increased risk for liveborns. Meanwhile, it is reasonable to offer prenatal diagnosis for couples in whom one parent has a paracentric inversion.

Interchromosomal Effects (Translocations and Inversions)

In addition to the abnormal gametes predictably resulting from normal meiotic segregation, translocations and inversions may predispose to aneuploidy for chromosomes other than those involved in the translocation or inversion in question. For example, a balanced reciprocal translocation between chromosomes Nos. 6 and 8 might predispose to trisomy 21. This is well proved in plants and lower mammals; the rationale is that abnormal meiotic configurations exert a generalized deleterious effect on chromosomal segregation. Many examples have been observed, but coincidental association of two independent phenomena is difficult to exclude. Using FISH probes, Estop and coworkers (2000) have now demonstrated the existence of an interchromosomal effect in male meiosis, using FISH probes for X, Y, 13, 18, and 21 chromosomes on spermatozoa derived from reciprocal translocations involving none of the above five chromosomes. Compared with controls, overall frequency of abnormalities for X, Y, 13, 18, and 21 was not increased in 9 cases. The overall disomy rate was 0.21% in controls and 0.19% in carriers. Disomy 21 was slightly higher in spermatozoa from carriers. In oocytes Cheng and associates (2000) observed an interchromosomal effect.

De Novo Structural Abnormalities

Of special relevance to prenatal cytogenetic diagnosis are de novo structural abnormalities. Suppose a fetus has a rearrangement but neither parent is abnormal. If the rearrangement is ascertained in a liveborn, the phenotype is known and the significance of the rearrangement is usually obvious (except for long-term development). However, the eventual phenotype cannot be predicted so confidently if a (de novo) rearrangement is unexpectedly ascertained at chorionic villus sampling or amniocentesis. Even if the de novo rearrangement *appears* balanced, submicroscopic deletions or duplications could exist. Empirical data reveal an abnormal outcome in 6.7% fetuses with a de novo reciprocal rearrangement detected in villi or amniotic fluid cells (Warburton, 1991). Given that telomeric and subtelomeric probes reveal subtle detections in about 8% of children with an IQ of <50 (Knight et al., 1999; Slavotinek et al., 1999), such probes are becoming invaluable ancillary tests. These probes may reveal balanced translocation in some cases.

The risk for a de novo robertsonian translocation is 3.7% (Warburton, 1991). Uniparental disomy could explain these cases, especially if trisomy 14 is involved (Berend et al., 2000).

REFERENCES

Aran B, Blanco J, Vidal F, et al.: Screening for abnormalities of chromosomes X, Y and 18 and for diploidy in spermatozoa from infertile men participating in an in vitro fertilization-intracytoplasmic sperm injection program. Fertil Steril 72:696, 1999.

Berend SA, Horwitz J, McCaskill C, et al.: Identification of uniparental disomy following prenatal detection of robertsonian translocations and isochromosomes. Am J Hum Genet 66:1787, 2000.

Bielanska M, Tan SL, Ao A: Fluorescence in-situ hybridization of sex chromosomes in spermatozoa and spare preimplantation embryos of a Klinefelter 46,XY/47,XXY male. Hum Reprod 15:440, 2000.

Bonduelle M, Wilikens A, Buysse A, et al.: A follow-up study of children born after intracytoplasmic sperm injection (ICSI) with epididymal and testicular spermatozoa and after replacement of cryopreserved embryos obtained after ICSI. Hum Reprod Suppl 1:196, 1998.

Bosch M, Rajmil O, Martinez-Pasarell O, et al.: Linear increase of diploidy in human sperm with age: A four-colour FISH study. Eur J Hum Genet 9:533, 2001.

Boué A, Gallano P: A collaborative study of inherited chromosome structural rearrangements in 1356 prenatal diagnoses. Prenat Diagn 4:45, 1984.

Bronson SK, Smithies O, Mascarello JT: High incidence of XXY and XYY males among the offspring of female chimeras from embryonic stem cells. Proc Natl Acad Sci USA 92:3120, 1995.

Brook JD, Gosden RG, Chandley AC: Maternal ageing and aneuploid embryos—evidence from the mouse that biological and not chronological age is the important influence. Hum Genet 66:41, 1984.

Castilla EE, Simpson JL, Queenan JT: Down syndrome is not increased in offspring of natural family planning users (case control analysis) Am J Med Genet 59:525, 1995.

Chadwick RB, Prior TW, Pyatt R, et al.: Absence of germline MSH6 mutations in hereditary nonpolyposis coloretal cancer (HNPCC) and endometrial cancer kindreds. Am J Hum Genet 65:639, A121, 2000.

Cheng EY, Storek C, Bonnet G, et al.: Evidence for an interchromosomal effect in human oogenesis. Am J Hum Genet In press, 2000.

Cunniff C, Jones KL, Benirschke K: Ovarian dysgenesis in individuals with chromosomal abnormalities. Hum Genet 86:552, 1991.

Daniel A, Boue A, Gallano P: Prospective risk in reciprocal translocation heterozygotes at amniocentesis as determined by potential chromosome imbalance sizes. Data of the European Collaborative Prenatal Diagnosis Centres. Prenat Diagn 6:315, 1986.

Daniel A, Hook EB, Wulf G: Risks of unbalanced progeny at amniocentesis to carriers of chromosome rearrangements: Data from European, USA and Canadian laboratories. Am J Hum Genet 43:A230, 918, 1988.

Delhanty JD, Harper JC, Ao A, et al.: Multicolor FISH detects frequent chromosomal mosaicism and chaotic division in normal preimplantation embryos from fertile patients. Hum Genet 99:755, 1997.

Dewhurst J: Fertility in 47,XXX and 45,X patients. J Med Genet 15:132, 1978.

Estop AM, Cieply K, Munne S, et al.: Is there an interchromosomal effect in reciprocal translocation carriers? Sperm FISH studies. Hum Genet 106:517, 2000.

Evans EP, Beechey CV, Burtenshaw MD: Meiosis and fertility in XYY mice. Cytogenet Cell Genet 20:249, 1978.

Freeman SB, Yang Q, Allran K, et al.: Women with a reduced ovarian complement may have an increased risk for a child with Down syndrome. Am J Hum Genet 66:1680, 2000.

Gardner RJM, Sutherland GR: Chromosome Abnormalities and Genetic Counseling. New York: Oxford University Press, 1989.

Gartler SM, Liskay RM, Campbell BK, et al.: Evidence of two functional X chromosomes in human oocytes. Cell Differ 1:215, 1972.

Grass F, McCombs J, Scott CI, et al.: Reproduction in XYY males: Two new cases and implications for genetic counseling. Am J Med Genet 19:553, 1984.

Griffin DK, Abruzzo MA, Millie EA, et al.: Non-disjunction in human sperm: Evidence for an effect of increasing paternal age. Hum Mol Genet 4:2227, 1995.

Guttenbach M, Köhn FM, Engel W, et al.: Meiotic nondisjunction of chromosomes 1, 17, 18, X, and Y in men more than 80 years of age. Biol Reprod 63:1727, 2000.

Guttenbach M, Michelmann HW, Hinney B, et al.: Segregation of sex chromosomes into sperm nuclei in a man with 47,XXY Klinefelter's karyotype: A FISH analysis. Hum Genet 99:474, 1997.

Hassold TJ: A cytogenetic study of repeated abortions. Am J Hum Genet 32:723, 1980.

Hassold TJ, Burrage C, Chan ER, et al.: Maternal folate polymorphisms and the etiology of human nondisjunction. Am J Hum Genet 69:434, 2001.

Hassold T, Pettay D, May K, et al.: Analysis of non-disjunction in sex chromosome tetrasomy and pentasomy. Hum Genet 85:648, 1990.

Henderson SA, Edwards RG: Chiasma frequency and maternal age in mammals. Nature 217:22, 1968.

Hobbs CA, Sherman SL, Yi P, et al.: Polymorphisms in genes involved in folate metabolism as maternal risk factors for Down syndrome. Am J Hum Genet 67:623, 2000.

Hook EB: Rates of chromosome abnormalities at different maternal ages. Obstet Gynecol 58:282, 1981.

Iitsuka Y, Bock A, Nguyen DD, et al.: Evidence of skewed X-chromosome inactivation in 47,XXY and 48,XXYY Klinefelter patients. Am J Med Genet 98:25, 2001.

ISCN: An international system for human cytogenetic nomenclature. Basel, Switzerland: S Karger, 1985.

ISCN: An international system for human cytogenetic nomenclature. Mitelman F (ed): Basel, Switzerland: S Karger, 1995.

James SJ, Pogribna M, Pogribny IP, et al.: Abnormal folate metabolism and mutation in the methylenetetrahydrofolate reductase gene may be maternal risk factors for Down syndrome. Am J Clin Nutr 70:495, 1999.

Kaneko N, Kawagoe S, Hiroi M: Turner's syndrome—Review of the literature with reference to a successful pregnancy outcome. Gynecol Obstet Invest 29:81, 1990.

Kinakin B, Rademaker A, Martin R: Paternal age effect of YY aneuploidy in human sperm, as assessed by fluorescence in situ hybridization. Cytogenet Cell Genet 78:116, 1997.

Kline J, Kinney A, Levin B, et al.: Trisomic pregnancy and earlier age at menopause. Am J Hum Genet 67:395, 2000.

Knight SJ, Regan R, Nicod A, et al.: Subtle chromosomal rearrangements in children with unexplained mental retardation. Lancet 354:1676, 1999.

Lamb N, Freeman S, Savage-Austin A, et al.: Susceptible chiasmate configurations of chromosome 21 predispose to nondisjunction in both maternal meiosis I and meiosis II. Nature Genet 14:400, 1996.

Lyons MF: Gene action in the mammalian X-chromosome of the mouse (Mus musculus L.) Nature (London) 190:372, 1961.

MacDonald M, Hassold T, Harvey J, et al.: The origin of 47,XXY and 47,XXX aneuploidy: Heterogeneous mechanisms and role of aberrant recombination. Hum Mol Genet 3:1365, 1994.

Martin RH, Spriggs E, Ko E, et al.: The relationship between paternal age, sex ratios, and aneuploidy frequencies in human sperm, as assessed by multicolor FISH. Am J Hum Genet 57:1395, 1995.

McGowen KD, Weiser JJ, Horwitz J, et al.: The importance of investigating for uniparental disomy in prenatally identified balanced acrocentric rearrangements. Prenat Diagn 22:141–143, 2002.

McInnes B, Rademaker AW, Martin RH: Donor age and the frequency of disomy for chromosomes 1, 13, 21 and structural abnormalities in human spermatozoa using multicolor fluorescence in-situ hybridization. Hum Reprod 13:2489, 1998.

Moosani N, Pattinson HA, Carter MD, et al.: Chromosomal analysis of sperm from men with idiopathic infertility using sperm karyotyping and fluorescence in situ hybridization. Fertil Steril 64:811, 1995.

Mroz K, Hassold T, Hunt P: Meiotic aneuploidy in the XXY mouse: Evidence that a comprised testicular environment increases the incidence of meiotic errors. Hum Reprod 14:1151, 1999.

Nicolaidis P, Petersen MB: Origin and mechanisms of nondisjunction in human autosomal trisomies. Hum Reprod 13:313, 1998.

Okada H, Fujioka H, Tatsumi N, et al.: Klinefelter's syndrome in the male infertility clinic. Hum Reprod 14:946, 1999.

Petersen MB, Karadima G, Samaritaki M, et al.: Association between presenilin-1 polymorphism and maternal meiosis II errors in Down syndrome. Am J Med Genet 93:366, 2000.

Phillips OP, Cromwell S, Rivas M, et al.: Trisomy 21 and maternal age of menopause: Does reproductive age rather than chronological age influence risk of nondisjunction? Hum Genet 95:117, 1995.

Phillips OP, Tharapel AT, Shulman LP: Segregation analysis and genetic counseling when both partners carry balanced translocations. Fertil Steril 56:646, 1991.

Reubinoff BE, Abeliovich D, Werner M, et al.: A birth in non-mosaic Klinefelter's syndrome after testicular fine needle aspiration, intracytoplasmic sperm injection and preimplantation genetic diagnosis. Hum Reprod 13:1887, 1998.

Ron-El R, Strassburger D, Gelman-Kohan S, et al.: A 47,XXY fetus conceived after ICSI of spermatozoa from a patient with non-mosaic Klinefelter's syndrome: Case report. Hum Reprod 15:1804, 2000.

Sherman SL, Petersen MB, Freeman SB, et al.: Non-disjunction of chromosome 21 in maternal meiosis I: Evidence for a maternal age-dependent mechanism involving reduced recombination. Hum Mol Genet 3:1529, 1994.

Shi Q, Martin RH: Aneuploidy in human spermatozoa: FISH analysis in men with constitutional chromosomal abnormalities, and in infertile men. Reproduction 121:655, 2001.

Shi Q, Martin RH: Multicolor fluorescence in situ hybridization analysis of meiotic chromosome segregation in a 47,XYY male and a review of the literature. Am J Med Genet 93:40, 2000.

Simpson JL: Genetics of female infertility. In Filicori M, Flamigni C (eds): Proceedings of the Conference, Treatment of Infertility: The New Frontiers. Boca Raton, FL, Communications Media for Education, 1998, p 37.

Simpson JL: Pregnancies in women with chromosomal abnormalities. In Schulman JD, Simpson JL (eds): Genetic Diseases in Pregnancy: Maternal Effects and Fetal Outcome. New York: Academic Press, 1981, p 439.

Simpson JL, Gray R, Perez A, et al.: Fertilization involving aging gametes is not associated with major birth defects and Down syndrome. Lancet 359:1670, 2002.

Simpson JL, Gray RH, Perez A, et al.: Pregnancy outcome in natural family planning users: Cohort and case control studies evaluating safety. Adv Contracep 13:201, 1997.

Simpson JL, Gray RH, Queenan JT, et al.: Pregnancy outcome associated with natural family planning (NFP): Scientific basis and experimental design for an international cohort study. Adv Contracept 4:247, 1988.

Slavotinek A, Rosenberg M, Knight S, et al.: Screening for submicroscopic chromosome rearrangements in children with idiopathic mental retardation using microsatellite markers for the chromosome telomeres. J Med Genet 36:405, 1999.

Staessen C: Fertility and assisted reproduction in XXY–ICSI and ART. In Simpson JL, et al.: Klinefelter Syndrome Conference "Expanding the Phenotype and Identifying New Research Directions. in preparation, 2002.

Stoll C, Flori E, Clavert A, et al.: Abnormal children of a 47,XYY father. J Med Genet 16:66, 1979.

Sundequist U, Hellstrom E: Transmission of 47, XYY karyotypes. Lancet 2:1367, 1969.

Sutherland GR, Gardiner AJ, Carter RF: Familial pericentric inversion of chromosome 19, inv(19)(p13q13) with a note on genetic counseling of pericentric inversion carriers. Clin Genet 10:54, 1976.

Thomas NS, Collins AR, Hassold TJ, et al.: A reinvestigation of non-disjunction resulting in 47,XXY males of paternal origin. Eur J Hum Genet 8:805, 2000.

Thomas NS, Ennis S, Sharp AJ, et al.: Maternal sex chromosome non-disjunction: Evidence for X chromosome-specific risk factors. Hum Mol Genet 10:243, 2001.

Tournaye H, Camus M, Vandervorst M, et al.: Surgical sperm retrieval for intracytoplasmic injection. Int J Androl 20:69, 1997.

Van De Velde Staquet MF, Breynaert R, Walbaum R, et al.: Progenency of mothers with trisomy 21 (apropos of a case). J Genet Hum 21:187, 1973.

Warburton D: De novo balanced chromosome rearrangements and extra marker chromosomes identified at prenatal diagnosis: Clinical significance and distribution of breakpoints. Am J Hum Genet 49:995, 1991.

Warburton D, Kline S, Stein Z, et al.: Does the karyotype of a spontaneous abortion predict the karyotype of a subsequent abortion? Am J Hum Genet 41:465, 1987.

Warburton D, Twersky S: Risk of phenotypic abnormalities in paracentric inversion carriers. Am J Med Genet 69:219, 1997.

Yoon PW, Freeman SB, Sherman SL, et al.: Advanced maternal age and the risk of Down syndrome characterized by the meiotic stage of the chromosomal error: A population-based study. Am J Hum Genet 58:628, 1996.

CHAPTER 2

Molecular and Mendelian Genetics

Mendelian Inheritance

In mendelian inheritance, a gene mutation usually involves only a single genetic locus. A chromosome carrying a single mutant gene but no other abnormality appears structurally normal because the change involves only a minute deletion, insertion, or a change in a single nucleotide sequence. Analysis of a mutant gene is therefore not ordinarily facilitated by cytogenetic studies. Instead, pedigrees are studied, a gene product or its metabolite is measured, or the DNA coding for the gene is examined.

Molecular Basis of the Gene

DNA exists in the form of a double helix, which may be envisioned as a twisted ladder (Fig. 2–1). Each vertical column consists of alternating phosphate and deoxyribose carbohydrate residues. Carbohydrate and phosphate residues of opposite sides are connected by various nitrogenous bases called nucleotides. The DNA nucleotides consist of the purines, adenine (A) or guanine (G), and the pyrimidines, thymine (T) or cytosine (C). One purine is always connected to one pyrimidine, joined by hydrogen bonds (base pairing) (Fig. 2–2). Adenine is bound to thymine by two hydrogen bonds; cytosine is bound to guanine by three hydrogen bonds and is thus more stable. As a result, the two DNA strands are complementary. If the sequence of bases on the one strand is adenine—thymine—thymine—guanine—cytosine (ATTGC), the sequence on the opposite strand must be (TAACG). The ratio of adenine to thymine is always 1:1, as is the ratio of guanine to cytosine. However, the ratio of adenine–thymine (AT) pairs to guanine–cytosine (GC) pairs varies in different portions of even a single chromosome

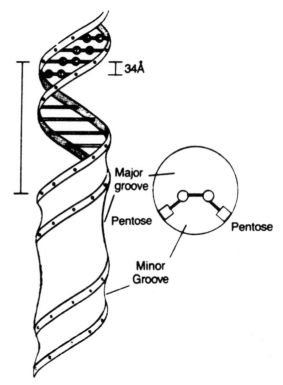

FIGURE 2–1 • Schematic representation of the double helical configuration of DNA. In (B) each vertical column is seen as consisting of alternating deoxyribose sugar residues (pentose) and phosphate residues. Pentose residues of opposite sides are connected transversely by nitrogenous bases: the purines adenine (A) or guanine (G) and the pyrimidines thymine (T) or cytosine (C). Each transverse connection consists of one purine and one pyrimidine, held together by hydrogen bonds represented here by dotted lines. (From Ford EHR: Human Chromosomes. New York: Academic Press, 1973.)

as well as among different chromosomes. The more GC pairs, the more stable the DNA. This variation is one basis for chromosomal banding. A region of a chromosome rich in GC pairs

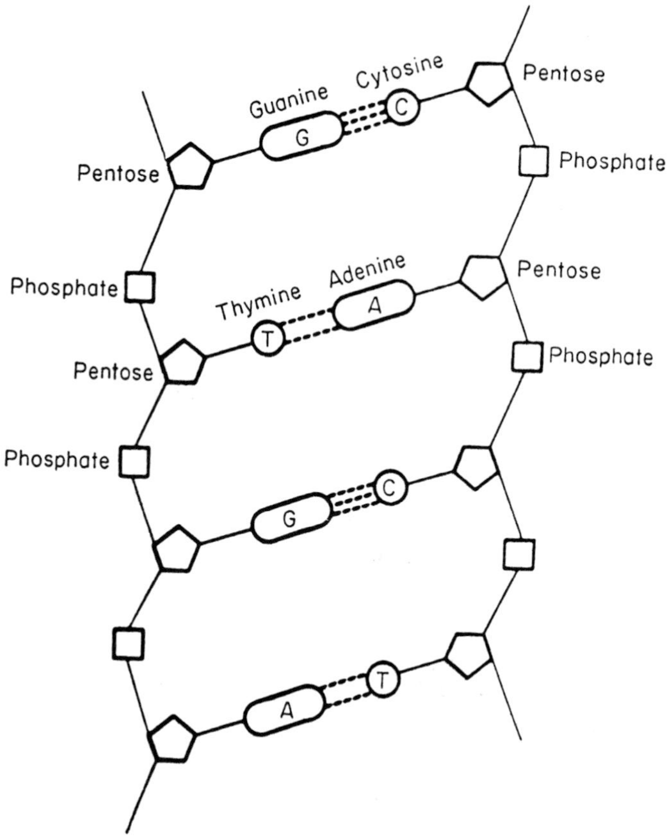

FIGURE 2–2 • Nucleic acid base pairing is controlled by hydrogen bonding (dotted lines) such that adenine always pairs with thymine and cytosine with guanine. (From Ford EHR: Human Chromosomes. New York: Academic Press, 1973.)

appears as a dark band, whereas a region rich in AT pairs appears as a light band.

Genetic information, specifically amino acid sequence, is determined by the sequence of nucleotides on one of the two DNA strands. A sequence of three bases forms a codon. A codon and its corresponding RNA signify one and only one of the 20 amino acids; however, some signals indicate cessation of transcription (Table 2–1). This table also shows abbreviations used in designating amino acid codons. UAA, UAG, and UGA are stop codons, serving as signs to terminate the message (protein). AUG is the start codon. The order (sequence) is read from the nucleotide with the carbon 5 phosphate (5′) to the nucleotide with the hydroxyl group on the carbon 3 (3′). Enzymes necessary for transcription and translation work in the 5′ to 3′ direction. The outer strand of the double helix reads 5′ to 3′ and is said to be the sense strand; the inner strand reads 3′ to 5′ and is said to be the antisense strand. The message is read from the *sense* strand; the *antisense* strand is complementary. The messenger RNA sequence corresponds to the strand, with the exception of uracil's replacing thymine.

STRUCTURAL ORGANIZATION OF THE GENE

Genes interspersed along chromosomes that are capable of coding for protein are characterized by *unique* sequences of DNA. By contrast, *repetitive* sequences of DNA are not capable of coding for protein. Not all nucleotides code for the amino acids. Sequences are discontinuous with respect to whether they do not code or do code for amino acids. Regions that code for amnio acids are called exons (Fig. 2–3). Interspersed between these sequences are repetitive sequences called intervening sequences or introns. There are also DNA distinct sequences essential for DNA transcription, RNA translation, and regulatory functions.

Upstream from the nucleotide sequence that will code for amino acids lie base sequences assumed to be involved in transcription regula-

▼ **Table 2–1.** TRIPLET NUCLEOTIDE SEQUENCES AND THE SIGNAL (AMINO ACID OR STOP) FOR
• WHICH THEY ENCODE*

First Nucleotide Base	Second Nucleotide Base				Third Nucleotide Base
	Uracil (U)	Cytosine (C)	Adenine (A)	Guanine (G)	
Uracil (U)	Phenylalanine (Phe; F)	Serine (Ser; S)	Tyrosine (Try; Y)	Cysteine (Cys; C)	U
	Phenylalanine (Phe; F)	Serine (Ser; S)	Tyrosine (Try; Y)	Cysteine (Cys; C)	C
	Leucine (Leu; L)	Serine (Ser; S)	*Stop*	*Stop*	A
	Leucine (Leu; L)	Serine (Ser; S)	*Stop*	Tryptophan (Trp; W)	G
Cytosine (C)	Leucine (Leu; L)	Proline (Pro; P)	Histidine (His; H)	R Arginine (Arg)	U
	Leucine (Leu; L)	Proline (Pro; P)	Histidine (His; H)	R Arginine (Arg)	C
	Leucine (Leu; L)	Proline (Pro; P)	Glutamine (Gln; Q)	R Arginine (Arg)	A
	Leucine (Leu; L)	Proline (Pro; P)	Glutamine (Gln; Q)	R Arginine (Arg)	G
Adenine (A)	Isoleucine (Iie; I)	Threonine (Thr; T)	Asparagine (Asn; N)	Serine (Ser; S)	U
	Isoleucine (Iie; I)	Threonine (Thr; T)	Asparagine (Asn; N)	Serine (Ser; S)	C
	Isoleucine (Iie; I)	Threonine (Thr; T)	Lysine (Lys; K)	Arginine (Arg; R)	A
	Start; M (Methionine) (Met)	Threonine (Thr; T)	Lysine (Lys; K)	Arginine (Arg; R)	G
Guanine (G)	Valine (Val; V)	Alanine (Ala; A)	Aspartic acid (Asp; D)	Glycine (Gly; G)	U
	Valine (Val; V)	Alanine (Ala; A)	Aspartic acid (Asp; D)	Glycine (Gly; G)	C
	Valine (Val; V)	Alanine (Ala; A)	Glutamic acid (Glu; E)	Glycine (Gly; G)	A
	Valine (Val; V)	Alanine (Ala; A)	Glutamic acid (Glu; E)	Glycine (Gly; G)	G

* Letters in front of signal designate the symbol for each amino acid (or stop). As an example, if the codon reads uracil (left or first column); uracil (horizontal); guanine (right or third column), the amino acid coded is leucine (Leu or L).

tion. The 5' region contains various promoters and enhancers, still not completely characterized. However, one consistent feature is that the nucleotide sequence TATA ("TATA box") is consistently found in about 30 base pairs (bp) prior to (5' side) the site at which transcription begins (see Fig. 2–3). The TATA box is thought to be the site at which transcription is initiated by RNA polymerase II, the enzyme actually responsible for transcribing mRNA from DNA. The TATA box helps properly align RNA polymerase II with DNA through interactions involving various transcription factors. The other pivotal sequence 5' to the coding region is CAAT, located 50–75 bp upstream from the TATA transcription site (see Fig. 2–3). The CAAT box is the site at which RNA polymerase II actually binds, again facilitated by transcription initiation factors. Transcription proceeds in the 5' to 3' direction, extending beyond the region of unique-sequence DNA.

The signal terminating transcription is not precisely known, but the sequence AATAAA is consistently observed 15–30 bases 5' to that site at which a 50 to 300 residue polyadenylated [poly(A)] tail will be added. The function of the

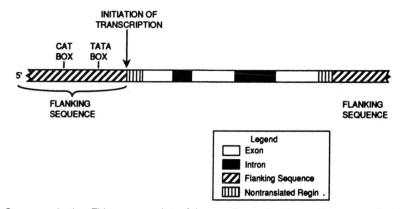

FIGURE 2–3 • Gene organization. This gene consists of three coding regions (exons) interspersed with two intervening sequences (introns). Upstream (5') to the coding region lie sequences necessary for gene regulation (so-called CAT box and TATA box, for example).

tail presumably relates to stabilizing mRNA. This "poly A tail" is also invaluable analytically, providing a ready method for recovering mRNA among other cellular components.

POST-TRANSCRIPTIONAL EVENTS

Figure 2–4 shows the sequence of events by which DNA is first transcribed into messenger RNA (mRNA) and then translated into protein. After an entire sequence is transcribed into mRNA in a 5' to 3' direction, post-transcriptional processes are necessary before the protein can be synthesized (translated). As noted throughout the genome unique-sequence, DNAs (exons) are interspersed among repetitive DNA sequences.

A precise splicing mechanism exists to excise introns prior to translation. The nucleotides GT on the 5' end of the intervening sequence are removed along with the entire intron and nucleotides AG on the 3' end. Mutations involving splice junction are common mechanisms producing mendelian disorders, one example being Tay-Sachs disease.

TRANSLATION

Once introns are excised, the transcribed mRNA can direct polypeptide synthesis (translation). This process takes place in the cytoplasm. The first step in translation is that mRNA moves into the cytoplasm to associate with ribosomes, structures consisting of both protein and a special high-molecular-weight RNA called ribosomal RNA (rRNA). Adenosine triphosphate next reacts with the carboxyl end of a specific amino acid to form an amino acid–specific transfer tRNA, which then lines up on the ribosome complex at that point signified by its appropriate codon (see Table 2–1). The amino acids that make up the polypeptide chain are thus brought into correct sequence.

CELLULAR TRANSPORT OF PROTEINS

After being synthesized on ribosomes, proteins must be transported to the appropriate location, either inside the cell (e.g., lysosome) or outside the cell (e.g., extracellular fluid). Specific pathways exist to accomplish this purpose. Certain amino acids bind to a receptor on the endoplasmic reticulum, allowing the still-growing polypeptide sequence to be transferred across the endoplasmic

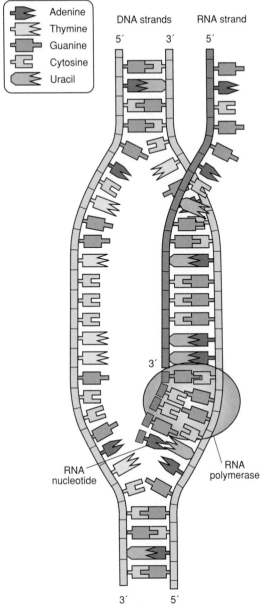

FIGURE 2–4 • Transcription of DNA to mRNA. RNA polymerase II proceeds along the DNA strand in the 3' to 5' direction, assembling a strand of mRNA nucleotides that is complementary to the DNA template strand. (From Jorde LB, Carey JC, Bamshad MJ, et al.: Medical Genetics, 2nd ed. St. Louis: Mosby, 2000.)

reticulum. Additional processes direct the polypeptide to more distant locations.

Transmission of Mutant Genes in Families

The familial patterns followed by mendelian traits depend not only on whether the mutant gene is dominant or recessive but also on whether the gene is located on an autosome or a sex chromosome. There are five potential patterns of transmission: autosomal dominant, autosomal recessive, X-linked dominant, X-linked recessive, and Y-linked.

DEFINITIONS

Chromosomes exist in pairs, one maternally derived and one paternally derived. Chromosomes contain genes; thus, genes exist in pairs. Stated more properly, alleles—different states of a single gene—exist in pairs. Alleles occupy identical places on homologous chromosomes and can become interchanged during meiotic recombination.

If alleles are identical, *homozygosity* exists (Fig. 2–5). If alleles are dissimilar, *heterozygosity* exists. An allele capable of expression in its heterozygous state is dominant, whereas an allele capable of expression only in homozygous form is recessive. The preceding definitions apply cleanly to autosomal loci. However, different circumstances exist for X-linked loci. A recessive trait whose allele is located on the X chromosome is expressed by all males (46,XY) carrying the recessive allele. Affected males are said to be *hemizygous*.

An important concept of particular relevance to autosomal recessive inheritance is *compound heterozygosity* (see Fig. 2–5). In compound het-

erozygosity, two alleles are dissimilar, but both are abnormal (dysfunctional). They need not necessary produce dysfunction to an identical extent. Homozygosity for ΔF508 cystic fibrosis (see Chapters 4 and 8) results in virtually no gene product (CFTR). Compound heterozygosity may occur in which one allele is ΔF508 and the other is a less deleterious allele capable of producing some functioning gene product (e.g., 10 to 20% of expected). Overall, the 5 to 10% of expected CFTR (ΔF508 contributes zero) may be enough to mitigate against the most severe CF phenotype. In other circumstances, compound heterozygosity may be clinically indistinguishable from homozygosity for a single mutant allele. By molecular techniques, it is clear that compound heterozygosity is the rule rather than the exception for autosomal recessive disorders. (The exception arises in consanguineous matings.) In cystic fibrosis heterozygotes, some affected individuals are homozygous for deletion of three nucleotides at position 508 (ΔF508), but others have one such mutant allele and one other dysfunctional allele at the same locus. The various disorders of sexual differentiation (see Chapters 10 to 12) also illustrate this concept.

AUTOSOMAL DOMINANT INHERITANCE

An autosomal dominant allele is recognized by its ability to be expressed in more than one generation (Fig. 2–6). In autosomal dominant traits, equal numbers of males and females are usually affected. The likelihood is 50% that an individual carrying a mutant autosomal dominant gene (allele) will transmit that allele to any given offspring, male or female. If penetrance (see later for definition) is complete, no unaffected individual will have an affected offspring.

Autosomal dominant patterns are not always associated with the idealized characteristics defined earlier. Some individuals may be more severely affected than others, a phenomenon known as *variable expression*. This characteristic has been known clinically for decades, but the molecular basis has only been elucidated more recently. In a given gene, the exact mutation may vary—deletion or single nucleotide substitution, for example. This is called molecular heterogeneity. Some molecular changes are more deleterious than others. A mutation resulting in no gene product (protein) is likely to be more serious than a mutation in which a single amino acid substitution has occurred. Variable expression occurs not only among families but also among different

Allelic forms of a single autosomal gene

A = normal ; a or b = mutation

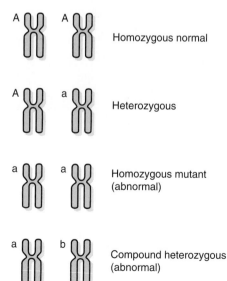

Homozygous normal

Heterozygous

Homozygous mutant (abnormal)

Compound heterozygous (abnormal)

FIGURE 2–5 • Allelic forms of a single autosomal gene. (A) = normal; (a or b) = mutation.

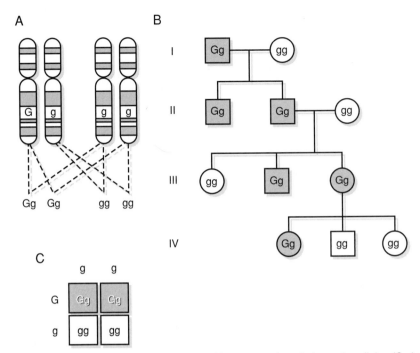

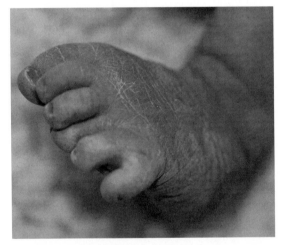

FIGURE 2–6 • Autosomal dominant inheritance produced by segregation of alternative alleles (G,g) at a single autosomal locus (A) as predicted using a Punnett square (C). An idealized pedigree is shown (B). (From Wilson GN: Clinical Genetics: A Short Course. New York: Wiley, 2000.)

affected members of a single family (intrafamilial *variability*). A single mutant gene may also be responsible for several ostensibly distinct phenotypical effects (*pleiotropy*). Occasionally an autosomal dominant allele may exert its effect only on individuals of one sex (*sex limitation*). Another characteristic of autosomal dominant inheritance is that some individuals may be phenotypically normal yet carry a mutant autosomal dominant allele. Such a mutant allele is said to show *lack of penetrance* in the phenotypically normal individual. Actually, the clinical observation of *lack of penetrance* probably reflects only our inability to study a given gene product directly. If molecular analysis were possible in all disorders, many "nonpenetrant" individuals probably would show an abnormality in the gene product or certainly in DNA itself.

In the absence of ability to measure DNA or its gene products, an autosomal dominant gene in humans must be recognized clinically. Usually one of the following clinical characteristics must exist for dominant inheritance to be recognized:

1. Lack of interference with reproductive ability (e.g., polydactyly) (Fig. 2–7).
2. Manifestation only after reproduction is completed (e.g., Huntington disease)

FIGURE 2–7 • Postaxial polydactyly. This common autosomal disorder does not adversely affect reproductive fitness (F) and thus is readily transmitted from generation to generation. (From Jorde LB, Carey JC, Bamshad MJ, et al.: Medical Genetics, 2nd ed. St. Louis: Mosby, 2000.)

3. Lack of penetrance or variable expressivity, resulting in a minimally affected parent potentially having a severely affected progeny.

Dominant disorders do not always have to be transmitted from an affected parent. The disorder may have arisen de novo, as result of a fresh mutation in a sperm or oocyte. An important principle is that the more severe the trait, the more likely it is that an affected individual has a new mutation. That is, as reproductive fitness (F) decreases, the proportion of cases due to a fresh mutation increases. As F approximates zero, all cases would reflect new mutations. Relatively few cases of polydactyly represent new mutations, but 90% of achondroplasia cases do. All individuals with a dominant trait conferring sterility must represent a new mutation. Thus, a reasonable hypothesis would be that conditions like müllerian aplasia could in part represent a fresh dominant mutation (see Chapter 8).

AUTOSOMAL RECESSIVE INHERITANCE

An autosomal recessive trait is expressed only when an individual is homozygous for the mutant allele. At a given genetic locus, both alleles show an identical mutation. As noted, different yet equally dysfunctional alleles could also exist (compound heterozygosity). For most disorders, this is more often than not the case.

However, an individual with a recessive trait is usually the product of a mating between parents who are both heterozygous (carriers) for mutation at the same locus. If two heterozygotes mate, the likelihood is 25% that a given offspring will be affected (Fig. 2–8). If multiple affected siblings of both sexes exist, autosomal recessive inheritance should be considered. Consanguineous parents (designated by double lines in Fig. 2–8) are more likely to have an affected child because they are more likely to carry identical alleles (mutant or normal) than nonconsanguineous parents. Thus, an individual with a recessive trait is relatively more likely to arise from a consanguineous than from a nonconsanguineous union. The rarer a trait, the higher the proportion of affected individuals who arise from consanguineous unions. For common traits (e.g., cystic fibrosis, sickle cell anemia), parents of affected offspring usually are not consanguineous. For very rare traits the only reported cases may have been derived from consanguineous unions (highly inbred communities).

Autosomal recessive inheritance can also occur if a homozygous individual mates with a heterozygous individual. Half (50%) of the offspring would be affected (pseudoautosomal

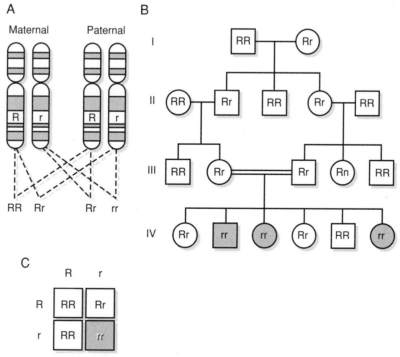

FIGURE 2–8 • Autosomal recessive inheritance. Allele R is dominant to r. Potential genotypes in offspring are shown in (A) and in (C) (Punnett square), illustrating the outcome of a mating between two clinically normal heterozygotes for the mutant allele. An idealized pedigree is shown in (B). (From Wilson GN: Clinical Genetics: A Short Course, 2nd ed. New York: Wiley, 2000.)

dominant inheritance). This phenomenon is becoming more frequent for serious traits, as survival to reproduction is becoming less unusual for those with serious autosomal recessive traits (e.g., cystic fibrosis, sickle cell anemia).

HARDY-WEINBERG EQUILIBRIUM

The mathematical relationship between the frequencies of homozygotes and heterozygotes is clinically important. This relationship is expressed by the Hardy-Weinberg equilibrium (Table 2–2). Suppose the normal allele is A and the mutant allele is a. The normal allele A is said to have the frequency p, and the mutant allele is said to have the frequency q. The frequencies of alleles at a given locus add up to 1, $p + q = 1$; after squaring both sides of the equation, $p^2 + 2pq + q^2 = 1$. Under binomial expansion, p^2 becomes the frequency of individuals homozygous for allele $A(AA)$; q^2 is the frequency of individuals homozygous for allele $a(aa)$; $2pq$ is the frequency of the heterozygote (Aa). Important clinically is that the frequency of a mutant allele (q) is usually much less than the frequency of a normal allele (p). If q is much less than 0.5, q^2 is very much less than $2pq$ because p is nearly equal to 1. Given the relative magnitudes of $2pq$ and q^2, it is clear that the "load" for deleterious recessive traits is carried mostly by heterozygotes; relatively few homozygotes exist (see Table 2–2). To illustrate, suppose the incidence of a trait is 1/10,000. Thus, q^2 = 1/10,000; q = 1/100. It follows that p = 99/100, or almost 1; $2pq = 2 \times 1 \times 1/100 = 1/50$. That is, 2pq (1/50) is much more frequent than 1/10,000 (q^2).

Clinically unaffected individuals who have a sibling with an autosomal recessive disorder often inquire about risks of their own offspring's having that disorder. Assuming that neither they nor their mate are related, the risk of having affected offspring can usually be shown to be low. If heterozygote detection tests are not available, the *a priori* likelihood that the unaffected individual is a heterozygote can be calculated if the incidence of the trait is known. If no tests exist to determine heterozygosity, the unaffected sib will have one of three equally likely genotypes: two connote heterozygosity and one connotes homozygosity for the normal allele; the fourth possibility (homozygous mutant) is excluded on clinical grounds. The likelihood of heterozygosity is thus 2 in 3. The likelihood of the individual's mate being heterozygous for the same mutant gene will reflect gene frequency in the general population, as determined by the Hardy-Weinberg equilibrium. If incidence of the trait is 1/8100 births, the heterozygote frequency is 1/45 (q^2 = 1/8100; q = 1/90; 2pq = 1/45). The likelihood that any given offspring will be affected is thus 2/3 × 1/45 × 1/4 = 2/540 = 1/270. If the trait is rarer (q^2 = 1/30,000), risk is correspondingly lower. Most couples are surprised to find that their risk is so low. Risks for other family members can be calculated on the basis of assuming that a heterozygous individual has equal likelihood of either transmitting or not transmitting a mutant gene. Thus, a normal individual whose uncle was affected would have a likelihood of only one third of being heterozygous (i.e., 2/3 × 1/2 = 2/6 = 1/3).

X-LINKED RECESSIVE INHERITANCE

A mutant recessive gene located on the X chromosome is expressed by all males (46,XY) who carry the mutation. Such individuals are said to be hemizygous. In the usual situation, X-linked recessive alleles are transmitted through phenotypically normal yet actually heterozygous females (Fig. 2–9). If an X-linked recessive mutant is segregating, affected individuals might have affected

▼ **Table 2–2.** RELATIONSHIP OF HETEROZYGOTE AND HOMOZYGOTE FREQUENCIES TO INCIDENCE
• OF AN AUTOSOMAL RECESSIVE TRAIT*

Disease	Disease Frequency	Allele Frequency		Genotype Frequency			Ratio of Heterozygotes to Homozygotes Aa/aa ($2pq/q^2$)
		A(p)	a(q)	AA(p^2)	Aa(2pq)	aa(q^2)	
Alkaptonuria	1/1,000,000	0.999	0.001	0.998	0.002	0.000001	2000
Oculocutaneous albinism *(OCA 1)*	1/40,000	0.995	0.005	0.990	0.010	0.000025	400
Phenylketonuria *(PKU)*	1/10,000	0.990	0.010	0.980	0.020	0.0001	200
Tay-Sachs disease *(TSD)*	1/3,600	0.983	0.017	0.966	0.033	0.0003	110
Cystic fibrosis *(CF)*	1/2,000	0.978	0.022	0.956	0.044	0.0005	88
Sickle cell anemia *(SCA)*	1/400	0.950	0.050	0.902	0.095	0.0025	38

*The rarer a trait, the greater the genetic burden in the heterozygote (higher ratio of 2pq and q^2).

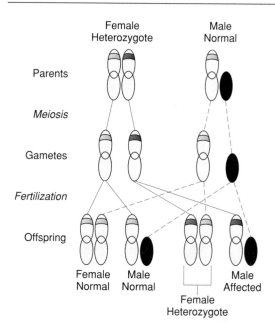

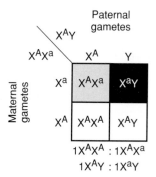

FIGURE 2–9 • X-linked recessive inheritance. The mating diagram and Punnett square illustrate the outcome of a mating between a clinically normal female heterozygous for the mutant allele (shown in red) and a normal male and between a homozygous normal female and a hemizygous affected male. (From Gelehrter TD, Collins FS, Ginsburg D: Principles of Medical Genetics, 2nd ed. Baltimore: Williams & Wilkins, 1998.)

male siblings, maternal uncles, maternal nephews, maternal male first cousins, and certain other maternal male relatives.

The probability is 0.5 that a heterozygous female will transmit an X-linked recessive allele to any given offspring. Males inheriting the allele will be affected, whereas females inheriting the allele will be heterozygous like their mother. An affected (hemizygous) male transmits the allele to all of his daughters but to none of his sons (Fig. 2–10). Male-to-male transmission thus excludes X-linked inheritance. All offspring of an affected male will be phenotypically normal, unless the female is heterozygous for the same mutant. In such a case, four genotypes are possi-

ble, and females may be affected. Although this is unlikely for severe traits (e.g., Duchenne muscular dystrophy), it is quite possible for mild traits (color blindness) or successfully treatable conditions (hemophilia).

Occasionally, phenotypical females may manifest X-linked recessive traits. 46,XX Individuals can be affected if they are homozygous, a circumstance that could result if their mothers were heterozygous and their fathers were hemizygous. This is not uncommon for nonlethal traits such as color blindness or treatable conditions like hemophilia A. Other situations resulting in affected females include vicissitudes of X inactivation (preferential inactivation of normal X) so extreme that phenotypical effects approximating those present in hemizygous males exist (see Fig. 2–10). More often, mild phenotypic consequences are observed in obligate heterozygotes. Heterozygotes for complete androgen insensitivity (see Chapter 11) may show scanty pubic hair and delayed menarche. There also exist mutant genes that show deviations in X-inactivation from the expected randomization between the maternal X and paternal X. This phenomenon is called skewed X-inactivation and could be relevant for recurrent abortions if one X contains a lethal allele (see Chapter 5). Finally, females with only one X chromosome (45,X) would obviously be affected if the sole X has a mutant allele (hemizygosity).

Although it has not yet been reported, clinically normal females heterozygous for an X-linked recessive mutation deleteriously affecting ovarian development could have a homozygous (affected) daughter as a result of mating with a hemizygous male, who could have the same mutant gene but be normal because the gene manifests only a sex-limited phenotype (males lack ovaries).

The possibility of new (gamete) mutations must always be considered. Thus, it cannot necessarily be assumed that the mother of a child with an X-linked recessive mutation is heterozygous. The child may represent a new mutation arising in the ovum. If the trait is lethal with respect to fertility and if no other relatives are affected, the likelihood of a new mutation is theoretically one in three (Table 2–3). For X-linked recessive traits that are genetically lethal in the sense of affected individuals being sterile (e.g., androgen insensitivity), this can actually be verified (Hiort et al., 1998).

X-LINKED DOMINANT INHERITANCE

X-linked dominant inheritance mimics autosomal dominant inheritance, except that male-to-

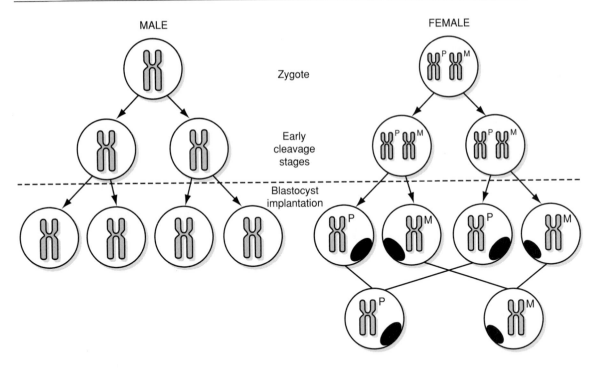

MALE

FEMALE

Zygote

Early
cleavage
stages

Blastocyst
implantation

MOSAICISM OF TWO TYPES OF CELLS

FIGURE 2–10 • Schematic diagram of the Lyon hypothesis. P represents the paternally derived X chromosome, and M the maternally derived X in the female; the single X in the male must be inherited from the mother. The inactive X is shown as the dark mass. (From Gelehrter TD, Collins FS, Ginsburg D: Principles of Medical Genetics, 2nd ed. Baltimore: Williams & Wilkins,1998.)

▼ **Table 2–3.** MUTATION RATES FOR
• AUTOSOMAL DOMINANT, AUTOSOMAL
RECESSIVE, AND X-LINKED RECESSIVE
GENES

Definitions: μ = mutation rate (locus/gamete/generation)
F = Fitness (reproductive efficiency as measured
in offspring versus general population)
X = Incidence of trait at birth

Formula: Autosomal dominant
$\mu = (1\text{-}F)\,X$
Autosomal recessive
$\mu = 1/2\,(1\text{-}F)\,X$
X–Linked recessive
$\mu = 1/3\,(1\text{-}F)\,X$

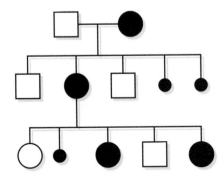

● Affected female
○ Unaffected female
□ Unaffected male
• Spontateous abortion

FIGURE 2–11 • X-linked dominant inheritance with male lethality. (From Scriver CR, Beaudet AL, Sly WS, et al.: The Metabolic and Molecular Bases of Inherited Disease, 8th ed. New York: McGraw-Hill, 2001.)

male transmission cannot occur (in the absence of Klinefelter syndrome caused by XY disomy). A male carrying an X-linked dominant allele transmits the mutant to all his daughters but to none of his sons (Fig. 2–11). The probability that a female with an X-linked dominant allele will pass that allele to any offspring, male or female, is 0.5. Relatively few X-linked dominant traits are known, one example being vitamin D–resistant rickets.

In X-linked dominant traits, the incidence of affected females is twice that of affected males.

However, females are usually less severely affected. In fact, some X-linked dominant traits are lethal in males. The only affected individuals would be females. A prenatal genetic diagnostic strategy might involve allowing only males to be delivered; males would either be normal or never survive until prenatal sampling. Females would have one chance in two of being affected.

BAYESIAN CALCULATIONS

In counseling individuals at risk for X-linked recessive traits, it is frequently helpful to utilize bayesian calculations. Conceptually simple but sometimes complex in application, bayesian calculations take into account all available data rather than merely being limited to *a priori* calculations. This might be called codified common sense. For example, logic dictates that a woman at theoretical risk for offspring having an X-linked recessive trait must be less likely to be heterozygous if multiple consecutive sons are to be unaffected. An example might arise if a woman (proband) relates that her two brothers have an X-linked disorder for which neither metabolic nor DNA analysis is currently possible. We can deduce that her own mother is an obligate heterozygote; thus, the prospective mother has a 50% likelihood of being heterozygous. This 50% likelihood (0.5 probability) is the proband's *a priori* risk (prior probability). If, on the other hand, a woman relates that she has had three unaffected males, she might still be heterozygous and simply fortunate enough to have had no affected sons; the probability is one in eight of a heterozygote's having three consecutive unaffected sons. However, the greater likelihood is that the woman is in fact not heterozygous. Table 2–4 illustrates how information concerning the three unaffected males can be taken into account. The newly calculated likelihood of being heterozygous is only one in nine, considerably lower than the one in two if one had counseling only on the basis of *a priori* expectations.

Bayesian calculations are also useful in other circumstances. Estimating likelihood of heterozygosity for a trait lacking a completely reliable assay is one example. Estimating risk for a trait with varying ages of onset is another. Clinical geneticists are familiar with their use, but in a genetic context obstetricians and gynecologists ordinarily need to be aware only of the existence of bayesian calculations.

Y-LINKED INHERITANCE

A male would pass a Y-linked gene to each of his sons but to none of his daughters. Y-linked inheritance for monogenic traits remains unproved in humans; however, several features are controlled

▼ **Table 2–4.** BAYESIAN CALCULATIONS IN A FAMILY AT RISK FOR AN X-LINKED RECESSIVE DISORDER.

	Proband Heterozygous	Proband not Heterozygous
Prior probability	$\frac{1}{2}$	$\frac{1}{2}$
Conditional probability	$(\frac{1}{2})^3 = \frac{1}{8}$	1
Joint probability (prior and conditional)	$\frac{1}{16}$	$\frac{1}{2}$
Posterior probability (joint and prior)	$\dfrac{\frac{1}{16} \text{ or } \frac{8}{16}}{\frac{1}{16} + \frac{1}{2} (\text{or } \frac{8}{16})}$ $=\dfrac{\frac{1}{16}}{\frac{9}{16}}$ $=\frac{1}{9}$	$\dfrac{\frac{1}{16} \text{ or } \frac{8}{16}}{\frac{1}{16} + \frac{1}{2}}$ $=\dfrac{\frac{8}{16}}{\frac{9}{16}}$ $=\frac{8}{9}$

This analysis calculates the likelihood of heterozygosity for a woman whose two brothers have Duchenne muscular dystrophy, an X-linked recessive disorder. The a priori risk (prior probability) of heterozygosity is 1/2, inasmuch as the woman's mother is an obligate heterozygote. Suppose the woman has three unaffected sons. What is the likelihood that she is nevertheless heterozygous? Multiplying prior by conditional probability yields joint probability. The newly derived heterozygosity risk, taking into account the three unaffected sons, is the posterior probability calculated as shown: 1/9 From Simpson JL: Principles of Human Genetics. *In* Reece EA, Hobbins JC (eds): Medicine of the Fetus and Mother. Philadelphia: Lippincott, 1992.

by factors on the Y chromosome, notably testicular determination and spermatogenesis. These topics are discussed in Chapter 10.

A male with a Y mutation, for example the Y long arm (Yq) deletion (DAZ) that causes azoospermia, *must* transmit that mutation to all his sons. In turn, DAZ (*Deleted AZoospermia*) cannot be transmitted to his daughters because by definition they fail to inherit his Y. Analogous to what occurs with autosomal dominant genes, it should not be assumed that all males who obligatorily inherit DAZ will have identical phenotypes. Variable expressivity exists. If DAZ or another Y gene conferring azoospermia or oligospermia were pleiotropic, offspring may or may not manifest the same spectrum of traits as the father.

SPONTANEOUS MUTATIONS

Gene mutations are individually rare, but overall 1% of all infants have a disorder resulting from a single mutant gene. Sometimes affected individuals inherit a mutant gene as described earlier, but at other times they are the first in their families to have the disorder. Spontaneous mutation rates average 10^{-5} to 10^{-6} per locus per gamete per generation. Overall, each gamete is estimated to contain 20 to 30 mutations. Most mutations are neutral or lethal. Otherwise, many more than 2 to 3% of liveborns would be abnormal.

Mutation rates increase with increasing paternal age. Fathers in their fifth and sixth decades have a greater likelihood of certain gene mutations arising in their germ cells. This applies to some but not to all X-linked recessive and autosomal dominant disorders. This increase is believed to reflect in some fashion the continued germ cell replication (spermatogenesis) that occurs throughout a male's fertile lifetime. The exact manner by which repeated replications lead to mutation remains obscure, but at the least it is known that there are more opportunities for errors with aging. Unlike the situation for chromosomal abnormalities, advanced maternal age is not associated with increased gene mutations.

There are many mutations, but it is often difficult to discern their role in an individual clinical case. Ionizing irradiation is one well-established mutagen. X-rays are the major source of ionizing irradiation, but ultraviolet light also causes mutations. Ultrasound and microwave radiation is not ionizing and probably not mutagenic. Exposure to a video display terminal is probably not mutagenic. Moreover, even x-ray exposures of 50–100 rad only double mutation rates; thus, the absolute risk following all except massive radiation exposure is relatively low.

Numerous chemicals cause mutations in animals and in vitro testing systems, and many of these would be plausible mutagens in humans. Well-known examples include alkylating agents, DNA base analogs (e.g., 5-bromouracil), antimetabolites, nitrous acid, and acridine dyes. Even inorganic salts, caffeine, nitrites, and other ubiquitous agents are mutagenic under certain circumstances. It is difficult to determine the likelihood of individual compounds being mutagenic in humans in a given circumstance. Retrospective clinical data cannot provide satisfactory information. Fortunately, even substantive exposure to alkylating agents or antimetabolites leads to little if any increase in abnormal liveborns. Individuals treated prior to pregnancy with chemotherapeutic agents show no increased abnormalities in subsequent progeny. This suggests that most induced mutations are lethal.

MOLECULAR BASIS OF MUTATIONS

The multitude of human mutations is the core of this volume. Fundamentally, however, only a few general types of DNA alterations exist. In point mutations only a single nucleotide is changed. The basis is either (1) a transition in which one pyrimidine is replaced by another or one purine is replaced by another (i.e., A to T or G to C), or (2) a transversion in which one pyrimidine is replaced by a purine, and vice versa. The latter is generally more deleterious, but in either case the altered nucleotide results in an altered codon. In missense mutation (Fig. 2–12), an altered protein is generated. The alteration could be deleterious (e.g., sickle cell anemia) or it could be innocuous (silent). Sometimes the mutation abolishes the capacity to synthesize an amino acid. If a transition or transversion results in transfer RNA's reading UAA, UAG, or UGA (DNA = TAA, TAG, TGA), the message now reads terminate or stop (X); thus, the gene product is truncated. These mutations are nonsense mutations.

A point mutation with major consequences is a frame shift mutation (Fig. 2–13). If three nucleotides are deleted, an entire amino acid is lost (e.g., ΔF508 cystic fibrosis). However, if only one nucleotide is deleted (or any number other than a multiple of three), the result is that the starting point for genetic transcription (i.e., codons) is altered; subsequent codons read a message differently from that previously transcribed, the result being that all codons distal (3') to the mutation are out of phase. The same situation arises with insertions of nucleotides other than a multiple of three. For example, a four base insertion (TATC) in the hexosaminidase A gene is the most common cause of Tay-Sachs disease.

Other molecular perturbations produce loss of large amounts of DNA. Deletions may arise from various mechanisms, common examples being α-thalassemia or Duchenne muscular dystrophy. The basis may be unequal crossing over during meiosis. Finally, mutations may involve splicing mechanisms necessary to excise introns (intervening sequences) from exons (coding sequences) (Fig. 2–14).

Volumes are written on the molecular details of mutations, to which we have alluded only briefly. Of note is that the same processes have been retained throughout evolution. The genetic code and molecular mechanisms underlying mutations are the same in humans as in lower species.

Imprinting and Uniparental Disomy

It is well known that X chromosomes in excess of one are inactivated. At a given time in embryogenesis, one of the two X chromosomes in a 46,XX cell is inactivated. Once the chromosome is inac-

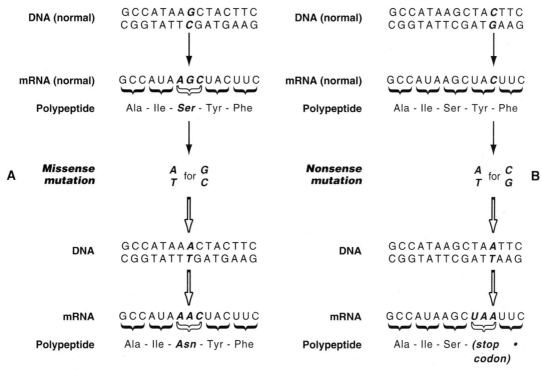

FIGURE 2–12 • Missense mutations (A) produce a single amino acid change, whereas nonsense mutations (B) produce a stop codon in the mRNA. Stop codons terminate translation of the polypeptide. (From Jorde LB, Carey JC, Bamshad MJ, et al.: Medical Genetics, 2nd ed. St. Louis: Mosby, 2000.)

tivated (presumably through processes relating to methylation), the process persists in perpetuity among descendants of a given cell, including gametes. The consequence of X inactivation is that X-linked genes in a given cell in normal females originate from a single parent, namely, the one from whom the active X was derived. This process is called imprinting.

Autosomal loci have historically been considered to display biallelic gene expression. In contrast to X-linked alleles, both autosomal alleles are active, one paternally and one maternally derived. It now develops that this expected symmetry is not always followed. Sometimes only a single allele is active (monoallelic expression). Further, the active allele must sometimes be obligatorily derived from only one or the other parent (male or female). If the allele is not inherited from the appropriate parent, an abnormal phenotype develops, even if the other parent transmits a normal allele. In monoallelic expression, the allele not required is inactivated, just as in X chromosomes in excess of one.

The prototypic disorders that helped elucidate autosomal imprinting in humans are Prader-Willi syndrome (PWS) and Angelman syndrome (AS), two well-recognized malformation syndromes controlled by contiguous regions on the long arm of chromosome No. 15. Paternally-derived genes in a given region must be expressed in order to avoid PWS; genes on the homologous maternally derived region do not suffice (Fig. 2–15). Maternally derived genes must be expressed in AS; the paternally derived region does not suffice. PWS and AS may arise under a variety of circumstances. Figure 2–16 shows how this deduction could be made for these or other imprinted conditions. In PWS (1) the paternally-derived critical region can be deleted, or (2) both (two) alleles may be inactive as result of both being maternal in origin. The latter circumstance can arise if the single paternal No. 15 chromosome is expelled from a trisomic zygote originally consisting of two maternal and one paternal 15 chromosomes. Uniparental disomy is then said to exist. By contrast, if one of the two maternal 15s had been expelled, a normal situation would have arisen (trisomic rescue).

Uniparental disomy is not necessarily rare or of small clinical relevance. In Chapter 14 it is shown that 2% of chorionic villi show trisomic cells, although usually in very low percentages. The frequency may be higher earlier in gestation. If the zygote had originally been trisomic and correc-

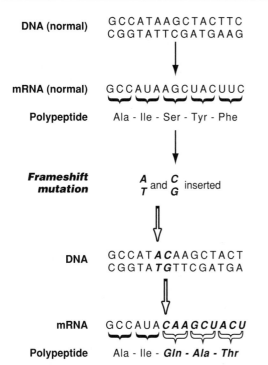

DNA (normal)
GCCATAAGCTACTTC
CGGTATTCGATGAAG

mRNA (normal)
GCCAUAAGCUACUUC

Polypeptide
Ala - Ile - Ser - Tyr - Phe

Frameshift mutation
$\frac{A}{T}$ and $\frac{C}{G}$ inserted

DNA
GCCAT*AC*AAGCTACT
CGGTA*TG*TTCGATGA

mRNA
GCCAUA*CAAGCUACU*

Polypeptide
Ala - Ile - **Gln - Ala - Thr**

FIGURE 2–13 • Frameshift mutations result from the addition or deletion of a number of bases that are not a multiple of three. This alters all of the codons downstream from the site of insertion or deletion. (From Jorde LB, Carey JC, Bamshad MJ, et al.: Medical Genetics, 2nd ed. St. Louis: Mosby, 2000.)

tion occurred through expulsion of one of the three chromosomes present in triplicate, uniparental disomy (UPD) could exist. (The likelihood of UPD would be one in three if expulsion occurs.) Two types of UPD exist: isodisomy and hetereodisomy (Fig. 2–17). In the former the two chromosomes contributed by the single parents are identical (one on the other homologue); in the latter two different chromosomes are contributed.

Whether UPD exerts a phenotypical effect depends on whether a given chromosome displays monallelic expression for any of its genes. UPD does not seem to have a deleterious effect for all chromosomes. A special concern is that UPD can follow asymmetric segregation in a parent having a balanced robertsonian translocation. However, this now seems less likely than once feared.

Imprinting may also involve entire haploid sets of chromosome. If both haploid sets in a diploid zygote are maternal in origin, the result is an ovarian teratoma (dermoid). If both haploid sets are paternal, the result is hydatidiform mole. Paternal chromosomes govern placental growth, whereas maternal chromosomes govern embryonic growth. If in triploidy two of the three haploid sets are paternal, hydatidiform mole

results. If two of the three sets are maternal, the placenta is small and intrauterine growth retardation results. This phenomenon of differential placental versus fetal growth is well established in rodents and seems to apply to humans as well.

Mitochondrial Genes

It is axiomatic that the number of human chromosomes is 46, but actually this refers only to the number of *nuclear* chromosomes. It would be more accurate to take into account that each cell also contains mitochondria, each of which contains a single circular chromosome. Mitochondrial DNA has the capacity to be translated into proteins, especially those of significance for oxidative phosphorylation (cytochromes).

The mitochondrial chromosome is more than 16,000 nucleotides long. The chromosome is circular, containing an outer H strand and an inner L strand (Fig. 2–18). The vital information is coded by the outer H strand. Minor differences exist between the mitochondrial and nuclear genetic codes, but these usually need not concern obstetricians and gynecologists. In mitochondrial DNA there are no intervening sequences and little noncoding DNA 5′ or 3′ to the actual coding sequence.

Mitochondrial DNA does not represent genetic esoterica; several human diseases result from abnormalities in mitochondrial DNA. Recall that females contribute almost all the cytoplasm present in a zygote; males contribute only a pronucleus. Inasmuch as mitochondria are located in the cytoplasm, mitochondrial disorders could be expected to be transmitted only through females to both female and male offspring. Transmission of mitochondrial mutations follows *cytoplasmic inheritance*, through exclusively maternal lineage (Fig. 2–19). If a mitochondrial mutation exists, it may or may not be transmitted because not all mitochondria will have the mutation. This phenomenon is known as heteroplasmy (Fig. 2–20).

Reflection reveals the dilemma mitochondrial mutations pose in prenatal diagnosis. Phenotype of offspring depends on the proportions of mutant and normal mitochondrial DNA in the oocyte participating in syngamy. Affected males could not transmit a disease coded by mitochondrial DNA. In females this can occur, but proportions may be almost unmeasurable.

The fact that mitochondrial genes are exclusively cytoplasmic and transmitted exclusively through the maternal lineage also raises an unexplored question in reproductive medicine. In intra-

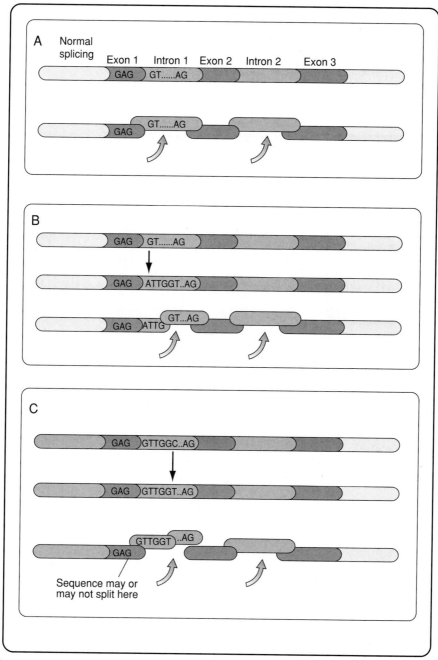

FIGURE 2–14 • The normal mechanism for splicing introns (intervening sequences) from exons (coding sequences) is shown in A. In the first splice site mutation shown here (B), the donor sequence, GT, is replaced with AT. This results in an incorrect splice that leaves part of the intron in the mature mRNA transcript. In the second mutation (C), a second GT donor site is created in the first intron, resulting in a combination of abnormally and normally spliced mRNA products. (From Jorde LB, Carey JC, Bamshad MJ, et al.: Medical Genetics, 2nd ed. St. Louis: Mosby, 2000.)

cytoplasmic sperm injection (ICSI) are cytoplasmic factors transmitted along with the sperm head necessary for syngamy? Could transmission of mutant maternal mitochondrial genes be obviated by nuclear transfer? For example, the Kearns-Sayre syndrome is a multisystem disorder caused (85%)

by deletions of a mitochondrial gene (Moraes et al., 1989). If a prospective mother were affected, one could transfer her pronucleus to an anucleated cell donated by an unaffected female, or transfer the zygote to an anucleated donor cell. Could cytoplasm from a younger, healthier donor contribute

Prader-Willi Syndrome

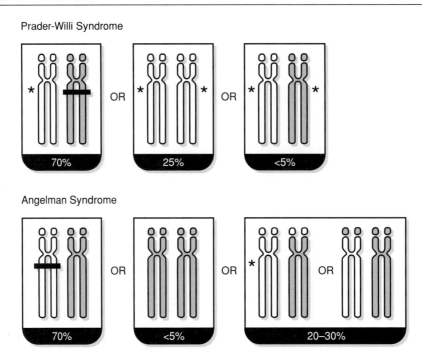

Angelman Syndrome

FIGURE 2–15 • Molecular basis for Prader-Willi syndrome (PWS) and Angelman syndrome (AS). Approximately 70 to 75% of patients with PWS have a detectable microdeletion (black bar) of a portion of the paternal chromosome 15 (gray). The maternal chromosome 15 (light shading) is methylated (asterisk) at several loci on 15q11–13. About 20 to 25% of PWS patients have maternal uniparental disomy with both maternal homologs methylated and transcriptionally silent. A small number of patients have biparental inheritance of chromosome 15 without a detectable deletion but show maternal methylation at several loci in the critical region on both chromosomes 15. In AS, 70% of patients have a detectable microdeletion of the maternal chromosome 15, but only less than 5% of patients have paternal uniparental disomy. Biparental inheritance of chromosome 15 with no deletion and with a normal methylation pattern is the most common situation in familial AS. It is assumed that these patients may have point mutations or other subtle abnormalities in the as yet unidentified AS gene on the maternal chromosome 15. Finally, some patients with AS have biparental inheritance with abnormal methylation (absence of normally methylated maternal allele). (From Gelehrter TD, Collins FS, Ginsburg D: Principles of Medical Genetics, 2nd ed. Baltimore: Williams & Wilkins, 2000.)

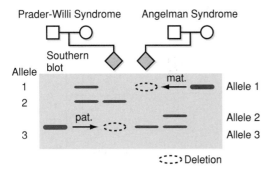

FIGURE 2–16 • Deducing parental origin of deletion in Prader-Willi syndrome and in Angleman syndrome. In Prader-Willi syndrome, the paternal allele (3) is not present in the affected child (shaded symbol). In Angelman syndrome, the maternal allele (1) is not present in the affected child. (From Passarge E: Color Atlas of Genetics. New York: Thieme Medical Publishers, Inc., 1995.)

growth factors or other substances lacking or deficient in a genetically abnormal or older women? This hypothesis was the basis underlying the ostensibly successful insertion of donor oocyte cytoplasm by Cohen and colleagues (1997).

Can Gene Frequency Be Altered?

Survival, treatment, and parenthood of homozygotes with formerly deleterious or lethal traits is now accepted. If homozygously affected individuals not only survive but reproduce as result of improved medical management, will the frequency of that abnormal allele in the population increase to a level that could prove disadvantageous for the general population? Fortunately, there is no cause for immediate concern.

Recall the relationship between the frequencies of heterozygotes and homozygotes in the population, as expressed by the Hardy-Weinberg equilibrium. Given that q is less than 0.5, q^2 is much less than $2pq$. That is, the frequency of heterozygotes is much greater than the frequency of homozygotes (affected individuals). If $q = 0.01$, $p = 0.99$; thus, the ratio of heterozygotes to homozygotes $(2pq/q^2)$ would be calculated as follows:

A Trisomy Rescue of a Robertsonian Translocation

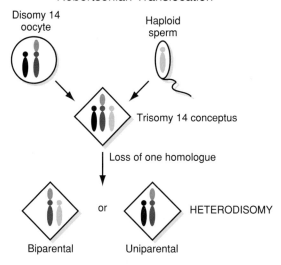

B Monosomy Rescue Through Isochromosome Formation

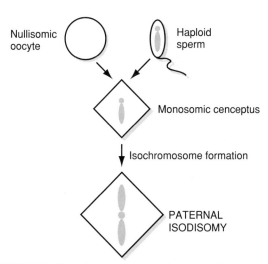

FIGURE 2–17 • Common mechanisms resulting in uniparental disomy involving acrocentric chromosome rearrangements. (A) Trisomy rescue of a trisomy conceptus from a robertsonian translocation carrier theoretically results in uniparental disomy (UPD) in 50% of cases. Since the nondisjunction must occur in meiosis I, the resulting UPD would be heterodisomic. (B) Monosomy rescue of a monosomic conceptus resulting from meiosis I nondisjunction and fertilization of a nullisomic gamete. Duplication (through isochromosome formation) of the only copy of a homologue would result in isodisomy in 100% of cases. Since the majority of nondisjunction occurs in maternal meiosis, most cases of isochromosomes arising through this mechanism would result in paternal isodisomy. (From Shaffer LG, Agan N, Goldberg JD, et al.: American College of Medical Genetics statement of diagnostic testing for uniparental disomy. Genet Med 3:206–211, 2001.)

$$\frac{(2)(0.99)(0.01)}{(0.01)(0.01)} \text{ or } \approx \frac{.02}{.0001} \text{ or } \approx 200/1$$

Reproduction by homozygotes (relaxed selection) would thus not greatly increase the number of abnormal alleles in the population because the numerical load rests in the heterozygotes (see Table 2–3). Conversely, eliminating homozygotes would change the gene frequency very little.

Mathematical improbabilities aside, there are valid scientific reasons against eliminating ostensibly deleterious recessive alleles. The rationale against eliminating heterozygotes is based upon such individuals having a theoretical selective advantage. If in homozygous form an allele is lethal, its frequency in the population would eventually decrease, although very slowly because the mean family size of matings involving two heterozygotes should theoretically be 25% less than the mean family size of couples in which two individuals are not heterozygous. The decreased family size reflects the 25% likelihood that any given offspring would be homozygous and, hence, die. Over many generations a gradual decrease in the frequency of that particular abnormal recessive allele would occur.

Yet in many autosomal recessive disorders the frequency of the abnormal recessive allele remains relatively high, often 1 in 20 to 30 in a given population. Maintenance in the population of a recessive allele deleterious in homozygous form could best be explained if heterozygotes possess an advantage over homozygously normal individuals that was responsible for maintaining the allele in the population. In sickle cell anemia, heterozygotes have an advantage over homozygously normal individuals in that they are less susceptible to malaria. It is estimated that each ostensibly normal individual has five or six mutant alleles that would be lethal if homozygous. Some mutant alleles must be advantageous for as yet unknown reasons. Proposals to eliminate abnormal alleles are thus not only mathematically impractical and obviously ethically unacceptable but also theoretically unwise. Individuals heterozygous for an ostensibly abnormal allele may possess an advantage over homozygously normal individuals that is useful to society. The alternative explanation for a high gene frequency is that the mutation arose by chance and simply persisted randomly or for reasons unrelated to fitness (genetic drift).

Linkage

Genes are located on chromosomes at given locations and in definite linear relationship to one

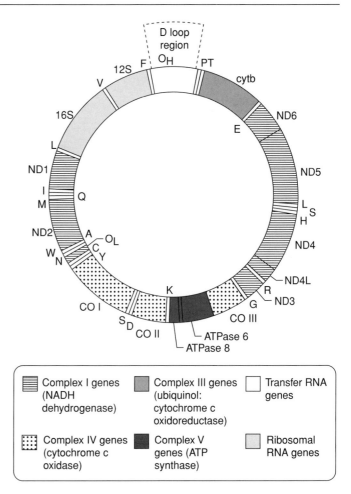

FIGURE 2–18 • The circular mitochondrial DNA genome. Locations of protein-coding genes (NADH dehydrogenase, cytochrome c oxidase, cytochrome c oxidoreductase, and ATP synthase) are shown, as are the locations of the two ribosomal RNA genes and 22 transfer RNA genes (designated by single letters). The replication origins of the heavy (O_H) and light (O_L) chains and the noncoding D loop (also known as the control region) are also shown. (Modified from Wallace DC: Mitochondrial genetics: a paradigm for aging and degenerative diseases? Science 256:628–632, 1992; From Jorde LB, Carey JC, Bamshad MJ, et al.: Medical Genetics, 2nd ed. St. Louis: Mosby, 2000.)

Complex I genes (NADH dehydrogenase)	Complex III genes (ubiquinol: cytochrome c oxidoreductase)	Transfer RNA genes	
Complex IV genes (cytochrome c oxidase)	Complex V genes (ATP synthase)	Ribosomal RNA genes	

another. Genes between homologous chromosomes also are exchanged, as discussed in Chapter 1. Genes on the same chromosome are said to be linked or to exhibit linkage (technically syntenic if further than 50 cm apart but still on the same chromosome). Genes show linkage if during meiosis, with its opportunity for recombination, they are more likely to remain on the same chromosome in parental combination than to behave as if they were on different chromosomes. Figure 2–21 shows a simple example of crossing-over.

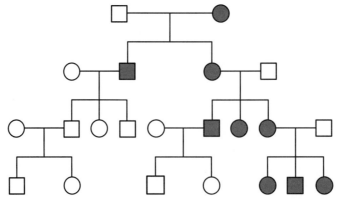

FIGURE 2–19 • A pedigree showing the inheritance of a disease caused by a mitochondrial DNA mutation. Only females can transmit the disease mutation to their offspring. (From Jorde LB, Carey JC, Bamshad MJ, et al.: Medical Genetics, 2nd ed. St. Louis: Mosby, 2000.)

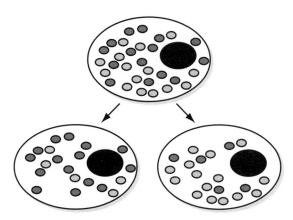

FIGURE 2–20 • Heteroplasmy with uneven distribution of mitochondria with mutated DNA (dark gray) and mitochondria with normal DNA (light gray).

If the frequency of recombination between two linked genes is 1%, those genes are defined to be 1 map unit or 1 centimorgan (cM) apart (percentage recombination equals centimorgans). Genes 50 cM apart on the same chromosome fail, by definition, to show linkage, because such genes segregate indistinguishably from genes on nonhomologous chromosomes. Linkage analysis is increasingly useful in prenatal diagnosis as a more complete map of the human genome becomes available.

Linkage analysis in prenatal diagnosis usually takes advantage of some polymorphic locus.

Polymorphism exists when two or more alleles are present at a given locus, such that the less frequent allele persists in at least 1% of the population. Polymorphisms used for linkage analysis were once gene products or a characteristic thereof, like electrophoretic mobility. Currently, polymorphisms used diagnostically are almost always DNA variants. These are discussed in the following sections. Figure 2–22 illustrates generation-measuring polymorphisms for restriction fragment length polymorphisms (RFLPs), and Figure 2–23 illustrates variable numbers of tandem repeats (VNTRs). In order to appreciate these applications, we first need to review pivotal analytical techniques.

Analytical Techniques in Molecular Analysis

Understanding several molecular genetics technologies is pivotal for appreciating molecular diagnosis of many disorders to be discussed. Brief explanations are provided here. The material covered is intended to provide only the minimal information necessary to understand general approaches in prenatal genetic diagnosis and general approaches to identifying and elucidating genes causing gynecologic diseases. These technologies are applied clinically throughout this volume.

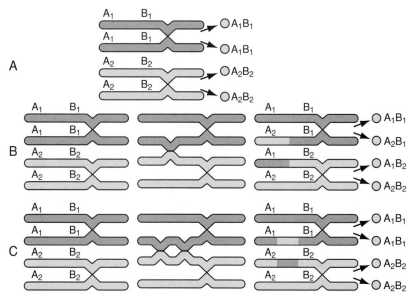

FIGURE 2–21 • Schematic diagram illustrating a single crossing-over event. (From Jorde LB, Carey JC, Bamshad MJ, et al.: Medical Genetics, 2nd ed. St. Louis: Mosby, 2000.)

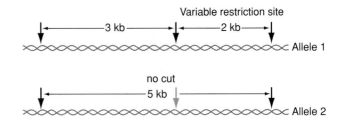

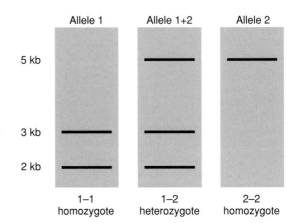

FIGURE 2–22 • Restriction fragment length polymorphism (RFLP) for linkage analysis. (From Passarge E: Color Atlas of Genetics. New York: Thieme Medical Publishers, Inc., 1995.)

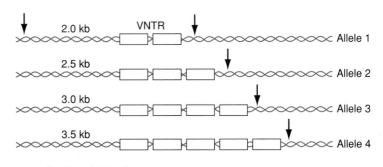

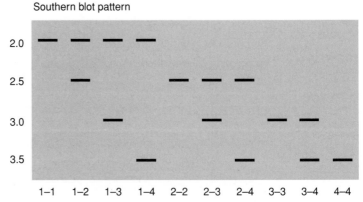

FIGURE 2–23 • Use of variable number tandem repeats (VNTR) to generate polymorphism for linkage analysis. Given four alleles connoted by 2.0, 2.5, 3.0 or 3.5 kb fragments, ten allelic contributions exist. (From Passarge E: Color Atlas of Genetics. New York: Thieme Medical Publishers, Inc., 1995.)

RESTRICTION ENDONUCLEASES

DNA can be digested by *restriction endonucleases*, enzymes present in bacteria and capable of recognizing and cutting certain sequences and that of 4–6 nucleotide. These enzymes are named from the bacteria in which they were found. For example, EcoRI was derived from *Escherichia coli*; Hind III was derived from *Haemophilus influenzae*.

Specificity of restriction endonucleases is very precise. A cut site exists for a given sequence and only for that sequence (Fig. 2–24). The closer together the recognition sites, the more DNA fragments exist. Some restriction recognition sequences are rare; thus, large fragments are produced ("rare cutters"). Others are more common and, conversely, yield shorter fragments. Not all individuals show the same spectrum of DNA fragments after exposure to a given restriction enzyme. This could indicate a missense or other mutation connoting a disease state. However, this could also merely reflect the innocuous differences in DNA sequences existing among the population (polymorphism). Polymorphic differences usually confer neither an advantage nor a disadvantage. However, the existence of polymorphisms means there may or may not be a restriction site for a specific restriction endonuclease.

The term *restriction fragment length polymorphism* (RLFP) connotes this phenomenon. Many RFLPs have been identified in the human genome, providing invaluable markers for linkage analysis. If a given RFLP is closely linked to a locus conferring a disease, the presence or absence of a disorder in a kindred at risk can be deduced. RFLPs exist every few centimorgans; thus, linkage analysis should permit prenatal diagnosis for almost all localized genes. RFLP linkage analysis forms the basis for prenatal diagnosis for many disorders in which either the molecular basis is not known or cannot practically be sought, as discussed in Chapter 14.

VARIABLE NUMBER TANDEM REPEATS (DINUCLEOTIDE REPEATS)

Principles of linkage analysis apply equally to other DNA polymorphisms, for example, variable number tandem repeats (VNTR) such as dinucleotide (cytosine-adenine) (CA) repeats. Figure 2–23 illustrates this principle. In other situations subgroups may exist in the population with differing numbers of CA repeats, for example 5, 7, 9, 11 $(CA)^n$. Analysis of polymorphic CA systems can be used for linkage analysis, just like RFLP linkage analysis. A further variant is a near unique polymorphism (single nucleotide polymorphism, SNP) that is innocuous per se but connotes some unusual phenotypical consequence, such as pharmacogenetic susceptibility to a given therapeutic agent.

CLONING AND GENE PROBES

For a specific gene—or more precisely a specific DNA sequence—to be located from among thousands of DNA fragments, DNA probes must be constructed. Probes are single-stranded and derived from cloned DNA. Probes of unknown sequences can be generated from genomic DNA (anonymous), but this is obviously not initially useful diagnostically. Rather, a known DNA sequence is the point of interest. For diagnostic work one can begin with purified mRNA. Single-stranded DNA, called complementary DNA (cDNA), can be generated by use of an enzyme called *reverse transcriptase* (RT) (Fig. 2–25). Present in viruses whose hereditary information is not DNA but *RNA*, RT can synthesize single-stranded DNA from a RNA template. The *complementary* (DNA) can then be injected into a vector that has the property of replicating the interloping DNA as well as its own. Plasmids are a common vector.

Under suitable laboratory conditions, plasmids can enter bacterial hosts, where a single

Restriction Endonucleases

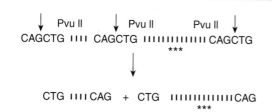

10 base pairs   20 base pairs

FIGURE 2–24 • Simplified diagram illustrating the manner in which a restriction endonuclease cuts DNA at a specific nucleotide sequence. PvuII recognizes the sequence CAGCTG and only that sequence. DNA is separated into fragments of different lengths on the basis of distances between restriction enzyme recognition sites. The farther the distance between sites, the longer the length of intervening DNA (i.e., 20 versus 30 base pairs). Shorter DNA fragments (e.g., 20 base pairs) show greater mobility and migrate farther in an agarose cell. (From Gabbe SG, Niebyl JR, Simpson JL: Obstetrics: Normal and Problem Pregnancies, 4th ed. New York: Churchill Livingstone, 2001.)

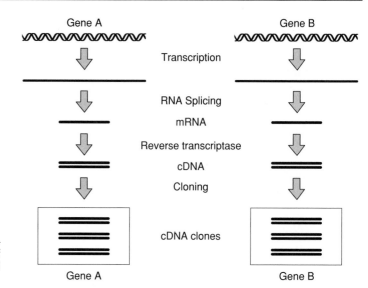

FIGURE 2–25 • Reverse transcriptase to generate cDNA. (From Passarge E: Color Atlas of Genetics. New York: Thieme Medical Publishers, Inc., 1995.)

plasmid can replicate along with its bacterium host (Fig. 2–26). The plasmid containing the DNA to be cloned usually contains a contiguous marker gene that confers antibiotic resistance, a characteristic that allows those bacterial clones containing the desirable plasmid to be identified from among the far more numerous bacterial clones in which the sequence in question was not successfully inserted. Bacteriophage and various synthetic systems—cosmids or yeast artificial chromosomes—can also be used as vectors. The various vectors have advantages and disadvantages applicable to specific circumstances, usually reflecting the size of sequences to be inserted.

POLYMERASE CHAIN REACTION FOR DNA AMPLIFICATION

A technique that truly revolutionized molecular biology is the *polymerase chain reaction* (PCR). In PCR, a target sequence of up to 1 kb can quickly be amplified 10^5 to 10^6 times (Fig. 2–27). With PCR there is no longer a necessity for a threshold number of cells (tissue) for DNA testing. Even a single cell can be amplified to produce sufficient DNA for testing. This technique allowed the field of preimplantation genetic diagnosis to develop. The DNA can even be ancient (mummies), as long as it is not completely degraded.

The prerequisite for PCR amplification is the ability to construct unique DNA primers that flank and are specific for the DNA region in question. The region in question may consist of a portion of a gene (e.g., that containing or not containing a mutation), a polymorphic DNA sequence (e.g., dinucleotide repeat or other repet-

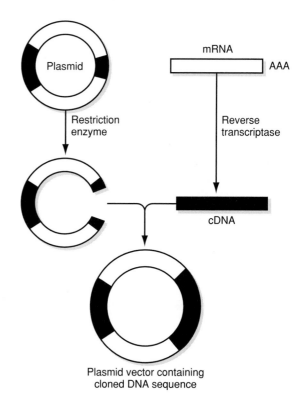

Plasmid vector containing cloned DNA sequence

FIGURE 2–26 • Principle underlying cloning DNA. A DNA fragment is inserted in a plasmid vector, which synthesizes many copies of itself as well as the inserted fragment. The clone can be labeled radioactively to constitute a gene probe. (From Gabbe SG, Niebyl JF, Simpson JL: Obstetrics: Normal and Problem Pregnancies. New York: Churchill Livingstone, 1986.)

itive DNA sequence characteristic of an entire chromosomal region). Heat-stable DNA polymerase extracted from *Thermas aquaticus* (a bacterium that thrives at very high temperatures) is traditionally used (thus, the term *Taq poly-*

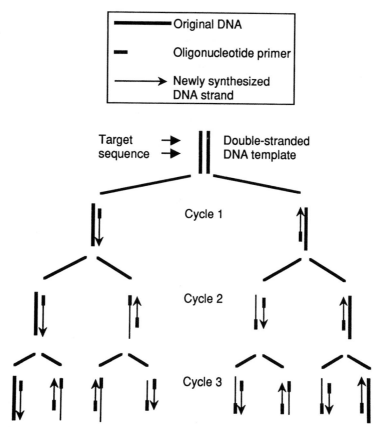

FIGURE 2–27 • Polymerase chain reaction. Placing the DNA in question, unique primers, and Taq polymerase together results in amplification (cycle 1). When the temperature is raised, denaturation into single-stranded DNA occurs. After cooling, a second amplification cycle begins. Continued amplification increases the amount of DNA located between primers in logarithmic fashion. (From Simpson JL: Principles of human genetics. In Reece EA, Hobbins JC (eds): Medicine of the Fetus and Mother, 2nd ed. Philadelphia: Lippincott, 1999.)

merase); other enzymes are sometimes used. In a single tube the DNA in question, the unique primers that flank the sequence to be amplified, deoxynucleotide triphosphates (dNTPs) dATP, dCTP, dGTP, dTTP, and Taq polymerase are placed. When the temperature is raised, native double-stranded DNA is denatured into single-stranded DNA (see Fig. 2–27). On cooling, primers anneal and amplification proceeds again, given that the remaining Taq polymerase is impervious to heat. The next round of heating again results in denaturation, but now an exponential amplification of single-stranded DNA follows because $2^2 = 4$ strands are now available for amplification. Repetition of this cycle results in DNA between primer increasing in logarithmic fashion (2^n). Some DNA on either side of the flanked regions is concomitantly amplified, but these sequences only increases arithmetically (linearly); thus, they are inundated by the more numerous exponential increases in the sequences flanked *within* the primers. Usually 20 to 30 rounds of amplification are performed. As more rounds of amplification are performed, the risk of including spurious sequences as a result of contaminant ambient DNA is increased.

A modification of PCR can be applied when greater sensitivity is needed. If a single set of primers is subjected to 20 to 30 PCR rounds modification, sensitivity for detecting a DNA sequence does not ordinarily extend below 100 picograms (pq) DNA. Although this is sufficient for most diagnostic purposes, it is inadequate for single-cell analysis. A single cell contains only 6pq DNA; for this reason, a nested PCR approach must be employed. Using a second set of primers internal to the first, sensitivity can be achieved down to 1pq DNA (Fig. 2–28). This technique proved pivotal in permitting single-cell diagnosis of mendelian traits in preimplantation genetic diagnosis (see Chapter 16).

PCR FOR DIAGNOSIS AND SEQUENCING

PCR is not only pivotal for amplifying DNA but with modification is invaluable in diagnosis and

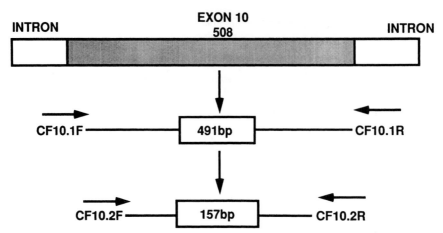

FIGURE 2–28 • Diagram illustrating nested-primer polymerase chain reaction (PCR), specifically of a type enabling detection of ΔF508 cystic fibrosis on the basis of analysis of a single cell. PCR is first initiated for a 491-bp fragment in exon 10, which contains the most common mutation in cystic fibrosis (ΔF508). After a given number of cycles (e.g., 30) with primers CD10.1F and CF10.1R, a 491-bp sequence is generated. A second set of primers (CF10.2F and CF10.2R), internal to the first, is then constructed to generate a 157-bp sequence. Nested-primer PCR allows far greater diagnostic sensitivity than possible on the basis of a traditional PCR. (From Simpson JL, Elias S: Essentials of Prenatal Diagnosis. New York: Churchill Livingstone, 1993.)

sequencing. The obvious extension is diagnosis per se. If a DNA sequence is absent (e.g., deletion as in α-thalassemia), no DNA exists with which the unique primers can anneal; thus, no hybridization (reaction) will be observed. The diagnosis is obvious. It is also possible to perform PCR concurrently for multiple sequences, overlapping or not in a given gene or exon. Analysis of more than one sequence (multiplex PCR) permits assessment of the presence or absence of deletions or mutations. An obvious application is the analysis of the Y long arm for deletions of DAZ, which cause azoospermia (see Chapter 10). Lack of a signal for any sequence provides an exact diagnosis.

PCR technology can also used for sequencing a chromosomal region. Starting 3′ to a known sequence, PCR can be allowed to proceed and generate a previously unknown region. This new region can then be sequenced. This approach can be used to sequence an entire region, gene, or genome. Amplified sequences of varying lengths are produced, and nested hierarchial analysis is used to order sequences correctly. This general approach was used to sequence the human genome.

SOUTHERN BLOTTING AND NUCLEIC ACID HYBRIDIZATION

A variety of approaches can be utilized for extracting DNA from any nucleated cell. The prototypical approach is called Southern blotting (Southern, 1975). A restriction endonuclease is first used to produce fragments of DNA varying in length, usually after amplifying DNA by PCR to yield a large amount of DNA. DNA is then denatured through heat or chemicals (sodium hydroxide). Single-stranded DNA fragments are allowed to migrate through an agarose gel, heavier DNA fragments being less mobile and remaining near the origin of the gel. Lighter fragments migrate faster and thus are further from the origin (Fig. 2–29). The sample-specific unique gel thus created can then be laid on nitrocellulose paper or nylon and buffer allowed to flow through the gel onto the nitrocellulose filter. DNA fragments concomitantly migrate from the gel and bind to the filter, thus creating a replica of the gel's DNA fragment pattern. The replica is used for ease of analysis. The entire process is called Southern blotting (Southern, 1975).

The next step is for the nitrocellulose or nylon replicate to be exposed to a single-stranded specific gene probe. The probe will search among innumerable fragments to hybridize only to that portion of the filter containing its complementary DNA sequence (or fragment). The size of the fragment in which the gene is question is contained is not necessarily important, reflecting only the specific restriction enzyme used. However, knowing the size of the fragment containing the relevant gene or sequence is important. To recognize the occurrence of hybridization, the probe is rendered radioactive or biotinylated. In this way a gene (or more specifically a DNA sequence that is part of a gene) can be identified among thousands of fragments, categorized according to relative

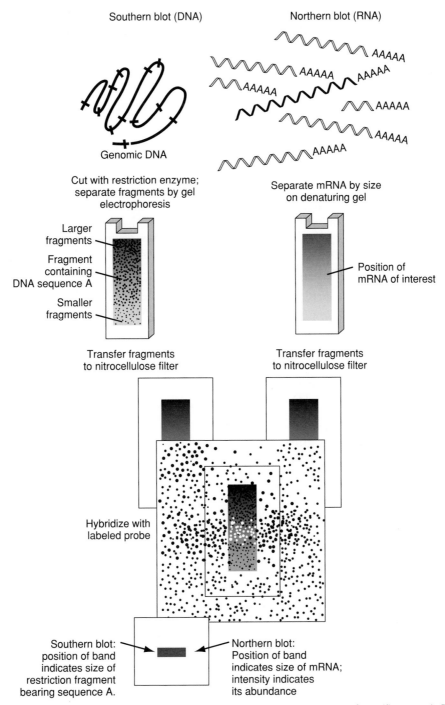

Southern blot (DNA)

Northern blot (RNA)

Genomic DNA

Cut with restriction enzyme;
separate fragments by gel
electrophoresis

Separate mRNA by size
on denaturing gel

Larger fragments

Fragment containing DNA sequence A

Smaller fragments

Position of mRNA of interest

Transfer fragments to nitrocellulose filter

Transfer fragments to nitrocellulose filter

Hybridize with labeled probe

Southern blot: position of band indicates size of restriction fragment bearing sequence A.

Northern blot: Position of band indicates size of mRNA; intensity indicates its abundance

FIGURE 2–29 • Southern and Northern blotting. These techniques allow detection of specific genomic DNA fragments or specific mRNA in complex mixtures. A Southern blot can visualize a specific, single genomic fragment (here denoted as gene A) in a mixture of about a million such fragments. The precise size of the fragment of interest can also be determined from how far it has migrated in the gel. In a Northern blot, a specific mRNA molecule (here denoted as B) can be detected in a complex mixture of 10,000 or more mRNAs derived from a tissue sample. The size of the mRNA can be determined by how far it has migrated in the gel and its abundance can be determined by the intensity of the band. (From Gelehrter TD, Collins FS, Ginsburg D, et al.: Principles of Medical Genetics, 2nd ed. Baltimore: Williams & Wilkins, 1998.)

size. Absolute size can be determined through concomitant use of markers of known size.

Binding of the probe to DNA is governed by various conditions. These include stability of the hybridization, which reflects ratio of GC to AT pairs; GC is more stable as a result of having three rather than two hydrogen bonds. Other variables include fidelity of hybridization (i.e., whether only an exact match yields hybridization or whether a limited number of mismatches are permitted). Stringency is another important concept. At high stringency (high temperature, low salt concentration, polar solvent), hybridization will occur only if the probe exactly corresponds to the DNA fragment. At low stringency some mismatches are tolerated. High stringency would typically be used for diagnostic work in which false-positive or false-negative results cannot be tolerated. Low stringency conditions might be used when searching for interspecies (partial) DNA homologies or for homologous sequences common among related groups of genes (e.g., homobox genes).

DNA LIBRARIES

A term frequently arising in the context of molecular investigation is the "library." A DNA library theoretically represents every gene that characterizes a given circumstance. There are several types of libraries. If the library is meant to encompass every gene of a given individual, it is said to be a *genomic library*. This library could be derived from any nucleated somatic cell because all contain the same DNA. The genomic library contains all 3 to 4 billion base pairs—introns, exons, promotor and regulatory regions, pseudogenes, and repetitive sequences of all types. Sequencing the entire genomic DNA was the accomplishment of the Human Genome Initiative (see later on).

A specific type of library is a cDNA library, initiated from multiple mRNAs. This principle has already been illustrated in Figure 2–25. The mRNAs alluded to must have been transcribed. Thus, only active genes were being identified. An advantage of a cDNA library is that it can be tissue- or organ (e.g., fetal ovary)-specific; another is that there is far less DNA to sequence. The disadvantage is that the library contains no information on promoter or regulatory sequences and lacks information concerning repetitive sequences. In turn, this may make it difficult to determine three-dimensional relationships among genes and their coding regions. Sequencing the genome on the basis of a cDNA library was the strategy of Venter and coworkers (2001) and the Celera Corporation (Rockville, MD), whereas the strategy of the Human Genome Research Institution (National Institutes of Health) was to sequence the entire genome—coding and noncoding regions (International Human Genome Sequencing Consortium, 2001). The latter involved producing many different DNA fragments, sequencing, and then ordering.

SCREENING FOR MUTATIONS

How does one screen a given chromosomal region, or even the entire genome, to detect the mutation responsible for a given condition? A variety of methods have been developed. All are capable of screening perhaps 1000 to 10,000 base pair segments of DNA to detect perturbations from normal mutations. No technique detects all mutations, but in aggregate perhaps 90% are detected. Still widely applied, these techniques may eventually become obsolete in the future as greater use of automated DNA sequencing becomes possible. In any case, a brief review of several techniques used to screen for mutations may be helpful.

Heteroduplex Analysis

Directly related in principle to single-stranded conformational polymorphism (see below) is heteroduplex analysis. However, heteroduplex analysis involves double-stranded DNA. The principle is based on the differential reannealing that occurs with two identical DNA sequences versus two dissimilar DNA sequences (Fig. 2–30). When two identical single-stranded fragments reanneal, the result is a homoduplex that is mobile and migrates easily. If nonidentical strands migrate, the resulting fragment is structurally less compact and migrates with less ease, thus appearing as if it were a heavier band (closer to the gel's origin). Heteroduplex could connote mutations or polymorphism, i.e., deviations from normal.

Heteroduplex analysis can either confirm or refute any given predicted genotype, normal or abnormal, as we shall illustrate in Chapter 16 when discussing preimplantation genetics. If one correctly predicts that the unknown DNA was ΔF508 CF, reannealing in the presence of ΔF508 CF DNA should produce only a single band (homoduplex). If one unexpectedly observes more than one band (i.e., a heteroduplex), the diagnosis of ΔF508 must have been incorrect, the unknown DNA instead being either heterozygous or homozygously normal.

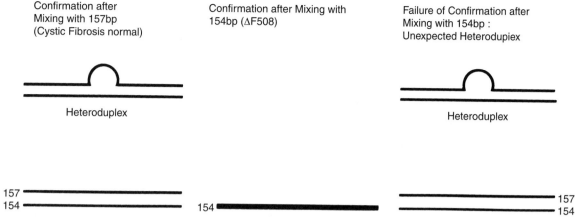

FIGURE 2–30 • Heteroduplex analysis illustrating approach necessary to diagnose ΔF508 cystic fibrosis on the analysis of a single cell, as would be accomplished for preimplantation genetics. If the DNA fragment does not show ΔF508, a 157-bp fragment (normal) is generated. If ΔF508 is present, the lack of three nucleotides results in a fragment that is only 154bp in length. Although distinguishing a 157-bp fragment from a 154-bp pair fragment is possible, it may be difficult. Determination is easier if the unknown sample is denatured and mixed with DNA from a normal individual (cystic fibrosis normal) or DNA from an individual known to show ΔF508. If DNA of the unknown individual (i.e., cell) is ΔF508, mixing with a 154-bp fragment results in a homoduplex (middle diagram). If the DNA ΔF508 is mixed with normal DNA (157-bp fragment), one observes not only the 157- and 154-bp fragments but also a heteroduplex resulting from incomplete reannealing when two dissimilar DNA fragments are placed together. The final figure (right) shows the presence of an unexpected heteroduplex, which would occur if the diagnosis of ΔF508 had been erroneous. (From Simpson JL, Elias S: Prenatal diagnosis of genetic disorders. In Creasy RK, Resnik R (eds): Maternal Fetal Medicine, 3rd ed. Philadelphia: WB Saunders, 1994, with permission.)

Single-Stranded Conformational Polymorphism (SSCP)

Single-stranded conformational polymorphism (SSCP) is one commonly applied technique to screen genomic DNA for sequence differences reflective of mutations (Fig. 2–31). The underlying principle is that fragments of single-stranded DNA migrate in a fashion directly related to their size and sequence. In turn, a mutation alters the DNA fragment's structural characteristics and, hence, its migration characteristics in gels. Even a single nucleotide alternation can alter the tertiary structure and, hence, mobility. Typically, the original sample is initially amplified by PCR. If RNA is available, reverse transcription can produce cDNA by reverse transcriptase and PCR (RT PCR). Resulting products are then run on an agarose gel. If a gel shift is detected, it is possible to elute (remove the specific portion of the gel) and directly sequence the amplified DNA to determine the exact change. Single-stranded conformational polymorphism is most effective if the PCR products are from 100 to 250 base pairs in length. When applied to fragments of larger size, SSCP is subject to decreased ability to recognize changes reflecting mutations.

Denaturing Gradient Gel Electrophoresis

Denaturing gel or gradient gel electrophoresis utilizes double-stranded DNA, like heteroduplex analysis (Fig. 2–31). Rather than analyzing denatured strands on the basis of their reannealing (heteroduplex analysis), denaturing gradient gel electrophoresis takes advantage of double-stranded DNA fragments denaturing differently as a function of differences in sequence. An agent like urea or temperature is first used to denature the native double-stranded DNA. Reannealing is then allowed. If the two single strands are perfectly matched, they anneal precisely (homoduplex). If the strands are not identical, mismatch upon annealing produces nonappositional conformation. A double-stranded product of dissimilar strands (e.g., heterozygosity) will denature more rapidly then the perfectly matched homoduplex formed by identical reannealed single strands (homozygosity). In turn, this will be reflected by a less mobile fragment, migrating with higher molecular weight homoduplexed.

Denaturing gradient gel electrophoresis is especially powerful in detecting heterozygous nucleotide (missense) mutations. It is applicable for DNA fragments larger than those used in single-stranded conformational polymorphism, perhaps up to 500 base pairs in length.

AUTOMATED SEQUENCING AND DNA MICROARRAYS

The techniques of SSCP, denaturing gradient gel electrophoresis, and heteroduplex analysis are

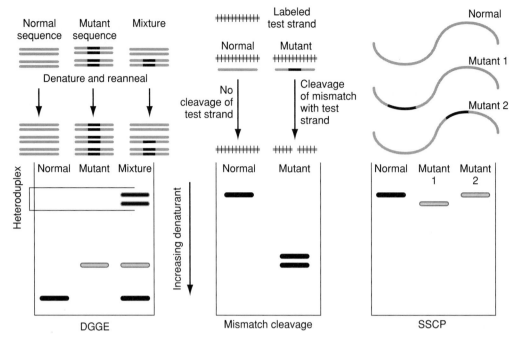

FIGURE 2–31 • Screening methods for mutation detection. DGGE, denaturing gradient gel electrophoresis; SSCP, single stranded conformational polymorphism. (From Gelehrter TD, Collins FS, Ginsburg D, et al.: Principles of Medical Genetics, 2nd ed. Baltimore: Williams & Wilkins, 1998.)

now widely used, but in the future automatic DNA sequencing may replace or largely supplant these techniques. This is illustrated in Figure 2–32. The speed and lowered costs of direct sequencing are likely to change the approach toward detecting mutations. The general principle of using sequencing to detect mutations is the same as that in which multiplex PCR is used to search for selected perturbations (mutant alleles or deletions) in a given gene. PCR can be performed for many sequences concurrently, each sequence initiated from a different site using an array of probes attached to a substrate. The array of DNA probes can be bound directly to small squares of silicon chips (hence, "microarray"), as shown in Figure 2–33. Each single-stranded probe can then be exposed to single-stranded DNA from an unknown DNA sample. If the sample contains a sequence corresponding to that of the probe, hybridization occurs, as signaled by a fluorochrome. If the sample does not contain the sequence, hybridization does not occur. Tens of thousands of different oligonucleotides (probes) can be placed on a single chip, allowing rapid analysis of large amounts of DNA. A microassay specific for a series of genes relevant to a given process (e.g., oogenesis) can be developed. This can be used to determine which genes are expressed or not expressed in a given biologic process (e.g., differentiation or oncogenesis).

ANALYZING RNA (NORTHERN BLOTTING)

Using the analytical techniques described above will tell us whether DNA is or is not present. However, this does not reveal whether the DNA actually is transcribed or translated. That is, no information is provided concerning whether messenger RNA is actually present or whether the gene product exists.

In order to determine whether a gene is transcribed, methods are needed to detect the presence of messenger RNA (mRNA). This can be done by methods analogous to Southern blotting. Like DNA, RNA can be recovered and separated from other cellular components on the basis of size (Fig. 2–29). In fact, messenger RNA (mRNA) is already single-stranded and already consists of fragments of differing length, based upon the length of the message having been transcribed when interrupted. Size differences can be visualized on an agarose gel. Analogous to the method of Southern blotting, a replica of the pattern of messenger RNAs can then be transferred to a membrane and challenged with a probe. The technique is termed "Northern" analysis (Fig. 2–29). The probe might be complementary DNA (cDNA), derived from known messenger RNA using reverse transcriptase PCR (RT-PCR). The term Northern blotting is not an eponym (unlike

A

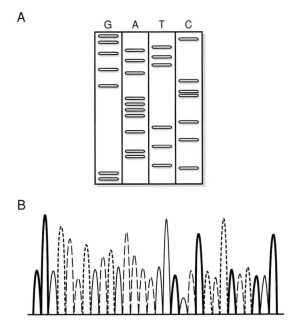

B

C

GGCTAATCATCAAAACCGCAGTATGATGCG

FIGURE 2–32 • DNA sequencing by the dideoxy-chain-termination method. The dideoxy-chain-termination sequencing method yields a population of DNA segments of different lengths, each terminated by a particular type of dideoxy nucleotide (i.e., G,A,T, or C) that marks the position of that base in the starting template. The resulting products are then separated by gel electrophoresis. (A) The detection of radioactively labeled DNA fragments by autoradiography. In this case, each band contains the DNA segments generated with a single type of dideoxy nucleotide, with the presence of a band at a particular rung position of the sequencing ladder reflecting the base at that position in the starting DNA template (the corresponding sequence is shown in C). (B) The automated detection of fluorescently-labeled DNA fragments. In this case, a laser is used to detect the migration of the fluorescently-labeled, dideoxy-terminated DNA fragments as they are electrophoresed through the gel. Each type of peak (indicated by thick, dotted, dashed, and thin lines) reflects the base (G,A,T, and C, respectively) at that position in the starting DNA template (the corresponding sequence is shown in C). (From Scriver CR, Beaudet AL, Sly WS, et al.: The Metabolic and Molecular Bases of Inherited Disease, 8th ed., vol. I. New York: McGraw-Hill, 2001.)

Southern) but rather was chosen to imply complementarity to Southern blotting.

The purpose of Northern analysis is to determine gene expression. Detecting messenger RNA verifies that transcription of the corresponding DNA sequence has occurred. Tissue and temporal specificity can thus be assessed. It may be necessary to obtain various modifications of Northern analysis from cDNA expression libraries; these can be used to create microarrays as discussed earlier. Using *in situ* hybridization, a cDNA probe

can be exposed to tissue *in situ* in order to determine if hybridization occurs at that site.

Of practical significance, messenger RNA is unstable. This contrasts with DNA, which is highly stable. (Recall that identifying DNA is possible for forensic or archeological purposes on long deceased specimens, even ancient specimens.) Thus, considerable attention must be given to preserving tissue if RNA assays (Northern analysis) are to be meaningful. One approach is to freeze specimens in liquid nitrogen or at very cold temperatures (–20° to 80°C) immediately after they have been obtained ("snap frozen").

More refined information on gene expression may be obtained from assays that determine rate of mRNA synthesis, effects of various factors on gene regulation, and rate of mRNA synthesis versus rate of protein synthesis. Assays can quantify the amount of translatable RNA or determine the stability of the message under various experimental conditions (RNA protection assays). In aggregate, these assays are less relevant to clinical genetics *per se* than to determining how genes act (translational analysis).

GENE EXPRESSION PROFILING

For decades, studies have been conducted to search for altered gene expression, comparing abnormal and normal tissues. The comparison could be between individuals (affected, unaffected) or between different tissues from the same individual. Either approach is based upon the hypothesis that differentially expressed genes connote or pinpoint causality. Until the molecular era the end point was the gene product, either protein itself or some indicator thereof (e.g., immunohistochemistry). Studies traditionally proceeded gene by gene, hypothesis by hypothesis.

ANALYZING GENE PRODUCTS (PROTEIN): WESTERN BLOTTING AND TRANSFECTION ANALYSIS

Even if a gene is present (as reflected by Southern analysis) or transcribed (as reflected by Northern analysis), messenger RNA must be translated into protein in order to produce the gene product. One may therefore wish to verify that a gene product is present.

Detecting a specific gene product from among many concurrent products (protein) is accomplished in a fashion completely analogous to that of Southern and Northern blotting. Proteins (gene products) can be separated on the basis of their size

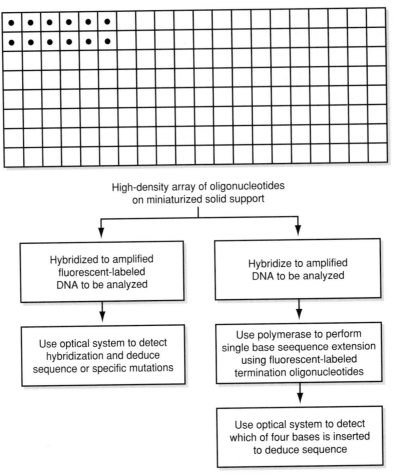

High-density array of oligonucleotides
on miniaturized solid support

Hybridized to amplified
fluorescent-labeled
DNA to be analyzed

Use optical system to detect
hybridization and deduce
sequence or specific mutations

Hybridize to amplified
DNA to be analyzed

Use polymerase to perform
single base seequence extension
using fluorescent-labeled
termination oligonucleotides

Use optical system to detect
which of four bases is inserted
to deduce sequence

FIGURE 2–33 • Use of DNA chips for molecular analysis. Large numbers of unique oligonucleotides are arrayed on a solid support and analyzed as indicated. (From Scriver CR, Beaudet AL, Sly WS, et al.: The Metabolic and Molecular Bases of Inherited Disease, 8th ed. New York: McGraw-Hill, 2001.)

and challenged with a suitable probe. Typically, the probe may be an antibody against the protein. This overall technique is called Western blotting. Western blotting largely serves a confirmatory role. Gynecologists are familiar with use of Western blotting as the definitive test for HIV.

Transfection analysis is a related, invaluable method for determining gene function. Through transfection analysis structure-function relationships can be assessed. The basic principle utilizes plasmid DNA, which is introduced into specialized cultured cells. Plasmids of different composition may be needed in transfection experiments, in which case the term cotransfection is applied. The basic principle is that one plasmid contains a reporter gene connected to a promotor sequence. If expression for the gene occurs, the reporter gene will signify this phenomenon. Activity can be quantified. Luciferase

is one commonly used reporter; antibody resistance (chloramphenicol toxicity or CAT) is another. Transfection analysis assesses *in vitro* the effects of missense or nonsense mutation. For example, does a particular androgen receptor mutation (see Chapter 11) completely abolish androgen binding or does residual activity remain? If so, how much—5%, 10%, or 20%?

Using transfection analysis can also determine whether a promoter region does or does not control a given gene. The precise portion of the promotor region responsible can be determined, sequentially deleting portions of the 5′ promoter region (deletion constructs) to localize the effect.

A pitfall of transfection analysis is the uncertain specificity of the requisite cultured cell line. This line is assumed to have characteristics reflecting the cell of origin. Actually this is a hazardous assumption, since established (immortalized) cell lines may dedifferentiate and differ considerably from their progenitors.

The Human Genome Project

The Human Genome Project is an international research effort that had located the estimated 30,000 human genes and sequenced the 3 billion nucleotide base pairs (bp) of the human genome. Identification of the human genome sequence will allow scientists and physicians to accurately study human genetic variation, especially in relation to genetic diseases. This information will be useful in the future for prevention and treatment of the estimated 4000 hereditary diseases and many other common diseases that are partially caused by an altered gene or genes such as cancer, heart disease, and diabetes.

In the United States, the National Human Genome Research Institute at the National Institutes of Health (NIH) and the Office of Biological and Environmental Research at the Department of Energy (DOE) sponsor the Human Genome Project (HGP). In 1990, the NIH and the DOE published a joint research plan entitled "Understanding Our Genetic Inheritance: the U.S. Human Genome Project. The First Five Years FY 1991-1995" (Department of Health and Human Services, 1990). The 1990 plan was updated in 1993 because the initial goals were accomplished more rapidly than anticipated as a result of technological improvements. The updated plan covered fiscal years 1994 to 1998 (Collins and Galas, 1993). Most recently, the NIH and DOE have presented their plan covering fiscal years 1998 to 2003 (Collins et al., 1998).

An important goal for 1998 to 2003 is the completion of entire human genome sequence by the end of 2003 (Collins, 1999), the 50th anniversary of the discovery of the double helix structure of DNA by Watson and Crick (1953). As readers know through enormous publicity, draft sequences were made available in 2001 (International Human Genome Sequencing Consortium, 2001). The human genome initiative data further collate nicely with cDNA-based draft generated from the private sector (Venter et al., 2001). The human genome draft is not derived from a single individual but from different cell lines that exist in laboratories around the world. Thus, the human genome will be a composite genome that serves as a reference sequence. In addition to the human genome sequence, the model organisms that the HGP is sequencing include *Escherichia coli*,

yeast, *Caenorhabitis elegans*, *Drosophilia melanogaster*, and mouse.

DNA MAPPING

Prior to the 1998 to 2003 plan, the HGP's major scientific goals were directed toward technology development and genome mapping. The first type of map, called a *genetic map*, consists of a series of sequence-based markers that can be used to identify the likely location of a mutated gene responsible for a disease phenotype (Fig. 2–34). The technology of marker production shifted rapidly from restriction fragment length polymorphisms to simple repeated microsatellites. These early genetic maps were important in identifying and isolating mendelian disorders by allowing a gene to be placed in a reasonably searchable interval (Collins, 1999). By 1994, a year ahead of schedule, an international consortium published a genetic map containing almost 6000 markers, spaced less than 1 million bases apart (Murray et al., 1994).

A second type of map, called a *physical map*, generates a set of overlapping cloned fragments of DNA (*contigs*) that represent regions of a chromosome or its entirety. Physical mapping provides information regarding the order of cloned pieces (see Fig. 2–34). Once genetic markers define the region containing a gene of interest, the cloned pieces provide a resource from which the gene can be isolated. Techniques used in physical mapping include PCR, pulsed field gel electrophoresis, fluorescence *in situ* hybridization, and yeast artificial chromosome (YAC) cloning, which permit only cloning of pieces of DNA from 100,000 to 1,000,000 bp (Fig. 2–35). To compare data from any of the above physical mapping techniques, "sequenced-tagged sites" (STS) were developed. Each mapped sequence contains a unique short DNA sequence: its sequenced-tagged site. The order and spacing of these sites from different mapping techniques are used to construct a physical map (Collins, 1999; Haddad et al., 1999).

CURRENT STATUS

The ultimate goal of the Human Genome Project is to obtain the entire 3 billion bp sequences of the human genome. A working draft of the complete DNA sequence is already available (International Human Genome Sequencing Consortium, 2001), and the full DNA sequence will be complete by

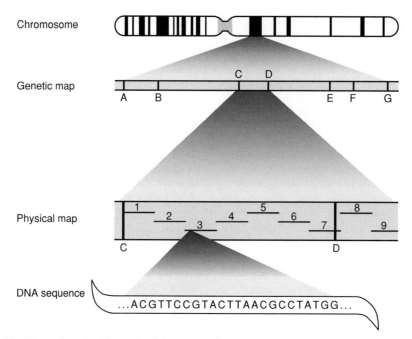

FIGURE 2–34 • The major scientific goals of the Human Genome Project are to develop genetic maps, physical maps, and DNA sequences. In the process, the entire 3 billion bp of the human genome, containing approximately 30,000 genes, has been determined. See International Human Genome Sequences Consortium (2001) and Venter et al. (2001). (From Gelehrter TD, Collins FS, Ginsburg D: Principles of Medical Genetics, 2nd ed. Baltimore: Williams & Wilkins, 1998.)

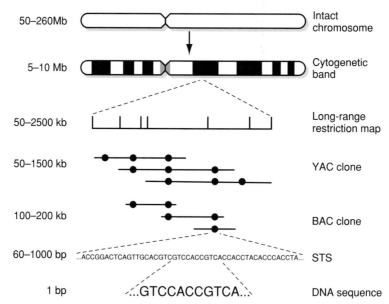

FIGURE 2–35 • Characteristic resolution ranges in human genome mapping. Individual human chromosomes range in size from about 50 to 260 million bases (Mb). When properly stained and examined microscopically, the characteristic cytogenetic banding pattern gives a unique appearance to each chromosome, with each band containing about 5 to 10 Mb of DNA. Physical mapping techniques, such as long-range restriction mapping by pulsed-field gel electrophoresis, yeast artificial chromosome (YAC) cloning, and bacterial artificial chromosome (BAC) cloning are associated with successively decreasing resolution ranges, as indicated. Individual DNA landmarks typically represent much smaller DNA segments (e.g., about 60 to 1000 bp for a sequence-tagged site [STS]). The highest level of resolution is the single base pair of DNA sequence. (From Scriver CR, Beaudet AL, Sly WS, et al.: The Metabolic and Molecular Bases of Inherited Disease, 8th ed, vol I. New York: McGraw-Hill, 2001.)

2003. The Celera draft is fundamentally compatible (Venter et al., 2001). The plan has been expanded to include anonymous markers as well as the genes themselves. As of February 2001, there are perhaps 1000 diseases for which information is available on the function of their gene product (Jimenez-Sanchez et al., 2001).

The biggest surprise is that there are only some 30,000 human genes. We humans differ very little (1 to 3%) from other primates and even mice. Differences among human ethnic groups are minuscule on this scale. An oversimplification but heuristically useful concept is that evolution occurred from lower organisms through a fourfold duplication in genes. Favorable mutants were selected, and unfavorable duplication and mutations were eliminated or rendered nonfunctional (pseudogenes). Pseudogenes are clinically relevant to several prominent genetic disorders that we will discuss, such as 21-hydroxylase deficiency (congenital adrenal hyperplasia; see Chapter 11).

Positional cloning is the application of human gene mapping techniques to clone disease-causing genes when no information is available about the biochemical basis of the disease. Such gene isolation allows understanding of human disease at its most fundamental level and provides the best hope for diagnosis, prevention, and therapy (Fig. 2–36). For example, the gene responsible for cystic fibrosis was identified by positional cloning without any chromosomal arrangement to indicate the specific region of the genome that contained the responsible gene. The genomic region of interest was localized to the long arm of chromo-

some 7 by linkage analysis that involved evaluation of inheritance patterns of genetic markers within families that had individuals with cystic fibrosis. Subsequently, a contig was developed within this chromosomal region, and open reading frames, representing coding sequences for genes, were identified. Mutations were found in a gene for a protein that had the features of a membrane channel, referred to as the cystic fibrosis transmembrane regulator (CFTR). CFTR was found to be involved in controlling the movement of chloride across the cell membrane (see Chapters 4 and 7). The same approach will continue to be used to elucidate the gene(s) responsible for other defined disorders. A host of heretofore unknown genes will also be identified, and in the process considerable scientific and medical information will be derived. The eventual goal is a complete map of gene and function. Figure 2–37 shows the current map of the X chromosomes.

IMPACT ON MEDICAL GENETICS

A major challenge is to define the interplay of environment, lifestyle, and the small effects of many genes in complex disorders of low penetrance in common gynecologic diseases (benign gynecologic and other cancers) and others such as diabetes mellitus, heart disease, autoimmune diseases, and mental illnesses. To this end, the Human Genome Project is initiating new studies of genetic variation in the human population enabling construction of a dense map of

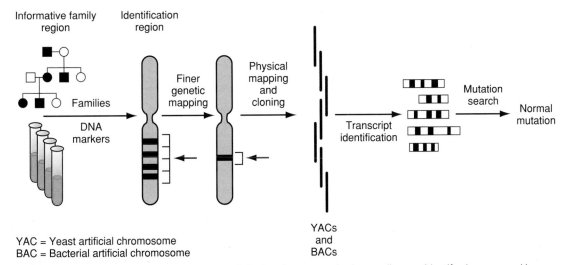

YAC = Yeast artificial chromosome
BAC = Bacterial artificial chromosome

FIGURE 2–36 • General approach to positional cloning. A cytogenetic abnormality may identify chromosomal location, or the disease gene may be mapped by linkage analysis or sequencing to a specific chromosomal region. YAC = yeast artificial chromosome; BAC = bacterial artificial chromosome. (From Gelehrter TD, Collins FS, Ginsburg D, et al.: Principles of Medical Genetics, 2nd ed. Baltimore: Williams & Wilkins, 1998.)

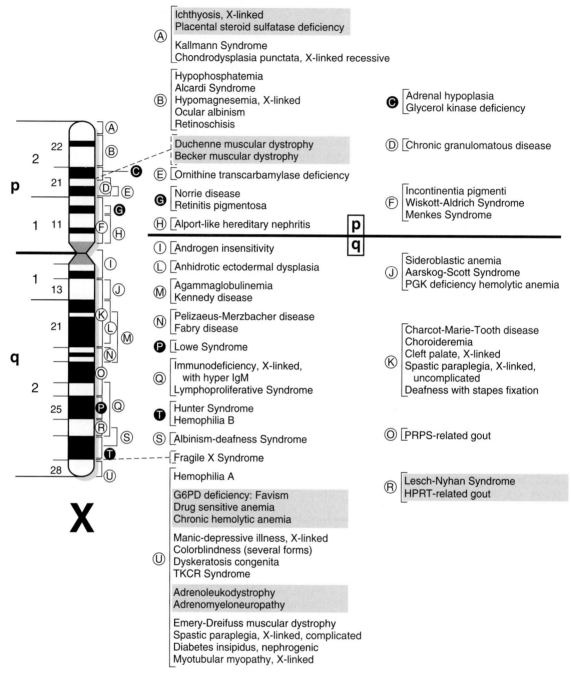

FIGURE 2–37 • Location of genes on the X chromosome responsible for genetic diseases. (http://www.ncbi.nlm.nih.gov/disease/.)

common polymorphic DNA variants (see Figs. 2–22 and 2–23). DNA sequence variations include not only difference in the number of repeat sequences but also a single-nucleotide polymorphism (SNP), which occurs in about 1 in every 300 to 500 bp in human DNA. Studies may point to an association between a variant and direct functional importance resulting in a disease. Alternatively, a variant may be used in linkage disequilibrium studies to map gene variants associated with disease. Work is already under way to develop a catalogue of 60,000 or more SNPs distributed over the entire human genome (Collins, 1999).

ETHICAL, LEGAL AND SOCIAL IMPLICATIONS

From the beginning, the U.S. Human Genome Project has been concerned about the ethical, legal, and social issues raised by genome information and technology. Among the most immediate and recurrent consequences of genome research are the development of new diagnostic and predictive tests from the localization and identification of specific disease-related genes. With the development of index and reference maker maps of the genome, the pace of gene localization and subsequent test development will accelerate. But a gene that can immediately serve as the basis for a test is only the first step in unraveling the pathogenesis of a disorder. Consequently, predictive genetic testing will typically be available well in advance of curative breakthroughs. The implications of acquiring and using genetic knowledge about individuals pose a number of choices for public and professional deliberation:

- Choices for individuals and families about whether to participate in testing, with whom to share the results, and how to act on them.
- Choices for health professionals about when to recommend testing, how to ensure its quality, how to interpret the results, and to whom to disclose the information.
- Choices for employers, insurers, the courts, and other social institutions about the relative value of genetic information to the kinds of decisions they must make about the individuals.
- Choices for governments about how to regulate the production and use of genetic tests and the information they provide, and how to provide access to testing and counseling services.
- Choices for society about how to improve the understanding of science and its social implications at every level and how to increase the participation of the public in science policy-making (Annas and Elias, 1992).

In 1990, the U.S. Human Genome Project established the Ethical, Legal and Social Implications (ELSI) Program to address these and other related issues. To finance the ELSI Program, the National Human Genome Research Institute at the NIH allocates 5% of its budget to study ELSI issues. The Office of Energy Research at DOE also reserves a percentage of its funding for ELSI research.

REFERENCES

Annas GJ, Elias SS: Gene Mapping: Using Law and Ethics as Guides. New York: Oxford Press, 1992.

Cohen J, Scott R, Schimmel T, et al.: Birth of infant after transfer of anucleate donor oocyte cytoplasm into recipient eggs. Lancet 350:186, 1997.

Collins, FS: Shattuck lecture—Medical and societal consequences of the Human Genome Project. N Engl J Med 341:28, 1999.

Collins FS, Patrinos A, Jordan E, et al.: New goals for the U.S. Human Genome Project: 1998–2003. Science 282:682, 1998.

Collins F, Galas D: A new five-year plan for the U.S. Human Genome Project. Science 262:43, 1993.

Department of Health and Human Services—Department of Energy: Understanding our genetic inheritance: The U.S. Human Genome Project: The first five years: FY 1991–1995. Washington, DC: Government Printing Office, 1990 (NIH Publication No. 90–1590).

Haddad FF, Yeatman TJ, Shivers SC, et al.: The Human Genome Project: A dream becoming a reality. Surgery 125:575, 1999.

Hiort O, Sinnecker GH, Holterhus PM, et al.: Inherited and de novo androgen receptor gene mutations: Investigation of single-case families. J Pediatr 132:939, 1998.

International Human Genome Sequencing Consortium: Initial sequencing and analysis of the human genome. Nature 409:921, 2001.

Jimenez-Sanchez G, Childs B, Valle D: Human disease genes. Nature 409:853, 2001.

Moraes CT, DiMauro S, Zeviani M, et al.: Mitochondrial DNA deletions in progressive external ophthalmoplegia and Kearns-Sayre syndrome. N Engl J Med 320:1293, 1989.

Murray JC, Buetow KH, Weber JL, et al.: A comprehensive human linkage map with centimorgan density. Cooperative Human Linkage Center (CHLC). Science 265:2049, 1994.

Southern EM: Detection of specific sequences among DNA fragments separated by gel electrophoresis. Biotechnology 24:122, 1975.

Venter JC, Adams MD, Myers EW, et al.: The sequence of the human genome. Science 291:1304, 2001.

Watson JD, Crick FC: Molecular structure of nucleic acids. Nature 171:737, 1953.

CHAPTER **3**

Polygenic-Multifactorial Inheritance

Not every congenital abnormality can be explained on the basis of a chromosomal abnormality or a single mutant gene. Nor can either of these mechanisms readily explain the heritability and genetics of normal anatomic and physiologic variations (e.g., stature, blood pressure, age at menarche). Yet the tendency of relatives to resemble one another in physical appearance is obvious, and most congenital anomalies show heritable tendencies. For example, after the birth of one child with a neural tube defect (anencephaly or spina bifida), the likelihood that any subsequent progeny will be similarly affected is 2% in the United States.

One possible explanation for familial aggregates is shared environmental factors among relatives. However, environmental factors are not solely responsible for familial aggregates, as can be deduced from twin studies. Monozygotic twins are much more likely to be concordant for any given anomaly than are dizygotic twins.

▼ **Table 3–1.** POLYGENIC-MULTIFACTORIAL
• TRAITS

Neural tube defects (anencephaly, spina bifida, encephalocele)
Hydrocephaly (except some cases of aqueductal stenosis
   and of Dandy-Walker syndrome)
Cleft lip, with or without cleft palate
Cleft lip (alone)
Cardiac defects (most types)
Diaphragmatic hernia
Omphalocele
Renal agenesis
Ureteral anomalies
Hypospadias (most forms)
Posterior urethral valves
Incomplete müllerian fusion
Hip dislocation
Limb reduction defect (most forms)
Talipes equinovarus (clubfoot)

Because monozygotic and dizygotic twins are exposed to the same intrauterine environmental factors, such factors alone cannot explain the concordance rates of the trait. Instead, genetic factors must be invoked for anomalies whose recurrence risks are greater than the population incidence but less than that expected on the basis of a single recessive or dominant gene (25% and 50%, respectively). Table 3–1 lists several anatomic defects, all of which show recurrence risks suggesting the necessity to postulate polygenic-multifactorial etiology. Unaffected parents have 1 to 5% risk of recurrence for subsequently affected progeny. An affected parent has a similar risk for passing his or her trait onto any given offspring, even if the other parent is unaffected.

Basis of Polygenic Inheritance

A logical explanation for familial resemblances is that anatomically variable traits are influenced by several genes. To illustrate this logic, let us consider the effect of progressively increasing the number of genes influencing a given trait.

Suppose only one gene controls a given trait, and that this gene has two alleles. If the frequency of allele A equals the frequency of allele a, 25% of the population is AA ($p = q = 0.5$; $p^2 = q^2 = 0.25$), 25% is aa, and 50% is Aa ($2pq = 0.50$) (Fig. 3–1). (See Chapter 2 for Hardy-Weinberg equilibrium.) Now suppose that not one but two genes influence a given trait. At the second locus, alleles B and b exist. Nine genotypes are now possible: AABB, AABb, AAbb, AaBB, AaBb, Aabb, aaBB, aaBb, and aabb (Table 3–2). The population will contain nine somatic classes if alleles A, B, a, and b each exert dissimilar influences. (If the alleles exert equal effect, there are only five classes, as seen in Fig. 3–2.) As the number of

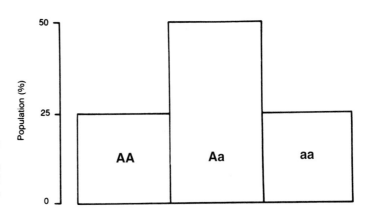

FIGURE 3–1 • Histogram showing the relative proportions of people with various genotypes (AA, Aa, aa) if a trait is influenced by a single gene that can exist in two allelic forms (A or a). If A = a = 0.5, then $A^2 = a^2 = 0.25$ and $2pq = 0.50$ (Hardy-Weinberg equilibrium). Thus, 25% of the population is AA, 25% is aa, and 50% is Aa. If A = 0.9, then 81% are AA, 18% are Aa, and 1% are aa. (From Simpson JL: Disorders of Sexual Differentiation: Etiology and Clinical Delineation. New York: Academic Press, 1976.)

		AAbb		
	AaBB	aaBB	aaBb	
AABB	AABb	AaBb	Aabb	aabb

FIGURE 3–2 • Histographs showing relative proportions in the population of individuals having the different genotypes that would be produced if two genes influence a trait, if each gene has two alleles, and if each gene is comparable in effect, i.e., A = B and a = b. Even with this simplest of examples, the histographic representation shows five genotypic classes of differing heights. As more alleles are added, the distribution more closely begins to approximate the normal distribution expected for traits showing continuous variation (e.g., height).

▼ **Table 3–2.** RELATIONSHIP BETWEEN
• NUMBERS OF GENES CONTROLLING A TRAIT AND NUMBERS OF GENOTYPES (CLASSES OF INDIVIDUALS) IN A POPULATION*

Number of Genes (Alleles)	Genotypes (Classes of Individuals)	Number of Genotype Classes
1 (Aa)	AA, Aa, aa	3
2 (Aa, Bb)	AABB, AABb, AAbb, AaBB AaBb, Aabb, aaBB, aaBb, aabb	9
n		3^n

* Assumes two alleles per locus, each of which exerts a differential phenotypic effect

▼ **Table 3–3.** RELATIONSHIP BETWEEN
• NUMBERS OF GENES CONTROLLING A TRAIT AND NUMBER OF GENOTYPES IN A POPULATION ASSUMING THREE ALLELES PER LOCUS

1 (A,a,á)	AA,Aa,Aá aa, aá, áá	6
2 (A,a,á; B,b,b´)		36
n		6^n

genes controlling a trait increases, the number of genotypes in the population increases rapidly. If three genes, each with two alleles, exist, there are 27 classes (3^n). There are also more genotype possibilities if a locus has more than two alleles. If there are three alleles per locus and two loci, 36 genotypes exist (Table 3–3). If one represents the proportion of individuals in each genotypic class histographically, a normal distribution will be approximated as more genotypes become possible. This is obvious with 27 different genotypes. Thus, continuous variation will be approximated in the population by the cumulative effect of only a few genes. Figure 3–3 illustrates this, assuming only two genes, each with two alleles, influence blood pressure. Table 3–3 shows that the number of genotypes is increased even further if three alleles exist at each loci.

Appreciating the general principles of polygenic inheritance helps explain why offspring usually but not always reflect parental origin. An example is height, well known to correlate with midparental height once corrected for sex. Suppose a given trait were controlled by only three genes, simplistically each with two alleles (A,a; B,b; C,c). Each dominant gene (A,B,C) might equally confer an additional 3 inches in height above some threshold, hypothetically 60 inches for males and 54 inches for females. Assume small case alleles (a,b,c) contribute nothing above the threshold. A father of genotype AaBBcC would be 72 inches tall (60 + 4 × 3 = 72); a mother of genotype AaBbCc would be 63 inches tall (54 + 3 × 3 = 63). On average one would expect the father to contribute two dominant alleles and the mother 1.5 (one or two).

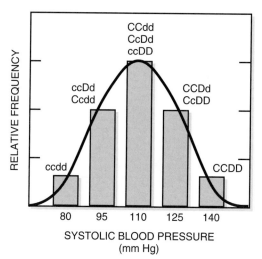

FIGURE 3–3 • Frequency distribution of systolic blood pressure determined by two-locus two-allele models. For each additional unfavorable allele (C or D), systolic blood pressure increases by 15 mm Hg, and the converse.

Thus, the child is likely to have three or four dominant alleles and resemble parental height. However, Table 3–4 shows that any given offspring could inherit between one and six dominant alleles, resulting in heights ranging from 63 to 78 inches in males or 57 to 72 inches in females. The likelihood of various possibilities' occurring is further shown in Table 3–4.

Polygenic Versus Multifactorial Inheritance

Additional details concerning the mathematic basis of polygenic inheritance are provided by Simpson (2002). A trait controlled by more than one gene is said to be inherited in polygenic fashion. Although the term polygenic inheritance is often used synonymously with continuous variation, the latter may also result from other mechanisms, namely, one multiple allele locus or interaction between a single locus and environmental factors. If environmental as well as genetic factors influence a trait, the term multifactorial is more appropriate. One usually cannot distinguish polygenic from multifactorial inheritance in humans, although comparisons between monozygotic and dizygotic twins theoretically permit such a distinction.

Geneticists are often guilty of loosely terming polygenic any trait whose inheritance is complex. Nonetheless, it is appropriate to invoke the concept of polygenic inheritance or multifactorial inheritance while being aware that the genetic complexities usually have not been precisely elucidated. Here we use the term polygenic-multifactorial inheritance to refer to the phenomenon described.

Polygenic-Multifactorial Inheritance in Discontinuous Variation

The term polygenic-multifactorial inheritance is invoked to explain the inheritance of normal anatomic and physiologic variables that display continuous variation—height, skin color, hair color, blood pressure, age at menarche, ability to metabolize a given drug or toxin. However, polygenic inheritance cannot readily explain discontinuous variation.

In discontinuous variation, the population consists of two discrete groups; in the current

▼ **Table 3–4.** HYPOTHETICAL EXAMPLE SHOWING PROBABILITY OF AN UNCOMMON GENOTYPE
• (TALL OR SHORT STATURE) ARISING FROM A MATING INVOLVING TWO AVERAGE PARENTS

Baseline Height Threshold
    Males: 60″
    Females: 54″
Calculation of Height Above Threshold:
    For each A,B, or C allele, add 3″
    For each a,b, or c allele, add 0
Examples:

			Parental Heights (inches)	
1. Parental genotypes and height:		Male AaBBCc	72	
		Female Aa Bb Cc	63	
2. Probabilities of selected genotypes in offspring and expected height	Genotype in Offspring	Probability of Genotype's Arising	Offspring Height (inches) Male	Female
	• Aa Bb Cc	1/2 × 1/2 × 1/2 = 1/8	69	63
	• AA BB CC	1/4 × 1/2 × 1/4 = 1/32	78	72
	• aa Bb cc	1/4 × 1/2 × 1/4 = 1/32	63	57

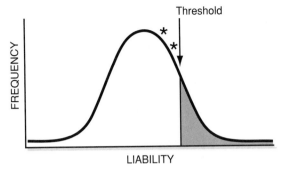

FIGURE 3–4 • Schematic representation of one model for polygenic-multifactorial inheritance, assuming a threshold beyond which liability is so great that an abnormality is manifested. Parents of affected offspring presumably have a greater liability (i.e., are closer to the threshold) than most of the population. Idealized parental genotypes would be near but not over the threshold, as designated by asterisks.

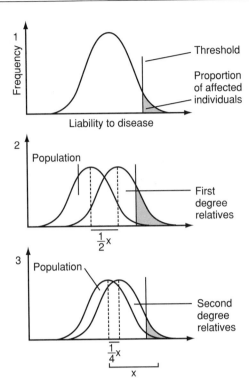

FIGURE 3–5 • Multifactorial threshold model shows how genetically determined liability is increased among relatives of an affected individual. Genetic liability in relatives of an affected proband is indicated by the shaded area. Genetic liability in first-degree relatives is increased because distribution of genotypes is shifted from that in the general population. The shift is greater for first-degree relatives than for second-degree relatives. (From Passarge E: Color Atlas of Genetics. New York: Thieme Medical Publishers, Inc., 1995.)

context they are affected (e.g., cleft palate) and unaffected. Either a person has cleft palate or does not. There is no continuum in the population. To explain such dichotomy (discontinuity) on a polygenic-multifactorial basis, a threshold is postulated beyond which the accrued genetic liability for developing a specific trait becomes so great that a malformation is manifested (Fig. 3–4). Phenotypically normal parents delivered of a child with a polygenic-multifactorial trait (anomaly) are assumed to have genetic liabilities nearer the threshold than most others in the general population, thus explaining the 1 to 5% risk for recurrence in any subsequent progeny. The distribution of their genotypes is closer to that in the normal population. By similar reasoning, a parent with a polygenic-multifactorial trait has 1 to 5% risk if having an affected offspring, assuming the other parent is normal. The risk is less for second-degree than for first-degree relatives (Fig. 3–5).

The threshold model becomes readily plausible biologically if "liability" reflects rate of embryonic growth. Growth at too slow a rate could prevent a key embryonic step from being achieved by a certain crucial time, thus leading to anomalous development. For example, if the paired palatine shelves reach the midline before a certain day of development, they fuse to form the secondary palate. After that day the shelves are too widely separated ever to fuse, thus resulting in cleft palate. Inherited factors (genes) contributing to the polygenic model might include velocity of growth, size of the mandible and tongue, and rapidity of palatine migration.

Characteristics of Disorders Inherited in Polygenic-Multifactorial Fashion

Several characteristics expected of a trait inherited in polygenic-multifactorial fashion can be cited. Traits fulfilling most or all of these criteria can be concluded to be inherited in polygenic-multifactorial fashion.

1. The disorder has an incidence of about 1 per 1000 live births.
2. The disorder usually involves a single organ system or embryologically related organ systems.
3. Frequency of similarly affected cotwins (concordance) is higher among monozygotic than dizygotic twins. Dissimilarly affected cotwins (discordance) is still observed among monozygotic twins, unlike expectations for mendelian traits (see Chapter 2).

4. Unlike in mendelian inheritance, the recurrence risk increases after more than one progeny is affected. However, the risk rarely approaches the 25% expected for recessive traits or the 50% expected for dominant traits. The potential exception for polygenic-multifactorial traits occur after three affected offspring.

5. The more serious the defect, the higher the recurrence risk. Bilateral cleft palate carries a higher recurrence risk than unilateral cleft palate. Long-segment aganglionosis (Hirschsprung disease) carries a higher recurrence risk than short-segment aganglionosis. The assumed model is that the more severe phenotype indicates a genotype further beyond the threshold than usual. In turn, the distribution of genotypes in first-degree relatives would also be shifted to the right (further away from the normal population).

6. If the trait occurs more frequently among members of one sex, the risk of relatives is higher if the proband (index case) is of the less frequently affected sex. Pyloric stenosis occurs more frequently in males; thus, the recurrence risk is higher if the proband is female. The converse is true for congenital hip dislocation.

7. As the degree of relation decreases, the recurrence risks for relatives decrease more rapidly than the risks observed for autosomal dominant traits.

Proportion of Genetic Control in Polygenic-Multifactorial Traits (Heritability)

The relative proportion of genetic and nongenetic factors responsible for multifactorial traits can be estimated. For this purpose, the term heritability (h^2) is invoked. This concept is used extensively in plant and animal breeding systems. Here systems, matings, and environment may be controlled, allowing that part of a disorder's variation resulting from additive genetic variation to be identified precisely.

Additive genetic variation, defined as heritability, is that genetic variation independent of dominance or epistasis. Dominance involves interaction between alleles at a single locus, whereas epistasis involves interaction of alleles at different loci. Dominance and epistasis are not additive genetic factors because their contributions are determined again with each successive generation. In contrast, additive factors are those that are always transmitted from generation to generation.

The concept of heritability has proved useful in plant and animal breeding. In humans, heritability for continuous variation traits such as height or blood pressure has often been calculated, usually on the basis of twin studies. However, in human populations neither matings nor environment can be controlled. Thus, heritability calculations represent only approximations, subject to variables that can be controlled in animals but not in humans. The phenomenon actually calculated in humans is more appropriately called genetic determination. This broader term connotes not only additive genetic factors but also dominance and epistasis. At any rate, the degree of genetic determination (H) can be formally estimated by the formula $H = (V_{DZ} - V_{MZ})/V_{DZ}$. V refers to the variance of the differences between pairs (MZ, monozygotic; DZ, dizygotic). This equation assumes, actually incorrectly, that environmental influences are equivalent for monozygotic and dizygotic twins. For heuristic purposes it is still appropriate to assume that MZ twins would be expected to differ less than DZ twins for any trait having a genetic component. Variance between DZ twins should be attributable to both genetic and environmental variation, whereas variance between MZ twins should reflect only environmental variation. The absolute value of heritability estimates in humans should not be accepted too rigidly, but relative values may help identify conditions in which it would be useful to pursue investigations using other methods.

Quantitative Linkage (QTL) Analysis

Even if no candidate genes exist, chromosomal regions that segregate with a given trait can be sought through linkage analysis using polymorphic loci. A common thread has been that a single gene has a major effect, with several additional genes having lesser effects. A search using linkage and clinical features could quickly reveal that many common disorders are etiologically heterogeneous. Table 3–5 shows a hypothetical example of what might become evident. Common disorders for which this stratification might be applicable include endometriosis, leiomyomas, and endometrial adenocarcinoma). We will explore this in detail in Chapters 8 and 9. Having stratified disorders on a genetic basis, subtle differences may become evident in treatment efficacy. Concurrently, the linked genes would point to chromosomal regions and candidate genes that could be causative.

▼ **Table 3–5.** HYPOTHETICAL EXAMPLES SHOWING HOW A COMMON DISORDER MIGHT BE
• STRATIFIED IN THREE DISTINCT SUBTYPES.

Subtype	Chromosomal Regions for Linked Genes	Clinical Features	Treatment (1, 2, or 3)
I	1p	A,B,C	1
II	3p	A,B,C,D,E	2
III	5p	A,B,D	3

Suppose first that three different patterns of genetic linkages are discerned (I, II, III) and shown to be localized to different chromosome regions (1p, 3p, 5p). Further, clinical features differ subtly. For example, all cases had clinical features A and B, but presence or absence of C, D, and E varied among subtypes. Linkage group and clinical features help define subtypes I, II, and III and consequently optimal treatment for a specific subtype.

More precise elucidation of the genetic basis of polygenic traits requires population and genetic studies that construct multiple gene models (quantitative traits). Identification of the several genes responsible for multifactoral-polygenic disorders requires methods such as (1) affected and unaffected sib-pair analysis, (2) multipoint linkage analysis, and (3) transmission disequilibrium studies. The underlying basis is that multiple gene regions (loci) exist and can be found at definable distances on each chromosome, measured in centimorgans (cM). Mapping the distance between loci (or between loci and an event or phenotype) is possible using DNA polymorphisms interspersed at known intervals. Polymorphisms usually utilized are characterized by nucleotide changes that include single base pair substitutions (SNIPs) variable number tandem repeats, namely, repetitive sequences like di-, tri-, or tetranucleotide repeats. The latter can be of variable length (i.e., CAT^n or CAG^n) and are easily assayed by molecular techniques that are widely available. When crossing over or recombination occurs during meiosis, a polymorphism can be found on the opposite homologous chromosome (see Chapter 2). The frequency of recombination is determined by the distance between loci (1cM = 1% recombination frequency). A polymorphic

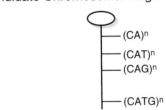

Candidate Chromosomal Region

Genotyping of Sibs

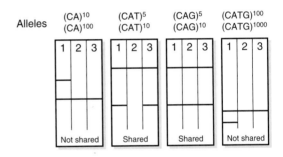

Interpretation: Most likely linkage between $(CAT)^n$ and $(CAG)^n$

FIGURE 3–7 • Principles of quantitative linkage analysis (GTL). Sibs 1 and 3 are similarly affected; sib 2 is normal. Genotyping of the two affected sibs shows maximal allele sharing for the CAT and CAG markers. The chromosomal region between these two alleles would be fruitful to explore for candidate genes. (Diagram prepared by Dr. Anthony Gregg, Baylor College of Medicine, Houston, Texas.)

marker near a disease (mutation) locus is more likely to be the same in two affected sibs than in a pair of sibs in which one is affected and the other is not. The specific methodology first involves performing a genome wide scan in order to establish candidate regions, traditionally known as quantitative trait loci (QTL). Starting with DNA obtained from thoroughly studied patients and their family members, DNA genotyping is obtained using the polymorphic DNA markers spaced 10 cM apart. There are tetranucleotide repeat polymorphic markers noted

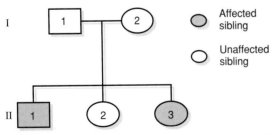

FIGURE 3–6 • One potentially informative affected sib-pair pedigree for quantitative linkage analysis (QTL). DNA from all five individuals would be desirable. The principle is that the two affected sibs would be more likely to share any given polymorphic allele than would any pair of affected and unaffected sibs.

above. Several methods of genome wide searching may be pursued. To illustrate one approach, Figure 3–6 shows an informative affected sib-pair pedigree. Figure 3–7 shows idealized results. In the illustration, the region of DNA located between the $CAG^{(n)}$ and the $CAT^{(n)}$ trinucleotide polymorphesis is worthy of further analysis.

One would seek to identify specific genes and their mutation through a search for candidate genes in a region within 5 cM of QTLs using the approach shown in Figure 3–7. Candidate genes within the QTLs can be sought through a careful search of the genome database (i.e., Genbank), utilizing widely available computer-based methodologies. Once specific candidate genes are identified, we will analyze them by direct (sequencing) and indirect (i.e., SSCP, single-strand conformational polymorphism) methods.

REFERENCE

Simpson JL: Polygenic/multifactorial inheritance. *In* Sciarra JJ (ed): Gynecology and Obstetrics, vol 5. New York: Lippincott-Raven, 2002.

CHAPTER 4

Genetic History-Taking and Genetic Counseling

The relative burden of major birth defects (2% to 3% of all deliveries) has increased as deaths caused by infection and prematurity decreased. Concurrent with this trend are the genetic advances of the last few decades. All this has increased public and professional awareness. Maternal and child health delivery systems must adapt to these trends, and integral to adaptation is a systematic approach for eliciting information about risks of genetic disorders.

This chapter discusses taking a genetic history. Those disorders amenable to genetic screening are enumerated, along with the principles underlying initiation of screening programs. Cystic fibrosis is used as an example of heterozygote carrier screening. Finally, the chapter addresses the psychological ramifications of genetic counseling.

The Routine Genetic History

Some obstetricians consider it useful to obtain genetic information through use of questionnaires or checklists. Figure 4–1 reproduces a form recommended by the American College of Obstetricians and Gynecologists (ACOG, 1987). Use of an earlier version of this form revealed that 21.4% of couples in a prenatal clinic gave at least one positive response, with 7.8% of the original sample requiring formal genetic counseling. Advanced maternal age is the most common indication (Simpson et al., 1981). For all pregnancies, it is standard practice to determine whether a couple or anyone in either of their families has a disorder that might prove heritable (Walker, 2002). The same holds true for gamete donors (ACOG, 1997; ASRM, 1998).

One should inquire about the health status of first-degree relatives (siblings, parents, offspring), second-degree relatives (uncles, aunts, nephews, nieces, and grandparents), and third-degree relatives (first cousins) (Kingston, 2002). Record any abnormal reproductive outcomes, such as repetitive spontaneous abortions, stillbirths, or anomalous liveborn infants. Couples with such histories should have chromosomal studies and other evaluations, as discussed in Chapters 5 and 14.

Subsequent genetic counseling may be sufficiently complex to warrant referral to a geneticist, or it may prove facile enough for the informed clinician to handle. If a birth defect is detected in a second- or third-degree relative, the likelihood of that anomaly recurring in a subsequent pregnancy is rarely significantly increased. Identification of a second- or third-degree relative with an autosomal recessive trait ordinarily places the couple at little increased risk for an affected offspring, the exception being if the couple is consanguineous (see Chapter 2). Nevertheless, one should inquire about the status of relatives as distant as first cousins (of the fetus), because identification of certain disorders in such relatives may be the only clue that the couple may be at increased risk for autosomal dominant disorders characterized by decreased penetrance or for X-linked recessive disorders.

In addition to identifying relatives with genetic disorders, any drug exposure of the woman and her partner should be recorded. Identify not only those agents currently taken but also any noxious agents to which exposure occurred before pregnancy that could be mutagenic.

Parental ages also should be recorded. Indeed, the most common indication for prenatal

Woman's Name _____   Identification # _____   Date _____

	Yes	No
1. Will you be 35 years or older when the baby is due?	Yes _____	No _____
2. Have you, the baby's father, or anyone in either of your families ever had any of the following disorders?	Yes _____	No _____
Down syndrome (mongolism)	Yes _____	No _____
Other chromosomal abnormality	Yes _____	No _____
Neural tube defect, e.g., spina bifida (meningomyelocele or open spine), anencephaly	Yes _____	No _____
Hemophilia	Yes _____	No _____
Muscular dystrophy	Yes _____	No _____
Cystic fibrosis	Yes _____	No _____
If yes, indicate the relationship of the affected person to you or the baby's father:		
_____		
3. Do you or the baby's father have a birth defect?	Yes _____	No _____
If yes, who has the defect and what is it? _____		
4. In any previous marriages, have you or the baby's father had a child born dead or alive with a birth not listed in question 2 above?	Yes _____	No _____
5. Do you or the baby's father have any close relatives with mental retardation?	Yes _____	No _____
If yes, indicate the relationship of the affected person to you or the baby's father: _____		
_____		
Indicate the cause, if known:_____		
6. Do you, the baby's father, or a close relative in either of your families have a birth defect, any familial disorder, or a chromosomal abnormality not listed above?	Yes _____	No _____
If yes, indicate the condition and the relationship of the affected person to you or to the baby's father: _____		
_____		
7. In any previous marriages, have you or the baby's father had a stillborn child or three or more first-trimester spontaneous pregnancy losses?	Yes _____	No _____
Have either of you had a chromosomal study?		
8. If you or the baby's father are of Jewish ancestry, has either of you been screened for Tay-Sachs disease and Canavan disease?	Yes _____	No _____
If yes, indicate who and the results: _____		
9. If you or the baby's father are African-American, has either of you been screened for sickle cell traits?	Yes _____	No _____
If yes, indicate who and the results: _____		
10. If you or the baby's father are of Italian, Greek, or Mediterranean background, has either of you been tested for β-thalassemia?	Yes _____	No _____
If yes, indicate who and the results: _____		
11. If you or the baby's father are of Philippine or Southeast Asian ancestry, has either of you been tested for α-thalassemia?	Yes _____	No _____
12. If you or the baby's father are Caucasian or of Jewish ancestry, has either of you been screened for cystic fibrosis?	Yes _____	No _____
If of other ethnic groups, has cystic fibrosis screening been made available?		
13. Excluding iron and vitamins, have you taken any medications or recreational drugs since becoming pregnant or since your last menstrual period? (include nonprescription drugs)	Yes _____	No _____
If yes, give name of medication and time taken during pregnancy: _____		
_____		

FIGURE 4–1 • Questionnaire for identifying couples having increased risk for offspring with genetic disorders. (Modified from American College of Obstetrics and Gynecology. Technical Bulletin Number 108, 1987.)

diagnosis is advanced maternal age. Advanced maternal age warrants discussion regardless of a patient's difficulties in achieving pregnancy and regardless of a physician's personal convictions regarding pregnancy termination. Offspring of fathers in their fifth or sixth decade are at increased risk for new dominant mutations but probably not significantly for chromosomal abnormalities (American College of Obstetricians and Gynecologists, 1997).

Ethnic origin should be recorded. This is relevant to the genetic screening issues to be discussed in more detail later in this chapter. Ashkenazi Jews are at increased risk for offspring with Tay-Sachs disease and Canavan disease and therefore should be screened to determine heterozygote status (ACOG, 1995, 1998). Additional carrier testing has been recommended by some, including familial dysautonomia, Gaucher disease-1, Niemann-Pick disease, and other disorders (Gilbert, 2001). As discussed later, offering cystic fibrosis carrier screening to individuals of Ashkenazi Jewish descent is also recommended. In the United States, Jewish people may be uncertain as to whether they are of Ashkenazi or Sephardic descent; thus, we recommend screening for all Jewish couples, including those in which only one partner is Jewish. Increasing availability of prenatal diagnostic techniques also makes advisable routine heterozygote screening for β-thalassemia in Mediterranean and Chinese people, sickle cell anemia in blacks, and α-thalassemia in Southeast Asians, Chinese, and Filipinos (ACOG, 2000). Cystic fibrosis screening is recommended for Caucasians and Ashkenazi Jews and is discussed in detail later in this chapter. In addition to Tay-Sachs disease, Canavan disease, and cystic fibrosis, some centers offer Ashkenazi Jews screening for even more disorders. This reasoning is based on efficiency screening in that ethnic group given that only a limited number of mutations are responsible for most in a given disorder. Overall, one in seven Ashkenazi Jews is heterozygozous for one of six disorders (Tay-Sachs disease, Gaucher disease, cystic fibrosis, Canavan disease, Niemann-Pick disease, dysautonomia).

Principles and Prerequisites of Genetic Screening

Genetic screening implies monitoring a population to identify clinically normal individuals who have genotypes that are associated with a detectable disease or that may lead to that disease in their offspring. Several aspects of genetic screening deserve emphasis, in particular the contrast between screening programs and case detection programs.

One principle is that genetic screening should be voluntary unless specifically mandated by law (National Academy of Science, 1975). Legal requirements usually dictate neonatal screening for phenylketonuria (PKU), hypothyroidism and other disorders in some states. Of course, voluntary screening does not mean that a physician must remain neutral or even fail to express his or her opinion. A given test should not be performed without a patient's knowledge, however, as the patient may not wish to be faced with the dilemma of deciding among options raised by the results of the screening process.

Second, in genetic screening one does not expect to detect all affected cases in a given population. This contrasts with case detection programs, an example of which is cervical cytologic screening. Yearly Papanicolaou smears are recommended to guard against laboratory errors and failed endocervical samplings. If such pitfalls did not exist, a normal smear would categorically exclude squamous cervical cancer for approximately 5 years, the interval required for a normal cervix to progress through dysplasia to carcinoma. In contrast, in neonatal screening for PKU, failure to detect 16% of affected infants is accepted if screening is performed on the first day of life, 3% if performed on the second day, and 0.3% if performed on the third day (Andrews, 1986).

Third, establishing technical feasibility for screening a given disorder alone does not justify screening. Indeed, many genetic disorders are amenable to screening. For example, all chromosomal abnormalities could be detected during the neonatal period, and almost all disorders of amino acid metabolism are amenable to screening. Conversely, screening is actually recommended only for those disorders that fulfill prerequisites essential for initiating screening programs. Five prerequisites must be fulfilled (Table 4–1).

CAPACITY TO ALTER CLINICAL MANAGEMENT

Although screening to achieve research objectives (e.g., determining the incidence of a disorder) is sometimes appropriate, widespread testing is ordinarily performed only if an abnormal finding could alter clinical management. Thus, neonates are screened for those metabolic disorders amenable to treatment (e.g., PKU and hypothyroidism) but not for untreatable disorders (e.g., Lesch-Nyhan syndrome). Neonatal screening for

▼ **Table 4–1. PREREQUISITES OF GENETIC**
• **SCREENING**

Capacity to alter clinical management of affected individuals
Ability to identify matings between two heterozygotes
Cost-effectiveness
Reliable methods of assessment of genetic status (reproducible assay)
Capacity to handle ancillary problems
   Variants not requiring action
   Potential stigmatization of heterozygote

sickle cell anemia was recommended only after it became clear that prophylactic antibiotics might prevent life-threatening infections. Relatively common disorders that are not treatable and, therefore, for which *neonates* should not be screened include chromosomal abnormalities, Tay-Sachs disease, and Duchenne muscular dystrophy.

If neonatal screening is undesirable for a given disorder, it may still be reasonable to screen adults to determine whether they are at increased risk for offspring with the same disorder. Identification of individuals heterozygous for an autosomal recessive disorder could alter reproductive choices and, thus, clinical management. The object is to identify matings between two individuals heterozygous for the same mutant allele and offer prenatal genetic counseling and diagnosis. Screening adults to determine heterozygote status is ordinarily applicable only if prenatal diagnosis is possible. The common mendelian disorders thus currently amenable to heterozygote determination include Tay-Sachs disease, Canavan disease, β-thalassemia, α-thalassemia, sickle cell anemia, and now cystic fibrosis. Ideally, screening should be performed before pregnancy; however, if the patient is already pregnant, screening should be completed as early in gestation as possible to allow maximum family planning options.

COST-EFFECTIVENESS

The ability to identify a heterozygote or even to detect an affected neonate with a treatable disorder does not necessarily dictate that screening be undertaken. The cost of screening justifies the monetary and emotional savings of detecting the rare affected case for only a few disorders. Indeed, technology now exists to screen for scores of mendelian disorders. Yet only a few disorders unequivocally fulfill the criteria of cost-effectiveness for screening: hypothyroidism, PKU, and arguably sickle cell anemia, galactosemia, maple syrup urine disease, adenosine deaminase deficiency, and adrenal 21-hydroxylase deficiency. Testing for other detectable disorders (e.g., rare metabolic traits) is not pursued. With the advent of mass spectrometry, a case can be made for screening additional disorders beyond the disorders listed, but only PKU and hypothyroidism are mandated in every state.

RELIABLE METHOD OF ASSESSMENT

The requisite assay must have a high predictive value. Although it is a general axiom of laboratory medicine, this statement is especially applicable to genetic diseases. Because genetic disorders are individually rare, even low false-negative rates could result in a greater likelihood that a given abnormal value represents a false-positive rather than a true positive value.

CAPACITY TO HANDLE UNANTICIPATED PROBLEMS

Fulfilling all the above prerequisites still does not mean that screening for a particular disorder should be initiated. A final requirement is the ability to handle difficulties that inevitably arise in screening programs. Sometimes inability to handle these problems obviates introduction of a screening program that would otherwise be desirable. Yet it should be anticipated that unexpected problems will arise. After screening programs for PKU were initiated, it became clear that elevated neonatal phenylalanine often was not the result of PKU but rather the result of other conditions that required no dietary treatment. Ability to separate "false-positive" from "true positive" testing for PKU proved crucial.

When screening normal populations to detect heterozygotes (sickle cell disease, Tay-Sachs disease, Canavan disease, α-thalassemia, β-thalassemia, cystic fibrosis), it must be ensured that individuals identified as heterozygotes do not become stigmatized or do not develop an erroneous impression that their own health is threatened.

Who Should Provide Genetic Counseling?

Genetic counseling cannot and should not be exclusively provided by a single specialist but is an interdisciplinary activity. There is also a growing recognition of the need to ensure that those providing genetic counseling are competent. Increasingly, genetic services are being provided by primary care physicians who are not necessarily trained in human genetics. In the clearest situations, the primary care physician may also be the most appropriate person to provide the counseling because he or she knows the family, their personal attitudes, and their socioeconomic background better than a consultant. However, in more complex situations, the primary care physician may lack the specific knowledge, time commitment, availability of necessary diagnostic tests, or skills required for genetic counseling.

Although there are no state or federal licensing bodies for genetic counselors, certification is provided by the American Board of Medical Genetics, Inc. To be eligible for certification, an individual must meet the criteria in the area of desired certification and pass a written examination. Areas in which certification is offered include clinical geneticists (M.D., D.D.S., D.M.D., or D.O.), clinical laboratory geneticists (M.D., Ph.D., D.D.S., D.M.D., or D.O.) and Ph.D. medical geneticists. Approximately 50 of the M.D. medical geneticists are also certified by the American Board of Obstetrics and Gynecology, Inc. The National Board of Genetic Counselors certifies individuals who hold postbaccalaureate degrees, most commonly a Masters of Science.

All who hold themselves out to the public as engaging in genetic counseling services must possess sufficient knowledge, training, and skill to provide these services in a reasonable manner. Practitioners must respect the limits of their individual competence and avoid acting beyond the scope of their abilities. The use of a genetics team approach has been endorsed as consistent with the notions of competence and appropriately shared responsibilities.

Principles of Genetic Counseling

Genetic counseling is the process whereby an individual or family is provided with information about a real or possible genetic problem. In educating and counseling about genetics, the counselor must provide information in an understandable way about the nature of genetic risks and our ability to predict such risks. This will depend on how a disease or condition is inherited, its severity, and other important factors, such as the interactions of environment and genetic background that must be present before a genetic susceptibility is expressed.

Genetic counseling is a dynamic communicative process that begins with trying to establish a diagnosis. This involves taking a medical and family history, performing clinical examinations, and obtaining relevant laboratory tests. The prediction of genetic risks based on laboratory tests depends on the sensitivity and specificity of the tests themselves and the quality of the laboratory performing the tests. The counselor must then provide information regarding risks of recurrence, genetic and medical implications of the disorder, prevention, family planning, and medically managing the condition. Because genetic counseling is directly concerned with human behavior, it must be based on an understanding of the psychological meanings of health and

illness, procreation, and parenthood. Genetic information can bring bad news, and the counselor must be a resource for individuals and families dealing with sadness, loss, anger, guilt, or anxiety. The counselor has a responsibility to help individuals and families adjust psychologically and socially to their genetic condition.

CONFIRMING THE DIAGNOSIS

Good genetic advice requires certainty of diagnosis; even the best counseling cannot compensate for an inaccurate diagnosis. In addition to taking a detailed family history, the proband (i.e., the family member through whom the family was identified) should be carefully examined, as should other family members at risk. If the proband is no longer living, the appropriate medical records should be sought and reviewed. The possibility of nonpaternity must also be considered.

Laboratory studies needed to establish the diagnosis often include chromosome analysis, DNA studies, or biochemical tests of blood, urine, or cultured cells. Improved techniques now permit DNA analysis of archival specimens (e.g., paraffin-embedded tissue blocks) in some cases. Nongenetic factors can mimic genetic factors in the production of disease (so-called phenocopies); a good history and various clinical and laboratory studies may help resolve questionable cases.

Despite the most intensive efforts, sometimes a precise diagnosis cannot be established. For some families, the answer "we do not know" leads to understandable frustration and dissatisfaction with the counseling experience. On the other hand, some families receive a measure of satisfaction and relief from the knowledge that all reasonable steps have been taken to answer their questions.

ESTIMATING AND INTERPRETING RISKS

The counselor must establish precisely what information the individual, couple, or family wants to know about their genetic situation. People often have less interest in the label of a disorder and its mechanism of action than in how tests may predict a disorder, what effect the disorder has on physical and mental functioning, and how intrusive, difficult, or effective an existing treatment or alternatives might be. Individuals generally remember the levels of risk they were told about counseling, not always in numerical form but whether it was high or low. However, how different people *perceive* their genetic risks varies widely from overly cautious to reckless. The counselor should strive to help the family understand the consequences of the genetic problem. Factual information must be conveyed concerning the problem's significance and natural history. Such explanations should be developed in small, discrete steps, with frequent pauses so that the patient or couple can ask questions. This may require several counseling sessions.

Perception of risk is highly dependent on individuals' subjective experiences and expectations and is related to the manner in which they receive the information and their experiential, emotional, religious, and situational concerns. For example, a cleft lip may be perceived as a major tragedy by some parents. On the other hand, some couples may readily accept a child with Down syndrome.

The manner in which risk numbers are presented has been an important influence on how they are interpreted. For example, telling a 35-year-old woman that her risk of having a child with Down syndrome is one in 385 might be interpreted differently than saying that she has a fourfold higher risk than a woman aged 20. Regardless of the actual risk, counselees often perceive risks as being "all or nothing," i.e., it will either happen or not happen. Although most counselors claim to use a nondirective approach (discussed further on), few deny that an element of counselor bias is always present. Risk figures might usefully be presented in several alternative ways; however, beyond near comprehension of numerical risks, genetic counseling must assist individuals in determining their own acceptable risks. Having said this, the counselor must always bear in mind that for the individual, couple, or family for whom the feared event actually occurs, the risk is now 100%—the gamble was lost.

All of this, of course, implies that the more accurate information the couple has, the more likely they are to make a final decision that is consistent with their own values. As a policy matter, this conclusion underlies the doctrine of informed consent in genetic counseling and its purpose: the promotion of self-determination and rational decision-making in situations that critically affect one's own life.

COMMUNICATION

At the heart of genetic counseling lies the necessity to educate patients about the genetic facts and issues relevant to their circumstances. One would assume that the higher an individual's educational level, the better he or she should be able to understand complicated and unfamiliar biologic and medical concepts. For common genetic counseling situations (e.g., advanced maternal age), prepared literature packets can be provided prior to the counseling session so that the patient can become familiar with the information to be discussed during the counseling session. Such printed materials not only initiate the education process but also serve as a resource to which the patient may wish to refer at a later time. They also have the advantage of emphasizing that a patient's problem is not unique and may standardize the informational content so that the counseling process is consistent.

NONDIRECTIVE APPROACH TO COUNSELING

In 1942 Carl Rogers, a clinical psychologist, coined the term "nondirectiveness" to describe his psychotherapeutic approach of not advising, interpreting, or guiding his clients. In 1969, the World Health Organization Expert Committee on Genetic Counseling endorsed the nondirective approach to genetic counseling, an attitudinal strategy that has become universally accepted by virtually all professionals providing genetic counseling services. The counselor makes clear from the onset that the process is educational and that no decisions will be made for the counselees. The counselor tries to remain impartial and objective in providing information that will allow the counselees to make their own rational decisions commensurate with their private concerns and desires. A variation on this theme is that some counselors will not comment on the decisions families suggest, whereas others will support any decisions families make. This is in contrast to the usual directive approach physicians take in dealing with patients who have medical problems. For example, a physician who detects a breast lump in a patient will usually give a strong recommendation as to what steps should or should not be taken next.

Completely nondirective counseling is probably unrealistic. The tendency for counselors to interject their own biases by either verbal or nonverbal messages always exists. Indeed, to provide counseling implies that it is necessary. Despite conscious efforts to provide nondirective counseling, counselors may unwittingly give directive signals. For example, a simple gesture (nonverbal body language), such as shifting in one's chair or raising one's eyebrows, may be interpreted as approval or disapproval of a decision. Repetition of certain points or their presentation in a louder voice may influence the way an individual weighs the information. Silence at certain crucial moments in a discussion may give the loudest message of all. These biases may reflect the attitudes of the genetic counselor about the nature and meaning of health and disease, the seriousness of the genetic condition in question, the perception of quality of life, and the appropriateness of decisions related to genetic counseling and testing, acceptance or rejection of advice, and other important issues.

Perhaps the most surreptitious directive signals occur in the managed care environment. For example, the availability of a test may be viewed as an endorsement of it and its unavailability as a condemnation of the test. The reality is that inclusion or exclusion of certain genetic services by a managed care organization may be more based on cost-efficiency determinations than on risk-benefit concerns and patient autonomy. Similar issues arise when one weighs decisions that follow genetic counseling with respect to reducing the societal burdens of genetic disease when they compete with the particular harm to an individual. This segues into societal stigmatization. For example, as prenatal diagnosis for advanced maternal age becomes more popular, there may now be less tolerance for an older woman's having a child with Down syndrome. This reduced tolerance may not only be directed toward the mother but also toward the affected child.

Psychological Considerations in Counseling Couples With A Previous Abnormal Pregnancy Outcome

Counseling couples who already have had an abnormal child requires additional appreciation for the psychological adaptations that such couples have undergone. Great sensitivity and considerable investment of time are necessary. Such couples are thus best managed by a geneticist who can efficiently set aside the necessary time. The role of most obstetricians/gynecologists is to recognize the problem and reinforce salient genetic data. Again, even if the diagnosis seems obvious, confirmation is obligatory. The clinician should not merely accept a patient's word or even accept a diagnosis made by a physician who is not highly knowledgeable

about the condition. If possible, the anomalous individual should be examined. If the affected relative is still alive, cells may need to be frozen in the event that diagnosis based on DNA studies is or will be feasible. Examining first-degree relatives also may be helpful if an autosomal dominant disorder such as neurofibromatosis needs to be excluded. Alternatively, one may need to rely on medical records or laboratory tests.

Psychological defenses are always operative in the couple receiving genetic counseling. Such defenses can impede the entire counseling process. Anxiety is often low in couples requesting genetic counseling because of parental age or because of an abnormality in a distant relative. As long as anxiety remains low, emotions are easily controlled and comprehension of information is not impaired. However, couples who have experienced a stillborn infant, an anomalous offspring, or multiple repetitive abortions are understandably more anxious. Their ability to retain information may be impaired.

STAGES OF PSYCHOLOGICAL RESPONSE

The psychological impact of a genetic diagnosis varies with its severity, treatability, and the unique responses of different individuals and families. Indeed, psychological defenses underlie all genetic counseling. If not appreciated, these defenses can impede communication and interfere with the entire counseling process.

The impact of diagnosing a genetic problem may be potentially devastating to an individual or family. Consider the delivery of an infant with multiple birth defects and predicted severe mental retardation or the discovery of a mutated gene that indicates a very high likelihood of cancer developing in an individual and other family members who inherit that gene. The physician or counselor needs to recognize that individuals receiving such bad news can be expected to manifest clearly identifiable sequential coping responses in dealing with such situations. Several distinct stages can be recognized in this process (Table 4–2).

▼ **Table 4–2.** PSYCHOLOGICAL (COPING)
· RESPONSES FOLLOWING BIRTH OF AN ABNORMAL CHILD

Denial
Anger
Depression
Bargaining (rationalization)

The first stage is shock and disbelief. *Denial* is a psychological mechanism whereby a person attempts to maintain the integrity of his or her personality simply by denying the stressful situation. This may take the form of the individual's insisting that a mistake has been made. Sometimes he or she appears not to comprehend the situation at all. The counselor must be alert to this coping response, because frequently such individuals appear to be composed on the surface and "very mature in handling the situation." If prolonged, such a response can be self-defeating and interfere with an understanding and acceptance of a genetic problem. It is also important for the counselor to recognize that during this period of time the counselee is usually not able to properly assimilate important information that is being given and must be acted upon.

In the second stage, *anger*, the individual begins to comprehend the reality of the situation and attempts to deal with it on an intellectual level. Anxiety may be manifested by nervousness, irritability, hyperactivity, fatigue, insomnia, loss of appetite, or other physical complaints such as headaches or indigestion. Sometimes this may precipitate a panic attack. Although the stressful event has been recognized at the intellectual level, the individual has not achieved a psychological equilibrium at the emotional level. The individual may become frustrated and angry. Fault may be assigned to others (e.g., spouse, affected child, physician, genetic counselor) without a rational basis. Alternatively, the anger may be self-directed and manifested by guilt.

The third stage of the coping reaction is *depression*. The symptoms of depression are feelings of worthlessness, uselessness, despair, and helplessness. Physical symptoms include loss of appetite, weight loss, fatigue, constipation, headaches, crying spells, and poor sleep patterns. Often individuals experience early morning awakening, a time when depressive symptoms are usually heightened. The counselor must be particularly aware of severe depression that may be associated with a high risk of suicide. In such cases, psychiatric referral and care are mandatory.

The fourth stage—*bargaining* or *rationalization*—occurs when an individual begins to abandon old modes of behavior and thought and reaches a new psychological homeostasis. The person actively tries adaptive changes. This is a critical time in the genetic counseling process because the individual is most receptive to new ideas. During this stage the role of the counselor should chiefly be supportive and the counselee should be encouraged to evaluate self-generated alternative courses of action with regard to decision-making and outcome.

Confidentiality

Genetic information may have an impact on health-care decisions for individuals and families and also result in social and legal problems, including stigmatization, discrimination in the workplace, and loss of or inability to obtain employment and health insurance. For these reasons, those entrusted with obtaining genetic information have a great responsibility to maintain it in strict confidence.

One such problem is whether a physician or counselor has an obligation to contact relatives potentially affected by a genetic finding. An analogy can be made to the legal obligation of informing sexual contacts when a venereal disease such as syphilis is diagnosed. Does the same hold true for genetic conditions? Suppose a mother learns through having an affected son that she is a carrier for Duchenne muscular dystrophy. Should the physician or counselor inform the mother's sisters, who are also at an increased risk of having affected sons? The mother should naturally be urged to notify her sisters herself, but if she refuses, what should be done? Unfortunately, there is not entirely satisfactory answer to this dilemma. Perhaps the most analogous situation is a case adjudicated in California involving a psychiatrist who failed to warn a woman that his patient, a disturbed graduate student from India who wanted to marry her, had threatened to kill her. When the woman was subsequently murdered, her parents sued the psychiatrist for failure to warn her (or them) of the danger. The court gave the following opinion: "Where a doctor ... in the exercise of his professional skill and knowledge, determines, or should determine, that a warning is essential to avert danger arising from the medical or psychological condition of his patient, he incurs a legal obligation to give that warning." The basis for this decision was the court's view that we live in an "interdependent" and "risk-infested" society, and that society cannot tolerate additional risks that physicians could eliminate by a simple act of communication. It is questionable whether this decision could be used to find a duty on the part of a physician or genetic counselor to warn other family members that their *offspring* might be in danger because of a genetic condition a family member *might* be carrying. However, in view of the public policy enunciated by the courts, a strong argument can be made that such a disclosure would be *legally* permissible even though not required.

It has been our opinion that a policy of strict nondisclosure without patient consent should be adhered to in the genetic counseling setting. Such a policy fosters patient self-determination and confidence in the integrity of the counseling process. On the other hand, we recognize the serious implications of many genetic disorders and understand the reasoning whereby one might want to breach confidentiality in certain instances. In any event, given the uncertainty in the law and the fact that this situation can be easily anticipated, we believe that individuals providing genetic counseling should have a clear written policy defining the circumstances, if any, under which they will disclose information or test results learned in the counseling program. Such a program should be spelled out *before* the counseling and genetic diagnosis process begins, so that the individual, couple, or family can opt out immediately if the policy is not acceptable.

Cystic Fibrosis: A Model for Genetic Screening

In this section we first discuss clinical implications of cystic fibrosis (CF) in adult women, followed by problems of molecular heterogeneity that had to be overcome to allow genetic screening for CF to become the standard. CF is a multisystem disease inherited in autosomal recessive fashion. In the white population approximately 1 in 2500 to 1 in 3300 individuals in North America and northern Europe are affected (Wright et al., 1996; ACOG, 2001). From the Hardy-Weinberg formula (see Chapter 2) it can be calculated that the frequency of heterozygous carriers is about 1 in 29 individuals in Caucasians (Northern European origin) and Ashkenazi Jews. The heterozygote is lower in Hispanic, Asians, and African-Americans.

CLINICAL CONSIDERATIONS

CF is a disease of the exocrine glands that results in viscid secretions; it most commonly and most severely affects the respiratory and gastrointestinal systems. In 1989, the CF gene was mapped to chromosome 7. Its gene product, a transport protein called cystic fibrosis transmembrane conductance regulator (CFTR), functions as a chloride channel activated by cAMP (adenosine monophosphate)-dependent protein kinase A phosphorylation. Over 1000 different mutations have been discovered that result in an abnormal

CFTR, the most common being ΔF508, which is a deletion of three base pairs that code for phenylalanine. The only other mutation present in high frequency in any ethnic group is W1282X, the most common mutant allele in Ashkenazi Jews.

The pathogenesis in CF involves a blocked or closed chloride channel in the epithelial cell membrane. As result, chloride ions are trapped inside the cell. This draws sodium ions and water into the cell, resulting in dehydration of mucus secretions. In the lungs, this can lead to airway obstruction and predisposition to infection, dyspnea, bronchiectasis, and pulmonary fibrosis. The major cause of morbidity and mortality in these individuals is progressive, chronic bronchopulmonary disease (Fig. 4-2). In the pancreas, the dehydrated secretions are also insufficiently alkalinized, causing not only duct obstruction but also a reduction in digestive enzymes and fibrosis. The fibrosis can involve the endocrine cells and may lead to pancreatic insufficiency and, hence, diabetes mellitus (Castellani et al., 1999). In the intestinal tract, the lack of digestive enzymes leads to malabsorption of fats and protein, and the altered mucus can lead to bowel obstruction. Infants born with meconium ileus as result of having CF have a significantly higher risk of subsequent malnutrition than unaffected infants (Lai et al., 2000). Sweat electrolytes are also abnormal in CF, with elevated concentrations of sodium and chloride. This, in turn, can lead to heat intolerance, hyponatremia, and a hypochloremic metabolic alkalosis (Gan et al., 1995; Boucher, 1998).

The clinical presentation and course of individuals affected with CF are highly variable. The median age at diagnosis is 6 to 8 months. Some individuals have severe pulmonary and/or gastrointestinal disease, whereas others have milder expression with presentation in adolescence and young adulthood. There is a close correlation of genotype with phenotype in relation to pancreatic function; however, identification of the specific CFTR mutation has not proved highly predictive of the severity of pulmonary disease. Modifier genes and environmental factors undoubtedly play roles in this varied expressivity.

With advances in medical treatment, the prognosis for individuals affected with CF has improved. In the United States, median survival has reached 31.1 years for men and 28.3 years for women. Data from the Cystic Fibrosis Foundation indicate that about a third of affected individuals are 18 years or older, and survival into the fourth or fifth decades is not uncommon (Cystic Fibrosis Foundation, 2000). Although neonatal screening for CF is being per-

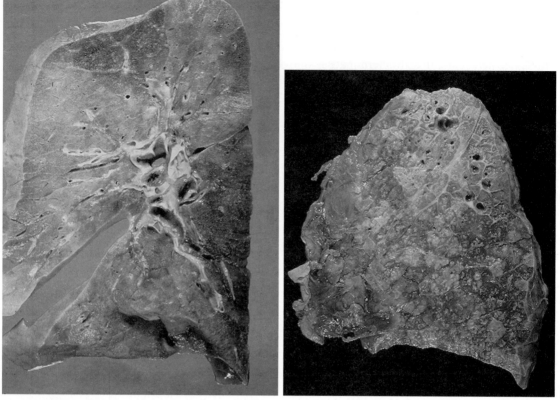

A   B

FIGURE 4–2 • *(A)* Normal lung tissue. *(B)* Lung tissue from a cystic fibrosis patient, showing extensive destruction as a result of obstruction and infection. (From Jorde LB, Carey JC, Bamshad MJ, et al.: Medical Genetics, 2nd ed. St. Louis, Mosby, 2000.)

formed in many locations, there is no evidence that early diagnosis is associated with improved survival (Rosenstein and Zeitlin, 1998).

Women with CF have compromised fertility. They show delayed onset of menarche; those with malnutrition and advanced lung disease often have anovulatory cycles with secondary amenorrhea. Dehydrated and thickened cervical secretions also may pose a physical barrier to sperm penetration of the cervical os. Nonetheless, as more women with CF enter reproductive age, they should be appropriately counseled about contraception, pregnancy, and the potential increased risks associated with CF (Hilman et al., 1996). Pregnancy rates among CF women have increased. During pregnancy these women are at risk for respiratory and cardiac compromise because their underlying lung disease has the potential to be further exacerbated by gestationally related hypoxemia and pulmonary hypertension. The changes in ventilatory drive, cardiac function, blood volume, and increased nutritional requirements all pose potential problems for the woman with CF (Frangolias et al., 1997).

Kent and Farquharson (1993) performed a literature review of CF and pregnancy from 1960 to 1991. They found 217 pregnancies reported in 162 women. Of these, 177 (81.6%) progressed beyond 20 weeks and 10 (4.6%) ended in spontaneous abortions. Forty-three (24.3%) of the deliveries were preterm, and 14 (7.9%) perinatal deaths occurred. Five of 43 preterm deliveries were secondary maternal complications associated with CF, and the remaining 88.4% were spontaneous preterm deliveries. This high preterm delivery rate was believed to be due to chronic hypoxia in the fetus, particularly in women who had poor pulmonary function. Another explanation could be related to inadequate maternal nutrition and/or pancreatic insufficiency, which would lead to malnutrition. The perinatal death rate was higher among infants of women with CF. Twelve of the 14 perinatal deaths were predominantly the result of prematurity. There were no congenital anomalies; only one infant had CF. There were 14 (7.9%) maternal deaths within 6 months after delivery and 24 (13.6) maternal deaths within 2 years after delivery. The maternal death rate did not exceed that among age-matched nonpregnant women with CF, and deaths occurred predominantly as a result of pulmonary complications. Maternal pulmonary status was found to be directly related to maternal death.

Most women with CF can complete a successful pregnancy. Kent and Farquharson (1993) recommend careful monitoring of lung function and ensuring adequate energy intake. Affected women should be counseled about the symptoms and signs of preterm labor, and routine cervical examinations should be considered. The authors suggest that women with a pregnancy forced vital capacity of 50% or less of the expected value or with evidence of cor pulmonale be discouraged from becoming pregnant, as they may be at greatest risk for complications. However, it was felt that these conditions should not necessarily be indications for pregnancy termination if the patient's lung function has been stable for some time.

Frangolias and coworkers (1997) reported a case-control study of seven pregnant women with CF who were compared with nonpregnant CF controls. They were matched using a 1-year preconception date in relation to age, height, weight, percentage of FEV_1, and pancreatic sufficiency status. All patients had pancreatic insufficiency and were dependent on enzyme supplementation. The patients were followed for 2 years postpartum. All patients survived pregnancy, although one died 6 months postpartum. A small, gradual, but significant decline in pulmonary function occurred in both groups over time. Pregnant women with CF demonstrated a lower rate of decline in FEV_1 (3.6%) versus controls (6.8%). There was no significant difference in the number of pulmonary exacerbations between the two groups. Most of the women gained approximately 5.2 kg through the pregnancy, but there was a 4–6 kg decline from preconception weight at 2 years postpartum. The authors concluded that pregnancy is a reasonable option for women with mild CF. Women who seem to be at higher risk for poor pregnancy outcome include those with poor nutritional status, insulin-dependent diabetes mellitus, colonization or infection with *Pseudomonas aeruginosa* and *P. cepacia*, and poor pulmonary status.

SCREENING FOR CYSTIC FIBROSIS

As mentioned above, over 1000 mutations have been identified in the *CFTR* gene. The ΔF508 mutation is represented in almost all populations, although its relative frequency varies among different geographic locations. The highest frequency for ΔF508 is observed in white populations, especially those of Northern European origin, where it accounts for 70 to 75% of the CF alleles. ΔF508 is present in 48% of CF alleles in African-Americans, 46% in Hispanics, 30% in Asian-Americans, and 30% in Ashkenazi Jews. About 15 to 20 other mutations account for 2 to 15% of the other CF alleles, depending on the ethnic group studied. Most remaining mutations are rare. A panel of 25 mutations will detect 87% in Caucasians and differing frequencies in other ethnic groups. In several populations the combination of ΔF508 with other ethnic-specific mutations allows for a 90 to 95% detection rate: Ashkenazi Jews, Celtic Britons, French Canadians from Quebec, and some Native Americans (Genetic Testing for Cystic Fibrosis, 1997). In Ashkenazi Jews ΔF508 and W1282X alone account for 85% of CF alleles.

An important implication of the various mutation detection rates among different populations is the number of couples in whom both partners can actually be identified as CF carriers, thereby enabling unequivocal prenatal diagnosis. For example, if the mutation detection rate is 75% and one partner is determined to be a carrier and the other is not, the risk of having an affected offspring is 1 in 400. By contrast, if the mutation detection rate is 90% and one partner is determined to be a carrier and the other is not, the risk for an affected offspring is 1 in 1000. If both partners are screen negative, the risk is 1 in 240,000 (Lemna et al., 1990).

If amniotic fluid analysis were possible for the CF gene product (protein), the inability to detect all mutations would not matter so much in situations in which one parent carries an identified CF mutation and the other is screen negative but still has a residual risk of carrying an unidentified CF mutation. Unfortunately, no such assay exists, meaning prenatal diagnosis is not possible except to exclude the fetus who inherited the mutation from the known heterozygous parent. Measuring microvillus intestinal enzymes in amniotic fluid is specifically not helpful, for a low value is more likely to connote a false-positive than a true-positive value.

Another issue with carrier screening is genotype-phenotype correlations. Predictions of the severity and course of pulmonary disease are variable for specific mutations, especially for fetuses detected to be compound heterozygotes; however, prediction for pancreatic function is substantial (Genetic Testing for Cystic Fibrosis, 1997). The issue of phenotype being different from CF with pancreatic and pulmonary insufficiency becomes most relevant when confronted with a male having two CF alleles resulting in congenital bilateral absence of the vas deferens (CBAVD).

Males with classic CF are virtually always sterile because of CBAVD. This disorder is discussed in Chapter 12. There is an increased frequency of CF mutations in otherwise healthy men with CBAVD. About 25% of these men with CBAVD are compound heterozygotes for two mutant alleles (one being a "mild" mutation); half have one identifiable mutation and the remainder have no identifiable mutation (Mercier et al., 1995). Eighty-four percent with no identifiable mutation carry this splice site variant for a CF mutation called the 5T allele and 25% with no identifiable mutation carry this splice site variant. The 5T refers to the number of thymines present at the end of intron 8, which alters the likelihood of proper splicing of exon 9. The 7T allele is associated with more normal splicing. The 5T allele is present in men with CBAVD at a fourfold higher frequency than in the general population (Kiesewetter et al., 1993; Chillon et al., 1995; Costes et al., 1995).

In March 1991 an NIH Workshop on Population Screening for the Cystic Fibrosis Gene concluded that CF screening should be offered to all individuals and couples with a family history of CF (e.g., a parent, sibling, uncle, aunt, niece, nephew, or cousin with CF). However, it was felt that population-based screening should not be recommended for individuals and couples with a negative family history. In April 1997, a second NIH Consensus Development Conference or Genetic Testing for Cystic Fibrosis recommended that CF carrier screening should be offered "... to adults with a positive family history of cystic fibrosis (CF), to partners of people with CF, to couples currently planning a pregnancy, and to couples seeking prenatal care" (Genetic Testing for Cystic Fibrosis, 1997). The addition of offering CF carrier screening to couples currently planning a pregnancy and to couples seeking prenatal care was a major change from previous recommendations by professional organizations. The conference concluded that "it is essential that the offering of CF carrier testing be phased in over a period of time in order to ensure that adequate education and appropriate genetic testing and counseling services are available to all persons being tested." This was followed by a workshop sponsored by NIH held on October 1997 to facilitate the recommendations of the Consensus Conference, which agreed that the next steps should include: (a) the development of

protocols on practice guides for CF screening; (b) the development of educational programs and materials for providers and consumers regarding genetic testing for CF as well as prototype informed consent protocols and documents; (c) the further development of laboratory standards (Mennuti et al., 1999). Implementation of these recommendations was undertaken by a collaborative effort between the American College of Obstetricians and Gynecologists (ACOG), the American College of Medical Genetics (ACMG), and the Ethical, Legal and Social Implications (ELSI) Research Program of the National Institute of Human Genome Research. Three working groups were formed with broad representation from professional organizations, consumer groups, and the public.

RECOMMENDATIONS FOR CYSTIC FIBROSIS SCREENING

Population-based programs offering CF carrier screening in the United States were introduced as the standard of care in the spring of 2001 (American College of Obstetricians and Gynecologists, 2001; Grody et al., 2001). The following guidelines and recommendations have been provided:

1. CF carrier screening should be offered to all couples with a positive family history of CF, all partners of individuals with CF, and all Caucasian couples of European or Ashkenazi Jewish descent planning a pregnancy or seeking prenatal care. Ideally screening is performed prior to conception or during the first or early second trimester. Information about CF screening should also be made available in other ethnic and racial groups. Counseling and screening should be provided and made available to individuals in the lower risk groups upon their request.
2. The clinician should identify couples to whom screening should be offered based on family history and ascertainment of the ethnicity and race of the partners during the initial history. Counseling and standardized written educational material or other formats such as videos, and interactive computer programs or both should be used to inform the woman and, whenever possible, her partner. In the event that her partner does not accompany the woman to a prenatal or preconception visit, written educational material should be provided for her to give to her partner. Women and their health care

▼ **Table 4–3.** RECOMMENDED CORE MUTATION PANEL FOR GENERAL POPULATION CF CARRIER
• SCREENING

Standard mutation panel					
ΔF508	Δ1507	G542X	G551D	W1282X	N1303K
R553X	621+1G→T	R117H	1717–1G→A	A455E	R560T
R1162X	G85E	R334W	R347P	711+1G→T	1898+1G→A
2184delA	1078delT	3849+10kbC→T	2789+5G→A	3659delC	I148T
3120+1G→A					

Reflex tests
  I506V,[a] I507V,[a] F508C[a]
  5T/7T/9T [b]

[a]Benign variants. This test distinguishes between a CF mutation and these benign variants. I506V, I507V, and F508C are performed only as reflex tests for unexpected homozygosity for ΔF508 and/or ΔI507.
[b]5T in *cis* can modify R117H phenotype or alone can contribute to congenital bilateral absence of vas deferens (CBAVD); 5T analysis is performed only as a reflex test for R117H positives.
From Grody WW, Cutting GR, Klinger KW, et al.: Laboratory standards and guidelines for population-based cystic fibrosis carrier screening. Genet Med 3:149, 2001.

providers may elect to use either a simultaneous or sequential carrier screening strategy for CF. Simultaneous testing may be particularly important when there are time constraints for making a decision regarding prenatal diagnosis or on the availability of termination of affected pregnancies.

3. The obstetric care provider should offer CF screening when appropriate and may choose to provide or refer the patient for pretest counseling. Post-test counseling for couples with positive-negative, positive-untested, or positive-positive screening results requires special knowledge of CF with regard to range of severity, prognosis, treatment options, and calculation of genetic risk. Referral to a geneticist or a provider with special expertise with CF testing may be considered in these situations. Referral to a geneticist or individual with special expertise with CF testing should also be considered when there is a family history of CF; when carriers are identified with CF mutations that may be associated with congenital absence of the vas deferens in the male offspring; or when an affected adult or an affected fetus is identified.

To implement these guidelines a minimum panel of 25 mutations to be included in CF screening is recommended (Table 4–3). It is planned that this mutation panel will change with increased experience in CF screening (Palomaki et al., 2002). Provider educational materials, patient pamphlets, and model informed consent forms are made available. Screening for this panel will result in the detection rates shown in Table 4–4. This table also shows the residual likelihood of an individual's still being a heterozygote despite having tested negative for all the alleles in the panel.

▼ **Table 4–4.** USEFUL DATA FOR GENETIC
• COUNSELING IN CYSTIC FIBROSIS CARRIER SCREENING IN DIFFERENT ETHNIC AND RACIAL POPULATIONS IN THE UNITED STATES

Ethnic Group	Carrier Detection rate	Estimated carrier risk	
		Before test	After negative test
Ashkenazi Jewish	97%	1/29	~1 in 930
European Caucasian	80%	1/29	~1 in 140
African American	69%	1/65	~1 in 207
Hispanic American[a]	57%	1/46	~1 in 105
Asian American	[b]	1/90	[b]

[a]This is a pooled set of data and requires additional information to accurately predict risk for specific Hispanic populations.
[b]No data available.
Note: Residual carrier risk after a negative test is modified by the presence of a positive family history of CF (i.e., having a first, second, or third degree relative affected with CF) and/or by admixture of various ethnic groups. For these specific situations, accurate risk assessment requires standard Bayesian analysis and genetic counseling. Data from Grody WW, Cutting GR, Klinger KW et al.: Laboratory standards and guidelines for population-based cystic fibrosis carrier screening. Genet Med 3:149, 2001.

Generic Consent for Genetic Screening

There is widespread ethical, legal, and medical agreement that genetic screening must be preceded by counseling about its purposes and followed by counseling about its results and their implications. The patient's choice is the centerpiece of legitimate screening. Even when a screening test becomes routine, it is not always performed; rather, it is routinely made available to patients who may accept or reject it. Such testing should not be performed without the patient's knowledge and informed consent. Some patients may not wish to be faced with the dilemma of deciding among options raised by the results of the screening process. However, voluntary screening does not mean that a physician or a genetic counselor must remain neutral or even fail to express his or her opinion.

Simply because it is technically possible to screen for a given genetic condition does not justify screening. For example, preconceptual screening of all couples for the remote possibility of being a carrier for a structural chromosome rearrangement that could predispose them to having a chromosomally abnormal offspring has not been advocated because it fails to meet many of the accepted prerequisites for establishing a screening program. These prerequisites include the capacity to alter clinical management, being economically justifiable, the availability of a reliable means of assessment, and the capacity to handle problems.

As mentioned earlier, in the United States, the American College of Obstetricians and Gynecologists and the American Academy of Pediatrics recommend that in relevant, ethnic, and racial populations carrier screening be offered for Tay-Sachs disease, sickle cell anemia, the thalassemias and cystic fibrosis (Table 4–5). As our ability to identify genes associated with

particular diseases increases, an additional screening of tests to identify carriers of numerous genes will surely be offered. It will then become increasingly difficult—if not impossible—to inform those offered screening or testing for reproductive purposes about all the genetic information that can be obtained and the implications of that information.

As we have said, our current model for screening and testing requires preset counseling, which serves as a method of obtaining informed consent. This obligation to counsel can be viewed as inherent to the fiduciary nature of the physician or counselor–patient relationship. In contrast to other medical procedures in which physical risks and treatment alternatives are the chief items of information that must be conveyed to patients, there are few physical risks in genetic screening. However, what must be conveyed in counseling regarding genetic screening is that the test may give new information that may ultimately force unwelcome choices such as whether to marry, abort, or adopt. Again, what is at stake is the right to decide whether or not to have a genetic test, with emphasis on the right to refuse if potential harm (in terms of stigmatization or unacceptable choices) outweighs potential benefits for the individual person or family. Here it should be emphasized that self-determination

▼ Table 4–5. GENETIC SCREENING IN VARIOUS ETHNIC GROUPS

Ethnic Group	Disorder	Screening Test	Definitive Tests
Ashkenazi Jews	Tay-Sachs disease	Decreased serum hexosaminidase-A, possibly molecular analysis	Chorionic villus sampling (CVS) or amniocentesis for enzymatic assays or molecular analysis to detect affected fetus for hexosaminidase-A
	Canavan disease	DNA analysis to detect most common alleles	CVS or amniocentesis for molecular analysis
African-Americans	Sickle cell anemia	Presence of sickle cell hemoglobin, confirmatory hemoglobin electrophoresis	CVS or amniocentesis for genotype determination (direct molecular analysis)
Mediterranean people	β-Thalassemia	Mean corpuscular volume (MCV) < 80%, followed by hemoglobin electrophoresis	CVS or amniocentesis for genotype determination (direct molecular analysis or linkage analysis)
Southeast Asians and Chinese (Vietnamese, Laotian, Cambodian, Filipino)	α-Thalassemia	MCV < 80%, followed by hemoglobin electrophoresis	CVS or amniocentesis for genotype determination (direct molecular studies or linkage analysis)
All ethnic groups	Cystic fibrosis In Caucasians and Ashkenazi Jews, should be offered; in other ethnic groups (Asians, Hispanics, African-Americans), should be made available	DNA analysis of specified panel of 25 CFTR mutations (those present in ≥ 0.1% of the general US population)	CVS or amniocentesis for genotype determination; definitive diagnosis of all fetuses is not possible; sensitivity varies by ethnic group

and rational decision-making are the central values protected by informed consent.

As fruits of the Human Genome Project are realized, tens if not hundreds of new genetic screening tests will become available for introduction into routine medical practice. Physicians and counselors who already worry about keeping up with new technology, providing good medical care, maintaining ethical standards, and avoiding malpractice suits will quickly be overwhelmed. Each new screening test will bring up the same questions: What information should be given to which patients, when should it be presented, who should present it, and how and by whom should the results be conveyed? Clearly we will come to a point where meaningful prescreening counseling about all available carrier tests will be impossible. Providing a surfeit of information ("information overload") can amount to misinformation and make the entire counseling process either misleading or meaningless. To prevent disclosure from being pointless or counterproductive, we believe that strategies based on general or "generic" consent should be developed for genetic screening. Their aim would be to provide sufficient information to permit patients to make informed decisions about carrier screening, yet avoid information overload that could lead to "misinformed" consent. An approach based on generic consent would emphasize broader concepts and common-denominator issues in genetic screening. We envision a situation in which patients would be told of the availability of the panel of screening tests that can be performed on a single blood sample. They should be told that the test could determine whether they carry genes that put them at increased risk of having a child with a birth defect that could involve serious physical abnormalities, mental disabilities, or both. Several common examples could be given to indicate the frequency and spectrum of severity of each type of category of condition for which screening was being offered. For example, screening could include tests for fetal conditions, such as neural tube defects (e.g., spina bifida), chromosome abnormalities (e.g., Down syndrome), and single gene disorders (e.g., CF). Important factors common to all genetic screening tests would be highlighted. Among these are the limitations of screening tests, especially the fact that negative test results cannot guarantee a healthy child; the possible need for additional, invasive tests, such as chorionic villus sampling or amniocentesis, to establish a definitive diagnosis; the reproductive options that might have to be considered, such as prenatal diagnosis, adoption, gamete donation, abortion, or acceptance of risks; the cost of screening; issues of confidentiality, including potential disclosure to other family members; and the possibility of social stigmatization, including discrimination in obtaining health insurance and employment.

This type of generic consent to genetic screening can be compared to obtaining consent to perform a physical examination and "routine" tests. Patients know that the purpose of the examination or test is to locate potential problems that are likely to require additional follow-up and that could present them with choices they would rather not have to make. The patient is not generally told, however, about all the possible abnormalities that can be detected by a routine physical examination or test, but only the general purpose of each. On the other hand, tests that may produce especially sensitive and stigmatizing information, such as screening of blood for the human immunodeficiency virus, should not be performed without specific consent. This would also apply to certain genetic conditions. For example, even in a generic model, tests for untreatable fatal conditions such as Huntington disease or breast cancer susceptibility genes should not be combined with other tests or performed without specific consent.

The concept of generic consent for genetic screening is not a waiver of the individual patient's rights to information. Rather, it reflects a decision that the most reasonable way to obtain informed consent to conduct a panel of genetic screening tests is to first provide basic general information and give much more detailed information on specific conditions only after they have been detected. Since in the vast majority of cases no such conditions will in fact be found, this method is also the most efficient and cost-effective. However, there are some limits to generic consent. It is essential to build into the screening program ample opportunity for patients to obtain all the additional information they need to help them make a decision. Counseling for generic consent for genetic screening could be provided in person by a physician, genetic counselor, or other health professional. Alternatively, audiovisual aids could be used to help ensure consistency in the information provided, be more efficient, and respond to the shortage of genetic counselors (Elias and Annas, 1994).

REFERENCES

American College of Obstetricians and Gynecologists and The American College of Medicine Genetics. Preconception and Prenatal Carrier Screening for Cystic Fibrosis. Washington DC: The American College of Obstetricians and Gynecologists, 2001.
American College of Obstetricians and Gynecologists: Committee Opinion Number 238, Genetic Screening for Hemoglobinopathies. Washington DC: ACOG, 2000.

American College of Obstetricians and Gynecologists: Committee Opinion Number 212, Screening for Canavan Disease. Washington DC: ACOG, 1998.

American College of Obstetricians and Gynecologists: Committee Opinion Number 192, Genetic Screening of Gamete Donors. Washington DC: ACOG, 1997.

American College of Obstetricians and Gynecologists: Committee Opinion Number 162, Screening for Tay-Sachs Disease. Washington DC: ACOG, 1995.

American College of Obstetricians and Gynecologists: Technical Bulletin Number 108, Antenatal Diagnosis of Genetic Disorders. Washington DC: ACOG, 1987.

American College of Obstetricians and Gynecologists: ACOG Committee Opinion Number 189, October 1997, Advanced Paternal age: risks of the fetus. Committee on Genetics. Washington DC: ACOG, 1997.

Andrews LB: State laws and regulations governing newborn screening. Chicago: American Bar Association, 1986.

Boucher RC: Cystic fibrosis. *In* Fauci AS, Braunwald E, Isselbacher KJ, et al. (eds): Principles of Internal Medicine, 14th ed. New York: McGraw-Hill, 1998, p 1452.

Castellani C, Bonizzato A, Rolfini R, et al.: Increased prevalence of mutations of the cystic fibrosis gene in idiopathic chronic and recurrent pancreatitis. Am J Gastroenterol 94:1993, 1999.

Chillon M, Casals T, Mercier B, et al.: Mutations in cystic fibrosis gene in patients with congenital absence of the vas deferens. N Engl J Med 332:1475, 1995.

Costes B, Girodon E, Ghanem N, et al.: Frequent occurrence of CFTR intron 8 (TG)n 5T allele in men with congenital bilateral absence of the vas deferens. Eur J Hum Genet 3:285, 1995.

Cystic Fibrosis Foundation: Patient Registry 1999 Annual Report. Bethesda, MD, September 2000.

Elias S, Annas GJ: Generic consent for gametic screening. N Engl J Med 330:1611, 1994.

Frangolias DD, Nakielna EM, Wilcox PG: Pregnancy and cystic fibrosis: A case-controlled study. Chest 111:963, 1997.

Gan KH, Geus WP, Bakker W, et al.: Genetic and clinical features of patients with cystic fibrosis after age 16 years. Thorax 50:1301, 1995.

Genetic Testing for Cystic Fibrosis: NIH Consensus Statement 15:No 4, April 14–16, 1997.

Gilbert F: Familial dysautonomia and the expansion of the Ashkenazi Jewish carrier screening panel. Genet Testing 5:83, 2001.

Grody WW, Cutting GR, Klinger KW, et al.: Laboratory standards and guidelines for population-based cystic fibrosis carrier screening. Genet Med 3:149, 2001.

Hilman BC, Aitken ML, Constantinescu M: Pregnancy in patients with cystic fibrosis. Clin Obstet Gynecol 39:70, 1996.

Kent NE, Farquharson DF: Cystic fibrosis in pregnancy. Can Med Assoc J 149:809, 1993.

Kiesewetter S, Macek M, Davis C, et al.: A mutation in CFTR produces different phenotypes depending on chromosomal background. Nat Genet 5:274, 1993.

Kingston HM: Genetic assessment and pedigree analysis. *In* Rimoin DL, Connor JM, Pyeritz RE, Korf BR (eds): Principles and Practice of Medical Genetics, 4th ed. Philadelphia: Churchill Livingstone, 2002, p 635.

Lai HC, Kosorok MR, Laxova A, et al.: Nutritional status of patients with cystic fibrosis with meconium ileus: A comparison with patients without meconium ileus and diagnosed through neonatal screening. Pediatrics 105:53, 2000.

Lemna WK, Feldman GL, Kerem B, et al.: Mutation analysis for heterozygote detection and the prenatal diagnosis of cystic fibrosis. N Engl J Med 322:291, 1990.

Mennuti MR, Thomson E, Press N: Screening for cystic fibrosis: Follow-up on Workshop to the NIH Consensus Development Conference. Obstet Gynecol 93:456, 1999.

Mercier B, Verlingue C, Lissens W, et al.: Is congenital bilateral absence of the vas deferens a primary form of cystic fibrosis? Analyses of CFTR in 67 patients. Am J Hum Genet 56:272, 1995.

National Academy of Science: Genetic Screening: Programs, Principles and Research. Washington DC: National Academy of Sciences, 1975.

Palomaki GE, Haddow JE, Bradley LA, et al.: Update assessment of cystic fibrosis mutation frequency in non-Hispanic Caucasians. Genet Med 4:90, 2002.

Rosenstein BJ, Zeitlin PL: Cystic fibrosis. Lancet 351:277, 1998.

Simpson JL, Martin AO, Elias S, et al.: Cancers of the breast and female genital system: Search for recessive genetic factors through analysis of a human isolate. Am J Obstet Gynecol 141:629, 1981.

Walker AP: Genetic counselling. *In* Rimoin DL, Connor JM, Pyeritz RE, Korf BR (eds): Principles and Practice of Medical Genetics, 4th ed. Philadelphia: Churchill Livingstone, 2002, p 842.

World Health Organization Expert Committee. Genetic Counseling. WHO Tech Rep 1:416, 1969.

Wright D, Gold R, Schwartz D: Maternal gastrointestinal disorders. *In* Isada ND, Drugan A, Johnson MP, et al. (eds): Maternal Genetic Disease. Stamford, CT: Appleton and Lange, 1996, p 159.

Clinical Genetics

CHAPTER 5

Genetics of Pregnancy Loss

Pregnancy loss is very common, both preclinically and clinically. Many embryos never implant and are lost even before clinical recognition of pregnancy. Of clinically recognized pregnancies, approximately 10 to 12% are lost (Wilcox et al., 1988). Among married women in the United States, 4% have experienced two recognized pregnancy losses (U.S. Department of Health and Human Services, 1982). At least 1% of women experience three or more losses. By far the most common etiologies of such losses are genetic and cytogenetic. In addition to these topics, this chapter discusses the likelihood of loss resulting from nongenetic causes.

Frequency and Timing of Pregnancy Losses

PRECLINICAL

Embryos implant 6 days after conception but are not generally recognized clinically until 5 to 6 weeks after the last menstrual period. Prior to this time, β-human chorionic gonadotropin (hCG) assays can detect preclinical pregnancies. To determine the frequency of losses prior to clinical recognition, Wilcox and coworkers (1988) performed daily urinary hCG assays beginning around the expected time of implantation (day 20 of gestation). Of pregnancies detected in this fashion, 31% (61/198) were lost; the preclinical loss rate was 22% (43/198). The clinically recognized loss rate in this cohort was 12% (19/155). These rates are consistent with data gathered by us and colleagues (Mills et al., 1988) in a National Institute of Child Health and Human Development (NICHD)

collaborative study using serum β–hCG assays performed 28 to 35 days after the previous menses. That cohort was ascertained approximately 10 days later than the date of ascertainment in the sample of Wilcox and coworkers (1988). The total loss rate (preclinical and clinical) in the NICHD cohort was approximately lower at 16%.

In couples with prior losses, abortion rates seem lowest when conception occurs in days other than the date of ovulation or day prior (optimal interval) (Gray et al., 1995). Moreover, conceptions occurring on days other than the date of ovulation day or the day prior are not associated with increases in liveborn Down syndromes, which might have occurred had the etiology of the lower abortion not been chromosomal abnormalities (Simpson et al., 2002). To assess this question, Wilcox and coworkers (1999) recently reanalyzed their cohort of 221 pregnancies. Of 189 pregnancies for which sufficient data existed, 141 lasted beyond 6 weeks. Assuming implantation to correspond with first appearance of hCG, 84% of implantations leading to a clinical pregnancy did so on day 8, 9, or 10 after ovulation. None occurred beyond day 12. Loss rate was 13% if implantation occurred by day 9, rising to 26%, 52%, and 82% on the next three days, respectively. These data relate to natural ovulatory cycles. Successful implantation has occurred up to 14 days after ovulation in *in vitro* fertilization cycles (Liu et al., 1991).

CLINICAL

Clinically recognized first-trimester fetal loss rates of 10 to 12% are well documented in both retrospective and prospective cohort studies (Simpson and Carson, 1993). The higher clinical loss rates reported in some older studies may have reflected misclassification, unwittingly including surreptitious illicit abortions. The latter were common during the era in which legal termination was proscribed in most of the United States (prior to the Supreme Court decision, Roe v. Wade, 1973).

Timing of pregnancy loss is also clinically important. Until perhaps 20 years ago, clinical pregnancy loss was not often appreciated until 9 to 12 weeks' gestation, at which time bleeding and passage of tissue (products of conception) occurred. Once ultrasonography became widely available, it was shown that fetal demise can actually occur weeks prior to the time overt clinical signs are manifested. This conclusion was first reached on the basis of cohort studies showing that only 3% of viable pregnancies are lost after 8 weeks' gestation (Simpson et al., 1987). Studies involving obstetric registrants were very similar (Christiaens and Stoutenbeek, 1984; Wilson et al., 1984; Gilmore and McNay, 1985; Cashner et al., 1987). Given the accepted clinical loss rate of 10 to 12%, fetal viability must cease weeks before maternal symptoms appear; thus, most fetuses aborting clinically at 9 to 12 weeks have died weeks previously. Almost all losses are retained *in utero* for an interval prior to clinical recognition, meaning that most losses are "missed abortions." This term is probably archaic.

RECURRENCE RISKS

Most pregnancy losses after 8 weeks occur in the next 2 gestational months. This can be deduced from loss rates being only 1% in women confirmed by ultrasound to have viable pregnancies at 16 weeks. Loss rates decline steadily through gestation (Hoesli et al., 2001).

Recurrence risks reflect many factors, but two associations that affect absolute rate loss are especially worth emphasizing at the onset. First, maternal age is positively correlated with risk of pregnancy loss. A 40-year-old woman has twice the risk of a 20-year-old woman. This increase occurs in euploid as well as aneuploid pregnancies (Stein et al., 1980). Second, prior pregnancy history is important. Among nulliparous women who have never experienced a loss, the rate is low—5% (4/87) in primiparous and 4% (3/73) in multiparous (Regan et al., 1989) (Table 5–1). The loss rate increases to 25 to 30% for women with three or more losses (Warburton, 1984;

▼ **Table 5–1.** APPROXIMATE RECURRENCE RISK
• FIGURES USEFUL FOR COUNSELING WOMEN WITH REPEATED SPONTANEOUS ABORTIONS:[*]

	Prior Abortions	Risk (%)
Women with liveborn infants	0	5
	1	20–25
	2	25
	3	30
	4	30
Women without liveborn infants	3	30–40

[*] Recurrence risks are slightly higher for older women; for those who smoke cigarettes or drink alcohol; and for those exposed to high levels of selected chemical toxins.
Based on data from Warburton D and Fraser FC (1964), Poland BJ, et al. (1977), and others.

Regan, 1989). Whitley and colleagues (1999) derived an odds ratio of 3.19 for another loss in women with two prior losses. Parazzini and coworkers (1997) reached similar findings. These risks apply not only to women whose losses were recognized at 9 to 12 weeks' gestation but also to those whose pregnancies were ascertained in the 5th week of gestation (Simpson et al., 1994).

The converse of these recurrence risk factors should be kept in mind, that is, the likelihood of maintaining pregnancy is 70% despite two or three prior losses (Warburton and Fraser, 1964). This high success rate has been confirmed often in cohort trials. Vlaanderen and Treffers (1987) reported successful pregnancies in each of 21 women having unexplained prior repetitive losses but subjected to no intervention. Similar findings were reported by others (Houwert-de Jong et al., 1989; Liddell et al., 1991). Most recently, 325 consecutive United Kingdom women with idiopathic recurrent abortions were followed. Of the 222 (70%) who conceived, 167 (75%) pregnancies persisted beyond 24 weeks. Most losses occurred before 6 to 8 weeks (Brigham et al., 1999). With a history of losses in an NIH collaborative immunotherapy trial, the success rate in 92 untreated women (placebo) was 65% (Ober et al., 1999). Regan and coworkers (2001) found the livebirth rate in couples with a balanced translocation was 50% (20 of 40).

To be judged efficacious in preventing spontaneous abortions, therapeutic regimens must therefore demonstrate success rates demonstrably higher than 70%, corrected for maternal age and other confounding variables. Essentially no therapeutic regimen is capable of making this claim for first-trimester losses, indicating that a proposed therapy should virtually never be promised as efficacious in treating women with two or three first-trimester losses. The situation could differ if 5 or more losses occur, but this is unproved.

Etiology of Preimplantation Losses

MORPHOLOGIC AND CHROMOSOMAL ABNORMALITIES

Establishing an etiology for preimplantation and preclinical losses is not easy, but morphologic and cytogenetic abnormalities are proven explanations in the early embryo. Initial advances were made decades ago by Hertig and coworkers (1956, 1959; Hertig and Rock, 1973), who examined the fallopian tubes, uterine cavities, and endometria of women undergoing elective hysterectomy. Women studied were of proven fertility, with a mean age of 33.6 years. Coital times were recorded prior to hysterectomy. Eight preimplantation embryos (less than 6 days from conception) were recovered. Four of these eight embryos were morphologically abnormal. The four abnormal embryos presumably would not have implanted, or, if implanted, would not have survived long thereafter. Nine of twenty-six implanted embryos (6 to 14 embryonic days) were morphologically abnormal (Fig. 5–1).

The first evidence that morphologically abnormal embryos in humans were likely to result from genetic causes came from elegant mouse studies performed in the 1970s and 1980s by Gropp (1975). Mice heterozygous for a variety of robertsonian translocations were selectively mated to generate monosomies and trisomies for each chromosome. By sacrificing pregnant animals at varying gestational ages, survival and phenotypical characteristics of the abnormal complements could be determined. In mice, as in humans, autosomal monosomy proved inviable. Monosomes aborted around the time of implantation (4 to 5 days after conception) (Fig. 5–2). Trisomies usually survived longer but rarely to term. These findings are analogous to those observed in aneuploid human fetuses.

In humans, a high frequency of chromosomal abnormalities began to be observed as soon as it became possible to perform cytogenetic studies on human preimplantation embryos. These were initially available from clinical *in vitro* fertilization programs (Plachot et al., 1987; Papadopoulos et al., 1989) studying embryos fertilized *in vitro* but neither transferred nor cryopreserved. (Technology for the latter was not initially available.) Of morphologically normal embryos, the consensus is that 25% show abnormal chromosomal number as determined by metaphase. A 25% aneuploidy rate in morphologically normal embryos is consistent with the occurrence of aneuploidy in 6% of sperm from ostensibly normal males (Egozcue et al., 1997) and in perhaps 20% of oocytes (Martin, 1991; Plachot, 1992).

Chromosome abnormalities as assessed by metaphase analysis are observed more frequently in morphologically abnormal than in morphologically normal embryos. Plachot and colleagues (1987) found chromosomal abnormalities in 78% of fragmented embryos compared with in 12.5% of morphologically normal embryos. Pellestor and associates (1994) reported 90% abnormalities in 118 poor quality embryos. Bongso and coworkers (1991) found 31.9% abnormalities in 91 poor quality embryos. Given the above, it has been accepted for over a decade that chromosomal abnormalities are the likely explanation for the morphologically abnormal embryos recovered by Hertig and colleagues (1956, 1959) and Hertig and Rock (1973).

Complete chromosomal (metaphase) analysis of preimplantation embryos provides the same information as obtained in chorionic villus or amniotic fluid cells, as would comparative genome hybridization (CGH). However, obtaining an interpretable metaphase on a single cell is a formidable task. For this reason, studies in the 1990s began to utilize fluorescence in situ hybridization (FISH) with chromosome-specific probes (Fig. 5–3). Probes are now available for all chromosomes, and with innovative hybridization schedules as many as nine or ten probes can be studied on a single cell. One caveat when comparing results of FISH studies with results of earlier studies using metaphase analysis is the differing composition of the sample in vitro fertilization (IVF) embryos available for study. Embryos obtained prior to modern cyropreservation techniques were relatively more normal morphologically. At present, these embryos are frozen, often leaving only nontransferable embryos for study.

From the onset FISH studies on preimplantation embryos showed a predictable positive relationship between aneuploidy and maternal age (Munné et al., 1995). Expectedly, morphologically abnormal embryos proved more likely to be chromosomally abnormal (50 to 75%) than morphologically normal embryos (25 to 50%). Of fragmented embryos, 57% were shown to be chromosomally abnormal by Munné and coworkers (1995). This total was contributed by aneuploidy (23%), mosaicism (22%), and less often polyploidy (13%). More

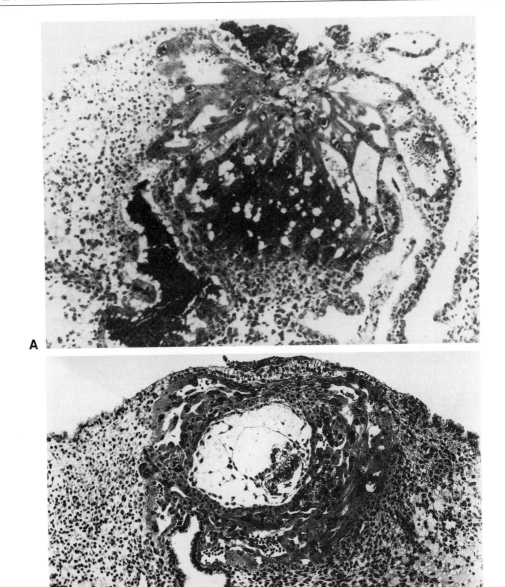

FIGURE 5–1 • Cross-section of endometrium containing an abnormal 14-day-old embryo (*A*) compared with a normal 11-day-old embryo. *B,* In the abnormal embryo no embryonic disk is present, and only syncytiotrophoblasts are identifiable. (*A,* Reprinted from Hertig AT, Rock J: On the development of the early human ovum, with special reference to the trophoblast of the previous stage. Am J Obstet Gynecol 47:149, 1944. *B,* From Hertig AT, Rock J: A series of potentially abortive ova recovered from fertile women prior to the first missed menstrual period. Am J Obstet Gynecol 58:968, 1949.)

than half of slow-growing embryos at the 2- to 4-cell stage or of arrested embryos are aneuploid (Almeida and Bolton, 1996).

Limited correlations can be made between specific morphologic abnormalities and chromo-somal status (Munné and Cohen, 1998). Tripronuclear embryos result from dispermy and are triploid or mosaic triploid (Staessen and Van Steirteghem, 1997). If three pronuclei and a single polar body are present, triploidy is the usual

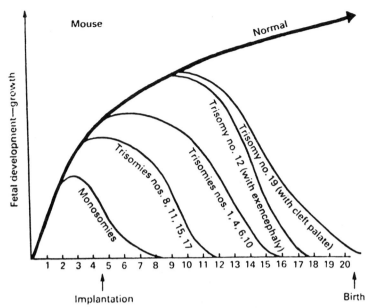

FIGURE 5–2 • Timing for loss of murine autosomal monosomy and murine autosomal trisomy. (From Gropp A: Chromosomal animal model of human disease: Fetal trisomy and development failure. *In* Berry L, Poswillo DE (eds): Teratology. Berlin: Springer-Verlag, 1975.)

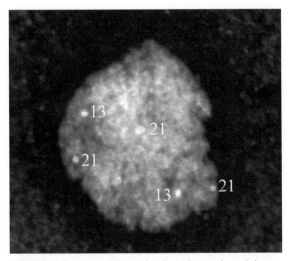

FIGURE 5–3 • Aneuploid preimplantation embryo (trisomy 21) showing signals for three chromosomes. In reality, probes for 13 and 21 are different in color (not evident here). (Prepared by Dr. Farideh Bischoff, Baylor College of Medicine, Houston, Texas.) *See Color Plate*

explanation (Staessen and Van Steirteghem, 1997). Pronuclei of uneven size almost always indicate mosaic triploidy (Sadowy et al., 1998). Multinucleated blastomeres show arrested development (Balakier and Cadesky, 1997) and extensive mosaicism or polyploidy (74%) (Kligman et al., 1996). Embryos with a single dominant cell are usually polyploid, whereas embryos developing from a large oocyte (>220 mm) are triploid (Munné et al., 1994).

Noted already is that the preimplantation embryos available for study are not necessarily reflective of the general population, either because of advanced maternal age or morphologic abnormalities. Of more general applicability, then, are the studies of Delhanty and associates (1997). This group sought aneuploidy by performing FISH for chromosomes X,Y, and 1 in embryos that were not transferred because preimplantation genetic diagnosis (PGD) had shown a mendelian mutation. These women were of relatively younger maternal age than the typical IVF cohort, more closely approximating the general population. Embryos were disaggregated and individual cells subjected to FISH for chromosomes X, Y, and 1. Of 95 disaggregated embryos, 48% proved chromosomally normal (diploid). Nonmosaic aneuploidy was present in 2%; the remaining 50% were mosaic, half showing only a single nonmodal cell (mosaicism) and the other half showing a variety of different chromosomal abnormalities in a single embryo. The former are probably normal, the single abnormal cell to be selected against and not surviving. However, the latter (chaotic embryos) are not likely to survive. Table 5–2 summarizes our impression of the distribution of preimplantation cytogenetic abnormalities.

Other studies on disaggregated embryos have tended to involve abnormal embryos and to come from older women, with predictably different results (Munné and Cohen, 1998). Marquez and

▼ **Table 5–2.** CHROMOSOMAL COMPLEMENTS IN SPONTANEOUS ABORTIONS RECOGNIZED
• CLINICALLY IN THE FIRST TRIMESTER

Complement		Frequency	(%)
Normal			54.1
46,XX or 46,XY			
Triploidy			7.7
69,XXX		2.7	
69,XYX		0.2	
69,XXY		4.0	
Other		0.8	
Tetraploidy			2.6
92,XXXX		1.5	
92,XXYY		0.55	
Not stated		0.55	
Monosomy X			8.6
Structural abnormalities			1.5
Sex chromosomal polysomy			0.2
46,XXX		0.05	
47,XXY		0.15	
Autosomal monosomy (G)			0.1
Autosomal trisomy			22.3
	Chromosome		
	No 1	0	
	No 2	1.11	
	No 3	0.25	
	No 4	0.64	
	No 5	0.04	
	No 6	0.14	
	No 7	0.89	
	No 8	0.79	
	No 9	0.72	
	No 10	0.36	
	No 11	0.04	
	No 12	0.18	
	No 13	1.07	
	No 14	0.82	
	No 15	1.68	
	No 16	7.27	
	No 17	0.18	
	No 18	1.15	
	No 19	0.01	
	No 20	0.61	
	No 21	2.11	
	No 22	2.26	
Double trisomy			0.7
Mosaic trisomy			1.3
Other abnormalities or not specified			0.9
			100.0

Pooled data from several series, as referenced elsewhere by Simpson JL and Bombard AT (1987).

coworkers (2000) studied 713 embryos judged not suitable for transfer in women undergoing IVF. The mean age was 37 years, a decade older than in the Delhanty and coworkers (1997) sample. In these 713 embryos 2998 blastomeres produced interpretacle results with fluorescent in situ hybridization (FISH); in aggregate the result was that 43.3% of embryos were chromosomally abnormal: aneuploidy (12.5%), polyploidy (11.4%), haploidy (3.1%), and mosaicism (33.7%). Abnormalities were lower in cleaving embryos with greater than 6 cells than in non-cleaving embryos or fragmented embryos. In women less than 40 years old, chaotic embryos were the most common abnormality. In cleaving embryos, aneuploidy (13, 16, 18, 21, X, Y) made up 19.3% of embryos; 14.7% additional were chaotic, 4.5% polyploid, and 4% haploid. Among all embryos (cleaving or not) in the 35- to 39-year-old group, 23.3% were aneuploid, 23.3% chaotic, 14.6% polyploid, and 3.6% haploid. Grossman and coworkers (1999) analyzed 27 normally developing, "discarded" embryos. Using probes for X,Y, and 18, 29.6% (8/27) were normal diploid, 3.7% (1/27) aneuploid, 37% (10/27) diploid mosaic, 18.5% (5/27) abnormal mosaic, and 11.1% (3/27) chaotic.

Of clinical relevance is the fact that given trends toward blastocyst transfer in IVF (Meldrum, 1999), mosaicism persists to the blastocyst stage. Thus, waiting until the blastocyst stage (5 to 6 days) for embryo transfer does not ensure selection against chromosomally abnormal embryos. Of 50 blastocysts studied by Sandalinas and associates (2000), 17 (13%) were cytogenetically abnormal when studied with FISH probes for X, Y, 13, 15, 16, 18, 21, and 22: 14 trisomies, 2 monosomy 21, and 1 monosomy X. Coonen and coworkers (2000) studied disaggregated blastocysts and found frequent mosaicism in ostensibly normal embryos. The mean percentage of normal diploid cells (2n = 46) was only 72% ± 17% in 199 blastocytes. A total of 69% of blastocysts were assumed diploid, defined on the basis of containing 70 to 90% diploid cells. The other 31% were considered abnormal because the basis of cells was not diploid. This included 15% mosaic, 11% chaotic, and 5% monosomic.

BIOLOGIC BASIS OF CHROMOSOMAL ABNORMALITIES

Two different phenomena seem to account for the mosaicism seen in preimplantation embryos. First, low-grade mosaicism exists, perhaps reminiscent of that occurring in chorionic villus sampling or amniotic fluid cells. If only one of six to eight cells fail to show the modal count (2n = 46), the finding may not be necessarily deleteriously affect survival. The developing embryo may simply be manifesting inevitable and not unexpected errors of cell division. The aberrant cells could be eliminated without long-term effect. Single cell aneuploidy could even be programmed (apoptosis). Otherwise, virtually every surviving embryo would be deduced statistically to be abnormal chromosomally. If FISH probes were applied for all chromosomes, the high rate of mosaicism noted on the basis of analyzing only a few chromosomes studied to date would surely increase further. If the above reasoning is correct, the significance of a single aneuploid cell may be less biologic than diagnostic, confusion generated in single-cell PGD or FISH analysis. However, not all six to eight cell embryos are mosiac.

The second phenomenon is different. In chaotic mosaicism the outcome is universally lethal. In these preimplantation embryos, almost every cell is cytogenetically abnormal. Unlike the

types of mosaicism encountered in prenatal genetic diagnosis (2n/2n+1 or 2n/2n-1), not just one but many different chromosomes are involved. There may be little consistency or pattern; trisomy for different chromosomes is observed in the same embryo. The chaotic situation may be a manifestion of generalized abnormalities of cell division, perhaps caused by perturbation of cell cycle check points.

In summary, the frequency of chromosomal abnormalities in preimplantation embryos is very high, as shown initially by metaphase analysis and more recently by larger studies using FISH with chromosome-specific probes. Nearly 50% of morphologically normal cleavage stage embryos are chromosomally abnormal, showing either single-cell (30%) mosaicism, chaotic multicell mosaicism (15 to 20%), or nonmosaic aneuploidy (2%). The frequency of aneuploidy is greater than 50% in fragmented, arrested, tripronuclear, multinucleated, and morphologically abnormal embryos.

CYTOGENETIC ABNORMALITIES IN PREIMPLANTATION EMBRYOS AND IVF SUCCESS

The very high frequency of aneuploidy, polyploidy, and mosaicism (particularly chaotic) in preimplantation embryos does not simply offer an explanation for early pregnancy loss. It also suggests clinical application to women undergoing IVF. In Chapter 16 we discuss the attractiveness of routine PGD for women over age 37 or 38 years. The strategy is to transfer only euploid embryos for chromosomes on the rationale that unwittingly transferring aneuploid embryos would decrease reproductive efficiency. Transferring only euploid embryos should increase the implantation rate, decrease the spontaneous abortion rate, and increase the live birth rate ("take home baby"). Indeed, several groups provide support for this conclusion (Ferraretti et al., 1999; Munné et al., 1999; Feliciani et al., 2000). Ferraretti and coworkers (1999) showed a higher cumulative IVF livebirth rate in 38- to 43-year-old women self-selecting PGD (FISH probes for X, Y, 13, 14, 15, 16, 18, 21, and 22). The rate in this group was 90% over three cycles versus 50% in 38- to 43-year-old women not undergoing PGD. This improvement was consistent with an increased implantation rate (26.6 versus 15.6%) and a decreased abortion rate (4.3 versus 14%). Munné and coworkers (1999) also found that the spontaneous abortion rate decreased, corresponding to improved ongoing and delivered babies (10.5% in controls versus 16.1% [57/354] in the PGD group). Feliciani and associates (2000) are now randomizing women ≥ 38 years into those having and not having PGD, using probes for nine chromosomes. In 70 women ≥ 38 years old who had PGD and in whom only two embryos were transferred, pregnancy and implantation rates were comparable to those of younger women; in women ≥ 38 years not having PGD, rates were much lower. Once embryo biopsy techniques are perfected (Munné et al., 1999) and experience is gained in individual centers, PGD could well become routine for older women undergoing assisted reproductive technique (ART). Latest evidence suggests that live birth rates are especially improved in older women who respond well to ovulation induction, having ≥ 6 embryos (Munné et al., 2002).

Preimplantation cytogenetic abnormalities are relevant for other phenomena, as discussed later in this chapter. Specifically, recurrent aneuploidy almost certainly encompasses clinical as well as preclinical and preimplantation conceptions. In turn, preimplantation embryonic abnormalities are also relevant to subfertility, which could be due to early unwitting losses.

Etiology of Clinically Recognized Pregnancy Loss

CHROMOSOMAL ABNORMALITIES

The major cause of clinically recognized pregnancy losses is chromosomal abnormalities, just as it is in preimplantation embryos that are either morphologically normal or morphologically abnormal. For decades it has been accepted that at least 50% of clinically recognized abortuses result from a chromosomal abnormality (Boué et al., 1975; Hassold, 1980; Simpson and Bombard, 1987). In fact, the proportion is probably even higher. If one analyzes chorionic villi after ultrasound diagnosis of fetal demise rather than relying upon recovery of spontaneously expelled products, the frequency of chromosomal abnormalities is 75 to 90% (Guerneri et al., 1987; Johnson et al., 1990; Sorokin et al., 1991; Strom et al., 1992). Sánchez and coworkers (1999) found 66% chromosomal abnormalities, even when including abortuses up to 14 weeks' gestation. Although maternal age is increased in the above samples, frequencies of first-trimester chromosomal abnormalities still seem to be 70% or higher.

Fritz and colleagues (2001) reached a similar conclusion after applying comparative genome hybridization (CGH) to 60 abortuses that could not be cultured and therefore studied by conventional cytogenetic methods. In the 57 successfully analyzed specimens, 72% were aneuploid and one was structurally imbalanced (2.4%). Their review of 4693 successfully karyotyped abortuses from prior publication resulted in the conclusion that first-trimester aberration rate was 64.8% prior to taking into account the above results; taking into account higher rates in abortuses not cultured led to the conclusion that the rate of chromosomal abnormalities was 70% in first-trimester abortuses.

Autosomal trisomies constitute the largest (approximately 50%) single group of chromosomal complements in cytogenetically abnormal spontaneous abortions. Monosomy X is the most common single chromosomal abnormality. The latter accounts for 20% of all abnormalities or at least 10% of all abortions. Trisomy for every chromosome except No. 1 has been reported, trisomy 1 being observed only in an eight-celled embryo (Watt et al., 1987). Polyploidy as a group accounts for 25 to 30%. Unbalanced chromosomal rearrangements occur in 5% or less of chromosomally abnormal embryos. Table 5–3 lists relative frequencies of the various chromosomal abnormalities found in abortions.

Among second-trimester losses, chromosomal abnormalities observed become more similar to those in liveborn infants: trisomies 13, 18, and 21; monosomy X; sex chromosomal polysomies. Among third-trimester losses (stillborn infants) the frequency of chromosomal abnormalities is approximately 5%. Their frequency is far less than observed in earlier abortuses but still much higher among liveborns (0.6%).

AUTOSOMAL TRISOMY

Cytologic Origins

Most trisomies show a maternal age effect, but the effect varies among chromosomes. Maternal age effect is especially impressive for double trisomies, the mean maternal age being 36 years (Reddy, 1997). Given the maternal age effect, autosomal trisomies are predictably more likely to arise cytologically in maternal meiosis than in paternal meiosis. Indeed, most autosomal trisomies (90%) arise during maternal meiosis, usually meiosis I.

Maternal meiotic errors predominantly occur at meiosis I, perhaps constituting 75 to 90% of

▼ **Table 5–3**. RECURRENT ANEUPLOIDY

Complement of First Abortus	Complement of Second Abortus					
	Normal	Trisomy	Monosomy	Triploidy	Tetraploidy	De Novo Rearrangement
Normal	142	18	5	7	3	2
Trisomy	31	30	1	4	3	1
Monosomy X	7	5	3	3	0	0
Triploidy	7	4	1	4	0	0
Tetraploidy	3	1	0	2	0	0
De Novo Rearrangement	1	3	0	0	0	0

The relationship between karyotypes of successive abortuses.
Tabulation by Warburton D, Kline J, Stein Z: Does the karyotype of a spontaneous abortion predict the karyotype of a subsequent abortion? Evidence from 273 women with two karyotyped spontaneous abortions. Am J Hum Genet 41:465, 1987.

all maternal meiotic errors . This generalization holds true for trisomy 15 (Robinson et al., 1998) and trisomy 21. Almost all trisomy 16 arises in maternal meiosis I (Hassold et al., 1995). A notable exception is trisomy 18, in which two thirds of the 90% of maternal meiotic cases arise at meiosis II (Fisher et al., 1995; Bugge et al., 1998).

A development of interest is newly initiated studies on the meiotic origin of trisomies in preimplantation embryos. Initial studies are surprisingly revealing distributions different from those in abortuses or liveborns. Verlinsky and coworkers (2001) and Kuliev (2002) found disomy 16 in polar bodies to have originated equally in meiosis I and meiosis II; similarly, trisomy 18 originated equally in maternal meiosis I and II.

The association between maternal meiosis I errors and advanced maternal age is in turn correlated with decreased to absent meiotic recombination in oogenesis (Fisher et al., 1995; Bugge et al., 1998; Hassold, 1998). Two cytologic hypotheses have been invoked to explain this relationship: (1) The production line hypothesis states that oocytes ovulated earlier in life are characterized by more recombinants and, hence, less nondisjunction (Henderson and Edwards, 1968); (2) nonspecific chiasmatic disruption may exist, secondarily leading to nondisjunction (Hassold et al., 1995). It has now become clear that cytologic errors involving meiosis II also show a maternal age effect (Yoon et al., 1996). Maternal meiosis II errors show an *increased* frequency of recombination, reflecting an initial perturbation in meiosis I that does not become manifest until meiosis II. Studying chromosome 21, meiosis II nondisjunction was restricted to proximal 21q. If recombination was absent, meiosis I nondisjunction existed (Lamb et al., 1996).

If errors of recombination are the primary pathogenesis in maternal meiotic I and II distur-bances leading to aneuploidy, it follows that periconceptional events such as exposure to toxins or fertilization involving gametes aged *in vivo* (delayed fertilization) are unlikely to play major etiologic roles in trisomies. This contrasts with a role expected for trisomies originating solely as a result of errors in maternal meiosis II, as occurs frequently (67%) and not uncommonly (10%) in trisomy 21. Thus, in retrospect our failure to find an increased frequency of Down syndrome in pregnancies conceived on days other than the day of ovulation or the day before is not surprising (Simpson et al., 1988; Castilla et al., 1995; Simpson et al., 2002).

Errors in paternal meiosis account for 10% of acrocentric (13, 14, 15, 21, and 22) trisomies (Zaragoza et al., 1994; Hassold et al., 1996; Koehler et al., 1996). In trisomy 21, paternal meiotic errors are equally likely to arise from meiosis I or II (Savage et al., 1998), in contrast to the meiosis I that predominates in maternal meiotic errors. Among nonacrocentric chromosomes, the paternal contribution is less common, virtually unobserved in trisomy 16 (Hassold et al., 1995).

Trisomy 2 is aberrant in that half of all cases are paternal in origin. Paternal errors also account for all 47,XYY cases and half the 47,XXY cases (Hassold et al., 1991; MacDonald et al., 1994; Hassold, 1998).

Morphologic Correlations

Attempts have been made, with arguable success, to correlate morphologic abnormalities with specific trisomies (Kalousek, 1991; Warburton et al., 1991). Schmidt-Sarosi and coworkers (1998) reported that empty gestational sacs characterize trisomies 2, 4, 7, 9, 14, 15, 20, and 22; discernible embryonic tissue was found in monosomy X and in abortuses trisomic for 12, 13, 15, 18, 20, and 22. Trisomies incompatible with life predictably show slower growth than trisomies compatible with life. The mean crown-to-rump length in abortuses trisomic for chromosomes 13, 18, or 21 is 20.65 mm, compared with 10.66 mm for trisomies that never survive until term (e.g., trisomy 10 or 16) (Warburton et al., 1991). The former may survive longer, or the latter may show greater intrauterine growth restriction, or both. Potentially viable trisomies are also more likely to show anomalies reminiscent of those found in full-term liveborn trisomic infants (Kalousek, 1991; Warburton et al., 1991). Malformations in trisomic abortuses have been said to be more severe than those found in abortuses induced after prenatal genetic diagnosis.

Polyploidy

Triploidy (3n = 69) and tetraploidy (4n = 92) account for 30% of chromosomally abnormal spontaneous abortuses. Triploid abortuses are usually 69,XXY or 69,XXX, the result of dispermy. An association exists between triploidy and hydatidiform mole, a "partial mole" said to exist if molar tissue and fetal parts coexist. "Complete" hydatidiform moles are most often 46,XX and androgenic origin (Beatty, 1978).

Pathologic findings in triploid placentas include disproportionately large gestational sac, cystic degeneration of placental villi, hemorrhage, and hydropic trophoblasts (pseudomolar degeneration) (Kalousek, 1991; Warburton et al., 1991). Malformations include neural tube defects and omphalocele, anomalies reminiscent of those observed in triploid conceptuses progressing to term. Facial dysmorphia and limb abnormalities have also been reported.

Tetraploidy rarely progresses beyond 4 to 5 weeks of gestation.

Monosomy X

Monosomy X is the single most common chromosomal abnormality among spontaneous abortions, accounting for 15 to 20% of all abortuses. Monosomy X usually (80%) occurs as result of paternal sex chromosome loss (Chandley, 1981; Hassold et al., 1985). If the remaining X is paternal in origin (X^p), the mean maternal age is 23.8 ± 6.1 years; if the remaining X is maternal (X^m), the mean maternal age is 29.6 ± 5.5 years (Hassold et al., 1988). That is, maternal age is *decreased* if 45,X arises through a maternal meiotic error (45,X^p). Spontaneously aborted monosomy X embryos may display only an umbilical cord stump, or anomalies characteristic of the Turner syndrome may exist. Later in gesta-

tion, cystic hygromas and generalized edema are typical. Liveborn 45,X individuals usually lack germ cells, but 45,X abortuses clearly show germ cells; however, germ cells rarely proceed beyond the primordial follicles. Pathogenesis of 45,X germ cell failure thus involves not so much failure of germ cell development as more rapid attrition in 45,X than in 46,XX embryos (Singh et al., 1966; Jirasék, 1976). This observation makes plausible the rare but well-documented pregnancies occurring in 45,X individuals (Simpson, 1981).

Structural Chromosomal Rearrangement

Structural chromosomal rearrangements are an important cause of repetitive spontaneous abortions but account for only 1.5% of abortuses (see Table 5–2). Rearrangements (e.g., translocation) may either arise *de novo* during gametogenesis or be inherited from a parent carrying a 'balanced' translocation or inversion. Phenotypical consequences depend upon the chromosomal segments that are duplicated or deficient.

Sex Chromosomal Polysomy

X and Y polysomies are only slightly more common in abortuses than in liveborns. The complements 47,XXY and 47,XYY each occur in about 1 per 800 liveborn male births; 47,XXX occurs in 1 per 800 female liveborn births.

In 47,XXX the cytologic origin is 59% maternal meiosis I, 16% maternal meiosis II, 6% paternal meiosis I or II, and 19% postzygotic (MacDonald et al., 1994; Thomas et al., 2000). In 47,XXY, half are paternal and half maternal in origin; the latter usually originate at meiosis I (MacDonald et al., 1994; Thomas et al., 2000). Almost all 47,XYY is paternal in origin (Hassold et al., 1991; Hassold, 1988).

RECURRENT ANEUPLOIDY

Complements of successive abortuses in a given family are more likely to be either recurrently normal or recurrently abnormal (Hassold et al., 1991) (see Table 5–3). If the complement of the first abortus is abnormal (Warburton et al., 1987; Hassold et al., 1991), successive abortuses are also likely to be abnormal. The recurrent abnormality usually is trisomy. It follows that numerical chromosomal abnormalities (aneuploidy) may be responsible for both recurrent and sporadic losses. Although it can be argued that corrections for maternal age actually render the ostensible nonrandom distribution marginally nonsignificant (Warburton et al., 1987), it seems far more likely to us that some couples are genuinely predisposed toward chromosomally abnormal conceptions. If recurrent aneuploidy is a genuine phenomenon, couples might logically be at increased risk not only for aneuploid abortuses but also for aneuploid liveborn infants. Consistent with this hypothesis is that Stern and colleagues (1998) found the same frequency of chromosomal abnormalities (57%) in abortuses from repetitively aborting women versus sporadically aborting women. Ogasawara and coworkers (1997) found the frequency among repetitively aborting women to be 51%, but Carp and coworkers (2000) found it to be only 29% (36/125). The lower rate found in the latter study could reflect ascertainment extending to women with losses before "20 weeks."

The recurrent trisomic autosome might not always confer lethality but rather might be compatible with life (e.g., trisomy 21). Liveborn recurrence risk of trisomy 21 following an aneuploidy is about 1%, based on ascertaining through a liveborn (Alberman, 1981). Recurrence risks more relevant to aneuploid abortuses are those based on ascertainment after detection of trisomy during pregnancy, such as by nuchal translucency or maternal serum analytes screening. In 2054 women with a previous trisomy 21 pregnancy, recurrence risk for trisomy was increased 0.75% over maternal and gestational-related expectations (Snijders et al., 1999). In 750 women with a prior trisomy 18 pregnancy, the increase was also 0.75%.

Data derived from preimplantation embryos support the validity of recurrent aneuploidy extending to earlier in gestation. Using disaggregated embryos, we described above how Delhanty and coworkers (1997) detected "chaotic" embryos. These chaotic embryos show recurrence in successive cycles in certain women; other women fail to show chaotic embryos in successive cycles. Similarly, preimplantation embryos of women experiencing repetitive abortions reveal consistently higher aneuploidy rates than women who do not have the same clinical problem. In 19 PGD cycles generating 136 embryos from 14 women, Rubio and coworkers (2000) found the percentage of chromosomal abnormalities to be 19.8%, 24.8, 11.0, 23.1, and 20.0%, respectively, for chromosomes 13, 16, 18, 21, and 22. PGD in 17 cycles generating 106 embryos from 10 control women yielded only 2.1%, 7.1, 4.6, 7.8, and 4.5% aneuploidies, respectively. Thus, women with unexplained abortions are far more likely to show chromosomally abnormal embryos.

Cryptic gonadal mosaicism in one parent is another explanation for recurrence of aneuploidy. Parental gametes could be aneuploid by secondary nondisjunction, through expected meiotic segregation. Another explanation is precocious chromatid segregation, which has been observed in a woman having several prior trisomy 21 conceptions. Of seven embryos studied by PGD, four showed trisomy 21.

Recurrent aneuploidy could be manifested as subfertility. This conclusion would be consistent with long recognized epidemiologic studies showing that subfertile women have increased rates of prior spontaneous abortions (Tietze, 1968; Rachootin et al., 1982; Baird and Wilcox, 1985). Gray and Wu (2000) recorded spontaneous abortion rates of 23% in pregnancies preceded by more than 1 year of attempts to become pregnant; rates were 14% in those achieving pregnancy without delay (OR, 1.7; 95% CI, 1.26, 2.94). Using hCG as an end point for subclinical pregnancy loss, Hakim and coworkers (1995) found higher losses in women with a history of impaired fertility.

If no karyotypic malformation exists on prior abortuses, recurrent aneuploidy may or may not have been the explanation. If the mother is age 30 to 34 years, the possibility of this being true is probably sufficient to justify prenatal cytogenetic diagnosis on statistical grounds. For younger patients, the recommendation is less clear. It may be possible to obtain information on prior abortuses from analysis of paraffin-embedded blocks of the products of conception. Specimens can be subjected to FISH with chromosome-specific probes or to CGH (Ozcan et al., 2000).

Whether prognosis is altered by karyotype of prior abortus is unclear. Carp and coworkers (2001) concluded that subsequent livebirths were more frequent (13 of 19 or 68.4%) when the abortus was aberrant versus euploid (16 of 39 or 41%).

IMPRINTING AND NOVEL CYTOGENETIC MECHANISMS CONTRIBUTING TO PREGNANCY LOSS

Mosaicism may be restricted to the placenta, the embryo *per se* being normal. This phenomenon is called confined placental mosaicism (CPM). Actually, losses caused by this mechanism may already have been reflected in existing data (e.g., see Table 5–2) because cytogenetic studies of abortuses usually involve analysis of only chorionic villus material. Although a relationship between CPM and intrauterine growth restriction (IUGR) also exists, this probably does not furnish an explanation for many early abortions.

A related phenomenon that could explain increased loss with CPM is *uniparental disomy*. Recall that in uniparental disomy (UPD) (see Chapter 1) both homologues of a given chromosome are derived from a single parent, probably as a result of expulsion of a chromosome from a trisomic zygote. If the expelled chromosome were from the parent contributing only the one chromosome, the karyotype would appear normal (46,XX or 46,XY) but the embryo would lack a genetic contribution from that parent. Both chromosomes for a given autosome would be derived from the parent contributing the disomic (n = 24) gamete. The likelihood that expulsion of a chromosome from a trisomic embryo would lead to UPD is one in three.

UPD is deleterious for some chromosomes but not others, chromosome 14 in particular (Berend al., 2000; McGowan et al., 2002). UPD was detected in an abortus with chromosome 21 (Henderson et al., 1994). However, UPD was not found in 18 fetal losses studied by a genome-based approach (Shaffer et al., 1998). The consensus is that UPD is not responsible for substantive numbers of abortions.

CHROMOSOMAL TRANSLOCATIONS

Among couples who experience repeated losses, the most common structural rearrangement is a translocation (Simpson et al., 1981; Simpson et al., 1989; De Braekeleer and Dao, 1990). Individuals with balanced translocations are phenotypically normal, but chromosomal duplications or deficiencies may arise as a result of normal meiotic segregation (see Chapter 1). Imbalance can be manifested either solely as spontaneous abortuses or as a combination of abortuses and abnormal liveborns in a single kindred. About 60% of translocations found in couples experiencing repetitive abortions are reciprocal; 40% are robertsonian. Women are about twice as likely as men to show a balanced translocation (Simpson et al., 1981).

If a child has Down syndrome as result of a translocation, the rearrangement will have originated *de novo* in 50 to 75% of cases. That is, neither parent will have a balanced translocation. The likelihood of Down syndrome offspring's recurring in such a couple is minimal. On the other hand, the risk is substantive in the 25 to 50% of families in which individuals have

Down syndrome as result of a balanced parental translocation [e.g. 45,XX,– 14,–21,+(14q;21q)]. Among liveborns, the theoretical risk for a child with Down syndrome is 33%, but empirical risks are much lower. The likelihood is 10% if the mother carries the translocation and only 2% if the father carries the translocation (Boué and Gallano, 1984; Daniel et al., 1989). In these cases half of all products would be lethal. If robertsonian (centric-fusion) translocations involve chromosomes other than numbers 14 and 21, empirical risks are lower. In t(13q;14q), the risk for liveborn trisomy 13 is 1% or less.

Reciprocal translocations do not involve centromeric fusion. Empirical data are available for few specific translocations, but a few generalizations can be made on the basis of data pooled from different translocations. Theoretical risks for abnormal offspring (unbalanced reciprocal translocations) are far greater than empirical risks. The risk is 12% for offspring of either female heterozygotes or male heterozygotes (Boué and Gallano, 1984; Daniel et al., 1989). The frequency of unbalanced fetuses is lower if the parental balanced translocation was ascertained through repetitive abortions (3%) than if it was ascertained through an anomalous liveborn infant (nearly 20%) (Boué and Gallano, 1984). In theory, segregation studies utilizing sperm chromosomes or fluorescent *in situ* hybridization (FISH) with chromosome-specific probes should provide data relevant for a translocation in a specific family. Determining the relative number of balanced and unbalanced gametes (spermatozoa) should be an indication of the respective expected number of fertilizable gametes and, hence, embryos. However, meiotic studies are laborious and expensive, available only on an investigational basis.

A novel explanation for otherwise unexplained mental retardation has proved to be sub-telomeric translocations. These subtle arrangements are not detectable by traditional karyotypes, and require multi-subtelomer FISH analysis. Although 5 to 8% of mentally retarded dysmorphic infants have sub-telomeric translocations (Knight and Flint, 2000), sub-telomeric rearrangements do not appear increased in couples having repetitive abortions (Benzacken et al., 2002; Fan and Zhang, 2002).

Occasionally a parental translocation precludes the possibility of a normal liveborn infant. This occurs when translocations involve homologous chromosomes [e.g., t(13q13q) of t(21q21q)]. If the father carries a homologous translocation, artificial insemination may be appropriate. If the mother carries the rearrangement, donor oocytes or donor embryos (assisted reproductive technologies) should be considered.

CHROMOSOMAL INVERSIONS

A less common chromosomal rearrangement responsible for repetitive pregnancy is an inversion, in which the order of the genes is reversed. Individuals heterozygous for an inversion should be clinically normal if their genes are merely rearranged and do not interrupt the coding sequence of the genes present at the break points; however, adverse reproductive consequences could arise as result of normal meiotic phenomena. Pericentric inversions are detected in perhaps 0.1% of females and 0.1% of males experiencing repeated spontaneous abortions. Some inversions (e.g., centromeric region of chromosome 9) are merely variants without effect, whereas others may not be detected by routine cytogenetic studies utilizing fewer than 500 to 600 metaphase bands. Using prometaphase banding (1200 bands) should be more sensitive.

The cytologic basis of unbalanced gametes in inversions is crossing-over involving the inverted region. As discussed in Chapter 1, homologous chromosomes can pair in inversions only if a loop is formed. Crossing-over may or may not occur within an inversion loop, but it is likely to do so if the loop encompasses a relatively long length of chromosome. (Recombination normally occurs at least once per chromosome, providing a mechanism to keep homologues in close proximity in preparation for orderly disjunction to opposite poles.) A single cross-over at any site within a pericentric loop yields four types of gametes. Two of the four have the parental genetic composition (one normal, one inverted); the other two have combinations of genes not present in either parent (recombinants). In both the recombinants, crossing-over will have resulted in duplication for genes distal to one break point and deficiency for other genes.

In Chapter 1 we showed that the unbalanced genes in inversion recombinants are those in the chromosomal region *outside* the inverted segment. As result, the paradox exists that when crossing-over occurs within the inverted segment, the *smaller* inversion produces the *greater* genetic imbalance in recombinant gametes and, hence, the more deleterious phenotype. That is, crossing-over that occurs in inversions characterized by only a small portion of the total chromosomal length results in large duplications and deficiencies. Imbalances may be so great that lethality occurs, the clinical consequences thus being almost nil.

Counseling an individual couple with an inversion is complex. Inversions involving a very small portion of the total chromosomal length may be of little significance because the likelihood of crossing-over is low. Conversely, inversion involving a large portion of the chromosome may be the least significant clinically; the large duplications or large deficiencies resulting from crossing-over prove lethal. Inversions involving 30 to 60% of the total chromosomal length are most likely to be characterized by duplications or deficiencies compatible with survival (Sutherland et al., 1976; Gardner and Sutherland, 1996). Risks also reflect gender and mode of ascertainment, as for translocations. Females with a pericentric inversion carry a 7% risk of abnormal liveborn infants; males carry a 5% risk. Also analogous to translocations, pericentric inversions ascertained through phenotypically normal probands are less likely to result in abnormal liveborn infants. Finally, Shim et al. (2001) reported a women with two invented dup (15) chromosomes; both the pregnancies resulted in abortion.

Few data are available for paracentric inversions. These inversions should show less risk for unbalanced products than pericentric inversions because recombinants in the former should more often be lethal. However, both abortions and abnormal liveborn infants have been observed when a parent has a paracentric inversion. The risk for viable recombinant offspring has been estimated to be 4% (Pettenati et al., 1995).

LUTEAL PHASE DEFECTS

Implantation in an inhospitable endometrium is an entirely plausible explanation for spontaneous abortions. Progesterone deficiency in particular could result in the estrogen-primed endometrium's being unable to sustain implantation. Luteal phase deficiency (LPD) describes the condition in which the endometrium manifests an inadequate response to progesterone for any of a number of reasons. Progesterone secreted by the corpus luteum is necessary to support the endometrium until the trophoblast produces sufficient progesterone to maintain pregnancy, an event occurring around seven gestational (menstrual) weeks or five weeks after conception. The various pathogenic mechanisms postulated as explanations for LPD include decreased secretion of gonadotropin-releasing hormone (GnRH), decreased follicle-stimulating hormone (FSH), decreased luteinizing hormone (LH), inadequate ovarian steroidogenesis, endometrial receptor defects, or deficiencies of gene products induced by progesterone (e.g., glycodelin). It could be reasoned that endometrial abnormalities are the explanations for Wilcox and colleagues (1999) finding progressively increased loss rates beginning on day 9 after ovulation; no pregnancies occurred beyond day 12. However, later implantation losses could also reflect late implantation of slower growing genetically abnormal embryos.

Diagnosis

Once almost universally accepted by gynecologists as a common cause for fetal wastage, LPD is now generally considered an uncommon explanation. One major problem is lack of reproducible diagnostic criteria. Another is that endometrial histology identical to that observed with luteal phase "defects" exists in fertile women. When regularly menstruating fertile women with no history of abortions underwent endometrial biopsies in serial cycles, LPD was found in 51.4% in any single cycle and 26.7% in sequential cycles (Davis et al., 1989). Not only is diagnosis of LPD not specific but interobserver variation in reading endometrial biopsies is considerable. Biopsies read by five different pathologists resulted in one third of patients having differences of interpretation sufficient to alter management (Scott et al., 1988). Pathologists reading coded endometrial biopsy slides a second time agreed with their own initial diagnosis in only 25% of cases (Li et al., 1989). With the possible exception of daily serial progesterone assays in research settings, measuring serum hormone levels shows little improvement in sensitivity and specificity over that of endometrial biopsy results. A single low serum progesterone level in the luteal phase is only 71% predictive of a luteal phase defect, as defined on the basis of an abnormal endometrial biopsy (Daya et al., 1988). Soules and colleagues have long attempted to characterize gonadotropin and progesterone secretion in LPD (Soules et al., 1989a, b). This group believes that diagnosis is best made on the basis of a single assay of three pooled blood samples; a level of < 10 ng/ml defines LPD (Soules et al., 1977). Combining Doppler ultrasound and hormone assays has been considered an alternative to endometrial biopsy, but this approach was not verified as reliable by Sterzik and coworkers (2000).

Li and coworkers (2000) show a correlation between low plasma progesterone level (< 30 nmol/L) and endometrial dating two days behind that expected on the basis of LH surge; the biopsy was taken 7 days after the LH surge. Of 24 women with recurrent abortions, plasma progesterone was < 30 nmol/L) and eight showed endometrial delay; of 62 women with progesterone ≥ 30 nmol/L, only seven showed a delay

▼ **Table 5–4.** CORRELATION OF ENDOMETRIAL
• DATING WITH PLASMA PROGESTERONE IN THE MIDLUTEAL PHASE OF WOMEN WITH RECURRENT PREGNANCY LOSS

Plasma Progesterone	Endometrial Dating	
	Normal (N)	Delayed (N)
≥ 30 nmol/L	55	7
< 30 nmol/L	16	8

$\chi^2 = 5.8$; $P < 002$.
From Li TC, Spuljbroek MD, Tuckerman E: Endocrinology and endometrial factors in recurrent miscarriage. Br J Obstet Gynaecol 107:1471, 2000.

(Table 5–4). The same study further concluded that the prevalence of endometrial defect is higher (27%) than in a control group of 22 fertile women with no prior abortions (11%). As in similar studies voluminous endocrine data were gathered, but relatively few other potentially confounding variables (e.g., maternal age) were taken into account. See Li et al. (2002) for related factors that correlate with progesterone levels.

Molecular analysis for genes governing endometrial receptors, integrins, mmPs (matrix metalloproteinases), or other progesterone-induced factors might prove useful, either directly or indirectly, depending on whether their perturbation is an explanation for LPD.

Treatment

Efficacy of treatment is unproved. No randomized studies have validated LPD as a genuine entity. Studies by Tho and coworkers (1979) and by Daya and Ward (1988) have been cited as providing some evidence of efficacy, but their experimental designs can be criticized because concurrent control groups were not recruited. Li and colleagues (2001) identified 21 women with three or more consecutive first-trimester losses. Following their previously published protocol (Li, 1998), they obtained blood or urine daily for 9 days until the LH surge; 7 days later timed endometrial biopsy was obtained to detect LPD, diagnosed as > 2 days behind chronologic dating. Among 25 subsequent pregnancies by the women, 13 conceived without treatment and 12 conceived with ovarian stimulation (human menopausal gonadotropin followed by hCG). The two groups were apparently not randomized but rather self-selected of the 13 pregnancies conceived by ovarian stimulation, 11 continued ≥ 24 weeks; of the 12 who conceived without ovarian stimulation, only 5 continued ≥ 24 weeks. Results were statistically significant, but there were no corrections for small numbers (Yates) or for potentially confounding variables (e.g., maternal age). Meta-analysis by Karamardian and Grimes (1992) showed no beneficial effect of progesterone treatment. The consensus is that LPD is either an arguable entity or cannot be proved to be treated successfully with progesterone or progestational therapy.

Of relevance are observations suggesting a relationship between fetal loss and either oligomenorrhea (Quenby and Farquharson, 1993) or polycystic ovary disease (PCO) (Sagle et al., 1988). Such a relationship could reflect endometrial dyssynchrony as mediated through abnormalities of LH. In 20 women with elevated LH levels, Regan and coworkers (1990) reported increased pregnancy loss; however, treatment to lower LH levels failed to decrease pregnancy loss rate (Clifford et al., 1996). Using the St. Mary's (London) Early Pregnancy Assessment unit cohort, Rai and associates (2000) found that 11% (53/486) of unexplained recurrent aborters had elevated LH levels. However, neither Carp and coworkers (1995) nor Tulppala and coworkers (1993) observed elevated LH levels in women experiencing recurrent losses. Bussen and colleagues (1999) failed to find elevated LH levels among 42 women with recurrent losses, despite the fact that such women showed prolactin and androstenedione concentrations 40% higher than in 15 other women who showed normal LH and had two losses. Most recently, Nando et al. (2002) found no correlation between pregnancy outcome and either serum LH or testosterone as a cohort of 344 women with first trimester recurrent abortion. We conclude that LH elevations per se are not significant but could point to other underlying problems.

THYROID ABNORMALITIES

Decreased conception rates and increased fetal losses are associated with overt hypothyroidism or hyperthyroidism. However, subclinical thyroid dysfunction has in general not been considered an explanation for repeated losses (Montoro et al., 1981). The situation could be more complex, however. Bussen and Steck (1995) studied 22 women with recurrent abortions and a like number of nulligravid and multigravid controls. Thyroid antibodies were increased in the former. Stagnaro-Green and coworkers (1990) and Glinoer and coworkers (1991) concluded that antithyroid antibodies and mild thyroid disease were associated with spontaneous abortions, and Singh and coworkers (1995) advanced that thyroid antibodies were a useful marker for clin-

ical losses in the ART population. Earlier, Pratt and associates (1993a) reported increased antithyroid antibodies in euthyroid women experiencing first trimester losses, but the same group (Pratt et al., 1993b) concluded that the ostensible association was secondary to nonspecific organ antibodies.

Rushworth and colleagues (2000) prospectively studied 870 women in the St. Mary's (London) Early Pregnancy Assessment Unit; all women had ≥ three spontaneous abortions. Of these 162 or 19% had antibodies against thyroglobulin or thyroid microsomal factors. However, subsequent outcomes did not significantly differ whether women were thyroid antibody–positive or –negative.

Overall, asymptomatic thyroid antibodies would not seem to be a major cause of early pregnancy loss.

DIABETES MELLITUS

Women with poorly controlled diabetes mellitus clearly show increased risk for fetal loss. In the cohort best studied to address this question, women whose glycosylated hemoglobin was greater than four standard deviations above the mean showed higher pregnancy loss rates than either diabetic women showing lower glycosylated hemoglobin levels or euglycemic controls (Mills et al., 1988). Total pregnancy loss rates were twice as high if initial glycosylated hemoglobin was > 4 SD than if < 2 SD. Almost all these losses were early in pregnancy, by 8 weeks. Similar conclusions have been repeatedly reached in retrospective studies (Miodovnik et al., 1986). Poorly controlled diabetes mellitus should thus be considered one cause of early pregnancy loss. However, subclinical, gestational, or well-controlled diabetes is probably not a major etiologic factor because the number of insulin-dependent diabetic women who experience pregnancy loss and have poor control is too small to exert a large attributable effect.

INTRAUTERINE ADHESIONS (SYNECHIAE)

Intrauterine adhesions could interfere with implantation or with early embryonic development. Most often these adhesions arise after overzealous uterine curettage during the puerperium, intrauterine surgery (e.g., myomectomy), or endometriosis. Adhesions are most likely to develop if curettage is performed 3 or

4 weeks postpartum. Women with uterine synechiae usually manifest hypomenorrhea or amenorrhea, but 25 to 30% have repeated abortions. Adhesions surely cause early pregnancy failure in rare individuals, but the overall contribution to pregnancy loss is probably very small.

INCOMPLETE MÜLLERIAN FUSION

Müllerian fusion defects (see Chapter 8) are well-accepted causes of second-trimester losses and pregnancy complications. Low birth weight, breech presentation, and uterine bleeding are also commonly accepted correlates. However, the role of incomplete müllerian fusion in early (first-trimester) losses is less certain. Most studies lack controls (Stampe-Sorenson, 1988; Candiani et al., 1990; Stein and March, 1990; Makino et al., 1991; Michalas, 1991; Golan et al., 1992; Moutos et al., 1992), or uncritically pool early and later pregnancy losses.

The major problem in attributing pregnancy losses to uterine anomalies is that both phenomena occur so frequently that concurrent adverse outcomes could be coincidental. Stampe-Sorenson (1988) found unsuspected bicornuate uteri in 2 of 167 (1.2%) women undergoing laparoscopic sterilization; another 3.6% had septate uteri and 15.3% showed fundal anomalies. Simon and coworkers (1991) found müllerian defects in 3.2% (22/679) of fertile women; 20 of the 22 defects were septate. A more unbiased figure was arrived at by Byrne and coworkers (2000) who performed ultrasound in women not undergoing imaging for gynecologic reasons. The frequency of uterine anomalies was estimated to be 0.4% (8 per 2065).

Increased spontaneous abortions have been claimed in those with septate uteri (Moutos et al., 1992) or T-shaped uteri (Makino et al., 1991). Other studies showed no discernible differences among various subtypes (Stein and March, 1990). Grimbizis and coworkers (2001) reviewed several series, including Acien (1993) and Raga and associates (1997). The tabulation was stratified to determine the abortion rate by anomaly subtype. Overall, the authors concluded that uterine malformations were found in 13% of women with recurrent losses versus 4.9% of fertile women. These relatively high rates probably reflect biases of ascertainment and inclusion of women with midtrimester losses. The highest rates were for untreated septate defects (44.3%); rates were 36.0% for bicornuate uterus; 25.7% for arcuate uterus; 32.2% for uterus didelphys, and 36.5% for unicornuate uterus. In septate

uteri increased risk of pregnancy loss could plausibly reflect the occurrence of implantation on an inhospitable fibrous surface. There is less reason to believe early losses would be increased with bicornuate uteri or T-shaped uteri, but poor vascularization could still play a role.

We believe that first-trimester spontaneous abortions should be attributed to uterine fusion defects only if they occur after ultrasonographic confirmation of a viable pregnancy at 8 or 9 weeks. Losses occurring after 8 weeks but lacking confirmation of fetal viability are statistically more likely to represent missed abortions in which fetal demise actually occurred weeks earlier. Losses in the second trimester can more confidentially be attributed to uterine anomalies, as can premature births.

LEIOMYOMAS

Leiomyomas occur frequently and produce clinical problems well recognized by gynecologists. Leiomyomas plausibly could cause early pregnancy loss but probably do so only rarely. Like uterine fusion anomalies, the coexistence of uterine leiomyomas and reproductive losses need not necessarily imply a causal relationship. Location of leiomyomas is probably more important than size, submucous leiomyomas being most likely to cause abortion.

Plausible mechanisms increasing pregnancy loss rates might include thinning of the endometrium over the surface of a submucous leiomyoma, predisposing to implantation in a poorly decidualized site. Rapid growth of leiomyomas could occur as a result of the hormonal milieu of pregnancy, compromising blood supply and resulting in necrosis ("red degeneration"); this in turn leads to uterine contractions or infections that eventually lead to fetal expulsion. Clinically, it should be initially assumed that leiomyomas have no etiologic relationship to pregnancy loss. Surgery for this indication alone should be undertaken with reticence. Ideally, surgery should be reserved for women whose abortuses were both phenotypically and karyotypically normal and in whom fetal viability was documented until at least 9 to 10 weeks.

INCOMPETENT INTERNAL CERVICAL OS

A functionally intact cervix and lower uterine cavity are obvious prerequisites for a successful intrauterine pregnancy. Characterized by painless dilation and effacement, cervical incompetence usually occurs during the mid-second or early third trimester. This condition frequently follows traumatic events such as cervical amputation, cervical laceration, forceful cervical dilatation, or conization. There is little reason to postulate a relationship with first-trimester losses.

Intermittently, the question arises as to whether prior induced abortion is associated with subsequent losses. The long-term consensus is that little if any relationship exists between the two (Ludmir and Stubblefield, 2001); however, controversy exists (Levin et al., 1980; Linn et al., 1983). Not all studies have taken into account obvious potential confounding variables, such as increasing maternal age in subsequent pregnancies. Indeed, increased loss rate is observed as the number of prior terminations increases (Lumley, 1998). However, this increase merely parallels that seen with increasing numbers of *spontaneous* losses.

INFECTIONS

Infections are accepted causes of late fetal losses and logically could be responsible for early fetal losses as well. Among the many infectious agents reported to have been associated with spontaneous abortion are variola, vaccinia, *Salmonella typhi*, *Vibrio fetus*, malaria, cytomegalovirus, *Brucella*, *Toxoplasma gondii*, *Mycoplasma hominis*, *Chlamydia trachomatis*, and *Ureaplasma urealyticum*. Transplacental infection doubtless occurs with each of these microorganisms, and sporadic losses could logically be caused by any of them.

Proof that infections truly cause *repetitive* losses has been less forthcoming. One line of indirect evidence is that certain organisms (e.g., *Ureaplasma urealyticum* and *Mycoplasma hominis*) have been isolated from midtrimester placentas and abortuses but only rarely from induced (control) midtrimester abortions (Sompolinsky et al., 1975). Other evidence consists of studies in which empirical antibiotic therapy ostensibly has benefitted couples experiencing repeated losses. For example, repetitive aborters treated for 4 weeks with tetracycline prior to pregnancy had a subsequent fetal loss in only 10% (Toth et al., 1986); aborters who chose not to take tetracycline showed a 38% loss rate. However, the two groups (treated, untreated) were not randomized and therefore were not necessarily comparable. Other studies have not found any differences in outcome between women treated and not treated with antibiotics (Van Iddekinge and Hofmeyr, 1991).

Bacterial Vaginosis

Some studies have suggested a relationship between bacterial vaginosis, presumed caused by *Gardnerella vaginalis*, and abortion. There are few data specific to early losses. Most literature in this field has focused on relationships with pregnancy complications in the second and third trimesters. For example, Hay (1994) found a 5.5-fold increased risk for 16- to 24-week losses, and McGregor and coworkers (1995) found increased risk for losses < 22 weeks. One more relevant study of interest involved Belgian women seen at obstetric registration at < 14 weeks of pregnancy (Donders et al., 2000). At the initial visit an investigator knowledgeable about bacterial vaginosis performed vaginal fluid microscopy, searching for clue cells and leukocytes; vaginal and cervical cultures were initiated for *G. vaginalis*, *U. urealyticum*, and *M. hominis*, *Chlamydia trachomatis*, various other bacterial species, and herpes simplex. Of 218 pregnancies, 21 (10%) were aborted, and in this group bacterial vaginosis was five times more common (RR, 5.5, 95%; CI, 2.9 to 10); gestational age at pregnancy loss was usually less than 14 weeks (mean 11.3 ± 2.9 weeks). Relative risk for pregnancy loss was also increased for *U. urealyticum* (1.58) and *Mycoplasma hominis* (1.25) but not for herpes, *Chlamydia*, or enteric bacteria. Regression analysis led the authors to conclude that bacterial vaginosis was the likely explanation for pregnancy losses. It is uncertain, however, whether this study took into account key confounding variables such as maternal age, prior pregnancy history, or gestational age. The magnitude of the attributable risk found in this study also is considerably different from that of other studies. Findings could be applicable only to this particular sample population, could be explained on the basis of failing to take into account confounding variables, or could be applicable only to pregnancies of later gestational age (late first and early second trimesters). Recall that all but 3% of pregnancy losses have occurred by 8 weeks and all but 1% by 16 weeks.

Ureaplasma Urealyticum and Mycoplasma Hominis

Of the organisms implicated in repetitive abortion, *Ureaplasma* and *Chlamydia* seem most plausibly related to repetitive spontaneous abortions because they fulfill several crucial prerequisites: (1) the putative organism can exist in an asymptomatic state, and (2) virulence is not universally severe enough to cause infertility due to fallopian tube occlusion and, hence, to preclude the opportunity for pregnancy in which spontaneous abortions might occur. Kundsin and coworkers (1967, 1981) have long contended that *Ureaplasma* is associated with recurrent abortions. From 46 women with histories of three or more consecutive pregnancy losses of unknown etiology, Stray-Pedersen and coworkers (1978) recovered *Mycoplasma* significantly more often among women with repetitive abortions (28%) than among controls (7%). Infected women and their husbands (n = 43) were then treated with doxycycline. Subsequent cultures confirmed eradication of *Mycoplasma*. Nineteen of the 43 women became pregnant; of the 19, three experienced another spontaneous abortion, whereas 16 had normal full-term infants. Among 18 women with untreated *Mycoplasma* infection, only five full-term pregnancies occurred. A study showing a positive correlation between pregnancy loss < 14 weeks and infection with *U. urealyticum* or *M. hominis* was discussed earlier (Donders et al., 2000).

Herpes Simplex

Data are less compelling for other organisms. Women with a history of herpesvirus have shown a higher spontaneous abortion rate than controls: 34 versus 10.6% in an early study by Nahmias and coworkers (1971). Other reports substantiated this potential relationship (Gronroos et al., 1983). However, potential confounding variables were not taken into account in the above studies. Donders and coworkers (2000) found no correlation between herpesvirus and spontaneous abortion rate, despite such findings for several other organisms.

Chlamydia Trachomatis

Chlamydial antibodies have been sought in the sera of women who experienced repeated losses and an association claimed on the basis of high antibody titers (Quinn et al., 1987; Witkin and Ledger, 1992). Gronroos and associates (1983) studied a population of women with threatened abortions and concluded that cervical IgA (but not IgG) antibody titers were increased in women who actually aborted. Other data show no relationship between chlamydia and pregnancy losses (Olliaro et al., 1991; Rae et al., 1994). Rae and coworkers (1994) found no significant difference between frequency of IgG antichlamydial antibodies in sera of women with recurrent abortion (n = 106) and controls (n = 3890) 24.5 versus

20.3%, respectively. Paukku and coworkers (1999) reported no differences in frequencies of occurrence of *C. trachomatis* (IgG or IgA antibodies) in 70 Finnish women with histories of spontaneous abortions compared with 40 parous women and 94 asymptomatic sexually active women. Donders and colleagues (2000) also found no such relationship in their prospective Belgian study.

In conclusion, most studies indicate no significant role in spontaneous abortion for *Chlamydia trachomatis*. A caveat is the possibility that only certain strains of *Chlamydia* could confer embryotoxicity. The ability to detect such an effect would be limited.

Toxoplasma Gondii

Toxoplasma antibodies have been observed in Mexican and Egyptian women having repetitive pregnancy losses (Zavala-Velazquez et al., 1989; el Ridi et al., 1991). However, the ubiquitous nature of this organism makes it unclear whether antibody frequencies are higher than in the general Mexican or Egyptian populations in which *Toxoplasma* is endemic. Most recent studies have tended to conclude that toxoplasmosis is not a significant cause of reproductive loss (Sahwi et al., 1995).

Infection as an Epiphenomenon

A key question is whether an infectious agent *causes* fetal losses or merely arises following fetal demise resulting from other etiologies. Cohort surveillance for infections beginning in early pregnancy can help shed light on the true role of infections in pregnancy loss. To this end, the frequency of infections in pregnant women was prospectively determined in the multicenter United States NICHD Diabetes in Early Pregnancy Study (DIEP) alluded to earlier. Simpson and colleagues (1996) analyzed data collected prospectively on clinical infections in 386 diabetic subjects and 432 control subjects seen frequently (weekly or ever other week) during the first trimester. Infection occurred no more often in 112 subjects experiencing pregnancy loss than among 706 with successful pregnancies. This held both for the 2-week interval in which a given loss was recognized clinically as well as for the prior 2-week interval. Similar findings were observed in both control and diabetic subjects and further held when stratified to ascending genital infection only versus systemic infection only. These prospective data suggest that the attributable risk of infection in first-trimester spontaneous abortion is low.

Of course, a role for a specific organism (e.g., *Mycoplasma*) in selective women with repetitive abortions could still exist.

Conclusions

Infections surely explain some pregnancy loss, especially later in the first trimester and subsequently throughout pregnancy. However, the attributable risk is probably low for an early loss, even in sporadic cases, and lower yet among women experiencing repetitive abortions.

ANTIPHOSPHOLIPID AND ANTICARDIOLIPIN ANTIBODIES

An association between second- and third-trimester pregnancy loss and certain autoimmune phenomena is accepted (Branch and Ward, 1989; Cowchock, 1991). Antibodies found in women with pregnancy loss are diverse, encompassing nonspecific antinuclear antibodies (ANAs) as well as antibodies against such specific cellular components as phospholipids, histones, and double- or single-stranded DNA. Antiphospholipid antibodies (aPLs) in turn represent a broad category that encompasses lupus anticoagulant (LAC) antibodies and anticardiolipin antibodies (aCLs). The consensus has long been that midtrimester fetal death (second and third trimester) is increased in women with LAC or aCLs, perhaps dramatically so (Scott et al., 1987). Contemporary studies continue to show consistent results (Sarig et al., 2002). Controversy centers on the role these antibodies play in first-trimester losses.

Descriptive studies initially seemed to show increased aCLs in women with first-trimester pregnancy losses. However, frequencies of various antiphospholipid antibodies (LAC, aCLs, aPLs) soon were shown to be similar in women who experienced and those who did not experience first-trimester abortions (Petri et al., 1987; Carp et al., 1993; Mishell, 1993; Ergolu and Scopelitis, 1994). A major pitfall in assessing the role these antibodies play in first-trimester losses is the unavoidable selection bias in ascertaining and studying couples only after they have had spontaneous abortions. The possibility that antibodies did not arise until *after* the pregnancy loss cannot readily be excluded. To address this pitfall, a multicenter NICHD collaborative study cohort was used, analyzing sera prospectively obtained from insulin-dependent and nondiabetic women within 21 days of conception (Mills et al., 1988). A total of 93 women who later experienced pregnancy losses (48 diabetic; 45 nondiabetic) were matched 2:1 with 190 controls (93 diabetic and 97 nondiabetic) who subsequently had normal liveborn offspring (Simpson et al., 1997a). No association was observed between pregnancy loss and presence of either aPLs or aCLs. Neither aCLs nor aPLs would thus seem to contribute greatly, if at all, to first-trimester pregnancy losses in the general population.

However, in the opinion of some the issue is not closed. It has been stated that results would be different if more specific assays were performed, such as antiphosphatidylethanolamine (Sugi et al., 1999). The marked variation in aPLs occurring during pregnancy is another confusing factor (Topping et al., 1999). Could antibodies connote significance only in selected clinical subsets, such as in women attempting to achieving pregnancy by *in vitro* fertilization? This is plausible given that some reports show increased prevalences of aCLs in women requiring *in vitro* fertilization (Egbase et al., 1999). The possibility of an effect's being restricted to the group experiencing only many repetitive abortions cannot be excluded. Power calculations are not adequate to categorically exclude an effect operative only in the 1 to 3% of women with three or more repetitive losses or especially in the few having five or more losses. However, one third of women in the cohort study of Simpson and coworkers (1997b) had experienced at least one prior loss, and in that group the frequency of aCLs and aPLs was still no greater than among women without prior losses (Simpson et al., 1998).

It has also been claimed that even if aCLs and aPLs are not present, antibodies to β2 glycoprotein (ab2 GP-1) might still be increased and relevant to repetitive aborters. However, Balasch and coworkers (1999) found no increase. Only 1 of 100 women having repetitive abortions and not having LAC or aCLs showed aβ2 GP-1. Any possible association between aβ2 GP-1 and spontaneous abortions is also unlikely to be independent of the association with aPLs and aCLs. No relationship is likely to exist between the aβ2-GP-1 and implantation failure in the IVF population, despite earlier claims of Stern and coworkers (1998).

In conclusion, a relationship between first-trimester loss and aPLs and aCLs seems unlikely to be generally applicable. Treatment regimens should thus be embarked upon with reticence and initiated only with relatively nontoxic agents (e.g., aspirin and heparin, but not steroids). Specifically giving aspirin to women who had only prior first-trimester abortions has shown no improvement in outcome compared with those not given aspirin (68% or 251/367 versus 64% or 278/438) (Rai et al., 2000). These results contrast with the beneficial effect observed in women who had a previous *second*-trimester loss (65% versus 49%). Administering intravenous immunoglobulin is not recommended (ASRM, A Practice Committee Report, 1999; ACOG, Practice Opinion, April 27, 2000).

ANTISPERM ANTIBODIES

Antisperm antibodies (ASAs) are another group of antibodies in which a relationship to fetal loss was once claimed. After vasectomy, approximately 50% of males show ASAs. In males, the presence of these antibodies connotes difficulty in impregnating women even after vasectomy is surgically reversed. Women manifesting antisperm antibodies could have their fertilization adversely impacted. Several studies show an increased frequency of antisperm antibodies among women experiencing repeated abortions (Hass et al., 1986; Witkin and Chaudhry, 1989; Erguven et al., 1990; Zhang, 1990). Others reached opposite conclusions (Yan, 1990; Clarke and Baker, 1993). The biologic basis for an association might be cross-reaction with paternally derived whole-body antigens essential for embryonic survival.

Again seeking to obtain prospective data on the relationship between the presence of antisperm antibodies (ASA) in maternal sera and first-trimester pregnancy losses, first-trimester sera from the NICHD DIEP cohort were studied. Recruiting within 21 days of conception, a total of 111 women who experienced pregnancy loss (55 diabetic, 56 nondiabetic) were matched 2:1 with 104 diabetic and 116 nondiabetic women (controls) who subsequently had a normal liveborn infant (Simpson et al., 1996). No differences were observed with respect to IgG, IgA, or IgM binding when a positive ASA test was defined as 50% of sperm showing antibody binding. At 20% binding, no association was found with IgG and IgM ASA antibodies, although a significant difference was observed for IgA ASA. This single positive finding probably reflects multiple comparisons.

In conclusion, antisperm antibodies contribute little to pregnancy loss in the general population. A role in the selective subset of couples experiencing repeated losses is not excluded.

HYPERCOAGULABLE CONDITIONS

Any relationship between fetal loss and aCLs or aPLs could reflect placental thrombosis. If so, other maternal hypercoagulable states could be associated with increased fetal losses. Currently observed associations include factor V Leiden (1691G→A), prothrombin (Factor II) 20210G→A and homozygosity for the 677C→T polymorphism in the methylene tetrahydrofolate reductase gene (*MTHFR*).

Studying sera from women previously experiencing repetitive losses, Rai and coworkers (1996) found an association between activated protein C resistance and second-trimester losses. The prevalence of factor V Leiden was 7.1% in women with abortions (Rai et al., 1999a) versus 4 to 5% in the general population; no association was observed between factor V Leiden and aPLs or aCLs. Women with histories of repetitive abortions who had factor V Leiden and then became pregnant had a lower likelihood (4/11 or 30%) of delivering a livebirth than women who lacked factor V Leiden (77/177 or 60%) (Rai et al., 1999b). This group also found thromboelastographic abnormalities to be more common in repetitive abortees than in controls (Rai et al., 1999c), offering a way to identify high-risk women. In a later contribution (Rai et al., 2001), they showed that acquired activated protein C resistance but not congenital (factor V Leiden) activated protein C resistance was more common in aborters. To evaluate acquired activated protein C resistance, they studied 904 women with three or more consecutive losses less than 12 weeks and 207 women with at least one loss after 12 weeks. *Acquired* activated protein C resistance Leiden mutation was more common in both groups (8.8% early losses, 8.7% late losses) than in 150 controls (3.3%). By contrast, factor V Leiden (the congenital form of acquired activated protein C resistance) was similar among all three groups (3.3% of 1808 women with recurrent early loss, 3.9% of 414 women with late loss, and 4.0% of 300 controls). In Brazilian women, Souza and coworkers (1999) found factor V Leiden in 4 of 56 (7.1%) aborters compared with 6 of 384 controls (1.6%). Factor II G20210A (prothrombin) was found in 2 of the 56 (3.6%) versus 1% of controls.

Not all authors agree that a relationship is established (Preston et al., 1996; Dizon-Townson et al., 1997). Pauer and colleagues (1998), and Balasch and colleagues (1997) failed to find a relationship between early losses and factor V Leiden. Deficiencies of antithrombin, protein C, or protein S were not found by Kutteh and coworkers (1999) to be any more frequent in 50 women with three or more losses than in 50 controls. Coumans and coworkers (1999) assessed 52 women with two or more losses before 12 weeks' gestation for markers, and found no relationship with any of these same hemostatic markers. An increased frequency of hyperhomocystinemia was observed in women with repeated losses (6 of 35 patients tested or 17.1%) compared with controls (4.5%). Such a relationship was also shown by Grandone and coworkers (1997) and Ridker and colleagues (1998).

Overall, hypercoagulable states, or at least factor V Leiden and prothrombin 20120G→A, seem plausible causes of repetitive losses. Additional studies would be helpful.

ANTIFETAL ANTIBODIES, EMBRYOTOXIC ANTIBODIES, AND ABERRANT Th1 CYTOKINE PRODUCTION

An otherwise normal mother may produce antibodies against her fetus on the basis of genetic dissimilarities. Obstetricians are familiar with late pregnancy loss caused by Rhesus-negative women having anti-D antibodies. More relevant for *early* pregnancy loss is isoimmunization resulting from anti-P antibodies, a phenomenon that adheres to the same principles as Rh(D) isoimmunization. Most individuals are genotype Pp or PP, but homozygosity for p exists (pp). If a woman of genotype pp has a Pp or PP husband, her offspring may or must be Pp. If the mother develops anti-P antibodies, pp fetuses will be rejected (aborted) early in gestation.

Hill and colleagues (1995) proposed that aberrant cytokines can cause repetitive abortions in women acting through T-helper cell perturbations. The rationale centers on the belief that T-helper 1 (Th1) cytokines are deleterious, whereas Th2 cytokines are not. The former include tumor necrosis factor (TNF), interleukin (IL)-2, and interferon (IFN)-α; the latter include IL-4, IL-5, IL-6, and IL-10, all secreted by activated T cells expressing the CD4 phenotype. Natural killer cells expressing CD56 also produce these salutary cytokines. In women with recurrent losses, immune cell responsiveness is activated to produce increased IFN-α and TNF (Hills et al., 1995). In support of the hypothesis that Th1 cytokines are deleterious, downregulation of Th1 cytokine in rodents improves pregnancy outcome (Wegmann et al., 1993; Raghupathy, 1997). Progesterone therapy is sometimes stated to ameliorate deleterious effects.

The presence of embryotoxic antibodies and aberrant cytokines is a reasonable hypothesis, but their existence prior to human recurrent embryonic loss has not been conclusively established. Prospective population-based studies in women without a prior history of abnormal outcomes are needed.

The contribution of this phenomenon to pregnancy loss in the general population remains uncertain.

Unfried and coworkers (2001) reported an increased frequency of polymorphic allele 2 of IL-IRA in 105 women having recurrent abortions compared with 91 controls (OR, 7.4; CI, 2.9, 10.8). However, women homozygous for allele 2 (IL-1RA[22]) were able to achieve successful pregnancies.

ALLOIMMUNE DISEASE (SHARED PARENTAL ANTIGENS)

A longstanding biologic puzzle is why the fetus is not rejected by its mother on the grounds of having foreign (paternal) antigens. The maternal immunologic response must be mitigated against through blocking or suppressive factors unique to pregnancy. Paradoxically, the protective mechanism could involve maternal-paternal differences (i.e., compatibilities).

Parental (and, hence, maternal-fetal) histo*in*compatibility has been proposed as salutary (counterintuitively) for pregnancy maintenance. Evidence in support of a beneficial effect for maternal-fetal incompatibility can be cited. Increased placental size exists in mice arising from matings in which paternal and maternal histocompatibility antigens differ, with higher implantation frequencies occurring in histoincompatible (H2) murine zygotes. It follows that human HLA antigens shared between mother and father could lead to maternal-fetal homozygosity for a given allele, potentially exerting a deleterious effect. Whether human HLA sharing per se is a mechanism underlying pregnancy loss in humans is unclear. Initially studies showed greater parental HLA sharing in aborters than in controls (Coulam, 1992; Laitinen et al., 1993). However, couples sharing HLA-DR antigens may experience no spontaneous abortions despite ten or more pregnancies (Ober et al., 1983). Thus, the story was destined to be complex.

Rigorous population-based studies have been conducted by Ober and colleagues (Ober et al., 1998; Ober, 1999), who studied the relationship of pregnancy losses and parental HLA-b sharing in the Hutterites. The Hutterites are a genetic isolate; their inbreeding produces a high rate of homozygosity by descent and, hence, opportunities for manifesting recessive alleles. These studies involved high-resolution HLA typing (alleles at 16 loci) in 31 Hutterite colonies in South Dakota. Pregnancy outcome was followed through a calendar diary and home pregnancy test kits, utilized if menses had not begun 1 month after prior menstrual bleeding. Data were available on 251 pregnancies in 111 couples (Ober et al., 1993, 1998). HLA genotyping was performed on surviving offspring to determine if losses selectively occurred with a specific genotype. Comparisons involved offspring homozygous for the shared antigen and who had inherited the maternal allele versus offspring heterozygous for the shared antigen who had not inherited the maternal allele shared with the spouse. Loss rates were greatest if couples shared alleles at all 16 loci, presumably reflecting inheritance of a common HLA haplotype (OR, 4.39). Sharing was greater for HLA-B (OR, 2.54) than for either HLA-C (OR, 2.20) or complement C4 (OR, 2.11). All pair-wise comparisons with controls were statistically significant, but only when couples sharing the entire haplotype were excluded. No deficiency of homozygous children was observed. If offspring were heterozygous but identical to the mother, 13.6% fewer than expected living children were observed ($P = 0.095$); however, sample size for this comparison was small.

Parental Sharing for Loci Other Than HLA

Genetic explanations other than HLA sharing per se could explain why only some couples who share HLA antigens show untoward outcomes. Any deleterious effect could reflect maternal-fetal histoincompatibility but not for HLA. The causative locus could be closely linked, specifically to HLA-B. This hypothesis would be consistent with HLA-G's being the only HLA antigen expressed on trophoblasts.

Genes responsible for deleterious effects exerted through shared parental alleles may not even be immunologically mediated. A lethal recessive gene, again perhaps closely linked to HLA, could exist. Murine embryos homozygous for certain alleles at the T/t locus die at early stages of embryogenesis. A T/t-like complex in humans could help explain the rare kindreds in which multiple family members have repeated pregnancy losses (Christiansen et al., 1990). Postulating a mutant gene in heterozygous form in parents implies autosomal recessive inheritance. If only homozygous offspring were lethal, the ratio of abortuses to liveborns should be 1:3 (25%:75%); however, in families in which the mechanism might usually be presumed opera-

tive, the clinically observed ratio seems closer to 1:0.

Immunotherapy

If fetal rejection occurs as result of diminished fetal-maternal immunologic interaction (alloimmune factors), immunotherapy to stimulate beneficial blocking antibodies generated at the few potentially differing loci is a reasonable hypothesis. The rationale was originally based on observations that blood transfusions prior to kidney transplantation decreased allograft rejection (Norman et al., 1986). Women lacking blocking antibodies but sharing HLA antigens with their spouses were immunized with paternal leukocytes, third-party leukocytes, or trophoblast membranes. The first prospective randomized trial yielded impressive results (Mowbray et al., 1985), but later studies were universally less impressive. A multicenter U.S. effort pooling the results of immunotherapy by injection of paternal leukocytes showed only an 11% increased pregnancy rate in the immunized group (Recurrent Miscarriage Immunotherapy Trialist Group, 1994). Meta-analysis by Fraser and coworkers (1993) found the odds ratio only 1.3 in favor of a beneficial effect.

In 1999, Ober (1999) reported the definitive study. This NICHD collaborative study involved six U.S. and Canadian centers, which identified women with three or more spontaneous abortions of unknown cause. Subjects were aged 40 years or younger, had no anti-HLA antibodies, and had no evidence of known or suspected causes of spontaneous abortion (parental chromosomal translocations, LPD, uterine anomalies, aCLs, LAC). Women were randomized into one arm (n = 91) that underwent immunization with paternal mononuclear cells and another arm in which women were given saline (controls) (n = 92). Pregnancy beyond 28 weeks occurred in 46% (31/68) in the immunized group versus 65% (41/63) in the nonimmunized group (P = 0.26). These findings were the opposite of expectation if immunotherapy was to have been salutary. Adjustments for potential confounding variables (e.g., maternal age, prior pregnancy) failed to alter conclusions. Importantly, success rate was nearly identical in immunized women who developed (31%) and failed to develop (30%) HLA antibodies. The sole puzzle was the relatively higher frequency of chromosomally abnormal abortuses or fetuses in the immunized group. This was explained by the authors on the basis of losses in their treatment group occurring later in pregnancy, a time when recovering products of conception for cytogenetic analysis was easier.

Conclusion

Parental HLA sharing leading to fetal rejection remains an attractive hypothesis, with HLA-B the locus showing the strangest association. However, the attributable role of HLA sharing in pregnancy losses in the general population is uncertain and probably low. The phenomenon could play a role in a subset of repetitive aborters, but in any case immunotherapy cannot be recommended. However, contrary opinions exist (Clark et al., 2001).

DRUGS, CHEMICALS, AND NOXIOUS AGENTS

Many exogenous agents have been implicated in fetal losses, but relatively few have been accepted scientifically. The difficulty is that pregnant women are frequently exposed to relatively low doses of ubiquitous toxic agents.

Outcomes are usually assessed through case control studies conducted after prior exposure to exogenous agents. Case control studies have considerable power to detect any associations present but suffer the inherent bias of the control sample's having less incentive to recall antecedent events than women experiencing an abnormal outcome (recall bias). Another experimental pitfall is that exposure to potentially dangerous chemicals is usually unwitting and, hence, poorly documented. Even when exposure unequivocally occurs (e.g., industrial accidents or residence near toxic waste sites), quantifying exposure and enumerating the multiple toxic agents present may be difficult if not impossible. Exposure to many agents concurrently makes it difficult to attribute adverse effects to a single agent.

Given these caveats, one must be cautious about attributing pregnancy loss to exogenous agents. On the other hand, common sense dictates that exposure to potentially noxious agents be minimized.

Environmental Chemicals

Many chemical agents have been claimed to be associated with fetal losses (Barlow and Sullivan, 1982; Fija-Talamanaca and Settimi, 1984), but consensus now seems to be settling around only a few (Savitz et al., 1994). These include anesthetic gases, arsenic, aniline dyes, benzene, solvents, ethylene oxide, formaldehyde, pesticides, and certain divalent actions (lead, mercury, and cadmium). Workers at greatest risk are those in rubber industries, battery factories, and chemical production plants. Many reports continue to be generated concerning specific agents, a recent example being selenium, an element considered relevant to fertilization (Kocak et al., 1999).

Scialli (1995) and Shephard (1998) have catalogued animal and human relevant references. On-line listings are available. The clinical difficulty lies in defining the effects of lower level exposures and in quantifying a risk that can be communicated to patients. Fortunately, most patient queries can be answered with reassurance that the pregnancy is not at increased risk.

Overall, the attributable contribution of environmental chemicals to pregnancy loss is probably low.

X-Irradiation

External irradiation and internal radionuclides in high doses are proved abortifacients. Of course, therapeutic x-rays or chemotherapeutic drugs are administered during pregnancy only to seriously ill woman whose pregnancies often must be terminated for maternal indications. Pelvic x-ray exposure up to perhaps 0.1 Gy (10 rad) places a fetus at little to no increased risk. In fact, most exposures are usually far smaller, 0.01–0.02 Gy (1–2 rad). The attributable contribution of X-irradiation to clinically recognized losses is thus small.

Chemotherapeutic Agents

Similar to x-irradiation, chemotherapeutic agents in high doses are proved abortifacients; however, high doses are encountered only in dire circumstances. Low doses may sometimes be medicinally important for non-neoplastic conditions, and ambient exposures can occur. A potential for deleterious effects on hospital personnel handling chemotherapeutic agents exists; thus, pregnant hospital workers must minimize exposure.

CAFFEINE

Consensus has long existed that no deleterious effects on pregnancy exist with caffeine. Most studies investigating pregnancy losses have been retrospective, and cohort data showed the odds ratio for an association between abortion and caffeine (coffee and other dietary forms) to be only 1.15 (95% CI; 0.9 to 1.45) (Mills et al., 1993). Additional data on women exposed to higher levels (>300 mg) of daily caffeine would be useful, but in general reassurance can be given concerning the lack of relationship between moderate caffeine exposure and pregnancy loss.

CIGARETTE SMOKING

An association between smoking and spontaneous abortion is accepted, but the effect is probably very modest. It could be explained entirely on the basis of confounding variables. Kline and associates (1980) reported increased abortion rates in smokers independent of maternal age and alcohol consumption. A modest dose—response curve was found by Alberman and coworkers (1976). Ness and coworkers (1999) compared tobacco use as assessed by urinary cotinine levels, comparing 400 women with spontaneous abortions to 570 who had ongoing pregnancies. Women with urinary cotinine had an increased risk of abortion, but the odds ratio only reached 1.8 (95% CI, 1.3–2.6).

ALCOHOL

An association between alcohol consumption and fetal loss was once well accepted but this claim now seems less certain. In 1980 Kline and coworkers compared 616 women experiencing spontaneous abortions to 632 women who delivered at less than 28 weeks' gestation. Among women whose pregnancies ended in spontaneous abortion, 17% drank alcohol at least twice per week; 8.1% of controls drank similar quantities. Harlap and Shiono (1980) also found an increased risk for abortion in women who drank during the first trimester. However, Halmesmäki and coworkers (1989) later found that alcohol consumption was nearly identical in women who did and those who did not experience an abortion. In that study, 13% of aborters and 11% of control women drank an average of three to four drinks per week. Parazzini and colleagues (1990) reached similar conclusions, as did Ness and coworkers (1999).

Alcohol consumption should be avoided or minimized during pregnancy for many reasons, but alcohol probably contributes little to rate of pregnancy loss. Given the high frequency of alcohol ingestion in the general population, however, even a small effect could have epidemiologic significance. Clinically, women will need to be reassured, especially after inadvertent drinking prior to their realizing they are pregnant.

CONTRACEPTIVE AGENTS

Contraception with an intrauterine device in place clearly increases the risk of fetal loss, and in the second trimester it is especially hazardous. If the device is removed prior to pregnancy, there is no increased risk of spontaneous abortion. Use of oral contraceptives before or during pregnancy is not associated with fetal loss nor is spermicide exposure prior to or after conception (Simpson, 1985; Phillips and Simpson, 2001).

TRAUMA

Women commonly attribute pregnancy losses to trauma, for example, a fall or a blow to the abdomen. However, fetuses are actually well protected from external trauma by intervening maternal structures and amniotic fluid. Any contribution of trauma to early pregnancy loss is quite small.

PSYCHOLOGICAL FACTORS

Impaired psychological well-being has been claimed to predispose to early fetal losses. The first investigations to show a benefit to psychological well-being were those of Stray-Pedersen (1984). One group consisted of 16 pregnant women who had previously experienced repetitive abortions and who received increased attention but no specific medical therapy. They proved more likely (85%) to complete their pregnancies than women (n = 42) who were not provided with such close attention (36% successful outcome). One pitfall was that only women living close to the university were eligible to be placed in the increased attention group. Women living farther away served as "controls" by default, and their differences from the experimental group in ways other than geographic proximity were not excluded from the study. In 811 subsequent couples, the same high success rate (86%) has been observed in women given "tender loving care" (Stray-Pedersen, 2000). Again, the expected background in this series is uncertain, making it difficult to assess significance. Other studies have also reported a beneficial effect of natural psychological well-being (Houwert-de Jong et al., 1989; Liddell et al., 1991; Rai and Regan, 1995; Bergant et al., 1997).

The biologic explanation for any salutary effect remains obscure. Unanswered is whether the ostensible positive effect of psychological well-being is real or secondary to other factors.

Confounding factors were not taken into account, making it difficult to determine if the outcome was truly better than the expected background rate of 70%. Given that no ostensible harm is caused, psychological support can be recommended but not at the expense of eschewing other potential causes.

SEVERE MATERNAL ILLNESS

Many symptomatic maternal diseases causing early pregnancy loss show increased frequency of spontaneous abortion. Potential confounding variables have been assessed in few disorders other than diabetes mellitus. Nonetheless, Wilson disease, phenylketonuria, cyanotic heart disease, hemoglobinopathies, and inflammatory bowel disease seem implicated in early abortion. Not every study claims that a maternal disease is associated with increased fetal loss rates; celiac disease is one example lacking a proven effect (Kolho et al., 1999).

Pathogenesis of losses in these disorders presumably involves one or more of the mechanisms discussed previously, more often endocrinologic or immunologic. Overall, relatively few fetal losses in the general population are the result of severe maternal disease.

ROLE OF OTHER MENDELIAN AND POLYGENIC FACTORS

Recurrence Abortions Due to Mendelian Genes

Consecutive abortuses in a given family usually show nonrandom distribution with respect to chromosomal complements. If the complement of the first abortus is abnormal, the likelihood is approximately 80% that the complement of the second abortus also will be abnormal (Warburton et al., 1987). These data suggest that certain couples are predisposed toward chromosomally abnormal conceptions, most of which result in spontaneous abortions. Genes exerting this effect could act by perturbing spindle formation, centromere stability, recombination, or orderly disjunction of homologues.

The converse is that other couples show repetitive losses of chromosomally normal abortuses. In these cases, mendelian mutations could be causing recurrent euploid losses. Mendelian (single-gene) or polygenic factors could mediate many of the processes alluded to above that cause spontaneous abortion. One obvious example is the alloimmune conditions. These mutations may be common. Recall that 1% of liveborns have an abnormality attributable to a single-gene (mendelian) mutation, whereas another 1% have a polygenic-multifactorial condition. In contrast, only 0.6% have a chromosomal abnormality (Chapter 1). Thus, the 30 to 50% of abortuses with normal chromosomes need not necessarily require explanation by such nongenetic causes as infections, luteal phase insufficiency, or uterine anomalies. These losses might more likely be caused by a mutant gene. The scientific task will be to enumerate the many genes whose perturbations result in pregnancy loss. A host of attractive candidate genes already can be envisioned, such as those in the developmental gene families PAX, HOX, or Oct.

The existence of mutant genes acting in novel fashion and causing spontaneous abortions has already been deduced. An example is the observations of Lanasa and coworkers (1999), Sangha and coworkers (1999), and Nelson and coworkers (2000) that highly skewed X-inactivation is associated with recurrent abortions (Table 5–5). For example, of 48 women having two prior unexplained pregnancy losses, 7 (14.6%) had highly skewed X-inactivation, defined as 90% of X chromosomes originating from one specific parent; only 1 of 67 controls (1.5%) showed skewed X-inactivation) (Lanasa et al., 1999). Kristiansen and colleagues (1999) found less skewed X-inactivation in both aborters and controls and no significant differences.

The most obvious hypothesis is that all male offspring of a woman with skewed X-inactivation would be aborted (male lethals). A pedigree consistent with this idea has been reported (Pegoraro

▼ **Table 5–5.** SKEWED X-INACTIVATION IN REPETITIVE ABORTERS

Study	Aborters	Controls	P-value
Robinson et al., 2001	140 (16%)	111 (5%)	< .01 Chi-square
Lanasa et al., 1999	48 (15%)	67 (1%)	< .01 Fisher's test
Kristiansen et al., 1999	87 (2%)	148 (0.7%)	NS
Nelson et al., 2000	57 (30%)	29 (3%)	< .005 Fisher's test

Definition of skewed X-inactivation was 90% in all studies except for that of Nelson et al. (2000), in which a cut-off of 85% was used.

et al., 1997), but other expectations inherent in this mechanism have not been met (Robinson et al., 2001). Other potential biologic explanations including reduction in precursor nuclei at the time of X-inactivation. In turn, this could result from trisomy mosaicism followed by selection favoring diploid cells or poor early growth in general. In other words, skewed X-inactivation per se may be less likely to cause abortions than to be a surrogate for genetic factors like trisomy mosaicism or mutant-generated X.

RELATIVE PROPORTION OF GENETIC AND NONGENETIC CAUSES OF SPONTANEOUS ABORTIONS

Many potential and plausible explanations for pregnancy losses have been considered. Some authors are fond of offering charts or tables enumerating the proportion of losses resulting from the various causes. In our opinion this is both unwise and naive. Data without confounding variables taken into account can be misleading. In reality cytogenetic and mendelian causes alone probably explain the overwhelming majority of losses. There is little need to invoke nongenetic causes, especially those not mediated by genes.

Doubtless some sporadic and repetitive losses are caused by nongenetic mechanisms either reviewed above as witness the anectodal experience of extraordinary numbers of losses. Success after embryo transfer to a surrogate uterus in a woman with 24 prior abortions suggests a deleterious condition that must not involve the embryo per se (Raziel et al., 2000). Nonetheless, the attributable percentage to "nongenetic" causes is low.

REFERENCES

Acien P: Incidence of müllerian defects in fertile and infertile women. Hum Reprod 12:1372, 1997.

ACOG Practice Opinion: Management of recurrent early pregnancy loss. No. 24, 2000.

Alberman ED: The abortus as a predictor of future trisomy 21. *In* De La Cruz FF, Gerald PS (eds): Trisomy 21 (Down Syndrome). Baltimore: University Park Press, 1981, p 69.

Alberman E, Creasy M, Elliott M, et al.: Maternal factors associated with fetal chromosomal anomalies in spontaneous abortions. Br J Obstet Gynecol 83:621, 1976.

Almeida PA, Bolton VN: The relationship between chromosomal abnormality in the human preimplantation embryo and development *in vitro*. Reprod Fertil Dev 8:235, 1996.

ASRM: A Practice Committee Report: Antiphospholipid antibodies do not affect IVF success, 1999. Birmingham, AL.

Baird DD, Wilcox AJ: Cigarette smoking associated with delayed conception. JAMA 253:2979, 1985.

Balakier H, Cadesky K: The frequency and developmental capability of human embryos containing multinucleated blastomeres. Hum Reprod 12:800, 1997.

Balasch J, Reverter JC, Creus M, et al.: Human reproductive failure is not a clinical feature associated with beta(2) glycoprotein-I antibodies in anticardiolipin and lupus anticoagulant seronegative patients (the antiphospholipid/cofactor syndrome). Hum Reprod 14:1956, 1999.

Balasch J, Reverter JC, Fabregues F, et al.: First-trimester repeated abortion is not associated with activated protein C resistance. Hum Reprod 12:1094, 1997.

Barlow S, Sullivan FM: Reproductive hazards of industrial chemicals: An evaluation of animal and human data. New York: Academic Press, 1982.

Beatty RA: The origin of human triploidy: An integration of qualitative and quantitative evidence. Ann Hum Genet 41:299, 1978.

Benzacken B, Carbillon L, Dupont C, et al.: Lack of submicroscopic rearrangements involving telomeres in reproductive failures. Hum Reprod 17:1154, 2002.

Bergant AM, Reinstadler K, Moncayo HE, et al.: Spontaneous abortion and first and second trimester. Lancet 2:173, 1980.

Boué J, Boué A, Lazar P: Retrospective and prospective epidemiological studies of 1500 karyotyped spontaneous human abortions. Teratology 12:11, 1975.

Boué A, Gallano PA: A collaborative study of the segregation of inherited chromosome structural rearrangements in 1356 prenatal diagnoses. Prenat Diagn 4:45, 1984.

Bongso A, Ng SC, Lim J, et al.: Preimplantation genetics: Chromosomes of fragmented human embryos. Fertil Steril 56:66, 1991.

Branch DW, Ward K: Autoimmunity and pregnancy loss. Semin Reprod Endocrin 7:168, 1989.

Brigham SA, Conlon C, Farquharson RG: A longitudinal study of pregnancy outcome following idiopathic recurrent miscarriage. Hum Reprod 14:2868, 1999.

Bugge M, Collins A, Petersen MB, et al.: Non-disjunction of chromosome 18. Hum Mol Genet 7:661, 1998.

Bussen S, Steck T: Thyroid autoantibodies in euthyroid nonpregnant women with recurrent spontaneous abortions. Hum Reprod 10:2938, 1995.

Bussen S, Sutterlin M, Steck T: Endocrine abnormalities during the follicular phase in women with recurrent spontaneous abortion. Hum Reprod 14:18, 1999.

Byrne J, Nussbaum-Blask A, Taylor WS, et al.: Prevalence of müllerian duct anomalies detected at ultrasound. Am J Med Genet 94:9, 2000.

Candiani GB, Fedele L, Parazzini F, et al.: Reproductive prognosis after abnormal metroplasty in bicornuate or septate uterus: A life table analysis. Br J Obstet Gynecol 97:613, 1990.

Carp HJ, Hass Y, Dolicky M, et al.: The effect of serum follicular phase luteinizing hormone concentrations in habitual abortion: Correlation with results of paternal leukocyte immunization. Hum Reprod 10:1702, 1995.

Carp HJ, Menashe Y, Frenkel Y, et al.: Lupus anticoagulant. Significance in habitual first-trimester abortion. J Reprod Med 38:549, 1993.

Carp H, Toder V, Aviram A, et al.: Karyotype of the abortus in recurrent miscarriage. Fertil Steril 75:678, 2001.

Carp HJA, Toder V, Orgad S, et al.: Karyotype of the abortus in recurrent miscarriage. XVI World Congress of Gynecology and Obstetrics FIGO, International Journal of Obstetrics, Supplement 1, Thursday 70: Abstract, 2000, p 44.

Cashner KA, Christopher CR, Dysert GA: Spontaneous fetal loss after demonstration of a live fetus in the first-trimester. Obstet Gynecol 70:827, 1987.

Castilla EE, Simpson JL, Queenan JT: Down syndrome is not increased in offspring of natural family planning users (case control analysis). Am J Med Genet 59:525, 1995.

Chandley AC: The origin of chromosome aberrations in man and their potential for survival and reproduction in the adult human populations. Ann Genet 24:5, 1981.

Christiaens GC, Stoutenbeek P: Spontaneous abortion in proven intact pregnancies. Lancet 2:571, 1984.

Christiansen OB, Mathiesen O, Lauritsen JG, et al.: Idiopathic recurrent spontaneous abortion: Evidence of familial predisposition. Acta Obstet Gynecol Scand 69:597, 1990.

Clark DA, Coulam CB, Daya S: Unexplained sporadic and recurrent miscarriage in the new millenium: A critical analysis of immune mechanisms and treatments. Hum Reprod Update 7:501, 2001.

Clarke GN, Baker HW: Lack of association between sperm antibodies and recurrent spontaneous abortion. Fertil Steril 59:463, 1993.

Clifford K, Rai R, Watson H, et al.: Does suppressing luteinising hormone secretion reduce the miscarriage rate? Results of a randomised controlled trial. BMJ 312:1508, 1996.

Coonen E, Dumoulin JCM, Derhaag JG, et al.: Genetic make-up of human embryos grown in vitro until the blastocyst state. Hum Reprod 15:P-212, 2000.

Coulam CB: Immunologic tests in the evaluation of reproductive disorders: A critical review. Am J Obstet Gynecol 167:1844, 1992.

Coumans AB, Huijgens PC, Jakobs C, et al.: Haemostatic and metabolic abnormalities in women with unexplained recurrent abortion. Hum Reprod 14:211, 1999.

Cowchock S: Autoantibodies and pregnancy wastage. Am J Reprod Immunol 26:38, 1991.

Daniel A, Hook EB, Wulf G: Risks of unbalanced progeny at amniocentesis to carriers of chromosome rearrangements: Data from United States and Canadian Laboratories. Am J Med Genet 33:14, 1989.

Davis OK, Berkeley AS, Naus GJ, et al.: The incidence of luteal phase defect in normal, fertile women, determined by serial endometrial biopsies. Fertil Steril 51:582, 1989.

Daya S, Ward S: Diagnostic test properties of serum progesterone in the evaluation of luteal phase defects. Fertil Steril 49:168, 1988.

Daya S, Ward S, Burrows E: Progesterone profiles in luteal phase defect cycles and outcome of progesterone treatment in patients with recurrent spontaneous abortions. Am J Obstet Gynecol 158:225, 1988.

De Braekeleer M, Dao TN: Cytogenetic studies in couples experiencing repeated pregnancy losses. Hum Reprod 5:519, 1990.

Delhanty JD, Harper JC, Ao A, et al.: Multicolour FISH detects frequent chromosomal mosaicism and chaotic division in normal preimplantation embryos from fertile patients. Hum Genet 99:755, 1997.

Dizon-Townson DS, Kinney S, Branch DW, et al.: The factor V Leiden mutation is not a common cause of recurrent miscarriage. J Reprod Immunol 34:217, 1997.

Donders GG, Van Bulck B, Caudron J, et al.: Relationship of bacterial vaginosis and Mycoplasmas to the risk of spontaneous abortion. Am J Obstet Gynecol 183:431, 2000.

Egbase PE, Al Sharhan M, Diejomaoh M, et al.: Antiphospholipid antibodies in infertile couples with two consecutive miscarriages after in-vitro fertilization and embryo transfer. Hum Reprod 14:1483, 1999.

Egozcue J, Blanco J, Vidal F: Chromosome studies in human sperm nuclei using fluorescence in-situ hybridization (FISH). Hum Reprod Update 3:441, 1997.

el-Ridi AM, Nada SM, Aly AS, et al.: Toxoplasmosis and pregnancy: An analytical study in Zagazig, Egypt. J Egypt Soc Parasitol 21:81, 1991.

Ergolu GE, Scopelitis E: Antinuclear and antiphospholipid antibodies in healthy women with recurrent spontaneous abortion. Am J Reprod Immunol 31:1, 1994.

Erguven S, Asar G, Gulmezoglu AM, et al.: Antisperm and anticardiolipin antibodies in recurrent abortions. Mikrobiyol Bul 24:1, 1990.

Fan YS, Zhang Y: Subtelomeric translocations are not a frequent cause of recurrent miscarriages. Am J Med Genet 109:154, 2002.

Feliciani E, Ferraretti AP, Gerin F, et al.: PGD for aneuploidy as a tool to avoid the need of transferring more than two embryos. Hum Reprod 15:P-219, 2000.

Ferraretti AP, Gianaroli L, Magli MC, et al.: The impact of preimplantation genetic diagnosis for aneuploidy on the implantation and abortion rates in patients over 37 years old. Hum Reprod 14:O-180, 1999.

Fija-Talamanaca I, Settimi L: Occupational factors and reproductive outcome. In Hafez ESE (ed): Spontaneous Abortion. Lancaster, PA: MTP Press, 1984, p 61.

Fisher JM, Harvey JF, Morton NE, et al.: Trisomy 18: Studies of the parent and cell division of origin and the effect of aberrant recombination on nondisjunction. Am J Hum Genet 56:669, 1995.

Fraser EJ, Grimes DA, Schulz KF: Immunization as therapy for recurrent spontaneous abortion: A review and meta-analysis. Obstet Gynecol 82:854, 1993.

Fritz B, Hallermann C, Olert J, et al.: Cytogenetic analyses of culture failures by comparative genomic hybridisation (CGH): Re-evaluation of chromosome aberration rates in early spontaneous abortions. Eur J Hum Genet 9:539, 2001.

Gardner RJM, Sutherland GR: Chromosome abnormalities and genetic counselling. New York: Oxford University Press, 1996.

Gilmore DH, McNay MB: Spontaneous fetal loss rate in early pregnancy. Lancet 1:107, 1985.

Glinoer D, Soto MF, Bourdoux P, et al.: Pregnancy in patients with mild thyroid abnormalities: Maternal and neonatal repercussions. J Clin Endocrinol Metab 73:421, 1991.

Golan A, Langer R, Neuman M, et al.: Obstetric outcome in women with congenital uterine malformations. J Reprod Med 37:233, 1992.

Grandone E, Margaglione M, Colaizzo D, et al.: factor V Leiden is associated with repeated and recurrent unexplained fetal losses. Thromb Haemost 77:822, 1997.

Gray RH, Simpson JL, Kambic RT, et al.: Timing of conception and the risk of spontaneous abortion among pregnancies occurring during the use of natural family planning. Am J Obstet Gynecol 172:1567, 1995.

Gray RH, Wu LY: Subfertility and risk of spontaneous abortion. Am J Public Health 90:1452, 2000.

Grimbizis GF, Camus M, Tarlatzis BC, et al.: Clinical implications of uterine malformations and hysteroscopic treatment results. Hum Reprod Update 7:161, 2001.

Gronroos M, Honkonen E, Terho P, et al.: Cervical and serum IgA and serum IgG antibodies to Chlamydia trachomatis and herpes simplex virus in threatened abortion: A prospective study. Br J Obstet Gynaecol 90:167, 1983.

Gropp A: Chromosomal animal model of human disease. Fetal trisomy and development failure. In Berry L, Poswillo DE (eds): Teratology. Berlin: Springer-Verlag, 1975, p 17.

Grossman M, Giménez C, Calafell JM, et al.: Mosaicism evaluation by FISH in normally fertilized and normally developing human embryos. Hum Reprod 14:O-O77, 1999.

Guerneri S, Bettio D, Simoni G, et al.: Prevalence and distribution of chromosome abnormalities in a sample of first trimester internal abortions. Hum Reprod 8:735, 1987.

Haas GGJ, Kubota K, Quebbeman JF, et al.: Circulating antisperm antibodies in recurrently aborting women. Fertil Steril 45:209, 1986.

Hakim RB, Gray RH, Zacur H: Infertility and early pregnancy loss. Am J Obstet Gynecol 172:1510, 1995.

Halmesmäki E, Valimaki M, Roine R, et al.: Maternal and paternal alcohol consumption and miscarriage. Br J Obstet Gynecol 96:188, 1989.

Harlap S, Shiono PH: Alcohol, smoking and incidence of spontaneous abortions in the psychosomatics. A prospective study on the impact of psychological factors as a cause for recurrent spontaneous abortion. Hum Reprod 12:1106, 1997.

Hassold TJ: Nondisjunction in the human male. Curr Top Dev Biol 37:383, 1998.

Hassold T: A cytogenetic study of repeated spontaneous abortions. Am J Hum Genet 32:723, 1980.

Hassold T, Abruzzo M, Adkins K, et al.: Human aneuploidy: Incidence, origin, and etiology. Environ Mol Mutagen 28:167, 1996.

Hassold T, Benham F, Leppert M: Cytogenetic and molecular analysis of sex-chromosome monosomy. Am J Hum Genet 42:534, 1988.

Hassold T, Benham F, Leppert M: Cytogenetic and molecular analysis of sex chromosome monosomy. Am J Hum Genet 42:534, 1985.

Hassold T, Merrill M, Adkins K, et al.: Recombination and maternal age-dependent nondisjunction: Molecular studies of trisomy 16. Am J Hum Genet 57:867, 1995.

Hassold TJ, Sherman SL, Pettay D, et al.: XY chromosome nondisjunction in man is associated with diminished recombination in the pseudoautosomal region. Am J Hum Genet 49:253, 1991.

Hay PE, Lamont RF, Taylor-Robinson D, et al.: Abnormal bacterial colonisation of the genital tract and subsequent preterm delivery and late miscarriage. BMJ 308:295, 1994.

Henderson SA, Edwards RG: Chiasma frequency and maternal age in mammals. Nature 217:22, 1968.

Henderson DJ, Sherman LS, Loughna SC, et al: Early embryonic failure associated with uniparental disomy for human chromosome 21. Hum Molec Genet 3:1373, 1994.

Hertig AT, Rock J: Searching for early fertilized human ova. Gynecol Invest 4:121, 1973.

Hertig AT, Rock J, Adams EC, et al.: Thirty-four fertilized human ova, good, bad and indifferent, recovered from 210 women of known fertility. A study of biologic wastage in early human pregnancy. Pediatrics 25:202, 1959.

Hertig AT, Rock J, Adams EC: Description of human ova within the first 17 days of development. Am J Anat 98:435, 1956.

Hill JA, Polgar K, Anderson DJ: T-helper and 1-type immunity to trophoblast in women with recurrent spontaneous abortion. JAMA 273:1933, 1995.

Hoesli IM, Walter-Göbel I, Tercanli S, et al.: Spontaneous fetal loss rates in a non-selected population. Am J Med Genet 100:106, 2001.

Houwert-de Jong MH, Termijtelen A, et al.: The natural course of habitual abortion. Eur J Obstet Gynecol Reprod Biol 33:221, 1989.

Jirásek JE: Principle of reproductive embryology. In Simpson JL (ed): Disorders of Sex Differentiation: Etiology and Clinical Delineation. New York: Academic Press, 1976, p 51.

Johnson MP, Drugan A, Koppitch F, et al.: Postmortem chorionic villi sampling is a better method of cytogenetic evaluation of early fetal loss than culture of abortous material. Am J Obstet Gynecol 163:1505, 1990.

Kalousek DK: Pathology of abortion: Chromosome anomalies and genetic correlations. In Kraus FT, Damjanov I, Kaufman N (eds): Pathology and reproductive failure. Baltimore: Williams and Wilkins, 1991, p 228.

Karamardian LM, Grimes DA: Luteal phase deficiency: Effect of treatment on pregnancy rates. Am J Obstet Gynecol 167:1391, 1992.

Kligman I, Benadiva C, Alikani M, et al.: The presence of multinucleated blastomeres in human embryos is correlated with chromosomal abnormalities. Hum Reprod 11:1492, 1996.

Kline J, Shrout P, Stein Z, et al.: Drinking during pregnancy and spontaneous abortion. Lancet 2:176, 1980.

Knight SJL, Fling J: Perfect endings: a review of subtelomeric probes and their use in clinical diagnosis. J Med Genet 37:401, 2000.

Kocak I, Aksoy E, Ustun C: Recurrent spontaneous abortion and selenium deficiency. Intl J Gynaecol Obstet 65:79, 1999.

Koehler KE, Boulton CL, Collins HE, et al.: Spontaneous X chromosome MI and MII nondisjunction events in Drosophila melanogaster oocytes have different recombinational histories. Nat Genet 14:406, 1996.

Kolho KL, Tiitinen A, Tulppala M, et al.: Screening for coeliac disease in women with a history of recurrent miscarriage or infertility. Br J Obstet Gynaecol 106:171, 1999.

Kristiansen M, Knudsen GP, Hagen C, et al.: X inactivation pattern in females with recurrent spontaneous abortions. International symposium on X-chromosome inactivation in mammals. Novosibirsk, Russia; September 6–12, 1999.

Kuliev A, Cieslak J, Ilkevitch Y, et al: Nuclear abnormalities in a series of 6733 human oocytes. Reprod BioMed Online 4:(Suppl)11, 2002. (Abstract)

Kundsin RB, Driscoll SG, Ming PL: Strain of mycoplasma associated with human reproductive failure. Science 157:1573, 1967.

Kundsin RB, Driscoll SG, Pelletier PA: Ureaplasma urealyticum incriminated in perinatal morbidity and mortality. Science 213:474, 1981.

Kutteh WH, Park VM, Deitcher SR: Hypercoagulable state mutation analysis in white patients with early first-trimester recurrent pregnancy loss. Fertil Steril 71:1048, 1999.

Laitinen T, Koskimies S, Westman P: Foeto-maternal compatibility in HLA-DR, -DQ, and -DP loci in Finnish couples suffering from recurrent spontaneous abortions. Eur J Immunol 20:249, 1993.

Lamb NE, Freeman SB, Savage-Austin A, et al.: Susceptible chiasmate configurations of chromosome 21 predispose to non-disjunction in both maternal meiosis I and meiosis II. Nat Genet 14:400, 1996.

Lanasa MC, Hogge WA, Kubik C, et al.: Highly skewed X-chromosome inactivation is associated with idiopathic recurrent spontaneous abortion. Am J Hum Genet 65:252, 1999.

Levin AA, Schoenbaum SC, Monson RR, et al.: The association of induced abortion with subsequent pregnancy loss. JAMA 243:2495, 1980.

Li TC: Guides for practitioners. Recurrent miscarriage: Principles of management. Hum Reprod 13:478, 1998.

Li TC, Ding S-H, Anstie B, et al.: Use of human menopausal gonadotropins in the treatment of endometrial defects associated with recurrent miscarriage: Preliminary report. Fertil Steril 75:434, 2001.

Li TC, Dockery P, Rogers AW, et al.: How precise is histologic dating of endometrium using the standard dating criteria? Fertil Steril 51:759, 1989.

Li TC, Spuijbroek MD, Tuckerman E, et al.: Endocrinology and endometrial factors in recurrent miscarriage. Br J Obstet Gynaecol 107:1471, 2000.

Li TC, Tuckerman EM, Laird SM: Endometrial factors in recurrent miscarriage. Hum Reprod Update 8:1:43, 2002.

Liddell HS, Pattison NS, Zanderigo A: Recurrent miscarriage—outcome after supportive care in early pregnancy. Aust N Z J Obstet Gynaecol 31:320, 1991.

Linn S, Schoenbaum SC, Monson RR, et al.: The relationship between induced abortion and outcome of subsequent pregnancies. Am J Obstet Gynecol 146:136, 1983.

Liu HC, Rosenwaks Z: Early pregnancy wastage in IVF (in vitro fertilization) patients. J In Vitro Fert Embryo Transf 8:65, 1991.

Ludmir J, Stubblefield PG: Surgical procedures in pregnancy. In Gabbe SG, Niebyl JR, Simpson JL (eds): Obstetrics: Normal and Problem Pregnancies, 4th ed. Edinburgh: Churchill Livingstone, 2001, p 607.

Lumley J: The association between spontaneous abortion, prior induced abortion and preterm birth in first singleton births. Prenat Neonat Med 3:21, 1998.

MacDonald M, Hassold T, Harvey J, et al.: The origin of 47,XXX and 47,XXX aneuploidy: Heterogeneous mechanisms and role of aberrant recombination. Hum Mol Genet 3:1365, 1994.

McGregor JA, French JI, Parker R, et al.: Prevention of premature birth by screening and treatment for common genital tract infections: Results of a prospective controlled evaluation. Am J Obstet Gynecol 173:157, 1995.

Makino T, Sakai A, Sugi T, et al.: Current comprehensive therapy of habitual abortion. Ann NY Acad Sci 626:597, 1991.

Marquez C, Sandalinas M, Bahce M, et al.: Chromosome abnormalities in 1255 cleavage-stage human embryos. Reprod BioMed 1:17, 2000.

Martin R: Chromosomal analysis of human spermatozoa. In Verlinsky Y, Kuliev A (eds): New York: Plenum Press, 1991, p 91.

Meldrum DR: Blastocyst transfer—a natural evolution. Fertil Steril 72:216, 1999.

Michalas SP: Outcome of pregnancy in women with uterine malformation: Evaluation of 62 cases. Int J Gynaecol Obstet 35:215, 1991.

Mills JS, Simpson JL, Driscoll SG, et al.: NICHD-DIEP Study: Incidence of spontaneous abortion among normal women with insulin-dependent diabetic women whose pregnancies were identified within 21 days of conception. N Engl J Med 319:1617, 1988.

Mills JL, Holmes L, Aarons JH, et al.: Moderate caffeine use and the risk of spontaneous abortion and intrauterine growth retardation. JAMA 269:593, 1993.

Miodovnik M, Mimouni F, Tsang RC, et al.: Glycemic control and spontaneous abortion in insulin dependent diabetic women. Obstet Gynecol 68:366, 1986.

Mishell DR: Recurrent abortion. J Reprod Med 38:250, 1993.

Montoro M, Collea JV, Frasier SD, et al.: Successful outcome of pregnancy in women with hypothyroidism. Ann Intern Med 94:31, 1981.

Moutos DM, Damewood MD, Schlaff WD, et al.: A comparison of the reproductive outcome between women with a unicornuate uterus and women with a didelphic uterus. Fertil Steril 58:88, 1992.

Mowbray JF, Gibbings C, Liddell H, et al.: Controlled trial of treatment of recurrent spontaneous abortion by immunization with paternal cells. Lancet 941:941, 1985.

Munné S, Alikani M, Cohen J: Monospermic polyploidy and atypical embryo morphology. J Hum Reprod 9:506, 1994.

Munné S, Alikani M, Tomkin G, et al.: Embryo morphology, developmental rates, and maternal age are correlated with chromosome abnormalities. Fertil Steril 64:382, 1995.

Munné S, Cohen J: Chromosome abnormalities in human embryos. Hum Reprod Update 4:842, 1998.

Munné S, Magli C, Cohen J, et al.: Positive outcome after preimplantation diagnosis of aneuploidy in human embryos. Hum Reprod 14:2191, 1999.

Munné S, Sadowy S, Walmsley R, et al.: PGD of aneuploidy for good responder IVF patients. Reprod BioMed Online 4:(Suppl)25, 2002. (Abstract)

Nahmias AJ, Josey WE, Naib ZM, et al.: Perinatal risk associated with maternal genital herpes simplex virus infection. Am J Obstet Gynecol 110:825, 1971.

Nardo LG, Rai R, Backos M: High serum luteinizing hormone and testosterone concentrations do not predict pregnancy outcome in women with recurrent miscarriage. Fertil Steril 77:348, 2002.

Nelson LM, Branch W, Ward K: Highly-skewed X-inactivation patterns are associated with many patients presenting with idiopathic recurrent pregnancy loss. Am J Hum Genet 67:43, 2000.

Ness RB, Grisso JA, Hirschinger N, et al.: Cocaine and tobacco use and the risk of spontaneous abortion. N Engl J Med 340:333, 1999.

Norman DJ, Barry JM, Fischer S: The beneficial effect of pretransplant third-party blood transfusions on allograft rejection in HLA identical sibling kidney transplants. Transplantation 41:125, 1986.

Ober C: Studies of HLA, fertility and mate choice in a human isolate. Hum Reprod Update 5:103, 1999.

Ober C, Hyslop T, Elias S, et al.: Human leukocyte antigen matching and fetal loss: Results of a 10 year prospective study. Hum Reprod 13:33, 1998.

Ober C, Karrison T, Odem RR, et al.: Mononuclear-cell immunisation in prevention of recurrent miscarriages: A randomised trial. Lancet 354:365, 1999.

Ober CL, Martin AO, Simpson JL, et al.: Shared HLA antigens and reproductive performance among Hutterites. Am J Hum Genet 35:994, 1983.

Ober C, Steck T, van der Ven K, et al.: MHC class II compatibility in aborted fetuses and term infants of couples with recurrent spontaneous abortion. J Reprod Immunol 25:195, 1993.

Ogasawara M, Kajiura S, Katano K, et al.: Are serum progesterone levels predictive of recurrent miscarriage in future pregnancies? Fertil Steril 68:806, 1997.

Olliaro P, Regazzetti A, Gorini G, et al.: Chlamydia trachomatis infection in "sine causa" recurrent abortion. Boll Inst Sieroter Milan 70:467, 1991.

Ozcan T, Burki N, Parkash V, et al.: Cytogenetical diagnosis in paraffin-embedded fetoplacental tissue using comparative genomic hybridization. Prenat Diagn 20:41, 2000.

Papadopoulos G, Templeton AA, Fisk N, et al.: The frequency of chromosome anomalies in human preimplantation embryos after in vitro fertilization. Hum Reprod 4:91, 1989.

Parazzini F, Bocciolone L, LaVecchia C, et al.: Maternal and paternal moderate daily alcohol consumption and unexplained miscarriages. Br J Obstet Gynecol 97:618, 1990.

Parazzini F, Chatenoud L, Tozzi L, et al.: Determinants of risk of spontaneous abortions in the first trimester of pregnancy. Epidemiology 8:681, 1997.

Pauer HU, Neesen J, Hinney B, et al.: Factor V Leiden and its relevance in patients with recurrent abortions. Am J Obstet Gynecol 178:629, 1998.

Paukku M, Tulppala M, Puolakkainen M, et al.: Lack of association between serum antibodies to Chlamydia trachomatis and a history of recurrent pregnancy loss. Fertil Steril 72:427, 1999.

Pegoraro E, Whitaker J, Mowery-Rushton P, et al.: Familial skewed X inactivation: A molecular trait associated with high spontaneous-abortion rate maps to Xq28. Am J Hum Genet 61:160, 1997.

Pellestor F, Dufour MC, Arnal F, et al.: Direct assessment of the rate of chromosomal abnormalities in grade IV human embryos produced by in-vitro fertilization procedure. Hum Reprod 9:293, 1994.

Petri M, Golbus M, Anderson R, et al.: Antinuclear antibody, lupus anticoagulant and anticardiolipin antibody in women with idiopathic habitual abortion. A controlled, prospective study of forty-four women. Arthritis Rheum 30:601, 1987.

Pettenati MJ, Rao PN, Phelan MC, et al.: Paracentric inversions in humans: A review of 446 paracentric inversions with presentation of 120 new cases. Am J Med Genet 55:171, 1995.

Phillips OP, Simpson JL: Contraception and congenital malformations. In Sciarra JJ (ed): Gynecology and Obstetrics, Vol. VI. Philadelphia: Lippincott Williams and Wilkins, 2001, pp 1–21.

Phung Thi Tho PT, Byrd JR, McDonough PG: Etiologies and subsequent reproductive performance of 100 couples with recurrent abortion. Fertil Steril 32:389, 1979.

Plachot M: Genetics of human oocytes. In Boutaleb Y, Gzouli A (eds): New concepts Reproduction. Lanes, England: Parthenon 88:36, 1992.

Plachot M, Junca AM, Mandelbaum J, et al.: Chromosome investigations in early life. II. Human preimplantation embryos. Hum Reprod 2:29, 1987.

Pratt DE, Kaberlein G, Dudkiewicz A: The association of antithyroid antibodies in euthyroid nonpregnant women with recurrent first trimester abortions in the next pregnancy. Fertil Steril 60:1001, 1993a.

Pratt DE, Novotny M, Kaberlein G, et al.: Antithyroid antibodies and the association with non-organ-specific antibodies in recurrent pregnancy loss. Am J Obstet Gynecol 168:837, 1993b.

Preston FE, Rosendaal FR, Walker ID, et al.: Increased fetal loss in women with heritable thrombophilia. Lancet 348:913, 1996.

Quenby SM, Farquharson RG: Predicting recurring miscarriage: What is important? Obstet Gynecol 82:132, 1993.

Quinn PA, Petric M, Barkin M, et al.: Prevalence of antibody to Chlamydia trachomatis in spontaneous abortion and infertility. Am J Obstet Gynecol 156:291, 1987.

Rachootin P, Olsen J: Prevalence and socioeconomic correlates of subfecundity and spontaneous abortion in Denmark. Int J Epidemiology 11:245, 1982.

Rae R, Smith IW, Liston WA, et al.: Chlamydial serologic studies and recurrent spontaneous abortion. Am J Obstet Gynecol 170:782, 1994.

Raga F, Bauset C, Remohi J, et al.: Reproductive impact of congenital müllerian anomalies. Hum Reprod 12:2277, 1997.

Raghupathy R: Th1-type immunity is incompatible with successful pregnancy. Immunol Today 18:478, 1997.

Rai R, Backos M, Chilcott I, et al.: Prospective outcome of untreated pregnancies amongst women with the factor V Leiden genotype and recurrent miscarriages. Hum Reprod 14:O-037, 1999b.

Rai R, Backos M, Rushworth F, et al.: Polycystic ovaries and recurrent miscarriage—a reappraisal. Hum Reprod 15:612, 2000.

Rai R, Chilcott I, Backos M, et al.: Prevalence of factor V Leiden genotype amongst 785 consecutive women with recurrent miscarriage. Hum Reprod 14:O-130, 1999a.

Rai R, Chilcott I, Tuddenham E, et al.: Computerized thromboelastographic parameters amongst women with recurrent miscarriage—evidence for a pro-thrombotic state. Hum Reprod 14:O-132, 1999c.

Rai R, Regan L, Hadley E, et al.: Second-trimester pregnancy loss is associated with activated C resistance. Br J Haematol 92:489, 1996.

Rai CK, Regan L: Future pregnancy outcome in women with unexplained recurrent miscarriage. Hum Reprod 10:19, 1995.

Rai R, Shlebak A, Cohen H, et al.: Factor V Leiden and acquired activated protein C resistance among 1000 women with recurrent miscarriage. Hum Reprod 16:961, 2001.

Raziel A, Friedler S, Schachter M, et al.: Successful pregnancy after 24 consecutive fetal losses: Lessons learned from surrogacy. Fertil Steril 74:104, 2000.

Recurrent Miscarriage Immunotherapy Trialist Group: Worldwide collaborative observational study and meta-analysis on allogenic leukocyte immunotherapy for recurrent spontaneous abortion. Am J Reprod Immunol 32:55, 1994.

Reddy KS: Double trisomy in spontaneous abortions. Hum Genet 101:339, 1997

Regan L, Braude PR, Trembath PL: Influence of post reproductive performance on risk of spontaneous abortion. Br Med J 299:541, 1989.

Regan L, Owen EJ, Jacobs HS: Hypersecretion of luteinising hormone, infertility, and miscarriage. Lancet 336:1141, 1990.

Regan L, Rai R, Backos M, et al.: Recurrent miscarriage and parental karyotype abnormalities: Prevalence and future pregnancy outcome. Hum Reprod 16:O-177, 2001.

Ridker PM, Miletich JP, Buring JE, et al.: Factor V Leiden mutation as a risk factor for recurrent pregnancy loss. Ann Intern Med 128:1000, 1998.

Robinson WP, Beever C, Brown CJ, et al.: Skewed X-inactivation and recurrent spontaneous abortion. Semin Reprod Med 19:175, 2001.

Robinson WP, Kuchinka BD, Bernasconi F, et al.: Maternal meiosis I non-disjunction of chromosome 15: Dependence of the maternal age effect on level of recombination. Hum Mol Genet 7:1011, 1998.

Rubio C, Vidal F, Mínguez Y, et al.: High incidence of chromosomal abnormalities in preimplantation embryos from recurrent spontaneous abortion patients. Hum Reprod 15:O-203, 2000.

Rushworth FH, Backos M, Rai R, et al.: Prospective pregnancy outcome in untreated recurrent miscarriers with thyroid autoantibodies. Hum Reprod 15:1637, 2000.

Sadowy S, Tomkin G, Munné S, et al.: Impaired development of zygotes with uneven pronuclear size. Zygote 6:137, 1998.

Sagle M, Bishop K, Ridley N, et al.: Recurrent early miscarriage and polycystic ovaries. Br Med J 297:1027, 1988.

Sahwi SY, Zaki MS, Haiba NY, et al.: Toxoplasmosis as a cause of repeated abortion. J Obstet Gynaecol 21:145, 1995.

Sánchez JM, Franzi L, Collia F, et al.: Cytogenetic study of spontaneous abortions by transabdominal villus sampling and direct analysis of villi. Prenat Diagn 19:601, 1999.

Sandalinas M, Sadowy S, Calderon G, et al.: Survival of chromosomal abnormalities to blastocyst stage. Hum Reprod 15:O-027, 2000.

Sangha KK, Stephenson MD, Brown CJ, et al.: Extremely skewed X chromosome-inactivation is increased in women with recurrent spontaneous abortion. Am J Hum Genet 65:913, 1999.

Sarig G, Younis JS, Hoffman R: Thrombophilia is common in women with idiopathic pregnancy loss and is associated with late pregnancy wastage. Fertil Steril 77:342, 2002.

Savage AR, Petersen MB, Pettay D, et al.: Elucidating the mechanisms of paternal non-disjunction of chromosome 21 in humans. Hum Mol Genet 7:1221, 1998.

Savitz DA, Sonnenfeld NL, Olshan AF: Review of epidemiologic studies of paternal occupational exposure and spontaneous abortion. Am J Ind Med 25:361, 1994.

Schmidt-Sarosi C, Schwartz LB, Lublin J, et al.: Chromosomal analysis of early fetal losses in relation to transvaginal ultrasonographic detection of fetal heart motion after infertility. Fertil Steril 69:274, 1998.

Scialli AR, Lione A, Padgett GK: Reproductive effects of chemical, physical, and biologic agents: Reprotox. Baltimore: The Johns Hopkins University Press, 1995.

Scott JR, Rote NS, Branch DW: Immunologic aspects of recurrent abortions and fetal death. Obstet Gynecol 70:645, 1987.

Scott RT, Synder RR, Strickland DM, et al.: The effect of interobserver variation in dating endometrial histology on the diagnosis of luteal phase defects. Fertil Steril 50:888, 1988.

Shaffer LG, McCaskill C, Adkins K, et al.: Systematic search for uniparental disomy in early fetal losses: The results and a review of the literature. Am J Med Genet 79:366, 1998.

Shepard TH: Catalog of teratogenic agents, 9th ed. Baltimore: The Johns Hopkins University Press, 1998.

Shim SH, Lee CH, Park YJ, et al.: Two inv dup(15) chromosomes in a woman with repeated abortions. Am J Med Genet 104:303, 2001.

Simon C, Martinez L, Pardo F, et al.: Müllerian defects in women with normal reproductive outcome, Fertil Steril 56:1192, 1991.

Simpson JL: PGD as part of pre-pregnancy genetic screening. Reprod BioMed Online 4:(Suppl)10, 2002. (Abstract)

Simpson JL: Ovarian maintenance determinants on the X chromosome and on autosomes. In Coutifaris C, Mastroianni L (eds): New Horizons in Reproductive Medicine. (Proceedings of the Ninth World Congress on Human Reproduction, Philadelphia, 1996). New York: Parthenon, 1997a, p 439.

Simpson JL: Genetics of oocyte depletion. In Lobo RA (ed): Perimenopause. Norwell, Mass: Springer, and New York: Serono Symposia USA, 1997b, p 36.

Simpson JL: Pregnancies in women with chromosomal abnormalities. In Shulman JD, Simpson JL (eds): Genetic Diseases In Pregnancy. New York: Academic Press, 1981, p 439.

Simpson JL: Relationship between congenital anomalies and contraception. Adv Contracept 1:3, 1985.

Simpson JL, Bombard AT: Chromosomal abnormalities in spontaneous abortion: Frequency, pathology and genetic counseling. In Edmonds K, Bennett MJ (eds): Spontaneous Abortion. London: Blackwell, 1987, p 51.

Simpson JL, Carson SA: Causes of fetal loss. In Gray R, Leridon L, Spira F (eds): Symposium on Biological and Demographic Determinants of Human Reproductio. NewYork: Oxford Press, 1993, p 287.

Simpson JL, Carson SA, Chesney C, et al.: Lack of association between antiphospholipid antibodies and first-trimester spontaneous abortion: Prospective study of pregnancies detected within 21 days of conception. Fertil Steril 69:814, 1998.

Simpson JL, Carson SA, Mills JL, et al.: Prospective study showing that antisperm antibodies are not associated with pregnancy losses. Fertil Steril 66:36, 1996.

Simpson JL, Gray R, Perez A, et al.: Fertilisation involving ageing gametes, major birth defects, and Down Syndrome. Lancet 359:1670, 2002.

Simpson JL, Gray RH, Queenan JT, et al.: Risk of recurrent spontaneous abortion for pregnancies discovered in the fifth week of gestation. Lancet 344:964, 1994.

Simpson JL, Gray RH, Queenan JT, et al.: Pregnancy outcome associated with natural family planning (NFP): Scientific basis and experimental design for an international cohort study. Adv Contracept 4:247, 1988.

Simpson JL, Meyers CM, Martin AO, et al.: Translocations are infrequent among couples having repeated spontaneous abortions but no other abnormal pregnancies. Fertil Steril 51:811, 1989.

Simpson JL, Mills JL, Holmes LB, et al.: Low fetal loss rate after ultrasound-proven viability in early pregnancy. JAMA 258:2555, 1987.

Simpson JL, Mills JL, Kim H, et al.: Infectious processes: An infrequent cause of first trimester spontaneous abortions. Hum Reprod 11:668, 1996.

Singh RJ, Carr DH: The anatomy and histology of XO embryos and fetuses. Anat Rec 155:369, 1966.

Singh A, Dantas ZN, Stone SC, et al.: Presence of thyroid antibodies in early reproductive failure. Biochemical versus clinical pregnancies. Fertil Steril 63:277, 1995.

Snijders RJ, Sundberg K, Holzgreve W, et al.: Maternal age and gestation-specific risk for trisomy 21: Effect of previous affected pregnancy. Ultrasound Obstet Gynecol, 13:167,1999.

Sompolinsky D, Solomon F, Elkina L, et al.: Infections with Mycoplasma and bacteria in induced midtrimester abortion and fetal loss. Am J Obstet Gynecol 121:610, 1975.

Sorokin Y, Johnson MP, Uhlmann WR, et al.: Postmortem chorionic villus sampling: Correlation of cytogenetic and ultrasound findings. Am J Med Genet 39:314, 1991.

Soules MR, Clifton DK, Cohen NL, et al.: Luteal phase deficiency: Abnormal gonadotropin and progesterone secretion patterns. J Clin Endocrinol Metab 69:813, 1989a.

Soules MR, McLachlan RI, Ek M, et al.: Luteal phase deficiency: Characterization of reproductive hormones over the menstrual cycle. J Clin Endocrinol Metab 69:804, 1989b.

Soules MR, Wiebe RH, Aksel S, et al.: The diagnosis and therapy of luteal phase deficiency. Fertil Steril 28:1033, 1977.

Souza SS, Ferriani RA, Pontes AG, et al.: Factor V leiden and factor II G20210A mutations in patients with recurrent abortion. Hum Reprod 14:2448, 1999.

Staessen C, Van Steirteghem AC: The chromosomal constitution of embryos developing from abnormally fertilized oocytes after intracytoplasmic sperm injection and conventional in-vitro fertilization. Hum Reprod 12:321, 1997.

Stagnaro-Green A, Roman SH, Cobin RH, et al.: Detection of at-risk pregnancy by means of highly sensitive assays for thyroid autoantibodies. JAMA 264:1422, 1990.

Stampe-Sorensen S: Estimated prevalence of müllerian anomalies. Acta Obstet Gynecol Scand 67:441, 1988.

Stein AL, March CM: Pregnancy outcome in women with müllerian duct anomalies. J Reprod Med 35:411, 1990.

Stein Z, Kline J, Susser E, et al.: Maternal age and spontaneous abortion. In Porter IH, Hook EB (eds): Human Embryonic and Fetal Death. London: Academic Press, 1980, p 107.

Stern C, Chamley L, Hale L, et al.: Antibodies to beta2 glycoprotein I are associated with in vitro fertilization implantation failure as well as recurrent miscarriage: Results of a prevalence study. Fertil Steril 70:938, 1998.

Sterzik K, Abt M, Grab D, et al.: Predicting the histologic dating of an endometrial biopsy specimen with the use of Doppler ultrasonography and hormone measurements in patients undergoing spontaneous ovulatory cycles. Fertil Steril 73:94, 2000.

Stray-Pedersen B: Psychological aspects. XVI FIGO World Congress of Gynecology and Obstetrics. Internal J Gynecol Obstet. Abstract. Suppl 70:16, 2000.

Stray-Pedersen B, Eng J, Reikvam TM: Uterine T-mycoplasma colonization in reproductive failure. Am J Obstet Gynecol 130:307, 1978.

Stray-Pedersen B, Stray-Pedersen S: Etiologic factors and subsequent reproductive performance in 195 couples with a prior history of habitual abortion. Am J Obstet Gynecol 148:140, 1984.

Strom C, Ginsberg N, Applebaum M, et al.: Analyses of 95 first trimester spontaneous abortions by chorionic villus sampling and karyotype. J Asst Reprod Genet 9:458, 1992.

Sugi T, Katsunuma J, Izumi S, et al.: Prevalence and heterogeneity of antiphosphatidylethanolamine antibodies in patients with recurrent early pregnancy losses. Fertil Steril 71:1060, 1999.

Sutherland GR, Gardiner AJ, Carter RF: Familial pericentric inversion of chromosome 19 inv (19) (p13q13) with a note on genetic counseling of pericentric inversion carriers. Clin Genet 10:54, 1976.

Tietze C: Fertility after discontinuation of intrauterine and oral contraception. Int J Fertil 13:385, 1968.

Topping J, Quenby S, Farquharson R, et al.: Marked variation in antiphospholipid antibodies during pregnancy: Relationships to pregnancy outcome. Hum Reprod 14:224, 1999.

Toth A, Lesser ML, Brooks-Toth CW, et al.: Outcome of subsequent pregnancies following antibiotic therapy after primary or multiple spontaneous abortions. Surg Gynecol Obstet 163:243, 1986.

Tulppala M, Stenman UH, Cacciatore B, et al.: Polycystic ovaries and levels of gonadotrophins and androgens in recurrent miscarriage: Prospective study in 50 women. Br J Obstet Gynaecol 100:348, 1993.

Unfried G, Tempfer C, Schneeberger C, et al.: Interleukin 1 receptor antagonist polymorphism in women with idiopathic recurrent miscarriage. Fertil Steril 75:683, 2001.

U.S. Department of Health and Human Services: Reproductive impairments among married couples. In U.S. Vital and Health Statistics Series 23, No.11. Hyattsville, MD: National Center for Health Statistics, 1982, p 5.

Van Iddekinge B, Hofmeyr GJ: Recurrent spontaneous abortion—aetiological factors and subsequent reproductive performance in 76 couples. S Afr Med J 80:223, 1991.

Verlinsky Y, Cieslak J, Ivakhnenko V, et al.: Chromosomal abnormalities in the first and second polar body. Mol Cell Endocrinol 183:547, 2001.

Vlaanderen W, Treffers PE: Prognosis of subsequent pregnancies after recurrent spontaneous abortion in first trimester. Br Med J 295:92, 1987.

Warburton D: Outcome of cases of de novo structural rearrangements diagnosed at amniocentesis. Prenat Diagn 4:69, 1984.

Warburton D, Byrne J, Canik N: Chromosome anomalies and prenatal development: An atlas. New York: Oxford University Press, 1991.

Warburton D, Fraser FC: Spontaneous abortion risks in man: Data from reproductive histories collected in a medical genetic unit. Am J Hum Genet 16:1, 1964.

Warburton D, Kline J, Stein Z, et al.: Does the karyotype of a spontaneous abortion predict the karyotype of a subsequent abortion? Evidence from 273 women with two karyotyped spontaneous abortions. Am J Hum Genet 41:465, 1987.

Watt JL, Templeton AA, Messinis I, et al.: Trisomy I in an eight cell human pre-embryo. J Med Genet 24:60, 1987.

Wegmann TG, Lin H, Guilbert L, et al.: Bidirectional cytokine interactions in the maternal-fetal relationship: Is successful pregnancy a Th2 phenomenon? Immunol Today 14:353, 1993.

Whitley E, Doyle P, Roman E, et al.: The effect of reproductive history on future pregnancy outcomes. Hum Reprod 14:2863, 1999.

Wilcox AJ, Baird DD, Weinberg CR: Time of implantation of the conceptus and loss of pregnancy. N Engl J Med 340:1796, 1999.

Wilcox AJ, Weinberg CR, O'Connor FJ, et al.: Incidence of early loss of pregnancy. N Engl J Med 319:189, 1988.

Wilson RD, Kendrick V, Wittmann BK, et al.: Risk of spontaneous abortion in ultrasonographically normal pregnancies. Lancet 2:920, 1984.

Witkin SS, Chaudhry A: Association between recurrent spontaneous abortions and circulating IgG antibodies to sperm tails in women. J Reprod Immunol 15:151, 1989.

Witkin SS, Ledger WJ: Antibodies to Chlamydia trachomatis in sera of women with recurrent spontaneous abortions. Am J Obstet Gynecol 167:135, 1992.

Yan JH: Evaluation of circulating antisperm antibodies and seminal immunosuppressive material in repeatedly aborting couples. Zhonghua Fu Chan Ke Za Zhi 25:343–344, 1990.

Yoon PW, Freeman SB, Sherman SL, et al.: Advanced maternal age and the risk of Down syndrome characterized by the meiotic stage of the chromosomal error: A population-based study. Am J Hum Genet 58:628, 1996.

Zaragoza MV, Jacobs PA, James RS: Nondisjunction of human acrocentric chromosomes: Studies of 432 trisomic fetuses and liveborns. Hum Genet 94:411, 1994.

Zavala-Velazquez J, Guzman-Marin E, Barrera-Perez M, et al.: Toxoplasmosis and abortion in patients at the O'Horon Hospital of Merida Yucatan. Salud Publica Mex 31:664, 1989.

Zhang XC: Clinical study on circulating antisperm antibodies in women with recurrent abortion. Zhonghua Fu Chan Ke Za Zhi 25:21, 1990.

CHAPTER 6

Mental Retardation and Multiple Malformation Patterns

Mental retardation represents a static encephalopathy with serious deficits in the cognitive realm (Accardo and Capute, 1994). Children with mental retardation may or may not have associated multiple malformations. In addition, multiple malformation patterns can occur in children without mental retardation as well as in stillborns. If a definitive diagnosis can be made, counseling can be given regarding treatment, prognosis, inheritance, and prenatal diagnosis. However, the obstetrician is often faced with a situation in which a specific diagnosis cannot be established. Under such circumstances genetic counseling must be based on empiric recurrence risks, which may show heritable tendencies (Crow and Tolmie, 1998). Also, obstetricians have a special incentive to become conversant with the topic of genetic influences in mental retardation and cerebral palsy. With the acceptance that intrapartum asphyxia is an infrequent cause of cerebral palsy (Nelson and Ellenberg, 1981, 1985, 1986; Niswander, 1988; ACOG Committee Opinion, 1994), it has become clear that genetic factors are of paramount importance in the etiology of conditions once thought attributable to obstetric factors, particularly *fetal distress* and *birth asphyxia*. It has been estimated that at least 10 to 15% of patients with mental retardation are caused by single-gene mutations (Turner, 1975; Laxova et al. 1977; Opitz, 1977).

Definition, Diagnostic Criteria, and Gradations of Mental Retardation

Intelligence shows continuous gradation with gaussian distribution that is skewed to the lower range. Such a distribution presumably results from the additive effect of many factors, environmental and genetic, each exerting a small influence. This is consistent with polygenic-multifactorial inheritance. According to the American Psychiatric Association (1994), mental retardation refers to substantial limitations in present functioning. It is characterized by significantly subaverage intellectual functioning, existing concurrently with related limitations in two or more of the following applicable adaptive skill areas: communication, self-care, home living, social skills, community use, self-direction, health and safety, functioning academics, leisure, and work. Mental retardation is manifested before age 18. Diagnostic criteria for mental retardation are given in Table 6–1.

Mental retardation consists of a clinically and etiologically heterogeneous group of conditions. A different spectrum of causes may be responsible for mild and moderate retardation than that for moderate or severe retardation (Knight et al., 1999). Many individuals with mild retardation are considered to represent the lower end of the normal distribution for IQ, and psychosocial factors are thought to be of primary etiologic importance. This concept is supported by observations that the IQ of sibs of persons with mild retardation often fall between those of the

▼ **Table 6–1.** DIAGNOSTIC CRITERIA FOR
• MENTAL RETARDATION

1. Significantly subaverage intellectual functioning: an IQ of approximately 70 or below on an individually administered IQ test (for infants, a clinical judgment of significantly subaverage intellectual functioning).
2. Concurrent deficits or impairments in present adaptive functioning (i.e., the person's effectiveness in meeting the standards expected for his or her age by his or her cultural group) in at least two of the following areas: communication, self-care, home living, social-interpersonal skills, use of community resources, self-direction, functional academic skills, work, leisure, health, and safety.
3. The onset is before age 18 years.
   Code based on degree of severity reflecting level of intellectual impairment:
   Mild mental retardation: IQ level 50–55 to approximately 70
   Moderate retardation: IQ level 35–40 to 50–55
   Severe mental retardation: IQ level 20–25 to 35–40
   Profound mental retardation: IQ level below 20 or 25
   Mental retardation, severity unspecified: when there is a strong presumption of mental retardation but the person's intelligence is untestable by standard tests.

From American Psychiatric Association: Diagnostic and Statistical Manual of Mental Disorders: DSM-IV, 4th ed. Washington DC: American Psychiatric Association, 1994.

retarded sibs and that of the population mean. In addition, there is a strong familial and presumably genetic tendency for mild mental retardation. Conversely, there are more individuals than would be expected at the extreme lower end of the curve on the basis of gaussian distribution (Penrose, 1938; Thapar et al., 1994). This excess of those individuals characterized by moderate or severe mental retardation is presumably due to gene mutations, chromosome abnormalities, and major environmental causes, including infections, teratogens, and trauma. In a significant number of retarded people, perhaps 40%, there is no readily apparent explanation.

Epidemiology

Depending on where one draws IQ and adaptive cutoff scores, the number of persons with mental retardation varies widely. The standard view is that approximately 3% of the population has an IQ less than two standard deviations below the mean. An estimated 80 to 90% of mentally retarded individuals function within the mild range, whereas only 5% of the population with mental retardation is severely to profoundly impaired (Shonkoff, 2000). More male than female individuals are found in the mentally retarded population (American Psychiatric

Association, 1994). The male excess has been seen worldwide and averages about 30% (Stevenson et al., 2000). Genes on the X chromosome have been considered responsible for a major part of this excess. Mental retardation is more prevalent among children who are of lower socioeconomic status and who are from disadvantaged minority groups.

GENETIC CAUSES OF MENTAL RETARDATION WITH OR WITHOUT MULTIPLE ANOMALIES

Recognized causes of mental retardation range from well-defined genetic conditions (e.g., Down syndrome) to conditions of clear nongenetic origin. Mental retardation can be congenital but not genetic, as in maternal phenylketonuria, in which biochemically normal fetuses can be adversely affected by the intrauterine environment. Severe mental retardation is more likely to have a genetic cause than is milder retardation (Knight et al., 1999). Approximately 50% of the cases of severe mental retardation are clearly genetic and are caused by single gene or major chromosomal abnormalities; half of the remainder may also have genetic components (Robinson and Linden, 1993; Crow and Tolmie, 1998). Other identifiable causes include encephaloclastic processes, such as infection, hypoxia-ischemia, trauma, and teratogens (e.g., fetal alcohol syndrome). A diagnosis or cause can be identified in 50 to 70% of all patients undergoing evaluation for mental retardation (McQueen et al., 1986; Anderson et al., 1996; Curry et al., 1996).

Chromosome Abnormalities

Chromosome abnormalities account for up to 40% of severe and 10 to 20% of mild mental retardation (Hagberg and Hagberg, 1984; Gostason et al., 1991). Indeed, the most common clinical feature of chromosomal abnormalities is intellectual impairment. Autosomal trisomies invariably cause severe or profound retardation, but some deletion or duplication syndromes may be associated with moderate or even mild retardation (see Chapter 1). The latter are also characteristic of certain sex chromosome polysomies (e.g., 48,XXXY) (see Chapter 11).

Down syndrome (Fig. 6–1) is the most common genetic cause of mental retardation and occurs in approximately 1 in 800 births (see Chapter 5). The genotype-phenotype relationship between Down syndrome and mental retardation

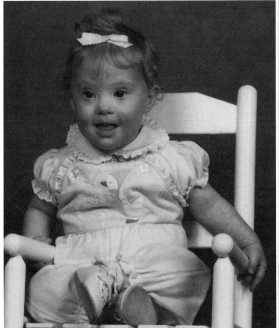
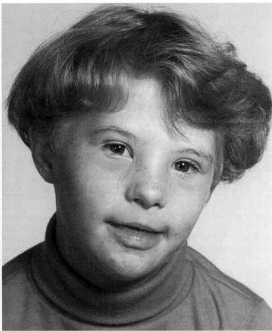

A   B

FIGURE 6–1 • (*A*) An infant with Down syndrome, illustrating typical features of this disorder: upslanting palpebral fissures, redundant skin of the inner eyelid (epicanthic fold), protruding tongue, and low nasal bridge. (*B*) Same girl as in (*A*) 7 years later. (From Jorde LB, Carey JC, Bamshad MJ, et al.: Medical Genetics, 2nd ed. St. Louis: Mosby, 2000.)

is not well understood. It has been known for more than a century that persons with Down syndrome experience a deterioration in memory, problem-solving, language, and adaptive self-care skills beginning in middle life (Brugge et al., 1994). Autopsy studies have documented the neuropathologic stigmata of Alzheimer disease, including senile plaques and neurofibrillary tangles, in the brains of approximately 95% of Down syndrome patients over the age of 40 and virtually all over the age of 50. It is of interest that some cases of familial early-onset Alzheimer disease are associated with mutations in a gene on chromosome 21 that encodes the amyloid precursor protein, a derivative that forms a major constituent of senile plaques (Goate et al., 1991). Those clinical and neuropathologic similarities between Down syndrome and Alzheimer disease suggest that these conditions may share similar genetic and pathophysiologic mechanisms.

In addition to Down syndrome, other chromosome abnormalities are estimated to cause 1 to 5% of cases of mental retardation (Robinson and Linden, 1993). The most common of these are trisomy 18, trisomy 13, 45,X; 47,XXX; 47,XXY; 47,XYY, and changes in chromosome structure such as deletions or translocations (Thapar et al., 1994). Cryptic subtelomeric chromosomal abnormalities have also been recognized as a cause of

mental retardation. Subtelomeric abnormalities occur in 1.9% of patients with idiopathic mental retardation/developmental delay and 4.1% of patients with dysmorphic features and/or malformations in the absence of a recognizable syndrome (Baker et al., 2002).

Contiguous Gene Syndrome

High-resolution chromosome banding and advanced molecular genetic techniques have made it possible to identify smaller, less obvious chromosome abnormalities, such as microdeletions and duplications, which result in an alteration of normal gene dosage. The term *contiguous gene syndrome* (CGS) has been used to describe such chromosome abnormalities that result in specific and complex phenotypes, which were recognized in some cases as a genetic syndrome prior to knowledge of their chromosomal etiology. The chromosomal segments involved in CGS are usually small from a cytogenetic perspective (less than three megabases); however, they involve multiple genes that independently contribute to the phenotype and often involve mental retardation (Fig. 6–2). Flint and coworkers (1995) have estimated that chromosome rearrangements in the telomeric regions (which have a high concentra-

Contiguous Gene Syndromes

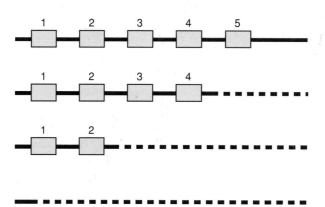

FIGURE 6–2 • A model for the contiguous gene syndromes. The boxes represent five genes that are adjacent to each other but could have unrelated activities. Loss of one of the five genes through a deletion (—) will produce a certain clinical phenotype. This phenotype will progressively become more deleterious as the number of deleted genes increases. An extensive deletion that removes all five genes will produce the complete syndrome. Other phenotypes are possible if interstitial deletions occur (genes 2 and 3). (From Trent RJ: Molecular Medicine and Introductory Text, 2nd ed. New York: Churchill Livingstone, 1997.)

tion of genes and are affected more commonly by chromosomal rearrangements than other part of the genome) cause 6% or more of idiopathic mental retardation. CGS may be caused by deletions of the X chromosome in males, with resulting structural and functional nullisomy or autosomal loci where deletions cause a reduction of gene dosage to structural and functional monosomy (Ledbetter and Ballabio, 1995). The major autosomal and X-linked contiguous gene syndromes are summarized in Table 6–2.

Autosomal Dominant Disorders

Autosomal dominant disorders account for about 5% of severely mentally retarded individuals. Some of the most common of these disorders are summarized in Table 6–3. Such conditions often represent new mutations, as expected (Chapter 2) given the lethality of the resulting phenotype. (The greater the severity, the higher the proportion of cases that result from a new mutation.) For example, in combining data from two etiologic surveys of mentally retarded children, 17 of 21 cases of tuberous sclerosis were found as new mutations (Laxova et al., 1977; Opitz, 1977). This is important for counseling because the recurrence risk would be essentially zero in such cases. To determine if a given condition is a new mutation, the affected person's sibs and parents must be carefully evaluated to exclude minimal expression of the disorder. As discussed in Chapter 2, new autosomal

dominant mutations are associated with advanced paternal age; thus, paternal age should be ascertained at the time of evaluation.

Autosomal Recessive Disorders

Five percent to ten percent of mentally retarded individuals have a known autosomal recessive condition (Turner, 1975). Examples of some of the most common conditions associated with mental retardation include ataxia-telangiectasia (mental deterioration after age 3 to 5, telangiectasia of the sclera, cerebellar ataxia, extrapyramidial signs, immune deficiency, and predisposition to malignancy); Laurence-Moon-Bardet-Biedl syndrome (mental retardation, obesity, hypogonadism, pigmentary retinopathy, and spastic paraplegia); Virchow-Seckel syndrome (mental retardation, short stature, dysmorphic facies); Marinesco-Sjögren syndrome (mental retardation, cerebellar ataxia, cataracts, skeletal abnormalities); and true microcephaly (mental retardation, small cranial vault). Texts by Jones (1997) and other dysmorphologists provide encyclopedic references.

Inborn Errors of Metabolism

The term "inborn errors of metabolism" was first coined by Archibald Garrod in 1902 (Garrod, 1908) to describe lifelong diseases that arise because the genetic deficiency of a specific enzyme causes a block in a normal metabolic

▼ **Table 6–2.** MAJOR CONTIGUOUS GENE SYNDROMES ASSOCIATED WITH MENTAL
• RETARDATION

Clinical Syndrome	Chromosome Location	Phenotypic Features
Langer-Giedion syndrome	del(8q24.1)	Sparse hair, pear-shaped nose, tricho-rhino-phalangeal syndrome, multiple cartilagenous exostosis, ± microcephaly, short stature, lax skin, variable mental retardation (20% normal, 17% retarded, 40% moderately retarded, 14% profoundly retarded)
Miller-Dieker syndrome	del(17p13.3)	Lissencephaly (absent gyri and sulci of the brain), prominent forehead, bitemporal hollowing, short upturned nose, small jaw, profound mental retardation
DiGeorge syndrome and Velocardio-facial syndrome	del(22q11.2)	Absent or hypoplastic thymus and hypoparathyroid glands, cellular immune deficiency, cardiac malformations (interrupted aortic arch or truncus arteriosus), hypertelorism, cleft lip and/or palate, bifid uvula, low-set ears, microcephaly, mild to moderate mental retardation
Smith-Magenis syndrome	del(17p11.2)	Brachycephaly with broad face and nasal bridge, flat midface, mental retardation associated with hyperactivity, and often self-destructive behavior
Alagille syndrome	del(20p11.2-p12)	Intrahepatic biliary hypoplasia with chronic cholestasis, broad forehead, deep-set eyes, mild hypertelorism, bulbous nose, pointed chin, peripheral pulmonary stenosis, vertebral anomalies, ocular embryotoxin, in mild mental retardation
Rubinstein-Taybi syndrome	del(16p13.3)	Microcephaly, broad nasal bridge, beaked or prominent nose, downward slant to palpebral fissures, micrognathia, broad thumbs and toes, moderate to severe mental retardation
Prader-Willi syndrome	del(15q11-q13) (paternal)	Hypotonia, hypogonadism, males with undescended testes, females with hypoplastic labia, hyperphagia leading to obesity (unless caloric intake is restricted) short stature, small hands and feet, almond-shaped palpebral fissures, strabismus, skin and hair hypopigmentation, mild to moderate mental retardation
Angelman syndrome	del(15q11-q13) (maternal)	Seizures, ataxia, wide mouth, protruding tongue, hypopigmentation, prominent jaw, thin upper lip, inappropriate laughter, hand flapping, severe mental retardation
Beckwith-Wiedemann syndrome	dup(11p15.5)	Macroglossia, omphalocele, visceromegaly and gigantism, predisposition to malignancy (Wilms tumor, adrenocortical carcinoma, hepatoblastoma, rhabdomyosarcoma), cryptorchidism in males, bicornuate uterus in females, neonatal polycythemia, diastasis mild to moderate mental retardation (may be secondary to untreated hypoglycemia)
WAGR syndrome	del(11p13)	Wilms tumor or nephroblastoma, aniridia, genitourinary abnormalities (ambiguous genitalia, undescended testes, hypospadia, fused kidneys, gonadoblastoma), hemihypertrophy, growth retardation, mental retardation
X-linked contiguous gene syndrome	Xp22.3	Variable including X-linked steroid sulfatase deficiency with ichthyosis, X-linked recessive chondrodysplasia punctata, Kallman syndrome, ocular albinism type 1, microphthalmia with linear skin defect, X-linked mental retardation
X-linked contiguous gene syndrome	Xq21	Variable including X-linked mixed deafness, hypergonadotropic hypogonadism, choroidpunctata, cleft lip and palate, X-linked mental retardation
X-linked contiguous gene syndrome	Xp21	Variable including dosage-sensitive sex reversal, congenital adrenal hypoplasia, glycerol kinase deficiency, Duchenne muscular dystrophy, McLeod phenotype (absent Kell blood group precursor substance), chronic granulomatous disease, retinitis pigmentosa, ± mental retardation

pathway. Most inborn errors of metabolism are inherited in autosomal recessive fashion. Children with metabolic disorders may appear normal at birth and deteriorate thereafter. Sometimes deterioration occurs in the nursery after feeding (Burton, 1987, 1998). In a few

metabolic disorders, dietary treatment corrects life-threatening neonatal acidosis and alters outcome substantially. Table 6–4 summarizes some autosomal recessive inborn errors of metabolism associated with mental retardation and other phenotypic abnormalities. The preva-

▼ **Table 6–3.**   SELECTED COMMON
• AUTOSOMAL DOMINANT DISORDERS
  ASSOCIATED WITH MENTAL RETARDATION

Disorder	Clinical Features
Neurofibromatosis 1 (NF$_1$)	Café-au-lait spots, central nervous system malformations (heterotopias, hamartomas), skeletal deformities (scoliosis), Lisch nodules of the iris, psychiatric disorders (depression, anxiety disorders), 10-40% mild to moderate mental retardation
Tuberous sclerosis	Adenoma sebaceum, calcified gliotic tumors in cortical and subependymal regions of the brain, shagreen patches and ash leaf depigmentation of the skin, periungual fibromas, cystic bone, seizures, 60% mental retardation (progressive in nature)
Apert syndrome	Craniosynostosis, midfacial hypoplasia, syndactyly (osseous and/or cutaneous), broad distal phalanx of thumb and big toe, variable mental retardation
Crouzon syndrome	Premature craniosynostosis, shallow orbits, maxillary hypoplasia, conductive hearing loss, variable mental retardation
Mandibulofacial dysostosis (Treacher Collins syndrome)	Molar hypoplasia with downslanting palpebral fissures, lower eyelid coloboma, malformed auricles, external ear canal defect, deafness, mental retardation (5% of cases)

lence of identified metabolic disorders among children with developmental delay or retardation is low, ranging from 0 to 5% (Allen and Taylor, 1976; Hunter et al., 1980; Majnemer and Shevell, 1995).

Nonmetabolic Syndromes of Unknown Cause

Some nonmetabolic syndromes of unknown causes are also considered autosomal recessive on the basis of multiple affected sibs and parental consanguinity. Therefore, it is important to obtain a pedigree and to examine all sibs in cases in which the cause of mental retardation is "unknown." The proportion of retarded patients with autosomal recessive conditions approximates 11%, even though a definitive diagnosis can be established in only 6%. Given available recurrence risks (see later on), the prevalence of recessive disorders can be assumed to be even higher. Chromosomal studies of

parents and offspring are indicated to exclude parental rearrangement (e.g., translocations) that could lead to multiple affected sibs.

X-linked Conditions

X-linked recessive conditions account for 10 to 20% of severely retarded children. It has long been recognized that there is an excess of approximately 30% of males over females among individuals in institutions for the mentally retarded (Lehrke, 1974; Turner, 1983; Knight et al., 1999). Although a variety of explanations have been put forth, including the probable ascertainment bias of mentally retarded males being institutionalized more frequently because of uncontrollable or violent behavior, it is now clear that X-linked loci contribute significantly to this gender inequity. Over 100 genes have been tentatively assigned to the X chromosome for which mutations lead to mental retardation as at least part of the phenotype (Schwartz, 1993). Examples of such conditions include the Lesch-Nyhan syndrome, X-linked hydrocephalus (aqueductal stenosis), and the Coffin-Lowry syndrome (coarse facies, short stature, down-slanting palpebral fissures, bulbous nose, hypodontia, tapering fingers, and severe mental retardation).

FRAGILE X SYNDROME

The most common inherited condition causing mental retardation is the fragile X syndrome. The incidence of fragile X syndrome is estimated to be approximately 1 per 1500 males and 1 per 2500 females (Webb et al., 1986). Among recognized X-linked mental retardation syndromes, it is the most common (Stevenson, 2000). Based on the incidence of disease and estimates of penetrance, the carrier frequency of fragile X syndrome in the population is approximately 1 in 866. Originally the diagnosis of fragile X syndrome was based on the expression of a folate-sensitive fragile site at Xq27.3 (FRXA) induced in cell culture under conditions of folate deprivation (Lubs, 1969).

In fragile X males, levels of fragile site expression in metaphase spreads from peripheral lymphocytes range from 5 to 50% of X chromosomes analyzed. The extent of expression in female heterozygotes is on the order of 1 to 30% (Sutherland, 1977, Sutherland et al., 1985). In normal controls, the levels of induced fragile sites expression in metaphase spreads are less than 1% (Jenkins et al., 1986). Initially, prenatal diagnosis and carrier testing relied upon scoring the fragile

▼ **Table 6–4.** SELECTED EXAMPLES OF AUTOSOMAL RECESSIVE INBORN ERRORS OF
• METABOLISM ASSOCIATED WITH MENTAL RETARDATION AND OTHER ASSOCIATED
PHENOTYPIC ABNORMALITIES

Disorders	Defect	Clinical Features
Galactosemia	Galctose 1-phosphate-uridyltransferase deficiency	Failure to thrive, vomiting, liver disease (hepatomegaly, jaundice, cirrhosis), cataracts, moderate mental retardation (85% IQ < 85)
Amnio acids Phenyletonuria	Phenylalanine hydroxylase deficiency	Untreated: vomiting in infancy, blue eyes, blond hair, eczematoid rash, seizures, unusual odor ("mose urine"), moderate to profound mental retardation. Maternal hyperphenylalanemia: growth retardation, microcephaly, heart malformations, moderate to profound mental retardation
Maple syrup urine disease (MSUD)	Branched chain α-keto acid dehydrogenase deficiency	Classic MSUD (untreated): hypertonia/hypotonia, ketosis, lethargy, "burnt-sugar" odor, seizures, bulging fontanel, pseudotumor cerebri, coma, death, survivors severely retarded, spasticity, cortical blindness
Homocystinuria	Cystathionine β-synthase deficiency	Dislocation of optic lens, osteoporosis, thinning and lengthening of long bones, epilepsy, thromboembolism, mental retardation (pyridoxine-responsive and unresponsive variants)
Methylmalonic acidemia	Methylmalonyl-CA mutase deficiency	Lethargy, failure to thrive, vomiting, hypotonia, hepatomegaly, coma, variable mental retardation (some responsive to vitamin B_{12} therapy)
Isovaleric acidemia	Isovaleryl-CA dehydrogenase deficiency	Acute form (untreated): vomiting, acidosis, hyperammonemia, bone marrow suppression, coma, seizures, foul odor ("sweaty feet"), death. Chronic intermittent form (untreated): recurrent episodes of vomiting, lethargy, acidosis, coma, developmental delay, mild to severe mental retardation
Lysosomal enzymes Tay-Sachs disease	Hexosaminidase A deficiency	Progressive weakness, hypotonia, macular pallor with prominent fovea (cherry-red spot), seizures, macrocephaly, decerebrate posturing, severe mental retardation, death
Metachromatic leukodystrophy	Arylsulfatase A deficiency	Various types from congenital to adult onset. Late infantile form: progressive ataxia, generalized weakness, loss of speech, optic atrophy, spastic quadriparesis, severe mental retardation, death
Niemann-Pick disease (Type A)	Acid sphingomyelinase deficiency	Failure to thrive, lymphadenopathy, microcytic anemia, hypotonia, muscular weakness, enlarged liver and spleen, pulmonary infiltration, cherry-red macula, spasticity, rigidity, severe mental retardation, death
Metals Menkes disease	Defect in copper transport	Premature delivery, hypothermia, hyperbilirubinemia, pili torti of hair, seizures, vascular complications (e.g., subdural hematoma), osteoporosis, skeletal fractures, diverticula of bladder or ureters, severe mental retardation, death

X marker in metaphase spreads; however, molecular advances have made cytogenetic tests supplementary (Sutherland et al., 1991; Warren and Nelson, 1994).

The fragile X syndrome was first clinically characterized as the Martin-Bell syndrome from early studies on kindreds segregating X-linked mental retardation (Martin and Bell, 1946). The major clinical features in adult males include mental retardation ranging from mild to severe; a long and narrow face with moderately increased head circumference (larger than the 50th percentile) (Fig. 6–3); prominence of the jaw and forehead; mildly dysmorphic ears; and macro-orchidism (enlarged testicular volume) in postpubescent affected males with volumes greater than 25 ml (Butler et al., 1991; Hagerman et al., 1991; Kaufmann and Reiss, 1999). It has been estimated that fragile X syndrome is present in many as 20% of all boys with IQ levels between 30 and 55 (Turner et al., 1980). With the obvious exception of macro-orchidism, all of the phenotypic changes of fragile X syndrome described in males may be exhibited by affected heterozygous females, although they tend to be less severe. In transmitting females, somatic signs may be absent or mild, although facies may tend to resemble those of affected males in middle-aged female patients. The mental retardation, in particular, is less severe, with most female patients falling in the mild-to-borderline range (Pennington et al., 1991). It has been suggested that the degree of somatic expression of the gene defect in females correlates with the severity of mental retardation (Fryns, 1986; Brainard et al., 1991).

In 1991, the fragile X gene (*FMR1*) was characterized and found to contain an expansion of

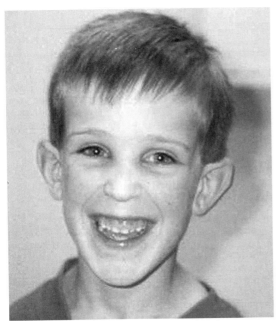

FIGURE 6–3 • A boy with fragile X syndrome: long face, prominent jaws, and large ears. (From Jorde LB, Carey JC, Bamshad MJ, White RL: Medical Genetics, 2nd ed. St Louis: Mosby, 2000.)

a tandemly repeated trinucleotide sequence (CGG) near its 5' end (Kremer et al., 1991; Oberle et al., 1991; Verkerk et al., 1991; Yu et al., 1991) (Fig. 6–4). Normal individuals have less than 12 CGG repeats. Affected males have from hundreds to thousands of CGG repeats (expansion). Full mutations are defined as having over 230 repeats (Maddalena et al., 2001). Although almost all males with the full expansion are clinically affected, approximately half of the females who carry the fully expanded repeat on one of their two X chromosomes are affected

(Rousseau et al., 1991). Presumably the other half of females are protected from the effect of the full mutation of the normal X chromosome as a result of random X-inactivation patterns. In some individuals, the number of CGG repeats is increased to between 55 and 200. Increases in this range are known to be clinically silent "premutations" that are characteristic of normal transmitting males and some mentally normal carrier females. The upper limit of premutation is 230 (Maddalena et al., 2001). Expansion of the number of repeats occurs during meiosis in females but not in males. Thus, a female may carry a premutation and be clinically unaffected. The CGG repeats in her *FMR1* gene can undergo expansion during meiosis to be passed on to a son, who will have the full mutation and an affected phenotype (Fig. 6–5). A male carrying the premutation is known as a "transmitting" male. Such a transmitting male will pass the premutation to all his daughters. Although the daughter who carries a premutation will have a normal phenotype, her *FMR1* gene may undergo an expansion that puts her at risk for having sons with the full mutation and an affected phenotype. Thus, the mutation responsible is a quantitative rather than qualitative alteration that can change drastically as it is passed from generation to generation in a single pedigree. In addition to the apparent instability of premutations when inherited, the length of a full mutation is also unstable during cell division, which results in marked mosaicism for the number of CGG repeats in the cells of a single affected individual (Nussbaum and Ledbetter, 1995; Kaufmann and Reiss, 1999).

In individuals expressing the fragile X phenotype, abnormal methylation of a CpG island located 250 base pairs upstream of the CGG

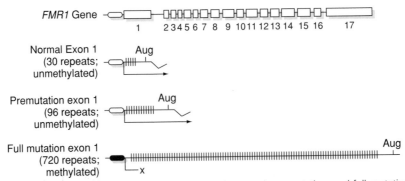

FIGURE 6–4 • Diagram of the *FMR1* gene and the first exon in normal, premutation, and full mutation alleles. The oval immediately to the left of the start site of transcription represents the promoter region of the *FMR1* gene. The open symbol represents active transcription, and the black symbol, silenced transcription. The vertical lines indicate CGG trinucleotides upstream of the methionine codon (AUG) at the translocational start site. (Reprinted with permission from Warren ST, Nelson DL: Advances in molecular analysis of fragile X syndrome. JAMA 271:536, 1994.)

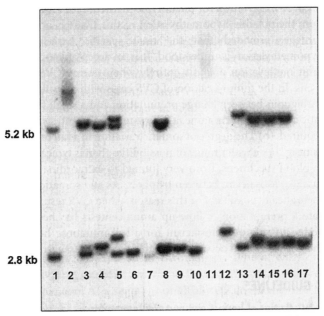

FIGURE 6–5 • Southern blot analysis using EcoR1 and Eagl digestion, probed with StB12.3, using extended electrophoresis to illustrate several subtle specimen types. (1) Normal female. (2) Full mutation male. Note the combination of a predominant band with a diffuse smear. (3) Female with 28 and 52 repeats, with the smaller allele predominantly active. (4) Female with 26 and 52 repeats, with the larger allele predominantly active. (5) Female with 18 and ~80 repeats, with equal X-inactivation. (6) Normal male. (7) Normal male, underloaded and smiling due to DNA degradation. (The apparent line between lanes 6 and 7 is a photographic artifact.) (8) Normal female. (9) Normal male. (10) Normal male. (11) Affected male, underloaded and very diffuse). (12) Premutation male. (13) Female with 20 and 70 repeats, with the smaller allele virtually exclusively active. The only evidence of abnormality is the slow migration of the "5.2 kb" band. (14) Female with 27 and 42 repeats, with the larger allele somewhat more active. (15-17) Unremarkable normal females and males. Figure provided by Genetics and IVF Institute. (From Maddalena A, Richards CS, McGinniss MJ, et al.: Technical standards and guidelines for fragile X. Genet Med 3:200, 2001.)

repeat of *FMR1* occurs in addition to the trinucleotide repeat expansion (Bell et al., 1991; Hansen et al., 1992). Methylation of the CpG island adjacent to the *FMR1* gene correlates with transcriptional silencing of *FMR1* and expression of the fragile X phenotype (Goody et al., 2002). Thus, most affected males have no detectable *FMR1* mRNA and have an absence of encoded protein.

Pedigree analysis shows that affected individuals appear to cluster in more recent generations, a phenomenon termed "anticipation." As the premutation is transmitted vertically to a family, it tends to increase in size, and therefore greater numbers of affected children are observed in later generations and greater numbers of carriers are seen in early generations. This increasing cumulative risk that a premutation will expand to a full mutation as it is passed on from earlier to later generations is responsible for anticipation (Sutherland and Richards, 1992). Genetic anticipation is a hallmark of certain diseases, such as myotonic dystrophy, which also has subsequently been demonstrated to be the result of trinucleotide repeat expansions. Guidelines have recently been

published for laboratory testing and reporting for fragile X syndrome (Maddalena et al., 2001).

Molecular diagnosis of fragile X syndrome has been developed using polymerase chain reaction (PCR) or Southern blot analysis approaches (see Fig. 6–5). PCR is useful for defining accurate premutation repeat lengths and for demonstrating instability (Warren and Nelson, 1994). Southern blot analysis allows both size of the repeat segment and methylation status to be assayed simultaneously. A methylation-sensitive restriction enzyme that fails to cleave methylated sites is used to distinguish between methylated and unmethylated alleles. PCR and Southern blot analysis thus complement each other to provide molecular diagnosis. The key to diagnosis using Southern blotting is a heavy fragment which is marked in affected individuals, subtly discernible (small signal) in premutation carriers and not evident in normal individuals.

DNA-based testing has considerably improved the prenatal diagnosis of fragile X syndrome and is currently the method of choice. Using DNA from amniotic fluid cells analyzed by PCR and Southern blotting for fragile X has been shown to be highly accurate for prenatal diagnosis (Murphy et al., 1992; Brown et al., 1993). Results from prenatal diagnosis using chorionic villi must be interpreted with caution because of abnormal fragment patterns caused by absent or partial methylation of the CpG island of the *FMR1* gene in this tissue, especially prior to 12 weeks' gestation (Castellvi-Bel et al., 1995; Decker Phillips et al., 1996).

Teratogenic Causes

Known environmental causes account for relatively few cases of mental retardation. Causes include chemical teratogens, infectious teratogens (e.g., rubella, toxoplasmosis, cytomegalovirus), postnatal infections (e.g., meningitis, encephalitis), birth injuries, and postnatal nutritional or stimulatory deprivation. The recurrence risk should be negligible.

Teratogenic causes of mental retardation, with or without cerebral palsy, is far lower in incidence than once believed (Nelson and Ellenberg, 1981, 1985, 1986; Niswander, 1988). Many cases attributed to "asphyxia" are in fact genetic. Not only is cerebral palsy usually preceded by no evidence of asphyxia but asphyxia does not usually lead to cerebral palsy. The term "asphyxia" should be reserved for the clinical context of damaging acidemia, hypoxia, and metabolic acidosis. In 1994, the Committee on Obstetric Practice of the American College of Obstetricians and Gynecologists concluded that a neonate who has had hypoxia proximate to delivery severe enough to result in hypoxic encephalopathy will show other evidence of hypoxic damage, including all of the following: (1) profound metabolic or mixed acidemia (pH less than 7.00) on an umbilical cord arterial blood sample if obtained; (2) a persistent Apgar score of 0–3 for longer than 5 minutes; and (3) evidence of neurologic sequelae (e.g., seizures, coma, hypotonia, and one or more of the following: cardiovascular, gastrointestinal, hematologic, pulmonary, or renal system dysfunction) (ACOG Committee Opinion, No. 137, 1994).

Genetic Counseling

The most important single prerequisite for genetic counseling is an accurate diagnosis. To accomplish this, one must consider prenatal and intrapartum records as well as the developmental history of the proband. A thorough physical examination with particular attention to minor developmental defects must be done. Cytogenetic studies are obligatory, and other studies are often necessary. In particular, an attempt should be made to exclude prenatal teratogens. Selected biochemical or DNA studies may be appropriate. If a diagnosis is made, counseling must be based on the condition found.

The recurrence risk of mild, idiopathic mental retardation unassociated with physical anomalies has been reported between 13 and 33% for first-degree relatives (20 to 25% for siblings) and between 5 and 9% for second-degree relatives (Nichols, 1984; Crow and Tolmie, 1998; Bundey et al., 1989). This compares with an expected rate of 20 per 1000. Evidence from twin studies is now dated and suffers from methodologic problems, in particular nonsystematic ascertainment. However, in one study concordance rates were 73% for monozygotic (MZ) twins and 29% for dizygotic (DZ) twins (Rosanoff et al., 1937). A higher concordance of MZ twins (100 %) compared with DZ twins (58%) was similarly found in another study (Gottesman, 1971). Thus, it can be concluded that idiopathic mental retardation appears to be familial, and the high recurrence risk suggests a relatively high proportion of recessive disorders.

Recall that developmental delay and mental retardation may be a part of a contiguous gene deletion syndrome caused by deletion of several physically contiguous yet functionally unrelated genes. For most microdeletion (or contiguous gene deletion) syndromes, the size of the deletion is below the level of cytogenetic resolution and can only be visualized using fluorescence in situ hybridization (FISH) analysis of the relevant chromosomes when a specific disorder is suspected. Using FISH analysis with a cocktail of probes that independently detect deletions in the Williams, Prader-Willi/Angelman, Smith-Magenis syndrome, and DiGeorge/velocardiofacial syndromes in 200 patients, Ligon and coworkers (1997) confirmed that ten patients had microdeletions by the multiprobe FISH analysis. Knight and colleagues (1999) studied 284 children with unexplained moderate to severe mental retardation and 182 children with unexplained mild mental retardation using FISH to examine the integrity of chromosome ends. Subtle chromosomal abnormalities also occur with a frequency of at least 10% in the children with moderate to severe mental retardation and of 1% in the children with mild retardation. Screening for subtle chromosomal rearrangements is thus warranted in children with unexplained moderate to severe mental retardation. Multiprobe cocktail FISH studies and telomeric probes can be used to identify microdeletions that may otherwise go undetected in a proportion of patients with idiopathic mental retardation or developmental delay. If a translocation is found, implications for offspring are significant.

Multiple Anomalies Without Mental Retardation

Some individuals have unusual facial features and multiple anomalies but no mental retardation. Such a pattern could result from a mutant gene but probably is not caused by a chromosomal aberration. For the clinician, the significance is that parents of an infant with multiple malformations should not always be counseled to expect their child to show mental retardation. Thorough diagnostic evaluation is obligatory. In a small series of 27 probands with multiple anomalies but normal intelligence, Bartley and Hall (1978) recorded no similarly affected sibs. Thus, empiric recurrence risks are low although not necessarily zero.

Genetic Counseling Following Stillborn Infants with Multiple Malformations

When parents seek genetic counseling after stillbirth or neonatal death, diagnosis is often impossible because no adequate description of the proband exists. Malformations may or may not have been obvious, and usually no information concerning mental status is known. If an autopsy was not performed, the counselor must rely totally on the memory of the couple and their physician concerning the infant's appearance. In our opinion, the only reliable diagnosis obtained this way is anencephaly.

If an accurate diagnosis cannot be obtained, counseling is obviously hazardous. To avoid such a dilemma, photography, full-body x-rays, autopsy, and chromosomal studies should ideally be performed on all stillborn infants. Storing DNA for future studies is also desirable. The options the clinician has for preserving tissue for future DNA studies include the following: (1) placing whole blood in ethylenediaminetetraacetic acid (EDTA) tubes and freezing; (2) collecting peripheral blood and using commercial kits (traditional methods to separate DNA); (3) establishing lymphoblast lines that provide a never-ending source for both DNA- and RNA-based tests (not readily available to many clinicians); (4) dried blood spots on filter paper (e.g.,

IsoCode Schleicher and Schull Number 903); (5) amniotic fluid cultures; (6) urine epithelial cells; (7) buccal mucosa; (8) culture of skin fibroblasts; (9) fibrous tissue obtained at autopsy (e.g., fascia); (10) hair bulbs (stored at room temperature). Such planning could greatly facilitate counseling before the next pregnancy (ACOG Committee Opinion, 1996). DNA from archival samples (e.g., paraffin-enbedded tissue) and cell fixation methods sometimes damage DNA and preclude the use of certain types of tests.

REFERENCES

ACOG Committee Opinion 178. Genetic Evaluation of Stillbirths and Neonatal Deaths. Washington DC: The American College of Obstetricians and Gynecologists, 1996.

ACOG Committee Opinion, No. 137: Fetal Distress and Birth Asphyxia. Washington DC: The American College of Obstetrics and Gynecology, 1994.

Accardo PJ, Capute AJ: Mental retardation. *In* Oski FA, De Angelis CD, Feigin RD, et al. (eds): Principles and Practices of Pediatrics, 2nd ed. Philadelphia: JB Lippincott, 1994, p 673.

Allen WP, Taylor H: Mental retardation in South Carolina VII. Inborn errors of metabolism. Proc Greenwood Genet Ctr 15:76, 1976.

American Psychiatric Association: Diagnostic and Statistical Manual of Mental Disorders: DSM-IV, 4th ed. Washington DC: American Psychiatric Association, 1994.

Anderson G, Schrorer RJ, Stevens RE: Mental retardation in South Carolina II, causation. Proc Greenwood Genetic Ctr 15:37, 1996.

Baker E, Hinton L, Callen DF, et al.: Study of 250 children with idiopathic mental retardation reveals nine cryptic and diverse subtelomeric chromosomal anomalies. Am J Med Genet 107:285, 2002.

Bartley JA, Hall BD: Mental retardation and multiple congenital anomalies of unknown etiology: frequency of occurrence in similarly affected sibs of the proband. Birth Defects 14(6b):127, 1978.

Bell MV, Hirst MC, Nakahori Y, et al.: Physical mapping across the fragile X: Hypermethylation and clinical expression of the fragile X syndrome. Cell 64:861, 1991.

Brainard SS, Schreiner RA, Hagerman RJ: Cognitive profiles of the carrier fragile X women. Am J Med Genet 38:505, 1991.

Brown WT, Houck GE Jr, Jeziorowska A, et al.: Rapid fragile X carrier screening and prenatal diagnosis using a nonradioactive PCR test. JAMA 270:1569, 1993.

Brugge KL, Nichols SL, Salmon DP, et al.: Cognitive impairment in adults with Down syndrome: similarities to early cognitive changes in Alzheimer's disease. Neurology 44:232, 1994.

Burton BK: Inborn errors of metabolism: The clinical diagnosis in early infancy. Pediatrics 79:359, 1987.

Burton BK: Inborn errors of metabolism in infancy: A guide to diagnosis. Pediatr 102:E69, 1998.

Bundey S, Thake A, Todd J: The recurrence risks for mild idiopathic mental retardation. J Med Genet 26:260, 1989.

Butler MG, Mangrum T, Gupta R, et al.: A 15 item checklist for screening mentally retarded males for the fragile X syndrome. Clin Genet 39:347, 1991.

Castellvi-Bel S, Mila M. Soler A, et al.: Prenatal diagnosis of fragile X syndrome: (cGG)$_n$ expansion and methylation of chorionic villus samples. Prenat Diagn 15:801, 1995.

Crow YJ, Tolmie JL: Recurrence risks in mental retardation. J Med Genet 35:177, 1998.

Curry CJ, Dandhu A, Frutos L, et al.: Diagnostic yield of genetic evaluations in developmental delay/mental retardation. Clin Res 44:130A, 1996.

Decker Phillips M, Kay H, Parks LR, et al.: Methylation studies of *FMR1* in paired fetal and extraembryonic tissue: Implication for prenatal diagnosis of fragile X syndrome using CVS. Am J Hum Genet 59:A41, 1996.

Flint J, Wilkie AO, Buckle VJ, et al.: The detection of subtelomeric chromosomal rearrangements in idiopathic mental retardation. Nat Genet 9:132, 1995.

Fryns JP: The female and the fragile X: A study of 144 obligate female carriers. Am J Med Genet 23:157, 1986.

Garrod A: Inborn errors in metabolism (Croonian lectures). Lancet 2:1, 73, 142, 214, 1908.

Goate A, Chartier-Harlin, MC, Mullan M, et al.: Segregation of a missense mutation in the amyloid precursor protein gene with familial Alzheimer's disease. Nature 349:704, 1991.

Gostason R, Wahlstrom J, Johannisson T, et al.: Chromosomal aberrations in the mildly mentally retarded. J Ment Defic Res 35:240, 1991.

Gottesman SJ II: An introduction to behavioral genetics of mental retardation. *In* Allen RM (ed): Role of Genetics in Mental Retardation. Coral Gables: University of Miami Press 1971, p 49.

Grody WW, Seligson DB, Telatar M: Diagnostic molecular genetics. *In* Rimoin DL, Connor JM, Pyeritz RE, Korf BR (eds): Principles and Practice of Medical Genetics, 4th ed. Philadelphia: Churchill Livingston, 2002, p 723.

Hagberg B, Hagberg G: Aspects of prevention of pre- and postnatal brain pathology in severe and mild mental retardation. *In* Dobbing J, Clarke AD, Corbett JA (eds): Scientific Studies in Mental Retardation. London: Macmilllan 1984, p 46.

Hagerman RJ, Amiri K, Cronister A: Fragile X checklist. Am J Med Genet 38:283, 1991.

Hansen RS, Gartler SM, Scott CR, et al.: Methylation analysis of CGG sites in the CPG island of the human *FMR1* gene. Hum Mol Genet 1:571, 1992.

Hunter AG, Evans JA, Thompson DR, et al.: A study of insitutionalized mentally retarded patients in Manitoba I: Classification and preventability. Dev Med Child Neurol 22:145, 1980.

Jenkins EC, Brown WT, Brooks J, et al.: Low frequencies of apparently fragile X chromosomes in normal control cultures: A possible explanation. Exp Cell Biol 54:40, 1986.

Jones KL: Smith's Recognizable Patterns of Human Malformations, 5th ed. Philadelphia: WB Saunders, 1997.

Knight SJ, Regan R, Nicod A, et al.: Subtle chromosomal rearrangements in children with unexplained mental retardation. Lancet 354:1676, 1999.

Kaufmann WE, Reiss AL: Molecular and cellular genetics of fragile X syndrome. Am J Med Genet 88:11, 1999.

Kremer EJ, Pritchard M, Lynch M, et al.: Mapping of DNA instability at the fragile X to a trinucleotide repeat sequence p $(CCG)_n$. Science 252:1711, 1991.

Laxova R, Ridler MA, Bowen-Bravery M: An etiological survey of the severely retarded Hertfordshire children who were born between January 1, 1965 and December 31, 1967. Am J Med Genet 1:75, 1977.

Ledbetter DH, Ballabio A: Molecular cytogenetics of continguous gene syndromes: Mechanisms and consequences of gene dosage imbalance. *In* Scriver CR, Beaudet AL, Sly WS, et al. (eds): The Metabolic and Molecular Basis of Inherited Diseases, 7th ed. New York: McGraw-Hill, 1995, p 811.

Lehrke RG: X-linked mental retardation and verbally disability. Birth Defects Orig Artic Ser 10(1):1, 1974.

Ligon AH, Beaudet AL, Shaffer LG: Simultaneous, multilocus FISH analysis for detection of microdeletions in the diagnostic evaluation of developmental delay and mental retardation. Am J Hum Genet 61:51, 1997.

Lubs HA: A marker X chromosome. Am J Hum Genet 21:231, 1969.

Maddalena A, Richards CS, McGinniss MJ, et al.: Technical standards and guidelines for fragile X: The first of a series of disease-specific supplements to the Standards and Guidelines for Clinical Genetics Laboratories of the American College of Medical Genetics. Quality Assurance Subcommittee of the Laboratory Practice Committee. Genet Med 3:200, 2001.

Majnemer A, Shevell MI: Diagnostic yield of the neurologic assessment of the developmentally delayed child. J Pediatr 127:193, 1995.

Martin JP, Bell J: A pedigree of mental defect showing sex-linkage. J Neurol Psychiatry 6:154, 1946.

McQueen PC, Spence MW, Winsor EJ, et al.: Causal origins of major mental handicap in the Canadian Maritime provinces. Dev Med Child Neurol 28:697, 1986.

Murphy PD, Wilmot PL, Shapiro LR: Prenatal diagnosis of fragile X syndrome: Results from parallel molecular and cytogenetic studies. Am J Med Genet 43:181, 1992.

Nelson KB, Ellenberg JH: Apgar scores as predictors of chronic neurologic disability. Pediatrics 68:36, 1981.

Nelson KB, Ellenberg JH: Antecedents of cerebral palsy. I. Univariate analysis of risks. Am J Dis Child 139:1031, 1985.

Nelson KB, Ellenberg JH: Antecedents of cerebral palsy: Multivariate analysis of risk. New Engl J Med 315:81, 1986.

Nichols PL: Familial mental retardation. Behav Genet 14:161, 1984.

Niswander K: Management of growth retardation with a view to preventing neuromotor dysfunction and mental handicaps. *In* Kabbi F, Patel N, Schmidt W, et al. (eds): Perinatal Events and Brain Damage in Surviving Children. Berlin: Springer-Verlag, 1988, p 108.

Nussbaum RL, Ledbetter DH: The fragile X syndrome. *In* Scriver CR, Beaudet AL, Sly WS, et al. (eds): The Metabolic and Molecular Basis of Inherited Disease, 7th ed. New York: McGraw-Hill, 1995, p 795.

Oberle I, Rousseau F, Heitz D, et al.: Instability of 550-base pair DNA segment and abnormal methylation in fragile X syndrome. Science 252:1097, 1991.

Opitz JM: Diagnostic/genetic studies in severe mental retardation. *In* Lubs HA, De La Cruz F (eds): Genetic Counseling. New York: Raven, 1977, p 417.

Pennington BF, O'Connor RA, Sudhalter V: Toward a neuropsychology of fragile X syndrome. *In* Hagerman RJ, Silverman AC (eds): Fragile X Syndrome: Diagnosis, Treatment and Research. Baltimore: Johns Hopkins University Press, 1991, p 173.

Penrose L: A clinical and genetic study of 1280 cases of mental defect. London: Her Majesty's Stationary Office MCR Special Report Series No. 229, 1938.

Robinson A, Linden MG: Clinical Genetics Handbook, 2nd ed. Boston: Blackwell Scientific Publications, 1993.

Rosanoff AJ, Handy LM, Plesset IR: The etiology of child behavior difficulties, juvenile delinquency and adult criminality with special reference to its occurrence in twins. Psychiatric Monographs 1:187, 1937.

Rousseau F, Heitz D, Bianacalana V, et al.: Direct diagnosis by DNA analysis of the fragile X syndrome of mental retardation. N Engl J Med 325:1673, 1991.

Schwartz CE: X-linked mental retardation: In pursuit of a gene map. Am J Hum Genet 52:1025, 1993.

Shonkoff JP: Mental retardation. *In* Behrman RE, Kliegman RM, Jenson HB (eds): Textbook of Pediatrics, 16th ed. Philadelphia: WB Saunders, 2000, p 125.

Stevenson RE: Splitting and lumping in the nosology of XLMR. Am J Med Genet 97:174, 2000.

Sutherland GR: Fragile sites on human chromosomes: Demonstration of their dependence on the type of tissue culture medium. Science 197:265, 1977.

Sutherland GR, Hecht F, Mulley JC, et al.: *In* Fragile Sites on Human Chromosomes. New York: Oxford, 1985.

Sutherland GR, Gedeon A, Kornman L, et al.: Prenatal diagnosis of fragile X syndrome by direct detection of the unstable DNA sequence. N Engl J Med 325:1720, 1991.

Sutherland GR, Richards RI: Anticipation legitimized: Unstable DNA to the rescue. Am J Hum Genet 51:7, 1992.

Thapar A, Gottesman SJ II, Owen MJ, et al.: The genetics of mental retardation. Br J Psychiatry 164:747, 1994.

Turner G: An aetiological study of 1,000 patients with an I.Q. assessment below 51. Med J Aust 2:927, 1975.

Turner G, Daniel A, Frost M: X-linked mental retardation, macro-orchidism and the Xq27 fragile site. J Pediatr 96:837, 1980.

Turner G: Historical overview. *In* Hagerman RJ, McBogg PM (eds): The Fragile X Syndrome: Diagnosis, Biochemistry, and Intervention. Dillon, CO: Spectra, 1983.

Verkerk AJ, Pieretti M, Sutcliffe JS, et al.: Identification of a gene (FMR-1) containing a CGG repeat coincident with a breakpoint cluster region exhibiting length variation of fragile X syndrome. Cell 65:905, 1991.

Warren ST, Nelson DL: Advances in molecular analysis of fragile X syndrome. JAMA 271:536, 1994.

Webb TP, Bundey SE, Thake AL, et al.: Population incidence and segregation ratios in the Martin-Bell syndrome. Am J Hum Genet 23:573, 1986.

Yu S, Pritchard M, Kremer E, et al.: Fragile X genotype characterized by an unstable region of DNA. Science 252:1179, 1991.

CHAPTER 7

Pregnancy in Women with Mendelian Disorders

With improving health care, a greater number of women with mendelian, i.e., single gene disorders, are surviving and reproducing. Women affected with mendelian disorders may have the expression of their condition altered by pregnancy. Conversely, the disorder may have adverse effects on pregnancy. Genetic counseling is particularly important in order for the couple to understand the heritability of the condition, reproductive options, possibilities for prenatal diagnosis, and medical issues that may impact the mother or fetus or both.

Over 9100 human mendelian disorders have been identified, and with progress in the Human Genome Project, the number continues to grow. Summaries with references of these disorders can be accessed on the Online Mendelian Inheritance in Man (OMIM) database developed by McKusick at Johns Hopkins University (http://www.ncbi.nih.gov/Omim/). Approximately 94% are autosomal entries, 5.8% X-linked, and 0.3% Y-linked.

In this chapter we discuss selected mendelian disorders that obstetricians may encounter in pregnant women. Mendelian inheritance patterns are reviewed in Chapter 2.

Cystic Fibrosis

Cystic fibrosis (CF) is a multisystem disease inherited in autosomal recessive fashion. In the white population, approximately 1 in 2500 to 1 in 3300 individuals in North America and northern Europe are affected (Wright et al., 1996). From the Hardy-Weinberg formula (see Chapter

2), it can be calculated that the frequency of heterozygous carriers is about 1 in 29 individuals.

CLINICAL CONSIDERATIONS

Women with CF have compromised fertility. They show delayed onset of menarche; those with malnutrition and advanced lung disease often have anovulatory cycles with secondary amenorrhea. Dehydrated and thickened cervical secretions also may pose a physical barrier to sperm penetration of the cervical os. Nonetheless, as more women with CF enter reproductive age, they should be appropriately counseled about contraception, pregnancy, and the potential increased risks associated with CF (Hilman et al., 1996). Pregnancy rates among CF women have increased. During pregnancy, these women are at risk for respiratory and cardiac compromise because their underlying lung disease has the potential to be further exacerbated by gestationally related hypoxemia and pulmonary hypertension. The changes in ventilatory drive, cardiac function, blood volume, and increased nutritional requirements all pose potential problems for the woman with CF (Frangolias et al., 1997).

Kent and Farquharson (1993) performed a literature review of CF and pregnancy from 1960 to 1991. They found 217 pregnancies reported in 162 women. Of these, 177 (81.6%) progressed beyond 20 weeks and 10 (4.6%) ended in spontaneous abortions. Forty-three (24.3%) of the deliveries were preterm, and 14 (7.9%) perinatal deaths occurred. Five of 43 preterm deliveries were secondary to maternal complications associated with CF, and the remaining 88.4% were spontaneous preterm deliveries. This high preterm delivery rate was believed to be due to chronic hypoxia in the fetus, particularly in women who had poor pulmonary function. Another explanation could be related to inadequate maternal nutrition or pancreatic insufficiency or both, which would lead to malnutrition. The perinatal death rate was higher among infants of women with CF. Twelve of the 14 perinatal deaths were predominantly the result of prematurity. There were no congenital anomalies; only one infant had CF. There were 14 (7.9%) maternal deaths within 6 months after delivery and 24 (13.6) maternal deaths within 2 years after delivery. The maternal death rate did not exceed that among age-matched nonpregnant women with CF, and deaths occurred predominantly as a result of pulmonary complications. Maternal pulmonary status was found to be directly related to maternal death.

Most women with CF can complete a successful pregnancy. Kent and Farquharson (1993) recommend careful monitoring of lung function and ensuring adequate energy intake. Affected women should be counseled about the symptoms and signs of preterm labor, and routine cervical examinations should be considered. The authors suggest that women with a pregnancy forced vital capacity (FEV$_1$) of 50% or less of the expected value or with evidence of cor pulmonale be discouraged from becoming pregnant, as they may be at greatest risk for complications. However, it was felt that these conditions should not necessarily be indications for pregnancy termination if the patient's lung function has been stable for some time.

Frangolias and coworkers (1997) reported a case-control study of seven pregnant women with CF who were compared with nonpregnant CF controls. They were matched using a 1-year preconception date in relation to age, height, weight, percentage of FEV$_1$, and pancreatic sufficiency status. All patients had pancreatic insufficiency and were dependent on enzyme supplementation. The patients were followed for 2 years postpartum. All patients survived pregnancy, although one died 6 months postpartum. A small, gradual, but significant decline in pulmonary function occurred in both groups over time. Pregnant women with CF demonstrated a lower rate of decline in FEV$_1$ (3.6%) versus controls (6.8%). There was no significant difference in the number of pulmonary exacerbations between the two groups. Most of the women gained approximately 5.2 kg through the pregnancy, but there was a 4- to 6-kg decline from preconception weight at 2 years postpartum. The authors concluded that pregnancy is a reasonable option for women with mild CF. Women who seem to be at higher risk for poor pregnancy outcome include those with poor nutritional status, insulin-dependent diabetes mellitus, colonization or infection with *Pseudomonas aeruginosa* and *P. cepacia*, and poor pulmonary status.

Phenylketonuria

Phenylketonuria (PKU) is among the most common disorders of amino acid metabolism, with an incidence of about 1 in 14,000 newborns in the United States (Veale, 1980). This disorder is attributable to an autosomal recessive trait usually caused by a deficiency of the liver enzyme phenylalanine hydroxylase (PAH), which allows too much phenylalanine to accumulate in the body. Affected infants appear normal at birth; however, within a few weeks elevated levels of phenylalanine begins to impair brain development. By 6 months of age, the infant has severe mental retardation. Untreated children have impaired synthesis of melanin and are almost always light haired and fair skinned. Facial dysmorphisms include microcephaly, prominent maxilla, widely spaced teeth, and abnormal dental enamel. These children often have eczema and neurologic abnormalities such as seizures, spasticity, and hypertonicity (Scriver et al., 1995).

PKU must be differentiated from other causes of hyperphenylalaninemia. A low phenylalanine diet in the first few days of life prevents most of the neurologic and intellectual damage. In fact, use of such diets in conjunction with the screening of newborns for PKU begun in the 1960s has allowed many of those with PKU to reach adulthood without experiencing any symptoms of the enzyme deficiency.

The *PAH* gene has been localized to chromosome 12q11-q24. More than 300 mutations have been found to be associated with PKU. The most common mutations are changes in donor splice sites of exon-intron junctions; however, missense mutations and deletions have also been found (Scriver and Kaufman, 2001). Unless the mutant alleles in the proband are known, prenatal diagnosis depends on restriction fragment length polymorphism studies, in gametic association with the *PKU* alleles (Chen et al., 1989; Scriver and Kaufman, 2001).

Newborn PKU screening programs and the initiation of phenylalanine-restricted diets in affected infants have virtually eliminated severe handicaps from this disease. As result, women affected with PKU, typically free of severe mental handicaps and with normal fertility, are reproducing. This has created a problem because their offspring are at high risk for fetal damage if they are exposed to high phenylalanine levels *in utero*. This condition has been referred to as mental PKU, and the resultant fetal damage includes intrauterine growth restriction, microcephaly, mental retardation, congenital heart disease, and dysmorphic facial features (Lenke and Levy, 1980; Lipson et al., 1984).

Lenke and Levy (1980) examined 524 pregnancies in 155 women with untreated PKU and found a high incidence of spontaneous abortions, mental retardation (95%), microcephaly (73%), birth weight <2500 g (56%), and congenital heart disease (17%). In 260 pregnancies, maternal phenylalanine levels > 1200 µmol (normal = < 100 µmol), and among their offspring, 92% were mentally retarded. The authors concluded that there was a dose relationship between phenylalanine levels and the frequency of occurence of microcephaly and mental retardation. They also suggested there was a threshold pattern for the incidence of low birth weight and congenital heart disease, as phenylalanine seemed to have severe teratogenicity at levels >600 µmol/L.

Peat (1993) reported a retrospective study of nine pregnancies in six women with PKU. Prepregnancy phenylalanine levels ranged from 710–1800 µmol/L, with a mean of 1347 µmol/L. All except one woman began dietary restriction between 4 and 12 weeks preconception. She did not present for treatment until 5 weeks' gestation with her first pregnancy and 12 weeks during her second. Phenylalanine levels were measured every 2 to 4 weeks and in all cases except one, phenylalanine levels were <1000 µmol/L. At term lower phenylalanine levels were observed, most likely a result of amino acid uptake by the fetus. The one woman with phenylalanine levels >1000 µmol/L throughout both her pregnancies was noncompliant with dietary restriction. Both her infants were born at 36 weeks and had microcephaly and low birth weight. In the remaining seven pregnancies, five women achieved phenylalanine levels <600 µmol/L at conception. One of the five pregnancies ended in a second trimester abortion, and this same woman completed a second pregnancy that produced a low birth weight, small for gestational age infant. There were no cases of microcephaly, congenital heart disease, or seizures in the adequately treated pregnant women. The author concluded that without good preconceptional control and especially good control in the first trimester, women with PKU put their offspring at risk for microcephaly, congenital cardiac anomalies, and fetal growth restriction.

Whitehead and coworkers (1996) performed a retrospective study of 11 women who had completed 17 pregnancies in which a phenylalanine-restricted diet was initiated preconceptionally. Once levels were consistently at <250 µmol/L, the women attempted to conceive. In eight unplanned continuing pregnancies, the diet was commenced at office visit, which was at 12 weeks in six out of eight; two out of eight were after 20 weeks. Serum phenylalanine and tyrosine levels were measured every 2 weeks, and tyrosine supplements were given as needed. There were 14 live births with median gestation at delivery of 38 weeks; one preterm delivery occurred at 28 weeks. There was one termination at 16 weeks for anencephaly in a planned pregnancy with good periconceptional phenylalanine levels. Two spontaneous abortions also occurred in this group (one with good control, the other an unplanned pregnancy with periconceptional phenylalanine values of 625 µmol/L). Among the eight infants born to mothers with periconceptional phenylalanine levels >250 µmol/L, three were below 3% for head circumference and length. Of the six infants born to mothers with a periconceptional phenylalanine level of <250 µmol/L, there were no cases of congenital cardiac abnormalities, and all were at or above 3% for head circumference, weight, and length.

In a study by Waisbren and associates (1998), neonatal neurologic assessments were administered within the first 8 days after birth and follow-up testing at 1 year of life in 56 offspring of women with PKU and 45 controls. The gestational age at which the mother attained metabolic control was an important factor in terms of subsequent developmental scores. Interestingly, these investigators found that home environment (i.e., close monitoring of diet and phenylanine levels) was a greater determinant of risk for a low Bayley Development Quotient than whether or not the mother attained metabolic control prior to pregnancy. They concluded that treatment strategies addressing both prenatal and postnatal factors will most effectively reduce risks of maternal PKU.

Fisch and coworkers (1993) suggested that because of the difficulty in maintaining strict dietary control, especially in patients who have been off their diets since childhood, women with PKU should be counseled about the option of using parental gametes and a surrogate mother to provide the best possible metabolic environment for the fetus.

Finally, Hanley and coworkers (1999) retrospectively reviewed 417 live-born children from 576 pregnancies being followed by the International Maternal Phenylketonuria Collaborative Study to ascertain cases of maternal PKU initially diagnosed during or after a pregnancy. Seventeen (4.1%) met their criteria; six of these mothers had their disease diagnosed after the birth of affected offspring, two as a result of transient hyperphenylalaninemia, and nine by prenatal screening. They estimated that undiagnosed maternal PKU occurs at a rate of 1 case per 100,000 births in North America and Europe. They suggested that physicians and midwives consider selective prenatal screening or case finding to detect undiagnosed PKU among their patients. They suggested a "draft protocol" for choosing such women, which is provided in Table 7–1.

In summary, preconceptional counseling and appropriate and early prenatal care are vital to reducing the incidence of congenital malformations and developmental disabilities in the offspring of PKU women. It is strongly recommended that these women be followed by a dietitian and that they receive L-tyrosine as a supplement to maintain blood tyrosine levels of higher than or equal to 0.5 mg/dL. Women with classic PKU should be placed on a diet that contains 250–500 mg/day of phenylalanine. To improve dietary compliance and neonatal outcome, it is important that these women receive adequate psychosocial support (Luke, 1994; Brown et al., 2002).

Hemoglobinopathies

SICKLE CELL DISEASE (HBSS AND HBSC)

Sickle cell disease is the most common mendelian disorder among African-Americans. This autoso- mal recessive disorder is defined as either the homozygous state of HbS or HbS in combination with another abnormal hemoglobin. Hemoglobin SS occurs in 1 in 625 and HbSC occurs in 1 in 833 African-Americans at birth. HbSS results from the substitution of valine, a neutral amino acid, for glutamic acid, which is negatively charged, at the sixth position from the N-terminus in the beta hemoglobin chain. In HbC lysine is substituted for glutamic acid at the sixth position.

HbS functions normally while oxygenated, but when deoxygenated, the valine forms hydrophobic bonds with adjacent globin chains. This results in the formation of insoluble tetramers, which polymerize into long strands in the red blood cell. These strands form cables with spicules, which deform the red blood cell membrane. With further deoxygenation, these cells become irreversibly sickled and obstruct the microcirculation.

This classic picture of HbSS is chronic anemia, childhood susceptibility to overwhelming infections, periodic painful vaso-oclusive crises, bone marrow or fat embolism, stroke, renal medullary infraction, papillary necrosis, retinopathy, splenic sequestration, leg ulcers, and asceptic necrosis of bone. The most common cause of death in early life is infection. The mortality in childhood is in the range of 1 to 2% in the United States, with higher rates in underdeveloped countries (Old, 1998). The median age of death is 48 years. HbSC disease generally is considerably milder than HbSS disease; the median age of death in this condition is 68 years. HbS is more common in people of African ancestry but also occurs in those with Mediterranean or East Indian ancestry. HbC is found in people with African and

▼ **Table 7–1.** A DRAFT PROTOCOL FOR CHOOSING WOMEN FOR SELECTIVE SCREENING OR CASE
• FINDING FOR MATERNAL PHENYLKETONURIA

Mandatory (High-Risk) Prenatal Maternal Phenylketonuria Screening

1. Women with a definite or suggestive personal or family history of phenylketonuria
2. Women whose previous offspring have microcephaly or mental retardation
3. Women whose intelligence has been measured within the retarded or borderline range

Prenatal Maternal Phenylketonuria Screening to Be Considered

1. Women born before neonatal screening was introduced in their county or jurisdiction or with uncertain screening results
2. Women whose previous offspring had congenital heart disease (especially left-sided heart outlet syndromes, tetralogy of Fallot, or coarctation of the aorta)

Prenatal Maternal Phenylketonuria Screening Usually Unnecessary

1. Women born after neonatal screening began in their jurisdiction*
2. Women with previous unaffected offspring
3. Women whose racial or ethnic background makes phenylketonuria very unlikely (blacks, Japanese, Finns)

*If the offspring of women with mild hyperphenylalaninemia are shown to be at significant risk at the conclusion of the International Maternal Phenylketonuria Collaborative Study, then the cost-effectiveness of including in this suggested protocol first-pregnancy screening of all women already (neonatally) screened will be considered (Hanley et al., 1999).

Mediterranean (especially southern Sicily) ancestry. Other examples of compound heterozygosity with HbS are HbS/HbD-Punjab, in which a moderate hemolytic anemia exists, and HbS/O-Arab, in which phenotype is indistinguishable from HbSS.

Pregnancy in women with these disorders is associated with increases in maternal oxygen consumption, blood viscosity, red cell mass, and other physiologic demands. It is therefore not surprising that women with sickle cell disease experience increased complications during pregnancy. Seoud and colleagues (1994) performed a retrospective analysis of pregnant women with sickle cell disease who received blood products when indicated for symptomatic anemia, severe anemia with hematocrit < 18%, sickle crisis, cardiovascular instability, or preoperative hematocrit of < 23%. Twenty-two pregnancies were complicated by HbSS disease and 36 by HbSC disease. In the HbSS group, there was one therapeutic abortion and one spontaneous abortion; one spontaneous abortion occurred in the HbSC group. Nine of the remaining 20 pregnancies (45%) in the HbSS group were complicated by preterm labor versus seven out of thirty-five (20%) in the HbSC group. The frequency of preterm premature rupture of the membrane was two out of ten (20%) in HbSS versus none in HbSC. Four of twenty (20%) women with HbSS suffered pregnancy-induced hypertension compared with three of thirty-five (8.6%) in the HbSC group. Two of twenty (10%) of pregnancies in women with HbSS were complicated by intrauterine growth restriction versus two of thirty-five (5.7%) of pregnancies in women with HbSC disease. Over two thirds of the HbSS group were transfused with an average of 3.6 units of blood. In the HbSC group, about 30% were transfused with an average of 1 unit of blood. In the HbSS group, 50% experienced bone/pain crisis, 30% hemolytic crisis, 5% pulmonary embolus, 20% pneumonia, 30% lower urinary tract infection, and 10% postpartum endometritis. In the HbSC group, about 34% suffered bone/pain crisis, 9% hemolytic crisis, 3% pulmonary embolus, 14% pneumonia, 40% lower urinary tract infections, and 11% postpartum endometritis. There were two maternal deaths (9.1%) among the HbSS group and none among the HbSC group. Cesarean delivery rate was 52.6% in HbSS disease patients and 37.1% in HbSC disease patients. One patient died from massive gastrointestinal bleeding and unavailability of matched blood. The second patient died from pulmonary embolism. The perinatal infant mortality was 10.5% in women with HbSS disease and 2.9% in women with HbSC disease.

Smith and associates (1996) reported the results of the U.S. Cooperative Study of Sickle Cell Disease, which is composed of 19 centers prospectively studying the clinical course of sickle cell disease. Among 445 reported pregnancies, 286 proceeded to delivery. Non–sickle-related antepartum and intrapartum complications rates were comparable with those of African-American women who did not have sickle cell disease. One of the two deaths observed during this study was directly related to the presence of sickle cell disease. Rates of maternal morbidity attributed to the presence of sickle cell disease were the same during pregnancy as during the nonpregnant state. Ninety-nine percent of those pregnancies carried to delivery resulted in a live birth. Twenty-one percent of the infants born to women with HbSS were small for gestational age. Preeclampsia and acute anemic events were identified as risk factors in these infants.

Howard and coworkers (1995) performed a retrospective study to determine the effect of prophylactic transfusions on maternal and fetal outcome. Among 39 women with HbSS, 22 were prophylactically transfused; 33 had HbSC and 7 of these were prophylactically transfused. The prophylactic exchange transfusion program was begun either following sickling crisis or to prevent subsequent crisis. All underwent prophylactic transfusion beginning in the first or second trimester. The authors concluded that there was no evidence that either first or second trimester prophylactic transfusions improved fetal outcome. Moreover, prophylactic transfusions create the potential for maternal antibody formation, with subsequent risk of hemolytic disease in the fetus and difficulty finding compatible blood for future transfusions.

Women with sickle cell disease should be evaluated frequently for evidence of sickling and infection. They should be monitored by measurements of hemoglobin and hematocrit and antibodies for asymptomatic bacteriuria. Pneumococcal pneumonia vaccination is important in preventing infection that may lead to crisis. Supplementation with 1 mg folic acid/day is recommended; however, iron therapy should only be given to those women demonstrating iron deficiency anemia because of the risk of iron overload and hepatotoxicity. Serial ultrasound evaluation is useful in assessing fetal growth and amniotic fluid volume. Routine scans are generally recommended beginning around 32 weeks' gestation, unless crisis or other signs or symptoms suggest beginning earlier.

Prophylactic blood transfusion regimens during pregnancy have been suggested using single transfusion or exchange transfusion. Morrison and colleagues (1991) reported using erythrocyta-pheresis every 4 to 6 weeks to achieve an HbA percentage of at least 50% and packed cell volume of at least 25%. This regimen reduced the number of vaso-occlusive crises during pregnancy.

Koshy and coworkers (1988) reported a randomized trial of 76 pregnant women comparing prophylactic red cell transfusion to transfusion for emergencies only. They showed a significant reduction in the number of painful crises among the group receiving transfusions to maintain their HbS levels below 35% and hemoglobin concentrations between 10 and 11 g/dL. However, this study showed no differences between the two groups in perinatal outcome.

This issue of prophylactic transfusion in pregnant women with sickle cell disease remains controversial. Keidan and associates (1988) proposed using a "sickle crit," which was the product of the hematocrit and percentage of hemoglobin, to identify which patients might benefit most from transfusion. If one chooses to perform prophylactic transfusion, the goal is to maintain a percentage of hemoglobin A above 20% at all times and preferably above 40% as well as to maintain the hematocrit above 25% (Samuels, 1996).

The role of blood transfusions in the treatment of chronic sickle cell disease is undergoing critical reappraisal, which has been prompted by the introduction of hydroxyurea therapy, improvements in allogenic bone marrow transfusions, and increasing attention to safety issues (e.g., infection, iron overload, and alloimmunization (Germain et al., 1999).

α-THALASSEMIA

Each chromosome 16 normally carries two functioning α-globin genes, leading to a total of four α-globin genes (Fig. 7–1). Four clinical types of α-thalassemia exist, depending on the number of genes affected. So-called "silent" carriers (α-thalassemia 2) have a single α-globin gene deletion (αα/α_ or α_/αα) and are asymptomatic because the reduction of αmRNA is insufficient to produce significant globin chain imbalance.

If two of the α-globin genes are inactivated, the condition is called α-thalassemia trait or α-thalassemia 1. This condition is characterized by a microcytic anemia with mild poikilocytosis and anisocytosis. The hemoglobin concentration is usually 10 to 12 g/dL and the mean corpuscular volume 70 to 80 fL. This condition is often misdiagnosed as iron deficiency and treated inappropriately. In individuals of Southeast Asian descent, both α-globin genes on one chromosome 16 are defective, whereas both α-globin genes on the other chromosome 16 are normal (αα/_ _). Blacks with α-thalassemia 1 usually have the alternative arrangement, with one functioning α-globin gene on each chromosome 16 (α_α_).

Hemoglobin H disease results from deletion of all but one of the α-globin genes. Although there is considerable variation in the severity of this condition, the predominant features are hypochromic microcytic anemia, with secondary jaundice and hepatosplenomegaly. Common complications include hypersplenism, infection, leg ulcers, gallstones, and folic acid deficiency (Weatherall et al., 1995). Hemoglobin H disease could arise, for example, if one parent carried an α-thalassemia 2 chromosome (αα/__). The net result is a four to one predominance of β-globin chain to α-globin chain ratio, leading to detectable levels of β4 tetramers.

The most severe form is α°-thalassemia (α-thalassemia₁ homozygote); no functioning α-globin genes present (__/__). This condition is almost

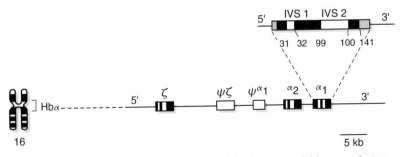

FIGURE 7–1 • Chromosomal location (16p) and organization of the human α globin gene cluster. ψ, pseudogene; IVS, introns (intervening sequences, white boxes). The numbers underneath the Hb α¹ gene—31, 32, 99, 100—refer to the codon numbers of the sequence at which a given intron interrupts the exon sequence. Intron 1 is interspersed between codons 31 and 32. (Only one pseudogene for Hb α is shown; newly discovered pseudogene 3′ of Hb α is not shown.) (From Vogel F, Motulsky AG: Human Genetics, 3rd ed. Berlin: Springer-Verlag, 1997.)

exclusively seen in individuals of Southeast Asian or Mediterranean origin. The predominant fetal hemoglobin is a tetramer of 8 β-chains known as hemoglobin Bart. The resulting severe fetal anemia leads to asphyxia, hydrops fetalis, and usually death *in utero* at 3 to 40 weeks' gestation or soon after birth. However, long-term survival has been recorded with aggressive transfusion therapy and iron chelation (Beaudry et al., 1986). Most recently, bone marrow transplantation has successfully been used for treatment as well (Ng et al., 1998). Pre-eclampsia is a frequent complication with hydrops fetalis (Old, 1998).

β-THALASSEMIA

The β-thalassemias are a clinically and molecularly heterogeneous group of disorders characterized by either a reduced rate of β-globin chain synthesis (β-) or absent β-globin chain systhesis (β°). There is only a single copy of the β-globin gene on each chromosome 11 (Fig. 7–2). The genetics of β-thalassemia are complicated by the large number (>300) and different mutations involving different sites (transcription, cap site, initiation codon, nonsense, splicing, insertion, deletion, frameshift, and poly A site) (Kazazian, 1990). Moreover, β° or β+-thalassemia mutations can exist in combination with β-chain or α-chain variants or α-thalassemia major or Colley anemia. No hemoglobin A is present when both β-globin genes are completely nonfunctional, whereas small amounts of hemoglobin A can be produced if one or both of the mutations still allow production of small amounts of β-globin chains.

At birth, infants with β-thalassemia major are asymptomatic because of the high amount of hemoglobin $F(\alpha_2/\delta_2)$ (Fig. 7–3). However, HbF decreases after birth, and by six months of age infants develop a severe microcytic hemolytic anemia with anisocytosis, poikilocytosis, polychromasia, and "teardrop" red cells. Precipitation of free α-chains results in inclusion bodies that damage red cell membranes and lead to destruction of red cells in the bone marrow. Affected children develop hepatosplenomegaly and a characteristic Asian facies due to excessive intramedullary hematopoiesis. The expanded bone marrow cavities predispose to pathologic fractures, and skull x-rays show a "hair-on-end" appearance. Affected individuals are also prone to cholelithiasis, infection, hypersplenism, and delayed growth and maturation (Nathan, 1972; Gay et al., 1997). Treatment involves frequent blood transfusions and iron chelation; otherwise, death results in the second or third decade from cardiac failure. Most recently, bone marrow transplantation has proved successful in patients showing deterioration with conventional therapy (Lucarelli et al., 1999).

Individuals with β-thalassemia trait (heterozygous β-thalassemia) are usually asymptomatic, although about half exhibit mild to moderate splenomegaly. They have a mild anemia (hemoglobin 10–11 g/dL), with decreased mean corpuscular volume (55-70 fL) and mean corpuscular hemoglobin (16–22 pg) (Gay et al., 1997).

Aessopos and coworkers (1999) reported 22 pregnancies in 19 women, including one twin pregnancy in twins with well-treated β-thalassemia major. Twenty-one healthy newborns were delivered. A spontaneous abortion and a case of omphalocele also occurred. Gestation, delivery, and recovery were uneventful, and no significant cardiac complications occurred. The authors concluded that pregnancy can be safe for mothers and infants with β-thalassemia major, provided that women are started early on intensive treatment and have a normal resting cardiac performance.

GENETIC SCREENING FOR HEMOGLOBINOPATHIES

Identifying individuals at increased risk for hemoglobinopathies is difficult. The American College

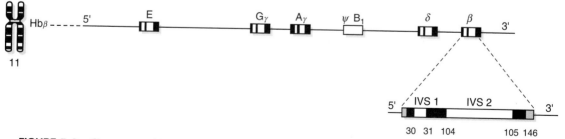

FIGURE 7–2 • Chromosomal location (11p) and organization of the human β globin gene cluster. Symbols and explanation identical to that for Figure 7–1. (From Vogel F, Motulsky AG: Human Genetics, 3rd ed. Berlin: Springer-Verlag, 1997.)

of Obstetrics and Gynecologists Committee on Genetics (1996) has stated that although universal screening of all couples of reproductive age is not recommended, the obstetrician should try to identify couples at increased risk for having offspring with sickle cell disease or the thalassemias. Ethnic groups considered at low risk are northern European, Japanese, Inuits (Eskimos), Native Americans, and individuals of Mexican and Korean descent. Although not explicitly stated, the assumption is that screening in all other ethnic or racial groups should be considered. When screening is indicated, both partners should have red cell indices and a hemoglobin electrophoresis as primary tests. Solubility tests (e.g., Sickledex) are inadequate because they fail to identify important transmissible hemoglobin gene abnormalities affecting fetal outcome, including HbC trait, β-thalassemia trait, HbE trait, Hbβ trait, and HbD trait. Determining mean corpuscular volume (MCV) is recommended for patients who are at increased risk for α-thalassemia and β-thalassemia. β-thalassemia is associated with elevated fetal hemoglobin and elevated HbA_2 levels (>3.5%). If MCV is below normal (<80 fL), iron-deficiency anemia is absent, and the hemoglobin electrophoresis is not consistent with β-thalassemia trait, DNA-based testing should be used to detect α-globin gene deletions characteristic of α-thalassemia.

Von Willebrand Disease

The most common inherited bleeding disorder is von Willebrand disease (vWD), with an estimated prevalence of up to 1 in 1000 individuals. There are more than 10 variants of vWD, most transmitted as autosomal dominant traits. The variants can be grouped into two major categories.

Types I and III vWD result from a decreased quantity of circulating von Willebrand factor (vWF), a heterogeneous multimeric plasma glycoprotein produced by endothelial cells and megakaryocytes. vWF is localized to chromosome 12. Seventy percent of all cases of vWD are type I, which shows autosomal dominant inheritance and is relatively mild. Type III is an autosomal recessive disorder and is characterized by extremely low levels of vWF and, thus, severe clinical manifestations.

Type II vWF constitutes about 10 to 15% of all cases and is the result of a qualitative defect in vWF. Point mutations or deletions in the vWF gene lead to abnormal multimeric structure of vWF. Affected individuals suffer from mild to moderate bleeding. Type II shows autosomal

dominant inheritance (Ginsburg and Bowie, 1992; Sorokin and Bardicef, 1996).

Individuals with vWD have a compound defect in platelet function and the coagulation pathway. Also, vWF serves as the plasma carrier for factor VIII, the antihemophilic factor, a critical blood coagulation protein. Clinical manifestations of vWD include easy bruising, spontaneous bleeding from mucous membranes, excessive bleeding from wounds, menorrhagia, and postpartum hemorrhage. Normally, levels of factor VIII vWF increase in response to stress, estrogens, and pregnancy. The most diagnostic patterns of laboratory tests are (1) a prolonged bleeding time, (2) a reduction in plasma vWF concentrations (normal vWF level is 10 mg/L), (3) a parallel reduction in biologic activity as measured with the ristocetin cofactor assay, and (4) reduction in factor VIII activity.

A woman with vWD should receive preconceptional counseling warning of the hemorrhagic complications she may encounter during pregnancy as well as the possibility of increased frequency of miscarriage, although no controlled studies have been performed. An international survey performed by Foster (1995) revealed that of 69 pregnancies in women with vWD, 15 (22%) ended in spontaneous abortions. There was a clustering, with miscarriages occurring in four women with type I disease. If the group was limited to only women with types II and III vWD, then the miscarriage rate was 11%. If miscarriage occurs, these women are at increased risk for severe hemorrhage. This increased risk is probably the result of insufficient protective effect of pregnancy on the factor VIII–vWF complex (Sorosky et al., 1980; Foster, 1995).

Prior obstetric history and response to medications such as desmopressin should be determined. During pregnancy, affected patients should be carefully monitored with periodic coagulation profiles and bleeding times. To avoid the risk of hemorrhage, factor VIII levels should be kept above 25% of normal, and the bleeding time should be kept under 15 minutes. Postpartum, the levels of vWF drop rapidly to their prepregnancy levels; thus, the risk of hemorrhage is increased during and after delivery (Kadir et al., 1998). The optimal mode of delivery is controversial, but it seems prudent to reserve vaginal deliveries for women with type I vWD and to offer cesarean delivery to women with types II and III so as to prevent any hemorrhagic complication (periventricular hemorrhage, cephalohematoma) in a potentially affected newborn.

Foster's (1995) international study revealed that among 24 deliveries or abortions, eight

(33%) were characterized by bleeding complications not attributable to surgical or anatomic causes. Twenty women who were known to be unresponsive to desmopression were treated prophylactically with blood products at the time of delivery or abortion. Factor VIII concentrate, cryoprecipitate, or fresh frozen plasma was used. Of these 20, 5 (25%) had bleeding complications. One case was a woman treated with factor VIII concentrate who suffered a 600-mL blood loss at delivery with no further blood loss postpartum. The other bleeding complications occurred 5 to 13 days postpartum and seemed to coincide with the cessation or reduction of therapy. The authors conclude that most women with type I disease can be successfully treated with desmopressin during the postpartum period, but for women with type III and those with types I and II disease who are resistant to desmopressin, prophylactic therapy with factor VIII concentrate or cryoprecipitate is recommended to mitigate against bleeding complications. Furthermore, the increased risk of postpartum hemorrhage mandates that these women be carefully monitored postpartum as to factor VII activity levels and bleeding times. These findings and conclusions were similar to those from a report of 31 women with vWD from the Royal Free Hospital in London during 1980–1996 (Kadir et al., 1998). The incidence of primary postpartum hemorrhage was 18.5%. None of the women who had prophylactic treatment during labor or the puerperium suffered any significant bleeding complications. Finally, preliminary evidence suggests that continuous infusion of a combined factor VIII–von Willebrand factor concentrate is superior to intermittent bolus injections to prevent bleeding at surgery and time of vaginal delivery (Lubetsky et al., 1999).

Factor V Leiden Mutation

A number of serious obstetric complications, including spontaneous abortion, pre-eclampsia, intrauterine growth restriction, and stillbirth, have been associated with abnormal placental vasculature and disturbances of hemostasis, leading to inadequate maternal-fetal circulation (Kupferminc et al., 1999). Several thrombophilic mutations are associated with an increased risk of thromboembolic complications (Seligsohn and Lubetsky, 2001). Among these is resistance to protein C caused by a missense mutation of the factor V gene (1691G→A), which results in an abnormal factor V protein called factor V Leiden. Factor V Leiden occurs in 2 to 4% of whites and 20 to 60% of individuals with a personal or family history of thrombosis (Bertina et al., 1994). This mutation predisposes carriers to thrombosis because the mutant protein is resistant to proteolytic inactivation by activated protein C (Svensson and Dahlback, 1994). Bertina and colleagues (1994) have shown that 80 to 100% of individuals with laboratory-confirmed activated protein C resistance are either heterozygous or homozygous for this mutation.

Dizon-Townson and coworkers (1996) studied 158 gravid women with severe pre-eclampsia and 403 normotensive controls for the factor V Leiden mutation. Fourteen of 158 women (8.9%) with severe pre-eclampsia were heterozygotes for the mutation compared with 17 of 403 normotensive women (4.2%) (χ^2 4.686, P = 0.03). No homozygotes were detected in either group. The authors concluded that carriers for the factor Leiden V mutation are at increased risk for severe pre-eclampsia and that testing for this mutation could serve as one component of a genetic screening profile for pre-eclampsia and other adverse pregnancy outcomes.

Recently, Kupferminc and coworkers (1999) studied 110 women who had severe pre-eclampsia, abruptio placentae, fetal growth restriction, or stillbirth and 110 women who had normal pregnancies and no history of thromboembolic complications during any pregnancy. Factor V Leiden mutation was detected in 22 of the women with pregnancy complications and in seven of the women with normal pregnancies (20% and 6%, respectively; P = 0.003). Among the women with complications, two were homozygous and 20 were heterozygous for factor V Leiden; all seven with this mutation who had normal pregnancies proved heterozygous. The authors suggests that women with severe complications of pregnancy should be tested for markers of thrombophilia, including the factor V Leiden mutation. By contrast, DeGroot and associates (1999) conducted a case-control study of 163 women with pre-eclampsia. Patients and controls were tested for the presence of factor V Leiden, prothrombin 2010A allele, protein C, protein S, and antithrombin deficiency. Surprisingly, they found no difference in the prevalence of these genetic risk factors of thrombosis in women with pre-eclampsia compared with control subjects.

Because these complications tend to recur (e.g., pre-eclampsia at a rate of 20%), the presence of thrombophilia in these women may be an important consideration in planning future pregnancies, surgical procedures, and oral contraceptive use (Bloomenthal et al., 2002).

Marfan Syndrome

Marfan syndrome is a hereditary connective tissue disorder with an estimated prevalence of four to six cases per 10,000. The disease results from mutations in the fibrillin-1 gene on chromosome 15q. Fibrillin-1 encodes the extracellular matrix component in microfibrils. Marfan syndrome demonstrates autosomal dominant inheritance. Of all cases, 65 to 75% are familial, and the remaining cases occur sporadically as result of new mutations. Clinical manifestations include musculoskeletal deformities (tall stature, scoliosis, chest wall deformities, arachnodactyly), cardiovascular disease (mitral valve prolapse, mitral regurgitation, aortic root dilatation, aortic incompetence), and an ocular feature (myopia and ectopia lentis) (Fig. 7–4). Cardiovascular manifestations are life-threatening. Individuals affected with Marfan syndrome have a shortened life-expectancy, with the mean age of death in the early thirties, most commonly the result of aortic dissection or rupture (Elias and Berkowitz, 1976; Elkayam et al., 1995; Rossiter et al., 1995; Lipscomb et al., 1997; Mayet et al., 1998).

Women with Marfan syndrome face two important risks during pregnancy: (1) the 50% chance that the child will inherit the disorder, analogous to other autosomal dominant conditions discussed in this chapter, and (2) the substantial cardiovascular stress imposed by pregnancy, which increases the risk of aortic dissection with potentially fatal consequences. In a retrospective study of 32 pregnant women with Marfan syndrome, Pyeritz (1981) found that 20 women (62.5%) suffered acute aortic dissection;

16 of the 20 died during or shortly after the pregnancy, and 4 died postpartum due to an aortic rupture or regurgitation. However, most of these women also had pre-existing cardiovascular abnormalities such as aortic dilatation, regurgitation, coarctation of the aorta, hypertension, and cardiomegaly. Pyeritz (1981) also noted that the women with minor cardiovascular involvement and an aortic root diameter of <40 mm had a relatively low risk of aortic dissection.

Rossiter and coworkers (1995) reported a prospective study of 21 pregnant women with Marfan syndrome whose manifestations ranged from mild to severe. He compared them to 18 nulliparous women with Marfan syndrome who were matched for age and clinical manifestations. Of 45 pregnancies, there were seven (16%) spontaneous abortions and ten (22%) elective abortions for secondary to maternal cardiovascular compromise (i.e., progressive aortic dilatation, mitral regurgitation, aortic dissection). There were 26 live births (58%): 48% were spontaneous vaginal deliveries, 30% forceps-assisted, and 22% cesarean deliveries for obstetric indications. There were two cases of aortic dissection; one had a dissection at 17 weeks' gestation, necessitating termination of the pregnancy. Her dissection occurred 1 week postpartum. Twenty-two of 28 women had echocardiographic measurements of the aortic root done approximately every 6 weeks throughout pregnancy and for 4 to 8 weeks postpartum. In the majority of women, there was little or no change in their aortic root diameter. Furthermore, 5-year follow-up revealed no worsening in their long-term cardiovascular prognosis compared with the nulliparous control group. The authors concluded that most Marfan patients with mild cardiovascular involvement (mild aortic dilatation without evidence of regurgitation or dissection) can safely undergo pregnancy. They

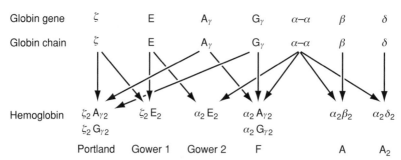

FIGURE 7–3 • Normal human globin genes. Single genes exist for Hb β, δ, ε and ζ. The genes for Hb α and Hb γ are duplicated. The products of the two hemoglobin γ genes (Hb ^{A}γ and Hb^{G}γ) differ from each other by a single amino acid residue, alanine (A) or glycine (G) at position 136. There are no known differences between the two Hb α genes. Tetrameric hemoglobin formation is shown in the lower portion of the figure. (From Vogel F, Motulsky AG: Human Genetics, 3rd ed. Berlin: Springer-Verlag, 1997.)

recommended that women with Marfan receive preconceptional cardiovascular assessment and be counseled regarding the risk of cardiovascular complications during pregnancy as well as the 50% risk of the newborn's inheriting their disease. If the woman has moderate or severe aortic regurgitation or an aortic root diameter of ≥40 mm, she should be advised that her risk of cardiovascular complications is greatly increased. However, if her aortic root is <40 mm and she has minor cardiovascular involvement, it is more than likely that she will tolerate pregnancy well. The authors also recommend the prophylactic use of beta blockers, at least from midtrimester onward, in order to prevent aortic dilatation. Patients should be closely monitored with echocardiograms every 6 to 10 weeks, depending on the initial findings. Delivery should be approached with attempts at minimizing maternal expulsive efforts as much as possible so as to reduce the rise in blood pressure. Most authors suggest liberal use of forceps or vacuum extraction to shorten the second stage of labor. Since the increased risk of dissection persists until 6 to 8 weeks postpartum, careful surveillance should continue throughout this time period. Antibiotic prophylaxis is suggested during labor and delivery.

Therapeutic abortion or surgical intervention should be considered if a pregnant woman with Marfan syndrome shows progressive dilatation of the aorta. Cola and Lavin (1985) reported successful aortic arch graft placement for an aortic dissection that occurred a few days postconception with normal fetal outcome. Smith and coworkers (1989) reported successful aortic valve replacement and aortic graft placement at 22 weeks' gestation for progressive aortic dilatation. However, maternal cardiac surgery does pose a risk to the fetus; thus, if fetal lung maturity can be confirmed, a cesarean delivery may be preferable before or concomitant with thoracic surgery.

If aortic dissection occurs during pregnancy, immediate treatment includes hydralazine (not nitroprusside because of the risk of thiocyanate toxicity in the fetus) and beta blockers to control blood pressure and decrease left ventricular contractility. This reduces ejection velocity and minimizes the shearing forces on the aorta. Hypotension follows if the dissection is large or if it ruptures. With ascending aortic arch involvement, a loud murmur of aortic insufficiency may be heard. In patients with progressive dissection, emergency surgical correction is required.

Lipscomb and associates (1997) performed a retrospective study of 36 women with Marfan syndrome. Of 91 pregnancies, there were 75 live births, eight miscarriages, seven therapeutic abortions, and one stillborn. There were seven cases of postpartum hemorrhages requiring blood transfusions. None of the women experienced cardiovascular compromise before pregnancy. Six of the thirty-six (16.7%) women suffered aortic events: dissection occurred in four women (one immediately fatal), and two developed progressive aortic root dilatation. For most women (82.7%), a safe delivery per vagina was possible, but for those with cardiovascular problems or obstetric indications (9.3%), a cesarean delivery was performed. The authors concluded that complication-free pregnancy cannot be guaranteed in women with Marfan syndrome. They agree with previous recommendations that women having an aortic root diameter ≥40 mm should be counseled that they are at significant risk of cardiovascular complications if they undergo pregnancy. The authors felt that women who demonstrate a steady increase in aortic dimension should also be informed of their increased complication risk during pregnancy. For women with a stable aortic measurement of <40 mm, delivery per vagina was advocated, preferably with epidural anesthesia (to prevent a labor-associated rise in blood pressure). Women who demonstrate progressive aortic dilatation or dimensions >40 mm should undergo an elective cesarean delivery to reduce the risk of cardiovascular complications. Women with Marfan syndrome should also be encouraged to complete their childbearing in their early 20s, since aortic events tend to occur in the fourth decade.

Ehlers-Danlos Syndrome

There are at least ten types of Ehlers-Danlos syndrome (EDS), all resulting in the abnormal production or secretion of collagens. Inheritance is typically autosomal dominant; however, some forms are autosomal recessive or X-linked recessive. The overall prevalence of EDS is 1 in 5000. Clinical manifestations include skin fragility, fragility of the dermal blood vessels, characteristic "papyraceous" scar, hyperextensible and transparent skin, and hypermobile joints. Severity of the symptoms varies with type (Fig. 7–5).

Type I is the most common and the most severe type, constituting 30 to 50% of the cases. The molecular defects in most patients with types I, II, and III forms of EDS are known. Type IV results from mutations in the COL3A1 gene, which encodes the polypeptides in type III procollagen (Milewicz, 1998). Blood vessels of the gastrointestinal tract and uterus are rich in type

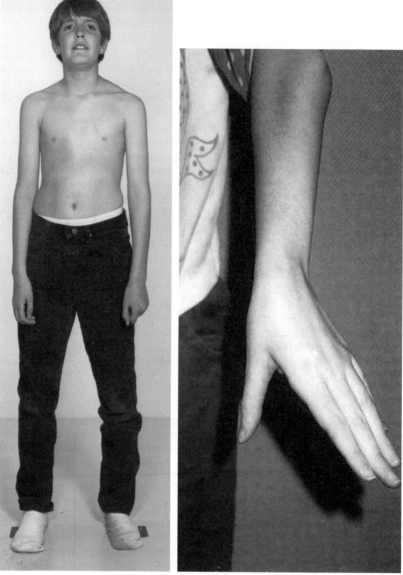

A   B

FIGURE 7–4 • (A) A young man with Marfan syndrome showing characteristically long limbs and narrow face. (B) Arachnodactyly in an 8-year-old girl with Marfan syndrome. (From Jorde LB, Carey JC, Bamshad MJ, et al.: Medical Genetics, 2nd ed. St. Louis: Mosby, 2000.)

III procollagen (Hordnes, 1994; Sorokin et al., 1994).

Pregnant women with EDS may experience numerous complications, including laxity with subluxations and separation of the symphysis pubis, varicose veins, and large abdominal hernias. Increased incidences of spontaneous abortion, stillbirth, and bleeding during pregnancy have been reported. A high preterm birth rate has also been found, believed to be due to a collagen abnormality in the chorionic membrane of the affected fetus (DeVos et al., 1999). This leads to premature rupture of the membranes and thus preterm labor. Cervical incompetence may also result in increased spontaneous abortions and preterm delivery (Barabas 1966; Beighton, 1969; Taylor et al., 1981; Peaceman and Cruikshank, 1987).

Sorokin and colleagues (1994) reviewed 43 women with EDS who had 138 pregnancies. The spontaneous abortion rate was 29% (40 out of 138). Among 95 women whose pregnancies continued, stillbirths occurred in 3.2%, preterm labor in 23.1%, cesarean delivery in 18.4%, small for gestational age infants in 15.7%, and antepartum and/or intrapartum hemorrhage in 14.8%. Other pregnancy complications included one case each of heart failure, hip pain, preeclampsia, and separation of the symphysis in a patient with EDS type IV. Five percent experienced a difficult or prolonged labor.

In type IV EDS, maternal mortality has been cited as high as 25%, typically the result of a gastrointestinal, uterine, or major blood vessel wall rupture (Rudd et al., 1983; Pepin et al., 2000). Maternal deaths have been reported from these complications (Barabas, 1972; Rudd et al., 1983; Snyder et al., 1983). Cardiovascular changes that occur during pregnancy (increased cardiac output and blood volume) may magnify the shear forces on the abnormal blood vessels, resulting in their rupture (Athanassiou and Turrentine, 1996). However, Gilchrist and coworkers (1999) studied a large French-Canadian kindred with EDS type IV caused by a point mutation (G571S) in the COL3A1 gene. They found few complications and no deaths in 37 pregnancies among eight affected women. The authors concluded that adverse pregnancy in some mutations of COL3A1 can be associated with lower pregnancy morbidity and mortality than the severe EDS type IV usually described.

In women with EDS, delivery per vagina can be complicated by hemorrhage, hematoma formation, severe lacerations of the vagina and perineum, and extension of episiotomies. Repair is difficult because of tissue fragility, sutures pulling through tissues, and wound dehiscence. Prolapse of the uterus and bladder may also occur. Use of forceps or vacuum extraction should be avoided, particularly if the fetus is affected with EDS, because operative obstetric procedures may increase the risk of severe fetal hematomas and lacerations. Cesarean delivery also carries the risk of weak scar formation and rupture in subsequent pregnancies (Georgy et al., 1997).

In summary, women with EDS should be counseled about the risks involved with pregnancy and to their offspring. Close follow-up is necessary throughout pregnancy and the postpartum period so that prompt intervention can be initiated in the event of a complication. Finally, there is no preferred mode of delivery cited in the literature, as both are associated with risks to the mother. The safest means of delivery for the patient with EDS must be determined on a case-by-case basis.

Myotonic Dystrophy

Myotonic dystrophy is the most common adult muscular dystrophy, having an incidence of 13.5 per 100,000 live births. This progressive systemic disease demonstrates autosomal dominant inheritance. The gene for myotonic dystrophy is on the long arm of chromosome 19 and is characterized by an unstable expansion of a CTG trinucleotide repeat sequence at 19q13.3 (Brook et al., 1992). The number of CTG trinucleotides on normal chromosomes ranges from 3 to 30; patients with mytonic dystrophy show amplifications of >45 repeats. Myotonic dystrophy demonstrates genetic anticipation; with successive generations, the severity of the phenotype increases in association with an increase in the number of trinucleotide repeats. Anticipation seems to be more pronounced with maternal transmission of the gene (Harper and Dyken, 1972). As result, the clinical expression of myotonic dystrophy varies widely. Manifestations include progressive muscle atrophy and weakness and myotonia that usually appears by age 5. It is demonstrable by slow relaxation of hand grip following a voluntary closure, cardiac disturbances (conduction system abnormalities, first-degree heart block, mitral valve prolapse), intellectual impairment, cataracts, gonadal atrophy, insulin resistance, decreased esophageal and colonic motility, and a "hatchet-faced" appearance owing to temporalis, masseter, and facial muscle atrophy and weakness (Fig. 7–6). Women with myotonic dystrophy often show infertility, particularly if they have severe disease (Lamon et al., 1981). Nonetheless, conception is possible, and most successfully when the woman is young.

Women with myotonic dystrophy need preconceptional counseling regarding the possible complications they may encounter during pregnancy. For instance, pregnancy may worsen the course of myotonic dystrophy. This has not been reported to be a regular occurrence, but when it does happen it is typically characterized by weakness and difficulty walking. An increased incidence of spontaneous abortions and preterm labor and delivery has also been reported (Besinger, 1993). A review of 60 pregnancies in 32 women with myotonic dystrophy revealed a spontaneous abortion rate of 13.3%, no higher than predicted in the general population (see Chapter 5). The authors noted that polyhydramnios complicated nine pregnancies, eight of which produced a child with congenital myotonic dystrophy. The ninth neonate died 2 hours after birth. He had severe muscular hypotonia and rupture of the tentorium (Esplin et al., 1998).

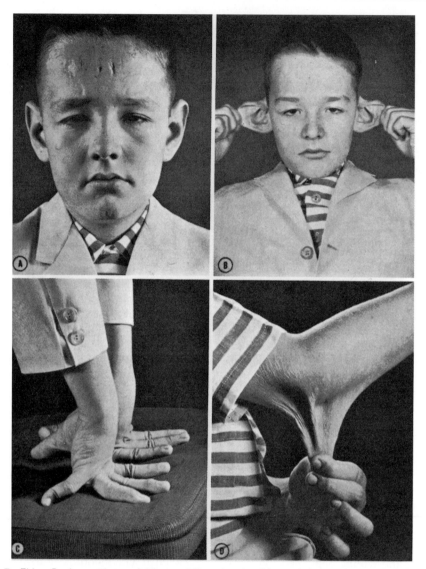

FIGURE 7–5 • Ehlers-Danlos syndrome. A 12-year-old boy showing thin persisting scars on his forehead (*A*), hyper-elasticity of auricles and skin (*B* and *D*), and hyperextensibility of joints (*C*). (From Jones KL: Smith's Recognizable Patterns of Human Malformation, 5th ed. Philadelphia: WB Saunders, 1997.)

Congenital myotonic dystrophy is a severe neonatal form of the disease. Occurring in approximately 25% of infants of affected mothers, this form is characterized by weak fetal movements during pregnancy, high neonatal death rate (35%), hypotonia, facial weakness, respiratory distress, and feeding difficulties (Vanier, 1960; Hojo et al., 1995). Those who survive develop the classic signs of adult type mytonic dystrophy in childhood.

Rudnik-Schoneborn and colleagues (1998) reported a retrospective study of 26 women with myotonic dystrophy who had a total of 67 gestations. Of 56 infants carried to term, 29 had or most likely had inherited the gene for myotonic dystrophy from their affected mothers. Perinatal loss rate was 11% and associated with congenital disease. Obstetric complications included preterm labor (55%) and polyhydramnios (21%). Eight women (31%) experienced a worsening of their symptoms during pregnancy. Failure to progress in the first or second stage of labor, often in combination with fetal distress, was documented in 13% of all pregnancies, mostly associated with an affected fetus.

Finally, regional anesthesia is preferred for operative delivery; however, general anesthesia is not contraindicated, provided that risks are anticipated and steps are taken to minimize complications (Boyle, 1999).

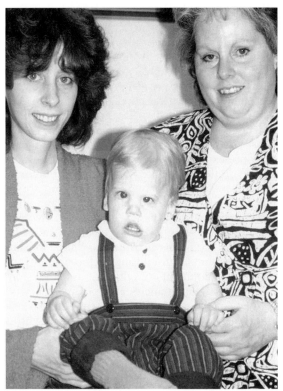

FIGURE 7–6 • A three-generation family affected with myotonic dystrophy. The degree of severity increases in each generation. The grandmother (right) is only slightly affected, but the mother (left) has a characteristic narrow face and somewhat limited facial expression. The baby is more severely affected and has the facial features of children with neonatal-onset myotonic dystrophy, including an open, triangle-shaped mouth. The infant has more than 1000 copies of the trinucleotide repeat, whereas the mother and grandmother each have approximately 100 repeats. (From Jorde LB, Carey JC, Bamshed MJ, White RL: Medical Genetics, 2nd ed. St. Louis: Mosby, 2000.)

Idiopathic Hypertrophic Subaortic Stenosis

Idiopathic hypertrophic subaortic stenosis (IHSS) is an autosomal dominant condition characterized by septal hypertrophy that obstructs left ventricular outflow and causes mitral valve regurgitation (Jelsema, 1996). Clinical manifestations vary, but the major complications include atrial fibrillation with mural thrombus formation, embolization from the mural thrombi, infective endocarditis on the mitral valve, intractable cardiac failure, and sudden death. The frequency of sudden death is 2 to 3% per year for adults and 4 to 6% per year for children (Schoen, 1994).

Linkage analysis studies have shown a statistically significant association between the disease

status and at least seven genetic loci, all coding for sacromeric proteins. The first identified disease gene was beta myosin heavy chain (BMHC). Epstein (1998) has identified 32 distinct gene mutations in 62 kindreds after screening representatives of over 400 kindreds. All but one of the 50 approximately known mutations are restricted to the head or head-rod junction of the molecule. Muscle biopsies with identified BMHC mutations show abnormal histology, and isolated myosin and skinned fibers.

The effects of pregnancy on IHSS are variable. The increased blood volume improves cardiac output, but the drop in systemic vascular resistance decreases it. The increased maternal heart rate reduces left ventricular filling time and increases outflow obstruction. Hypertrophic cardiomyopathy is indeed compatible with gestation, and most affected women complete their pregnancies without serious complications (Rothlin et al., 1995; Jelsema, 1996). However, postpartum congestive heart failure and severe left ventricular systolic dysfunction, as well as maternal death, have been reported (Oakley et al., 1979; Kazimuddin et al., 1998).

Autosomal Dominant Polycystic Kidney Disease

Autosomal dominant polycystic kidney disease (ADPKD) is a common condition with a high penetrance. The estimated prevalence is approximately 1 in 1000 individuals (Dalgaard, 1957). Mutations in at least three different genes can lead to ADPKD. The *PKD1* gene is on chromosome 16 (16p 13.3), covers about 52 kb of genomic DNA, and consists of 46 exons. The 4303 amino acid product appears to be related to polycystin-2 (Hateboer et al., 1999). At least one other gene is known to be associated with ADPKD; its chromosomal location remains unknown (Daoust et al., 1995). Among European patients with ADPKD, *PKD1* is the cause in about 85% of families, with *PKD2* the cause of about 15% (Peters and Sandkuijl, 1992).

ADPKD is characterized by the presence of multiple cysts in the cortex and medulla of both kidneys. These cysts enlarge the organs and interfere with function. Clinical manifestations typically begin in the third or fourth decade. These include flank pain, hematuria, nocturia, renal colic secondary to stones and blood clots, hypertension, and progression to chronic renal failure. Chronic renal failure is a very slow process in these patients and may persist for years, with azotemia slowly progressing to uremia. Forty percent also have hepatic cysts that are usually asymptomatic, and 10 to 30% have intracranial Berry aneurysms. Eventually, one third die of renal failure, one third of hypertensive complications, and the remaining one third of unrelated causes. Patients with *PKD1* have more severe disease, a higher risk of the disease's progressing to renal failure, a higher prevalence of hypertension, and a shorter life expectancy as compared with *PKD2* patients (Hateboer et al., 1999; Wilson and Guay-Woodford, 1999).

Chapman and associates (1994) reported the maternal and fetal outcomes of 235 women with ADPKD who had 605 pregnancies. Compared with a control group of 108 non-ADPKD women who had 244 pregnancies, the mean age at ADPKD diagnosis was 31 years, and fertility was equivalent to that in the control group. There were seven ectopic pregnancies in the ADPKD women compared to only one among the control group. Although they are not statistically significant, these data remain noteworthy since severe abdominal pain often occurs in women with ADPKD. Therefore, the possibility of an ectopic pregnancy needs to be kept in mind.

The spontaneous abortion rate among women with ADPKD is not significantly different from that of the control group (12 versus 13%, respectively) (Chapman et al., 1994). Of 12 therapeutic abortions performed in the ADPKD group, 10 were directly related to ADPKD (ectopic, worsening maternal hypertension, severe fetal polycystic kidney disease, and marked oligohydramnios). The rate of maternal complications was significantly higher in the ADPKD group (35 versus 19%). Fifteen percent of women with ADPKD developed new-onset hypertension during their pregnancies, a rate similar to that found in other studies. Seven percent developed worsening hypertension, and 11% developed pre-eclampsia (versus 4% in the control group). Twenty-five percent of women in the APKD group developed edema versus 15% in the control group. Women with ADPKD who developed pre-eclampsia had significantly higher rates of preterm delivery (26%) compared with their non–pre-eclampsia counterparts (10%). Perinatal mortality rates had a tendency to increase, although not significantly, in women with ADPKD who had hypertensive complications during pregnancy.

Chapman and associates (1994) also found that normotensive women with ADPKD who developed hypertension, pre-eclampsia, or eclampsia were at greater risk for developing chronic hypertension compared with their non–pre-eclamptic, non–hypertensive counterparts (83 versus 62%). Thus, hypertensive complications during preg-

nancy in women with ADPKD are a strong risk factor for the development of chronic hypertension in the future. Women with ADPKD also have a higher risk of acute renal failure during pregnancy. In this study, four affected women developed acute renal failure during pregnancy, a rate much higher than that of the general population (1 in 10,000).

Overall, the majority of women with ADPKD did not suffer fetal or maternal complications. Most had normal renal function prior to conception; pre-existing hypertension imposed the most negative effect on maternal and fetal outcome. Women with pre-existing hypertension are at higher risk for increased fetal loss and maternal complications such as pre-eclampsia. Women with ADPKD who develop pre-eclampsia are at higher risk for premature birth, perinatal mortality, acute renal failure during pregnancy, and the future development of chronic hypertension. Four or more pregnancies also put women with ADPKD at risk for loss of renal function.

In conclusion, a woman with ADPKD who is normotensive prior to conception can be reassured that her chances of a successful, uncomplicated pregnancy are good. However, if she has poor renal function or pre-existing hypertension or both, her pregnancy should be regarded as high risk and requires close surveillance. All women with ADPKD should receive appropriate preconceptional genetic counseling regarding the potential risks of pregnancy as well as the 50% chance of having an affected fetus.

Pre-eclampsia and Eclampsia

Pre-eclampsia is the development of hypertension with proteinuria or edema between the 20th week of gestation and the end of the 1st week postpartum. Incidence ranges between 3 and 7% in nulliparas (Knuist et al., 1998; Campbell and MacGillivray, 1999; Hauth et al., 2000; Sibai et al., 2000) and between 0.8 and 5.0% in multiparas (Long et al., 1979; Campbell and MacGillivray, 1999). The incidence is significantly increased in patients with twin pregnancies (Campbell and MacGillivray, 1999). Blood pressure must increase by at least 30 mm Hg systolic or 15 mm Hg diastolic. Readings of 140/90 mm Hg after 20 weeks' gestation, if prior blood pressure readings are unknown, are considered sufficiently elevated for the diagnosis of pre-eclampsia. Proteinuria is defined as 0.3 g in a 24-hour collection, and edema is diagnosed as clinically evident generalized swelling. In mild pre-eclampsia, the diastolic blood pressure remains below 110 mm Hg. The criteria for severe pre-eclampsia are given in Table 7–2. Eclampsia is when convulsive seizures or coma not

▼ **Table 7–2.** SELECTED MENDELIAN DISORDERS THAT OBSTETRICIANS MAY ENCOUNTER IN
• PREGNANT WOMEN

Disorders	Inheritance	Clinical Presentation and Complications of Pregnancy
Ornithine transcarbamylase deficiency	AR	Hyperammonemia associated with orotic aciduria. Low-protein diet required.
Acute intermittent porphyria	AD	Abdominal pain, nausea, vomiting, diarrhea, peripheral motor neuropathy, bulbar paralysis, muscle pain or weakness, hypertension, seizures, psychosis. Increased porphobilinogen and urine delta-aminolevulinic acid
Wilson disease	AR	Abnormal copper metabolism. Cirrhosis, neurologic deterioration, Kayser-Fleischer rings of cornea, hemolytic anemia, psychiatric disorders. Requires discontinuation of penicillamine during pregnancy (chelating agent)
Malignant hyperthermia	AD	Succinylcholine and/or general anesthesia may lead to fulminant and often fatal hyperthermia and muscle rigidity
Osteogenesis imperfecta–type I	AD	Blue sclerae, brittle bones with frequent fractures, hypocalcemia, contracted pelvis, uterine rupture, separation of the pubis, poor scar healing
Neurofibromatosis 1	AD	Café au lait spots, cutaneous and subcutaneous neurofibromas, scoliosis, pheochromocytomas, optic gliomas, seizures, deafness, increased intracranial pressure, hypertension
Achondroplasia	AD	Rhizomelic skeletal dysplasia, large head, midfacial hypoplasia, spinal cord compression with hyperflexion of head, uterine leiomyomas, diabetes mellitus, cephalopelvic disproportion requiring cesarean section
Thrombocytopenia with absent radius (TAR syndrome)	AR	Thrombocytopenia, bilateral absent radii, skeletal abnormalities, congenital heart defects, hemorrhagic manifestations
Tuberous sclerosis	AD	Seizures, mental retardation, adenoma sebaceum, renal hamartomas
Congenital chloride diarrhea	AR	Most commonly found among individuals from Finnish ancestry. Diarrhea with chloride loss, distended abdomen, hypokalemia, polyhydramnios
Noonan syndrome	AD	Valvular pulmonic stenosis, short stature, hypotelorism, micrognathia, webbed neck, skeletal anomalies, atrial septal defect, Ebstein anomaly, coarctation of aorta

AR, autosomal recessive; AD, autosomal dominant.

attributed to other causes occurs during the same time frame as pre-eclampsia.

The etiology of pre-eclampsia is unknown. Currently, four major areas are under investigation, and most certainly there are interactions between them. The first is endothelial cell dysfunction related to increased trophoblast deportation resulting from placental ischemia. The second is the reduction in nonesterified fatty acids during pregnancy in women with already low albumin concentrations, which may reduce albumin's antitoxic activity to a level at which very-low density lipoprotein toxicity occurs. Third, an increased release of cytokines, proteolytic enzymes, and free radicals may occur because of immune maladaptation leading to shallow invasion of spiral arteries by endovascular cytotrophoblast cells and endothelial cell dysfunction. The fourth area is genetic factors that may display considerable genetic heterogencity (Dekker and Sibai, 1998). Our discussion will focus on this last group.

FAMILY STUDIES

There is substantial evidence for a familial predisposition to pre-eclampsia, with virtually all modes of inheritance being invoked. In 1968, Chesley and coworkers (1968) reported a study in which there was a 26% incidence of pre-eclampsia in daughters of women with pre-eclampsia but only an 8% incidence in the daughter-in-law. Sibai and coworkers (1991) reported 108 women with severe pre-eclampsia that developed in the second trimester who subsequently had 169 pregnancies. Follow-up showed that 110 (65%) of these pregnancies were complicated by pre-eclampsia, 32% of these developing in the second trimester, 32% at 28 to 36 weeks, and 36% at 37 to 40 weeks.

Recent data continue to support a genetic susceptibility for pre-eclampsia. Cincotta and Brennecke (1998) studied 368 primigravid women, 34 (9.2%) of whom developed pre-eclampsia. Eighteen (4.9%) women of the total group reported a mother (12), sister (5), or both (1) who had pre-eclampsia. Of these women, five (27.8%) developed pre-eclampsia. Of the women who had no family history, 29 (8.3%) developed pre-eclampsia.

The pattern of inheritance for pre-eclampsia remains unclear. Autosomal recessive inheritance in mother or fetus, maternal-fetal genotype interaction (i.e., the same single recessive gene in mother and fetus), and polygenic-multifactorial inheritance have all been suggested (Chesley and

Cooper, 1986; Liston and Kilpatrick, 1991; Arngrímsson et al., 1997). In a recent review of the subject, Morgan and Ward (1999) opined that it is unlikely that any single genotype is necessary for pre-eclampsia to occur; rather, "pre-eclampsia genes" act as susceptibility loci that lower a woman's threshold for the disease. This model is consistent with polygenic-multifactorial inheritance. Difficulties in analyzing inheritance patterns include inconsistent definitions of the pre-eclampsia "phenotype" and few and inconclusive twin-concordance studies or consanguinity studies that can be used for inheritance pattern modeling.

CANDIDATE GENES

HLA Antigens

Conflicting data have been reported about the involvement of HLA antigens. Kilpatrick and colleagues (1989) studied 56 women who had pre-eclampsia and who had parous sisters. The frequency of HLA DR4 was higher in sisters with pregnancy-induced hypertension than in sisters with normotensive pregnancies (8 of 18 [44%] versus 10 of 54 [19%]) and more of them shared HLA DR4 with their spouses (4/14 [29%] versus 0/29). They concluded that genetic susceptibility to pre-eclampsia is associated with HLA DR4. Peterson and coworkers (1994) reported that women with HLA haplotypes A23/29, B44, and DR7 are at higher risk for developing pre-eclampsia. By contrast, Wilton and associates (1990) studied 10 families with multiple cases of pre-eclampsia/eclampsia and found no evidence of close linkage to the HLA region on chromosome 6. Others have come to similar conclusions (Hayward et al., 1992). Humphrey and colleagues (1995) failed to show any HLA-G deletion polymorphisms and pre-eclamptic families when compared with controls.

Angiotensinogen

Angiotensinogen is the precursor of the vasoconstrictive hormone angiotensin II, which plays an important role in blood pressure regulation, fluid volume, and vascular remodeling. Ward and coworkers (1993) found an amino acid substitution in the angiotensinogen gene on chromosome 1 (the presence of threonine rather than methionine at residue 235 [235T] in the protein) to correlate with pre-eclampsia. In their Caucasian population, 20% of women homozygous for the T235 variant developed pre-eclampsia compared with <1% in women homozygous for the normal M235 allele. Although similar findings were

reported from Japan (Kobashi et al., 1999), other groups have not shown such an association (Wilton et al., 1990; Morgan et al., 1995). More recently, a tightly linked mutation in the angiotensinogen promotor, A(-6) has been found (Inoue et al., 1997). This A(-6) mutation causes elevated angiotensinogen expression *in vitro* and *in vivo* (Morgan et al., 1995; Inoue et al., 1997). The renin-angiotensinogen reaction is the rate-limiting step in the generation of angiotensin II. Thus, any abnormal local elevation in angiotensinogen expression would result in elevated angiotensinogen levels (Morgan and Ward, 1999). Genetic alterations in angiotensin II receptor are currently under investigation because changes in their expression may be involved in regulating vasodilatation in uteroplacental and fetoplacental vessels (Cox et al., 1996).

Factor V Leiden Mutation and Other Coagulation Abnormalities

Abnormal placentation has been associated with an increased tendency toward thrombosis (Dizon-Townson et al., 1996; Kupferminc et al., 1999). Thus, it has been hypothesized that the tendency toward thrombosis in women with pre-eclampsia might be the result of the combination of an underlying genetic risk factor for venous thrombosis and pregnancy (DeGroot et al., 1999). The factor V Leiden mutation is discussed earlier in this chapter. Dizon-Townson and coworkers (1996) showed that 14 of 158 (8.9%) women with severe pre-eclampsia were heterozygous for the Leiden V mutation compared with 17 of 403 (4.2%) normotensive controls.

As discussed earlier, in the case-control study by DeGroot and colleagues (1999) of 163 women with pre-eclampsia in their first pregnancy matched for age and delivery date, patients and controls were tested for factor V Leiden mutation, prothrombin 20210A allele, protein C, protein S, and antithrombin deficiency. Logistic regression methods were used for data analysis. The prevalence of these genetic risk factors for thrombosis was similar in the patient group (12.9%) and in the control group 12.9%; odds ratio, 1.0; 95% confidence interval, 0.5–3.9.

Mitochrondrial DNA

Mutations and deletions in mitochondrial DNA and deficiencies in the enzyme complexes of the mitochondrial respiratory chain in placenta from women with pre-eclampsia have been postulated (Furui et al., 1994). Vuorinen and coworkers (1998) isolated mitochondria from the placentas of 17 women with pre-eclampsia and 25 controls. Neither large-scale deletions nor the common 5-kb and 7.4 kb deletions were detected, nor were the three most common point mutations found in either pre-eclamptic or eclamptic placental samples. Mitochondrial respiratory chain enzyme complex activities were also similar in the two groups. The authors concluded that although alterations in the energy state of the pre-eclamptic placenta remain a possibility, there was no evidence that mitochondrial DNA mutations or deletions or respiratory chain enzyme activities play a major role in the etiology of pre-eclampsia.

By contrast, an earlier study by Folgero and coworkers (1996) of two families with a high occurrence of pre-eclampsia showed mutations in mitochondrial + RNA (m + RNA) genes. In the first family, an A to G mutation at nucleotide 3243 was found. The mutation was heteroplasmic, meaning that both mutant and wild-type (normal) mitochondrial DNA were present. In the second family there was an A to G mutation at nucleotide 12,308. In this family the mutation was homoplasmic (i.e., only mutant DNA was present). The authors concluded that because mutations of mRNA genes are generally considered to have systemic consequences, they might explain the multiorgan involvement in pre-eclampsia. It was also suggested that a nuclear gene defect can predispose to mRNA mutations and might be inherited as an autosomal dominant trait (Folgero et al., 1996).

Endothelial Nitric Oxide Synthase

The nitric oxide synthases (NOS) are a family of enzymes capable of converting L-arginine to L-citrulline with the subsequent release of nitric oxide (NO). In rats, long-term inhibition of NOS during the middle to late pregnancy is associated with many pathologic changes similar to those observed in pre-eclampsia (Baylis et al., 1996; Novak et al., 1997). NO has been shown to have multiple biologic effects, depending on the isoform responsible for its production and its tissue of origin. NO derived from endothelial NOS (eNOS) is known to mediate vascular smooth muscle relaxation and has been considered an important molecular candidate in the pathogenesis of pre-eclampsia. Arngrímsson and coworkers (1997) studied allele sharing among sisters affected with pregnancy-induced hypertension in 50 families and showed a strong association and linkage with a microsatellite within intron 13 of the eNOS gene. They concluded that a familial pregnancy-induced hypertension susceptibility locus is present in the region of chromosome 7g 36 encoding the eNOS gene. Gregg

and associates (1998) reported creating a mouse strain deficient in eNOS by deleting the first exon of eNOS3. They showed that homozygous mutant mice displayed hypertension across all trimesters of pregnancy with increasing severity. However, Lade and coworkers (1999) studied 26 Australian families containing 11 eclamptics, 59 severe pre-eclamptics, and 27 mild pre-eclamptics to test for linkage between the eNOS gene region and pre-eclampsia. Two microsatellite markers (D7S483 and D7S505) in the proximity of the eNOS gene were used. No evidence was found for linkage between pre-eclampsia and the two markers. It was suggested that the linkage reported by Arngrímsson and coworkers (1997) for eNOS reflects its relationship with hypertension rather than with pre-eclampsia. Hypertension appears to be a consequence rather than a primary cause of pre-eclampsia.

Other Susceptibility Genes

Other candidate genes have been implicated in the etiology of pre-eclampsia-eclampsia. A genome-wide linkage study of 15 informative families was reported by Harrison and coworkers (1997). Using 90 polymorphic DNA markers from all autosomes, a region between D45450 and D4S610 on the long arm of chromosome 4 was identified as a strong candidate region for a pre-eclampsia-eclampsia locus. In a study from Iceland of 343 women affected with pre-eclampsia, Arngrímmson and colleagues (1999) detected a significant locus for pre-eclampsia on chromosome 2p13. In a study 54 women with a diagnosis of severe pre-eclampsia, 52 healthy pregnant women, and 101 nonpregnant healthy women, Nagy and coworkers (1998) found a higher frequency of the apolipoprotein E (ApoE) epsilon 2 allele among women with severe pre-eclampsia, suggesting that ApoE plays a role in the development of pre-eclampsia. Finally, a common missense mutation in the methylenetetrahydrofolate reductase (MTHFR) gene, a C to T substitution at nucleotide 677, was found by Sohda and coworkers (1997) to be significantly increased in 67 pre-eclamptic women compared with 98 healthy pregnant women.

Unifying Hypothesis

Although the etiology and pathogenesis of pre-eclampsia remain unknown, Dekker and Sibai (1998) have proposed a unifying hypothesis. Genetic factors are certainly involved; however, it is likely that no single major pre-eclampsia gene will be found but rather that several genetic factors are associated with maternal susceptibility.

This would be consistent with polygenenic-multifactorial inheritance. Endothelial cell dysfunction appears to be the final common pathway in pathogenesis. Genomic imprinting is an important area of future research. Graves (1998) has suggested that pre-eclampsia could be caused by a mutation in a paternally imprinted, maternally active gene that must be expressed by the fetus in order to establish a normal placenta in the first trimester.

Other Selected Disorders

Table 7–2 provides information about additional selected mendelian disorders that obstetricians may encounter in pregnant women.

REFERENCES

ACOG Committee Opinion: Committee on Genetics. Genetic Screening for Hemoglobinopathies, 168, February, 1996. Washington DC: The American College of Obstetricians and Gynecologists, 1996.

Aessopos A, Karabatsos F, Farmakis D, et al.: Pregnancy in patients with well-treated β-thalassemia: Outcome for mothers and newborn infants. Am J Obstet Gynecol 180:360, 1999.

Arngrímsson R, Hayward C, Nadaud S, et al.: Evidence for a familial pregnancy-induced hypertension locus in the eNOS-gene region. Am J Hum Genet 61:354, 1997.

Arngrímsson R, Sigurard ttir S, Frigge ML, et al.: A genome-wide scan reveals a maternal susceptibility locus for pre-eclampsia on chromosome 2p13. Hum Mol Genet 8:1799, 1999.

Athanassiou AM, Turrentine MA: Myocardial infarction and coronary artery dissection during pregnancy associated with type IV Ehlers-Danlos syndrome. Am J Perinatol 13:181, 1996.

Barabas AP: Ehlers-Danlos syndrome associated with prematurity and premature rupture of foetal membranes: possible increase in incidence. Br Med J 5515:682, 1966.

Barabas AP: Vascular complications in the Ehlers-Danlos syndrome with special reference to the "arterial type" or Sack's syndrome. J Cardiovasc Surg 13:160, 1972.

Baylis C, Slangen B, Hussain S, et al.: Relationship between basal NO release and cyclooxygenase products in the normal rat kidney. Am J Physiol 271:1327, 1996.

Beaudry MA, Ferguson DJ, Pearse K, et al.: Survival of hydropic infant with homozygous a-thalassemia-1. J Pediatr 108:713, 1986.

Beighton P: Obstetric aspects of the Ehlers-Danlos syndrome. J Obstet Gynaecol Br Commonw 76:97, 1969.

Bertina RM, Koeleman BP, Koster T, et al.: Mutation in blood coagulation factor V associated with resistance to activated protein C. Nature 369:64, 1994.

Besinger RE: Preterm labor, premature rupture of membranes, and cervical incompetence. Curr Opin Obstet Gynecol 5:33, 1993.

Bloomenthal D, Delisle MF, Tessier F, et al.: Obstetric implications of the factor V Leiden mutation: a review. Am J Perinatol 19:37, 2002.

Boyle R: Antenatal and preoperative genetic and clinical assessment in myotonic dystrophy. Anaesth Intensive Care 27:301, 1999.

Brook JD, McCurrach ME, Harley HG, et al.: Molecular basis of myotonic dystrophy: Expansion of a trinucleotide (CTG) repeat at the 3′ end of a transcript encoding a protein kinase family member. Cell 68:799, 1992.

Brown AS, Fernhoff PM, Waisbren SE, et al.: Barriers to successful dietary control among pregnant women with phenylketonuria. Genet Med 4:84, 2002.

Campbell DM, MacGillivray I: Preeclampsia in twin pregnancies: Incidence and outcome. Hypertens Pregnancy 18:197, 1999.

Castellani C, Bonizzato A, Rolfini R, et al.: Increased prevalence of mutations in cystic fibrosis gene in idiopathic chronic and recurrent pancreatitis. Am J Gastroenterol 94:1993, 1999.

Chapman AB, Johnson AM, Gabow PA: Pregnancy outcome and its relationship to progression of renal failure in autosomal dominant polycystic kidney disease. J Am Soc Nephrol 5:1178, 1994.

Chen SH, Hsiao KJ, Lin LH, et al.: Study of restriction fragment length polymorphisms at the human phenylalanine locus and evaluation of its potential in prenatal diagnosis of phenylketonuria. Hum Genet 81:226, 1989.

Chesley LC, Annitto JE, Cosgrove RA: Long-term follow-up study of eclamptic women. Fifth periodic report. Am J Obstet Gynecol 101:886, 1968.

Chesley LC, Cooper DW: Genetics of hypertension in pregnancy: Possible single gene control of pre-eclampsia and eclampsia in the descendants of eclamptic women. Br J Obstet Gynaecol 93:898, 1986.

Cincotta RB, Brennecke SP: Family history of pre-eclampsia as a predictor for pre-eclampsia in primigravidas. Int J Gynaecol Obstet 60:23, 1998.

Cola LM, Lavin JP Jr: Pregnancy complicated by Marfan's syndrome with aortic arch dissection, subsequent aortic arch replacement and triple coronary artery bypass grafts. J Reprod Med 30:685 1985.

Cox BE, Word RA, Rosenfeld CR: Angiotensin II receptor characteristics and subtype expression in uterine arteries and myometrium during pregnancy. J Clin Endocrinol Metab 81:49, 1996.

Dalgaard OZ: Bilateral polycystic disease of the kidneys. Acta Med Scand 328:1, 1957.

Daoust MC, Reynolds DM, Bichet DG, et al.: Evidence for a third genetic locus for autosomal dominant polycystic kidney disease. Genomics 25:733, 1995.

DeGroot CJ, Bloemenkamp KW, Duvekot EJ, et al.: Preeclampsia and genetic risk factors for thrombosis: A case-control study. Am J Obstet Gynecol 181:975, 1999.

Dekker GA, Sibai BM: Etiology and pathogenesis of preeclampsia: Current concepts. Am J Obstet Gynecol 179:1359, 1998.

DeVos M, Nuytinck L, Verellen C, et al.: Preterm premature rupture of membranes in a patient with the hypermobility type of the Ehlers-Danlos syndrome. A case report. Fetal Diagn Ther 14:244, 1999.

Dizon-Townson DS, Nelson LM, Easton K, et al.: The factor V Leiden mutation may predispose women to severe preeclampsia. Am J Obstet Gynecol 175:902, 1996.

Elias S, Berkowitz RL: The Marfan syndrome and pregnancy. Obstet Gynecol 47:358, 1976.

Elkayam U, Ostrzega E, Shotan A, et al.: Cardiovascular problems in pregnant women with the Marfan syndrome. Ann Intern Med 123:117, 1995.

Epstein ND: The molecular biology and pathophysiology of hypertropic cardiomyopathy due to mutations in the beta myosin heavy chains and the essential and regulatory light chains. Adv Exp Med Biol 453:105, 1998.

Esplin MS, Hallam S, Farrington PF, et al.: Myotonic dystrophy is a significant cause of idiopathic polyhydramnios. Am J Obstet Gynecol 179:974, 1998.

Fisch RO, Tagatz G, Stassart JP: Gestational carrier—A reproductive haven for offspring of mothers with phenylketonuria: an alternative therapy for maternal PKU. J Inher Metab Dis 16:957, 1993.

Folgero T, Storbakk N, Torbergsen T, et al.: Mutations in mitochondrial transfer of ribonucleic acid genes in preeclampsia. Am J Obstet Gynecol 174:1626, 1996.

Foster PA: The reproductive health of women with von Willebrand disease unresponsive to DDAVP: Results of an international survey. Thromb Haemost 74:784, 1995.

Frangolias DD, Nakielna EM, Wilcox PG: Pregnancy and cystic fibrosis: A case-controlled study. Chest 111:963, 1997.

Furui T, Kurauchi O, Tanaka M, et al.: Decrease in cytochrome c oxidase and cytochrome oxidase subunit I messenger RNA levels in preeclamptic pregnancies. Obstet Gynecol 84:283, 1994.

Gay JC, Phillips JA III, Kazazian HH Jr: Hemoglobinopathies and thalassemias. In Rimoin DL, Connor JM, Pyeritz RD (eds): Principles and Practice of Medical Genetics, 3rd ed. New York: Churchill-Livingstone, 1997, p 1995.

Georgy MS, Anwar K, Oates SE, et al.: Perineal delivery in Ehlers-Danlos syndrome. Br J Obstet Gynaecol 104:505, 1997.

Germain S, Brahimi L, Rohrlich P, et al.: Transfusion in sickle cell anemia. Pathol Biol (Paris) 47:65, 1999.

Ginsburg D, Bowie EJ: Molecular genetics of von Willebrand disease. Blood 79:2507, 1992.

Gilchrist D, Schwarze U, Shields K, et al.: Large kindred with Ehlers-Danlos syndrome type IV due to a point mutation (G571S) in the COL3A1 gene of type III procollagen: Low risk of pregnancy complications and unexpected longevity in some affected relatives. Am J Med Genet 82:305, 1999.

Gregg AR, Schauer A, Shi O, et al.: Limb reduction defects in endothelial nitric oxide synthase-deficient mice. Am J Physiol 275:H2319, 1998.

Graves JA: Genomic imprinting, development and disease—is pre-eclampsia caused by a maternally imprinted gene? Reprod Fertil Dev 10:23, 1998.

Hanley WB, Platt LD, Bachman RP, et al.: Undiagnosed maternal phenylketonuria: The need for prenatal selective screening on case finding. Am J Obstet Gynecol 180:986, 1999.

Harper PS, Dyken PR: Early onset dystrophia myotonica: Evidence supporting a maternal environmental factor. Lancet 2:53, 1972.

Harrison GA, Humphrey KE, Jones N, et al.: A genomewide linkage study of preeclampsia/eclampsia reveals evidence for a candidate region on 4q. Am J Hum Genet 60:1158, 1997.

Hateboer N, v Dijk MA, Bogdanova N, et al.: Comparison of phenotypes of polycystic kidney disease types 1 and 2. Lancet 353:103, 1999.

Hauth JC, Ewell MG, Levine RJ, et al.: Pregnancy outcomes in healthy nulliparas who developed hypertension. Calcium for Preeclampsia Prevention Study. Obstet Gynecol 95:24, 2000.

Hayward C, Livingstone J, Holloway S, et al.: An exclusion map for pre-eclampsia: Assuming autosomal recessive inheritance. Am J Hum Genet 50:749, 1992.

Hilman BC, Aitken ML, Constantinescu M: Pregnancy in patients with cystic fibrosis. Clin Obstet Gynecol 39:70, 1996.

Hojo K, Yamagata H, Mojo H, et al.: Congenital myotonic dystrophy: molecular diagnosis and clinical study. Am J Perinatol 12:195, 1995.

Hordnes K: Ehlers-Danlos syndrome and delivery. Acta Obstet Gynecol Scand 73:671, 1994.

Howard RJ, Tuck SM, Pearson TC: Pregnancy in sickle cell disease in the UK: Results of a multicentre survey of the effect of prophylactic blood transfusion on maternal and fetal outcome. Br J Obstet Gynaecol 102:947, 1995.

Humphrey KE, Harrison GA, Cooper DW, et al.: HLA-G deletion polymorphism and pre-eclampsia/eclampsia. Br J Obstet Gynaecol 102:707, 1995.

Inoue I, Nakajima T, Williams CS, et al.: A nucleotide substitution in the promotor of human angiotensinogen is associated with essential hypertension and affects basal transcription in vitro. J Clin Invest 99:1786, 1997.

Jelsema RD: Genetic and cardiac disease in pregnancy. In Isada NB, Drugan A, Johnson MP, et al. (eds): Maternal Genetic Disease. Stamford, CT: Appleton and Lange, 1996, p 97.

Kadir RA, Lee CA, Sabin CA, et al.: Pregnancy in women with von Willebrand's disease or factor XI deficiency. Br J Obstet Gynaecol 105:314, 1998.

Kazazian HH Jr: The thalassemia syndromes: Molecular basis and prenatal diagnosis in 1990. Semin Hematol 27:209, 1990.

Kazimuddin M, Vashist A, Basher AW, et al.: Pregnancy-induced severe left ventricular systolic dysfunction in a patient with hypertrophic cardiomyopathy. Clin Cardiol 21:848, 1998.

Keidan AJ, Marwah SS, Bareford D, et al.: Laboratory tests for monitoring prophylactic exchange transfusion in pregnancy complicated by sickle cell disease. Clin Lab Haematol 10:243, 1988.

Kent NE, Farquharson DF: Cystic fibrosis in pregnancy. Can Med Assoc J 149:809, 1993.

Kiesewetter S, Macek M, Davis C, et al.: A mutation in CFTR produces different phenotypes depending on chromosomal background. Nat Genet 5:274, 1993.

Kilpatrick DC, Liston WA, Gibson F, et al.: Association between susceptibility to pre-eclampsia within families and HLA DR4. Lancet 2:1063, 1989.

Knuist M, Bonsel GJ, Zondervan HA, et al.: Intensification of fetal and maternal surveillance in pregnant women with hypertensive disorders. Int J Gynaecol Obstet 61:127, 1998.

Kobashi G, Hata A, Shido K, et al.: Association of a variant of the angiotensinogen gene with pure type of hypertension in pregnancy in the Japanese: Implication of a racial difference and significance of an age factor. Am J Med Genet 86:232, 1999.

Koshy M, Burd L, Wallace D, et al.: Prophylactic red-cell transfusions in pregnant patients with sickle cell disease. A randomized cooperative study. N Engl J Med 319:1447, 1988.

Kupferminc MJ, Eldor A, Steinman N, et al.: Increased frequency of genetic thrombophilia in women with complications of pregnancy. N Engl J Med 340:9, 1999.

Lade JA, Moses EK, Guo G, et al.: The eNOS gene: A candidate for the preeclampsia susceptibility locus? Hypertens Pregnancy 18:81, 1999.

Lamon JM, Lenke RR, Levy HL, et al.: Selected metabolic diseases. In Schulman JD, Simpson JL (eds): Genetic Diseases in Pregnancy: Maternal Effects and Fetal Outcome. New York: Academic Press, 1981, p 1.

Lenke RR, Levy HL: Maternal phenylketonuria and hyperphenylalaninemia. An international survey of the outcome of untreated and treated pregnancies. N Engl J Med 303:1202, 1980.

Lipscomb KJ, Smith JC, Clarke B, et al.: Outcome of pregnancy in women with Marfan's syndrome. Br J Obstet Gynaecol 104:201, 1997.

Lipson A, Beuhler B, Bartley J, et al.: Maternal hyperphenylalaninemia fetal effects. J Pediatr 104:216, 1984.

Liston WA, Kilpatrick DC: Is genetic susceptibility to pre-eclampsia conferred by homozygosity for the same single recessive gene in mother and fetus? Br J Obstet Gynaecol 98:1079, 1991.

Long PA, Abell DA, Beischer NA: Parity and preeclampsia. Aust N Z J Obstet Gynaecol 19:203, 1979.

Lubetsky A, Schulman S, Varon D, et al.: Safety and efficacy of continuous infusion of a combined factor VIII-von Willebrand factor (vWF) concentrate (Haemate-P) in patients with von Willebrand disease. Thromb Haemost 81:229, 1999.

Lucarelli G, Cleft RA, Galimberti M, et al.: Bone marrow transplantation in adult thalassemic patients. Blood 93:1164, 1999.

Luke B: Maternal-fetal nutrition. Clin Obstet Gynecol 37:93, 1994.

Mayet J, Steer P, Somerville J: Marfan syndrome, aortic dilatation, and pregnancy. Obstet Gynecol 92:713, 1998.

Mennuti MR, Thomson E, Press N: Screening for cystic fibrosis: follow-up on Workshop to the NIH Consensus Development Conference. Obstet Gynecol 93:456, 1999.

Milewicz DM: Molecular genetics of Marfan syndrome and Ehlers-Danlos type IV. Curr Opin Cardiol 13:198, 1998.

Morgan L, Baker P, Pipkin FB, et al.: Pre-eclampsia and the angiotensinogen gene. Br J Obstet Gynaecol 102:489, 1995.

Morgan T, Ward K: New insights into the genetics of preeclampsia. Semin Perinatol 23:14, 1999.

Morrison JC, Morrison FS, Floyd RC, et al.: Use of continuous flow erythrocytapheresis in pregnant patients with sickle cell disease. J Clin Apheresis 6:224, 1991.

Nagy B, Rigo J, Fintor L, et al.: Apolipoprotein E alleles in women with severe pre-eclampsia. J Clin Pathol 51:324, 1998.

Nathan DG: Thalassemia. N Engl J Med 296:586, 1972.

Ng PC, Fok TF, Lee CH, et al.: Is homozygous alpha-thalassemia a lethal condition in the 1990s? Acta Paediatr 87:1197, 1998.

Novak J, Reckelhoff J, Bumgarner L, et al.: Reduced sensitivity of the renal circulation to angiotensin II in pregnant rats. Hypertension 30:580, 1997.

Oakley GD, McGarry K, Limb DG, et al.: Management of pregnancy in patients with hypertrophic cardiomyopathy. Br Med J 1:1749, 1979.

Old JM: Prenatal diagnosis of hemoglobinopathies. In Milunsky A (ed): Genetic Disorders and the Fetus. Diagnosis, Prevention and Treatment, 4th ed. Baltimore: Johns Hopkins University Press, 1998, p 581.

Peaceman AM, Cruikshank DP: Ehlers-Danlos syndrome and pregnancy: association of type IV disease with maternal death. Obstet Gynecol 69:428, 1987.

Peat B: Pregnancy complicated by maternal phenylketonuria. Aust NZ J Obstet Gynaecol 33:163, 1993.

Pepin M, Schwarze U, Superti-Furge A, et al.: Clinical and genetic features of Ehlers-Danlos syndrome Type IV, the vascular type. N Engl J Med 342:673, 2000.

Peters DJ, Sandkuijl LA: Genetic heterogeneity of polycystic kidney disease in Europe. Contrib Nephrol 97:128, 1992.

Peterson RD, Tuck-Muller CM, Spinnato JA, et al.: An HLA-haplotype associated with preeclampsia and intrauterine growth retardation. Am J Reprod Immunol 31:177, 1994.

Pyeritz RE: Maternal and fetal complications of pregnancy in the Marfan syndrome. Am J Med 71:784, 1981.

Rossiter JP, Repke JT, Morales AJ, et al.: A prospective longitudinal evaluation of pregnancy in the Marfan syndrome. Am J Obstet Gynecol 173:1599, 1995.

Rothlin ME, Egloff L, Flesch M, et al.: Acquired heart diseases and pregnancy. Schweiz Med Wochenschr 125:304, 1995.

Rudd NL, Nimrod C, Holbrook KA, et al.: Pregnancy complications in type IV Ehlers-Danlos syndrome. Lancet 1:50, 1983.

Rudnik-Schoneborn S, Nicholson GA, Morgan G, et al.: Different patterns of obstetric complications in myotonic dystrophy in relation to the disease status of the fetus. Am J Med Genet 80:314, 1998.

Samuels P: Hematologic complications of surgery. In Gabbe SG, Niebyl JR, Simpson JL (eds): Obstetrics: Normal and Problem Pregnancies, 4th ed. New York: Churchill Livingstone, 2002, p 1169.

Scriver CR, Kaufman S: Hyperphenylalaninemia: phenylalanine hydroxylase deficiency. In Scriver CR, Beaudet AL, Sly WS, Valle D (eds): The Metabolic and Molecular Basis of Inherited Disease, 8th ed. New York: McGraw-Hill, 2001, p 1667.

Schoen FJ: The heart. In Robbins SL, Kumar V, Cotran RS (eds): Pathologic Basis of Disease, 5th ed. Philadelphia: WB Saunders, 1994, p 517.

Seoud MA, Cantwell C, Nobles G, et al.: Outcome of pregnancies complicated by sickle cell and sickle-C hemoglobinopathies. Am J Perinatol 11:187, 1994.

Seligsohn U, Lubetsky A: Genetic susceptibility to venous thrombosis. N Engl J Med 344:1222, 2001.

Sibai BM, Mercer B, Sarinoglu C: Severe preeclampsia in the second trimester: Recurrence risk and long-term prognosis. Am J Obstet Gynecol 165:1408, 1991.

Sibai BM, Hauth J, Caritis S, et al.: Hypertensive disorders in twin versus singleton gestations. National Institute of Child Health and Human Development Network of Maternal-Fetal Medicine Units. Am J Obstet Gynecol 182:938, 2000.

Smith JA, Espeland M, Bellevue R, et al.: Pregnancy in sickle cell disease. Experience of the Cooperative Study of Sickle Cell Disease. Obstet Gynecol 87:199, 1996.

Smith VC, Eckenbrecht PD, Hankins GD, et al.: Marfan's syndrome, pregnancy, and the cardiac surgeon. Mil Med 154:404, 1989.

Snyder RR, Gilstrap LC, Hauth JC: Ehlers-Danlos syndrome and pregnancy. Obstet Gynecol 61:649, 1983.

Sohda S, Arinami T, Hamada H, et al.: Methylenetetrahydrofolate reductase polymorphism and pre-eclampsia. J Med Genet 34:525, 1997.

Sorokin Y, Bardicef M: Maternal hematology disorders. In Isada NB, Drugan A, Johnson MP, et al. (eds): Maternal Genetic Disease. Stamford, CT: Appleton and Lange, 1996, p 131.

Sorokin Y, Johnson MP, Rogowski N, et al.: Obstetric and gynecologic dysfunction in the Ehlers-Danlos syndrome. J Reprod Med 39:281, 1994.

Sorosky J, Klatsky A, Nobert GF, et al.: Von Willebrand's disease complicating second trimester abortion. Obstet Gynecol 55:253, 1980.

Svensson PJ, Dahlback B: Resistance to activated protein C as a basis for venous thrombosis. N Engl J Med 330:517, 1994.

Taylor DJ, Wilcox I, Russell JK: Ehlers-Danlos syndrome during pregnancy: A case report and review of the literature. Obstet Gynecol Surv 36:277, 1981.

Vanier TM: Dystrophia myotonia in childhood. Br Med J 1:1284, 1960.

Veale AMO: Screening for phenylketonuria. In Bickel H, Guthrie R, Hammerson G (eds): Neonatal Screening for Inborn Errors of Metabolism. Berlin: Springer, 1980, p 7.

Vuorinen K, Remes A, Sormunen R, et al.: Placental mitochondrial DNA and respiratory chain enzymes in the etiology of preeclampsia. Obstet Gynecol 91:950, 1998.

Waisbren SE, Chang P, Levy HL, et al.: Neonatal neurological assessment of offspring in maternal phenylketonuria. J Inherit Metab Dis 21:39, 1998.

Ward K, Hata A, Jeunemaitre X, et al.: A molecular variant of angiotensinogen associated with preeclampsia. Nat Genet 4:59, 1993.

Weatherall DJ, Clegg JB, Higgs DR, et al.: The hemoglobinopathies. *In* Scriver CR, Beaudet AL, Sly WS, Valle D (eds): The Metabolic and Molecular Basis of Inherited Disease, 8th ed. New York: McGraw Hill, 2001, p 5471.

Whitehead H, Holmes J, Roberts R, et al.: Maternal phenylketonuria 1987 to 1993, pregnancy outcome and early infant development: The Northern Ireland experience. Br J Obstet Gynaecol 103:1041, 1996.

Wilson PD, Guay-Woodford L: Pathophysiology and clinical management of polycystic kidney disease in women. Semin Nephrol 19:123, 1999.

Wilton AN, Cooper DW, Brennecke SP: Absence of close linkage between maternal genes for susceptibility to pre-eclampsia/eclampsia and HLA DR beta. Lancet 336:653, 1990.

Wright D, Gold R, Schwartz D: Maternal gastrointestinal disorders. *In* Isada ND, Drugan A, Johnson MP, et al. (eds): Maternal Genetic Disease. Stamford, CT: Appleton and Lange, 1996, p 159.

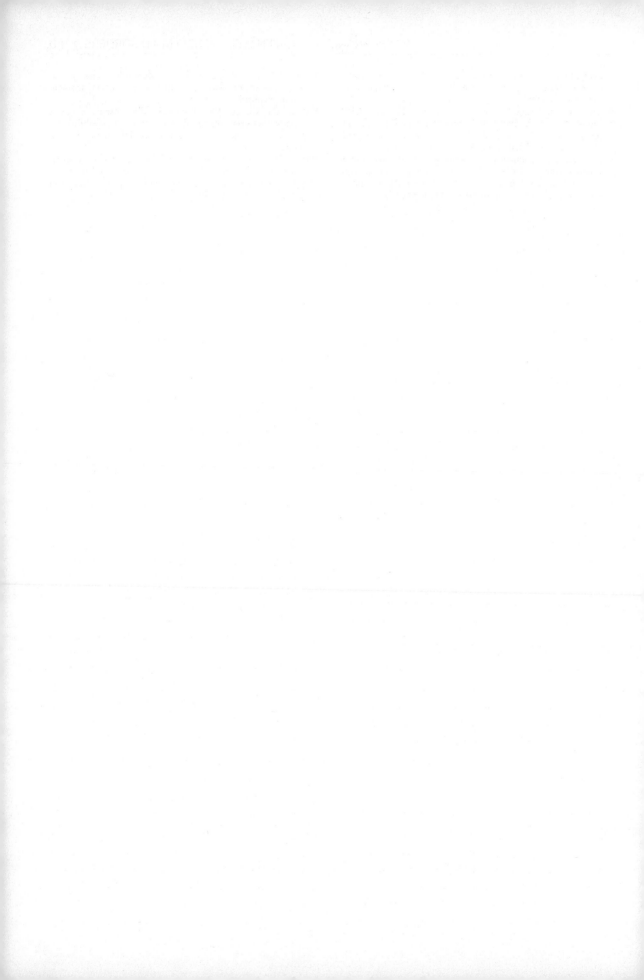

CHAPTER 8

Common Gynecologic Disorders

The genetics of common gynecologic disorders have until recently received relatively little attention. This neglect is striking compared with the considerably greater knowledge available concerning inherited tendencies in most other organ systems. There are several logical explanations for this relative lack of information. First, gynecologic disorders usually involve internal organ systems, which are visualized only infrequently. It is thus relatively more difficult to recognize heritable tendencies in gynecologic disorders than in more readily accessible organ systems. Second, gynecologic disorders occur only in members of one sex; thus, fewer familial aggregates would be expected than if both sexes were affected. Third, progress has been delayed by the relative paucity of gynecologists trained in genetics.

This chapter discusses some common conditions for which genetic data are available. Genetics of gynecologic cancers are discussed in Chapter 9, and the disorders of sexual differentiation in Chapters 10 to 12.

Bony Pelvis and Uterine Dystocia

Bone mass and shape are heritable in animals, and surely as well in humans. Consistent with this assumption are widely accepted clinical impressions that anthropoid and android pelvises are more characteristic of blacks than of whites. Naylor and Warburton (1974) recorded that the length of the diagonal conjugate is heritable in whites although not in blacks.

Several linked registries have provided evidence for familial tendencies (mother and daughter) in cesarean sections or operative deliveries, a correlation that could reflect either heritable abnormalities of the bony pelvis or abnormalities of uterine contractions. A study from Utah by Varner and colleagues (1996) defined an index case as a woman having been delivered by "cesarean section, midforceps or high forceps"; matched controls were identified. Women born by cesarean section (that is, affected mothers) showed an odds ratio of 1.41 for having a cesarean section themselves (95% CI 1.18–1.70). Odds ratio for cesarean section was higher when the index case had been delivered by mid- or high forceps (OR 1.72; 95% CI 1.20–2.47), had been born by cesarean section for cephalopelvic disproportion (OR 1.83, 95% CI 1.16–2.88), or been born by cesarean section as a result of dysfunctional labor (OR 5.97; CI 1.5–23.6). The higher odds ratio for the latter suggests that pertinent uterine factors are probably more heritable than are bony abnormalities. Uterine factors could involve oxytocin receptors, collagen, or gap junction proteins. On the other hand, heritable factors play only a small role in cesarean section in general. Varner and coworkers (1996) calculated the attributable risk of heritable factors to operative delivery at only 3.5%.

A study using a Swedish database confirmed that "dystocia" is familial (Berg-Lekas et al., 1998). The following International Classification of Disease (ICD) codes was used: (1) prolonged labor, uterine spasm, or rigid cervix (8th revision), or (2) uterine inertia, primary or secondary; hypertonic inordinate or prolonged uterine contractions; prolonged first- or second-stage labor or unspecific prolonged labor (9th revision). If a subject's mother had been delivered after dystocia, the odds ratio was 1.7 (95% CI 1.2–2.4) that her oldest daughter would also be delivered after dystocia. The odds ratios was 1.8 for recurrence if an operative delivery occurred in the mother. The odds ratio for an operative delivery among primiparous sisters was 3.5 and the risk was 24.0 among twins.

From these two studies, it is clear that familial tendencies and presumably to some extent surely genetic tendencies affect labor and delivery. Again, dysfunctional labor could be the result of disparate pathogenic factors—amounts of collagen in the cervix (Granstrom et al., 1989), abnormalities of the bony pelvis, and presence or absence of myometrial factors like the gap junction protein connexon-43.

Finding mutations that deleteriously affect uterine contractions has not been successful to date. Yet, there have been tantalizing clues, derived from animal data. In mice in which 5 α-reductase type 1 (SRD5A1) is null ("knockout"), the sole manifestation in females is absence of parturition—67% of cases (Mahendroo et al., 1996). However, human females homozygous for SRD5A1 deficiency seem normal (Chapter 11). Parturition is also abnormal in mice in which the prostaglandin F2α-receptor gene ($PGF2\alpha R$) is disrupted (Sugimoto et al., 1997). Algovik and colleagues (1999) studied women with "dystocia," operationally defined as "failure to progress in labor (prolonged or dysfunctional labor) as well as cephalopevic disproportions." The sample was composed of 23 women who had a cesarean section and in which no evidence of pelvic bone abnormalities was found. Single stranded confirmational polymorphism (SSCP) and DNA sequencing were performed for three candidate genes: $SRD5A1$, $PGF2\alpha R$, and endothelin-1 (ET-1). All three genes are expressed in human uteri, but they may not be pivotal in human parturition. No perturbations involving any of the three genes were detected.

Pelvic Relaxation and Urinary Incontinence (Stress, Detrusor)

In pelvic relaxation a variety of organs—uterus, bladder, rectum—lose their integrity and prolapse. This common gynecologic condition occurs in 15 to 30% of the population, depending upon precision of diagnostic criteria and nature of the population. Prevalence is increased in women of increased parity and advanced age. With the increasingly aging population, pelvic relaxation is a major health problem.

Clinical factors associated with pelvic organ prolapse are well known to gynecologists: multiple vaginal births, especially with large babies; pre-existing or secondary nerve damage; hormonal deficiency; obesity; and increased intra-abdominal pressure. There has been relatively little attention paid to potential genetic factors, but the hypothesis that defects or perturbations of connective tissue can play a role in determining which individuals develop pelvic relaxation is attractive. The fact that women with mendelian disorders (e.g., Ehlers-Danlos syndrome) caused by connective tissue abnormalities are showing pelvic relaxation favors this idea. It would be reasonable to expect that subtle abnormalities might exist in some women experiencing bladder or uterine prolapse.

Differences in Types of Incontinence Among Ethnic Groups

The first clue to genetic factors is differences in prevalence of a trait among different ethnic group. Several authors have found differences in frequency of incontinence among different ethnic groups. In South Africa, Knobel (1975) noted that stress incontinence was rare in black women, consistent with an earlier South African report stating that prolapse was far more common in whites than blacks (Heyns, 1956). Knobel (1975) compared an equal number (n = 20) of Asian Indian women also studied by cinefluorocystourethrography, cystometry, and perineometry, and found that black women had higher bladder necks, longer urethras, higher intraurethral resistance, higher pelvic floor contractile force, and greater intravesical pressure rise (55 versus 10%) at a bladder volume of 400 mL.

Both Bump (1993) and Graham and Mallett (2001) observed stress incontinence to be more common in whites than in blacks, whereas detrusor instability showed the converse. Neither study was populated-based, reflecting only patients at clinics in North Carolina and Michigan, respectively. Peacock and coworkers (1994) also found detrusor instability in a black population to be more common than stress incontinence or mixed incontinence. Bump (1993) reported pure stress incontinence to be 2.3 times more common in white women (n = 146) than in black women (n = 54) (95% CI 1.4–4.0). Studying 183 black and 132 white women, Graham and Mallett (2001) calculated the magnitude of white race as a predictor of stress urinary incontinence as 2.21 (95% CI 1.3–3.7); the magnitude of black race as a predictor of detrusor instability was 2.6 (95% CI 1.45–1.8).

Duong and Korn (2001) stratified 415 San Francisco women by ethnic group. African-American women (n = 59) had higher maximum urethral closure pressure than Hispanic (n = 195), white (n = 60), and Asian (n = 66) women. In the first group, mean was 58±23 cm H_2O versus 47 or 48 cm H_2O for other ethnic groups.

Graham and Mallett (2001) also found that a higher proportion of white women had a maximum urethral closing pressure of less than 20 cm H_2O. As in studies of Bump (1993) and Graham and Mallett (2001), detrusor instability was diagnosed by Duong and Korn (2001) more frequently in African-Americans (29%) than in Hispanics, whites, and Asians (8%, 15%, and 14%, respectively).

In summary, the studies cited above are consistent with white women being at greatest risk for stress urinary incontinence and black women being at increased risk for detrusor instability. There is no ethnic predilection for mixed incontinence. However, observations have not been population-based and could be biased by referral patterns and ascertainment biases based on socioeconomic factors and access to health care. Nonetheless, genetic factors seem to be present.

Familial Studies

One study has formally sought familial tendencies in urinary incontinence. Mushkat and associates (1996) studied Israeli women diagnosed with stress urinary incontinence. Diagnostic criteria included both clinical assessment and urodynamic testing (cystometry and urethral pressure profiles). Controls consisted of women attending the same gynecology clinic "who denied any kind of micturition disorders." Information was gathered on relatives of 259 subjects with incontinence and compared to that on relatives of 165 women with no micturition disorders. Age and parity were similar in the two groups, as was presence of various medical conditions. However, multivariate analysis was not performed. Queries were made concerning leakage upon exertion, with symptoms experienced at least twice weekly constituting the basis of a diagnosis (affected relative). The prevalence of incontinence was 20.3% (158/780) in first-degree relatives of subjects versus 7.8% (37/474) in first-degree relatives of controls (Table 8–1). To verify accuracy of diagnosis in relatives, urodynamic testing was offered to 195 newly detected affected relatives, 158 being

relatives of subjects and 37 relatives of controls. Of the 195 considered affected by history, the 48 studied all had urinary stress incontinence by urodynamic testing; 8 of the 48 had combined stress incontinence and detrusor instability. Thus, the diagnoses in relatives were probably accurate. Clearly, familial tendencies and probably genetic factors exist in urinary incontinence.

One explanation for familial tendencies or ethnic differences could be differences in collagen. Indeed, women with bladder neck prolapse and urinary stress incontinence show cross-link modification in their pubocervical fascia compared with patients who have stress incontinence alone (Sayer et al., 1990). Collagen content in the vaginal cuff is significantly reduced in premenopausal women who require vaginal hysterectomy for prolapse compared with controls who do not. In this same study, significant increases in gelatinases MMP2 (matrix metalloproteinase 2), MMP9, and cathepsin were consistent with loss of collagen fiber strength. Cross-linking and glycation cross-links were increased in prolapsed tissue. There was no change in the type I to type III collagen ratio. This initial attempt comparing tissue in women with and without prolapse suggests perturbation of collagen content in the former.

Circumstantial evidence supports a relationship between hypermobility of joints and fascial relaxation (Norton et al., 1995). Hypermobile joint syndrome is more common in West Africa and other populations (Birrell et al., 1994), suggesting that certain populations might be predisposed toward urinary incontinence. Also from Africa, Cox and Webster (1975) reported that genital prolapse was the most common operation performed in the Pokot, a tribe residing in Kenya.

Age at Menarche and Thelarche

Social and environmental confounding variables complicate human studies, but age at menarche is clearly heritable. Age at menarche has long been recognized by virtue of greater correlation

▼ **Table 8–1.** FREQUENCY OF WOMEN WHOSE RELATIVES SHOW OR DO NOT SHOW PELVIC
• RELAXATION

	N	Affected Relatives			
		Mothers	Sisters	Daughters	All First-Degree
Subjects	259	71/203(34.9%)	73/367(19.9%)	14/210(6.7%)	158/780(20.3%)
Control	165	19/149(12.7%)	15/220(6.8%)	3/105(2.9%)	37/474(7.8%)

From data of Mushkat Y, Bukovsky I, Langer R: Female urinary stress incontinence—does it have familial prevalence? Am J Obstet Gynecol 174:617, 1996.

▼ **Table 8–2.** INITIAL STUDIES SHOWING CORRELATION BETWEEN RELATEDNESS
• AND AGE OF ONSET OF FIRST MENSTRUATION: MEAN DIFFERENCES IN MONTHS

	Petri (1934)	Tisserant-Perrier (1953)	Fischbein (1977)
Identical twins	2.8 (n = 51)	2.2 (n = 46)	3.5 (n = 28)
Nonidentical twins	12.0 (n = 47)	8.2 (n = 39)	8.5 (n = 48)
Sibs	12.9 (n = 145)		
Mother-daughter	18.4 (n = 120)		
Unrelated	18.6 (n = 120)		

for monozygotic (MZ) twins than for dizygotic (DZ) twins (Petri, 1934; Tisserant-Perrier, 1953; Fischbein, 1977). Age at menarche has long been known to differ less among sisters than among unrelated women (Table 8–2). The magnitude of the observed difference is consistent with polygenic-multifactorial etiology.

In the last decade, several additional intergenerational and familial studies concerning age at menarche have been conducted (Table 8–3). These studies differ from those cited in Table 8–2 by taking into account various confounding factors, e.g., decreasing age at menarche over time in the general population. However, familial tendencies still continue to prove substantive. Despite mothers showing older mean ages at menarche than their daughters (usually 4 to 12 months), mother-daughter and sister-sister correlations persist for age at onset of menarche. Taking into account birth order and paternal occupation does not affect conclusions (Sanchez-Andres, 1997). These findings have been observed in Spanish women (Sanchez-Andres, 1997) and in South African Indians (Cameron and Nagdee, 1996) and can be presumed to be applicable in all populations. Heritability also remains high despite adjustments for weight, height, and skeletal maturation (Loesch et al., 1995). Studying 44 monozygotic (MZ) and 42 dizygotic (DZ) twins, Malina and coworkers (1994) confirmed a familial correlation for age at menarche. This persisted even when comparing women who were university athletes to sisters and mothers who were not. Using a Finnish twin registry, Kaprio and colleagues (1995) studied 468 MZ twin girls, 378

girls from like-sex DZ twin pairs, and 434 girls from unlike sex DZ twin pairs; correlation(s) for age at menarche were 0.75, 0.34 and 0.32, respectively. Variance for age at menarche was estimated at 37% for additive genetic factors (see Chapter 3) and 37% for dominance effects; the remaining 26% were attributed to "unique environmental factors." Correlation between body mass and age at menarche was 0.57, suggesting that factors relating to mass could help explain the genetic correlation. Based on 1177 MZ and 711 DZ twins, Treloar and Martin (1990) concluded that the phenotypic variance in age of menarche attributable to genes was 65%. Taking a different approach by studying a genetically isolated group (Hutteries), Ober and coworkers (2000) found heritability to be 63%, entirely due to additive factors without dominant or recessive components.

The heritability of age at menarche and pubarche was studied in a longitudinal study of 74 pairs of sisters in Croatia (Jakic and Prebeg, 1994). The onset of breast development showed greater correlation among sisters than among nonrelated individuals. The same held for age of onset of pubic hair development (pubarche). Premature thelarche not associated with hormone-producing neoplasia has been found in Rubinstein–Taybi syndrome (broad radially-deviated syndromes, polysyndactly of toes, facial dysmorphia, mental retardation) (Izumikawa et al., 1998; Kurosawa et al., 2002). This disorder is caused by haploinsufficiency for a gene (CRE BBP) at 16p13.3 (Breuning et al., 1993; Petrij et al., 1995).

▼ **Table 8–3.** TWIN-PAIR CORRELATION *(R)* FOR HERITABILITY IN AGE AT MENARCHE

	Monozygotic (MZ) Twins	Dizygotic (DZ) Twins	Heritable (H^2)
Snieder and colleagues (1998)	0.61 (n = 275)	0.18 (n = 353)	45%
Treloar and Martin (1990)	0.65 (n = 1177)	0.18 (n = 711)	61–68% (youngest to oldest)
Kaprio (1995)	0.75 (n = 468)	0.31 (n = 378 like sex) (sib-twin correlation 0.32)	37% (plus another 37% dominance)

Age at menarche does not necessarily correlate with age at menopause.

Age at Menopause

In humans, the age at menopause is familial. This is not surprising, given that germ cell (oocyte) number is normally distributed in mammals. Different rodent strains show a characteristic breeding duration, implying genetic control over either the rate of oocyte depletion or the number of oocytes initially present. It follows that some ostensibly normal (menstruating) women may have a decreased oocyte reservoir or increased oocyte attrition on polygenic or even stochastic grounds (Simpson, 2000).

In humans, proving heritability of age at menopause is complicated because of iatrogenic factors (e.g., hysterectomy) and other confounders (e.g., presence of leiomyomas). Cramer and coworkers (1995) took these into account in a case control study of 10,606 US women between the ages of 45 and 54. Women with an early menopause (40 to 45 years) were age-matched with controls who were either still menstruating or had experienced menopause after age 46 years. Of 129 early menopause cases, 37.5% had a similarly affected mother, sister, aunt, or grandmother. Only 9% of controls had such a relative (odds ratio after adjustment 6.1, 95% CI 3.9–9.4). As predicted on the basis of polygenic inheritance, the odds ratio was greatest (9.1) for sisters and greater when menopause occurred prior to 40 years. Incidentally, frequency of galactose 1-phosphate uridyltransferase (GALT) variants (N314D or Q188R) did not deviate from that expected in early menopause cases, in contrast to earlier studies by the same authors (Cramer et al., 1989). Results of Cramer and coworkers (1995) were confirmed by Torgerson and colleagues (1997), who studied women undergoing menopause during the 5-year centile ages 45 to 49 years. The likelihood was increased that menopause would occur in a similar 5-year centile in their daughters.

Twin studies have confirmed heritability of age at menopause—two studies showing similar results (Treloar et al., 1998a). Snieder and coworkers (1998) studied 275 MZ and 353 DZ United Kingdom twin pairs. For age at menopause, correlation (r) was 0.58 for MZ and 0.39 DZ twins; heritability (h^2) was calculated to be 63%. The study of Treloar and associates (1998b) involved 466 MZ and 262 DZ Australian twin pairs. For age at menopause, the correlation (r) was 0.49–0.57 for MZ and 0.31–0.33 for DZ twin pairs. Differences between MZ and DZ held when iatrogenic causes of menopause were taken into account. de Bruin et al. (2001) studied data collected from breast cancer screening projects (243 singleton women, 74 DZ twins, 44 MZ twins). Heritability (h^2) was 0.85–0.87 for singleton sisters.

Imperforate Hymen

Ordinarily the central portion of the hymen is patent (perforate), thereby allowing outflow of mucus and blood. If the hymen is imperforate, mucus and blood accumulate in the vagina or uterus (hydrocolpos or hydrometrocolpos). An imperforate hymen is not particularly rare. The anomaly is easily corrected by surgical incisions, preferably cruciform.

McIlroy and Ward (1930) reported affected siblings with imperforate hymens, and until recently no additional familial aggregates had been reported. Stelling and coworkers (1998a) reported concordant monozygotic twins; one of the twins had an affected daughter, who also had pyloric stenosis and possibly hip dislocation. In Schinzel-Giedion syndrome, an autosomal recessive tract, "hymenal atresia," was said to be present (Schinzel and Giedion, 1978).

Fusion of the Labia Minora

Fusion of the labia minora is often the sequela of infection or sexual abuse. However, congenital fusion apparently unassociated with these factors has been observed in sibs (Simpson, 1972) and in more than one generation (Sueiro and Piloti, 1964; Klein et al., 1987). In several syndromes labial hypoplasia has been found to be present (Simpson, 1999). In Schinzel-Giedion syndrome a prominent labial sulcus exists (Schinzel and Giedion, 1978).

Vaginal Atresia

The vagina is shortened or absent in many females whose external genitalia are ambiguous (pseudohermaphrodites). In the present context, however, we consider those females who lack a vagina but whose *external* genitalia are otherwise normal. Two groups of individuals fulfill these characteristics: (1) those lacking most of the vagina and all or almost all of the uterus (müllerian aplasia), and (2) those lacking a portion of the vagina but having a normal uterus (vaginal atresia). These two condi-

Müllerian Aplasia

Vaginal Atresia

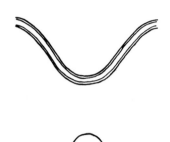
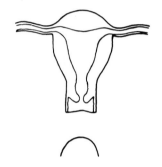

FIGURE 8–1 • Diagram showing differences between müllerian aplasia and vaginal atresia, both of which may have absence of the vagina.

tions are embryologically and anatomically distinct (Fig. 8–1). In müllerian aplasia the lower vagina is present, whereas in vaginal atresia only the upper vagina is present. Of individuals with an absent vagina, 80 to 90% have müllerian aplasia (Bryan et al., 1949; Turunen and Unnerus, 1967; Cali and Pratt, 1968; Leduc et al., 1968; Jones and Wheeless, 1969; Jones and Scott, 1971).

In vaginal atresia the urogenital sinus fails to contribute the caudal portion of the vagina. The lower fifth to third of the vagina is replaced by 2 cm to 3 cm of fibrous tissue, above which lie a well-differentiated upper vagina, cervix, uterine corpus, and fallopian tubes (see Fig. 8–1). Ultrasound, magnetic resonance imaging (MRI), or rectal examination may help verify the presence or absence of müllerian derivatives. Hydrometrocolpos can develop.

Familial aggregates of isolated vaginal atresia are rare if not nonexistent. However, vaginal atresia is often reported only as part of a larger series of patients having "absence of vagina." In such patients, müllerian aplasia (see following sections) is the most common diagnosis (see Fig. 8–1). Analysis of a heterogeneous sample of patients might obscure findings that would be evident if a distinct and less common component (i.e., vaginal atresia) were analyzed separately. Moreover, in the context of multiple malformation syndromes, vaginal atresia (see below) can be familial.

Vaginal Atresia in Multiple Malformation Syndromes

An etiologically distinct form of vaginal atresia in otherwise normal women is vaginal atresia present as one component of a multiple malformation complex. Table 8–4 summarizes salient features of several such syndromes. Winter and coworkers described four siblings with a probable autosomal recessive syndrome characterized by vaginal atresia, renal hypoplasia or agenesis, and middle ear anomalies (malformed incus, fixation of the malleus and incus) (Winter et al., 1968).

▼ **Table 8–4.** MULTIPLE MALFORMATION SYNDROMES ASSOCIATED WITH VAGINAL ATRESIA

Syndrome	Somatic Anomalies	Etiology
Antley-Bixler	Craniosynostosis, choanal atresia, humeroradial synostosis, gracile ribs, bowed femora, camptodactyly, renal anomalies	Autosomal recessive
Bardet-Biedl	Degeneration of retinal pigment (retinitis pigmentosa), polydactyly, obesity, mental retardation	Autosomal recessive
Fraser	Cryptophthalmia, nose and ear anomalies, stenotic larynx, skeletal defects, syndactyly, renal agenesis, large clitoris and labia majora, mental retardation (müllerian aplasia also reported)	Autosomal recessive
Winter	Lacrimal duct stenosis, external and middle ear anomalies, renal agenesis	Autosomal recessive
Cavalcanti	Tibial aplasia, triphalangeal thumb, microtia, scoliosis, clubfoot (incomplete müllerian fusion also reported)	Unknown

From Simpson JL: Genetics of the female reproductive ducts. Am J Med Genet 89:224, 1999.

The Fraser syndrome is characterized by vaginal atresia and cryptophthalmos, with resultant blindness (Fraser, 1962). In Bardet-Biedl syndrome the frequency of vaginal atresia is also relatively high. Other syndromes characterized less commonly by vaginal atresia are listed in Table 8–4.

Transverse Vaginal Septa and the McKusick-Kaufman Syndrome (MKS; MKKS)

Transverse vaginal septa (TVS) occur at several locations. Complete or incomplete, these septa are usually about 2-cm thick and located near the junction of the upper third and lower two thirds of the vagina (Lodi, 1951; Simpson, 1976; Jones and Rock, 1983). However, septa may be located in the middle or lower third of the vagina (Lodi, 1951) (Fig. 8–2). Usually central, perforations may be eccentric in location (Bowman and Scott, 1954; Kanagasuntheran and Dassanayake, 1958; White, 1966; Deppisch, 1972). If no perforation exists, mucus and menstrual blood obviously cannot egress; thus, hydrocolpos or hydrometro-

colpos may develop. Other pelvic organs are usually normal, although occasionally the uterus is bicornuate.

Vaginal septa presumably result from failure of urogenital sinus derivatives and the müllerian duct derivatives to meet or canalize. This explanation is deduced from the location of the septa, which are usually at the predicted sites of müllerian-urogenital sinus fusion. Consistent with this explanation is the histologic nature of the septa. Typically, cranial surfaces of septa are lined by columnar (müllerian) epithelium, whereas caudal surfaces are lined by squamous epithelium (urogenital sinus invagination).

For over 30 years it has been recognized that an autosomal recessive gene is responsible for transverse vaginal septum (hydrometrocolpos). First recognized in the Amish, multiple cases could be traced back to the same 16th century progenitors (McKusick et al., 1964, 1968). This condition has even been used as a genetic paradigm (McKusick, 1978). The major extant question is whether isolated TVS, especially in non-Amish populations, is caused by the same gene that results in TVS and selected somatic anomalies (i.e., McKusick-Kaufman syndrome).

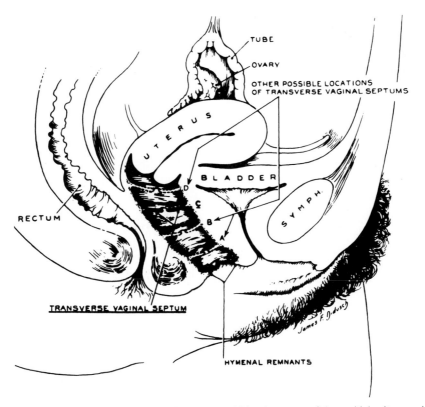

FIGURE 8–2 • Diagram showing transverse vaginal septa, which arise at any of the multiple sites as shown. Only a single septum is present in a given individual. (From Bowman JA, Scott RB: Transverse vaginal septum: Report of four cases. Obstet Gynecol 3:441, 1954.)

MCKUSICK-KAUFMAN SYNDROME (TVS AND POLYDACTYLY)

Transverse vaginal septa may be associated with polydactyly, cardiac defects, and other multiple defects (Kaufman et al., 1972). The name McKusick-Kaufman syndrome (MKKS or MKS) is applied. Familial aggregates are not restricted to Amish but found also in Italian, Puerto Rican, and other populations (Chitayat et al., 1987). In some MKKS cases the reproductive defect is vaginal atresia (Chitayat et al., 1987), suggesting overlap between vaginal atresia and TVS in the etiology of MKKS. However, usually the defect in MKKS is TVS, indistinguishable anatomically from isolated TVS. The presence of somatic anomalies could indicate merely that the TVS mutant in the Amish is pleiotropic (Pinsky, 1974). Alternatively, somatic anomalies could indicate the presence of a different mutant gene. A contiguous gene syndrome could also exist. Familial aggregates have apparently been detected, although uncommonly, in non-Amish kindreds (Chitayat et al., 1987).

Making the assumption that only a single pleiotropic gene exists, Chitayat and coworkers (1987) analyzed 54 Amish cases of vaginal septa. Hydrometrocolpos was estimated to be present in 95% of cases, polydactyly in 93%, and cardiovascular malformations in 9%. Individuals were identified having all three anomalies, various pairwise combinations, or only one (McKusick, 1978). Stone and associates (1998) estimated penetrance to be 70% for hydrometrocolpos in females, 60% for polydactyly in either sex, and 15% for cardiovascular defects. Accepting these probabilities, 9% of males and 3% of females would have the gene in the completely nonpenetrant state.

MOLECULAR BASIS OF MCKUSICK-KAUFMAN SYNDROME

Homozygosity mapping for short tandem repeat polymorphism (STRP) has been performed in two large Amish pedigrees, analyzing 385 markers (Stone et al., 1998). The McKusick-Kaufman gene was localized to chromosome 20p12; the peak two-point LOD score was 3.33, and the peak three-point LOD score was 5.21. Chromosome 20p12 includes the locus for Alagille syndrome, an autosomal recessive gene causing a multiple malformation syndrome characterized by cardiac anomalies, hepatic ductal hypoplasia, and abnormal (butterfly-shaped) vertebrae. Alagille syndrome is caused by perturbation of *jagged* 1 (Li et al., 1997). However, no DNA mutations in *jagged* 1 were found in two Amish cases of transverse vaginal septa (McKusick-Kaufman syndrome) (Stone et al., 1998).

The mutant gene seems to be a chaperonin, a representative of a class of proteins that facilitate protein folding in conjunction with adenosine triphosphate hydrolysis (Stone et al., 2000). That the causative gene was a chaperonin was deduced from analysis of ESTs (expressed sequence tags) generated from the 450 kb region of 20p12 in which the *MKS* locus was localized. A novel transcript generated by sequence comparison analysis revealed six exons and a predicted open reading of 570 amnio acids beginning in exon 3 (Fig. 8–3). A mouse homologue to *MKS* exists, with 76% amino acid identity and 88% similarity. No known homologue exists in *Drosophila* or *C. elegans*. Old order Amish showed two unusual chaperonin sequence differences (H84Y and A242S), each found 1 per 100 Amish "controls." Neither sequence difference was found in 100

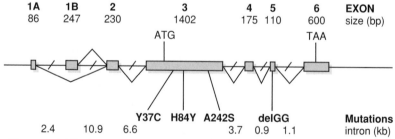

FIGURE 8–3 • Diagram of *MKKS* structure and mutations. Exons are shown as rectangles with alternate splicing of exons 1a and 1b as indicated. The sequence alterations on the Old Order Amish chromosome are shown (two alterations, H84Y and A242S, on the disease chromosome) as well as those of the sporadic patient (compound heterozygote for Y37C and 2111-2112delGG). We identified several polymorphisms when sequencing *MKKS*. In exon 3, G49V is present in 8.3% of normal chromosomes. In exon 6, R517C is present in 6.3% of normal chromosomes, and G532V in 6.4% of normal chromosomes. In exon 4, the frequency of polymorphism A369G was not estimated. (From Stone DL, Slavotinek A, Bouffard GG, et al.: Mutation of a gene encoding a putative chaperonin causes McKusick-Kaufman syndrome. Nature Genet 25:79, 2000.)

non-Amish controls. The 1% frequency in Amish is consistent with a heterozygote frequency (2pq) of that magnitude. H84Y/A242S also segregated with the disease in a large pedigree. All affected cases were homozygous, but three homozygous individuals were unaffected. The frequency of nonpenetrance was thus higher than the 3 to 9% estimated on clinical grounds by Stone et al. (1998).

An atypical non-Amish patient of northern European descent showed a frameshift mutation in the gene; this patient had a hypoplastic clitoris with prominent labia majora, small ears, uterine and skeletal anomalies, and atrioventricular septal defects. Five other *MKS* probands showed no perturbations in the chaperonin gene, and in these Stone and coworkers (2000) wondered if the diagnosis of Bardet-Biedl syndrome might not be more appropriate. Slavotinek and colleagues (2000) showed that Bardet-Biedl syndrome also results from disturbance of the *MKS* gene.

Other genes could play a role in MKKS, particularly in non-Amish cases. Attractive candidate genes include homologues of two mouse mutants showing urogenital and skeletal anomalies: dominant hemimelia (dh) and loop tail (lp) (Strong and Hollander, 1949; Snell et al., 1954; Searle, 1964). However, both genes map to mouse chromosome 1, a region not homologous to human 20p (Li et al., 1997). These two mouse mutants may not be ideal models for the McKusick-Kaufman syndrome. Another candidate gene is mouse ivp (imperforate vagina), an autosomal recessive mutant that has not yet been mapped (Eisen et al., 1989).

Longitudinal Vaginal Septa

Vaginal septa may be longitudinal (Fig. 8–4) as well as transverse (coronal or sagittal). Longitudinal septa probably result from abnormal mesodermal proliferation or persisting epithelium. Usually no clinical problems arise, but sometimes longitudinal septa impede the second

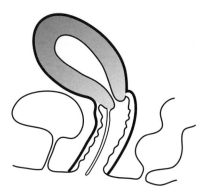

FIGURE 8–4 • Diagram illustrating longitudinal vaginal septum.

stage of labor. Heritable tendencies are not obvious, although no systematic studies have been reported.

Edwards and Gale (1972) reported an autosomal dominant syndrome characterized by longitudinal vaginal septum, hand anomalies, and urinary incontinence apparently related to a bladder neck anomaly (Edwards and Gale, 1972). Longitudinal vaginal septa may be the diagnosis in the Johanson-Blizzard syndrome ("septate vagina") an autosomal recessive disorder (Johanson and Blizzard, 1971) (Table 8–5). Uterine anomalies of the type expected in incomplete müllerian fusion (IMF) have not been documented.

Absence or Atresia of the Uterine Cervix

The cervix may be absent or markedly atretic despite a normal uterine corpus and a normal vagina. There have been no reports of multiple affected family members with this rare condition (Geary and Weed, 1973; Farber and Marchant, 1976; Fujimoto et al., 1997). The condition presumably results either from failure of müllerian duct canalization or from aberrant local epithelial proliferation after canalization. Hydrometrocolpos should be anticipated.

▼ **Table 8–5.** SYNDROMES ASSOCIATED WITH LONGITUDINAL VAGINAL SEPTA

Syndrome	Somatic Anomalies	Etiology
Edwards-Gale (camptobrachydactyly)	Flexion contractures of distal interphalangeal joints, brachydactyly, polydactyly, syndactyly, urinary incontinence	Autosomal dominant
Johanson-Blizzard	Scalp defects, deafness, hypoplastic alae nasi, microdontia, primary hypothyroidism, malabsorption, mental retardation, hypotonia, short stature	Autosomal recessive

From Simpson JL: Genetics of the female reproductive ducts. Am J Med Genet 89:224, 1999.

Of the cases reviewed by Fujimoto and associates (1997), approximately half had normal vaginas; the others had complete or partial vaginal atresia in addition to absence of the cervix (Fig. 8–5). Surgically created uterovaginal canalization was followed by menstruation in 60% of reported cases overall but more often if vaginoplasty was *not* required (68 versus 43%). Chakravarty and coworkers (2000) described a new surgical procedure (sequential vaginal and abdominovaginal approach) that resulted in each of 18 women's menstruating. Hovsepian and coworkers (1999) used a combined surgical and

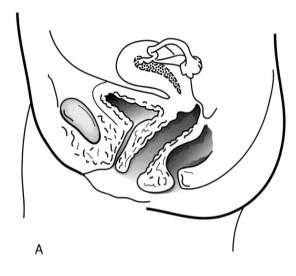

A

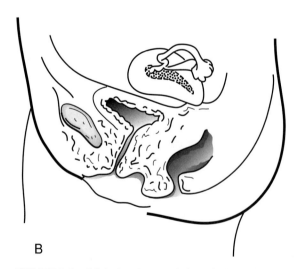

B

FIGURE 8–5 • (A) Isolated congenital cervical atresia with normal vaginal development. (B) Congenital cervical atresia with complete vaginal agenesis. (Adapted from Fujimoto VY, Miller JH, Klein NA, et al.: Congenital cervical atresia: Report of seven cases and review of the literature. Am J Obstet Gynecol 177:1419, 1997.)

radiologic technique. Pregnancies may occur in these women (Fraser, 1989). Although only 2 of the 18 women operated on by Chakravarty and associates (2000) were delivered of viable infants, Deffarges and coworkers (2001) reported that 10 of 12 undergoing uterovaginal anastomoses became pregnant; 4 of the 10 deliveries occurred after 30 weeks' gestation.

Given that the ovaries are normal, assisted reproductive technologies with use of a surrogate uterus might be the preferable option to achieve biologic offspring. Lai and coworkers (2001) achieved a successful pregnancy in a 33-year-old patient who had previously undergone two unsuccessful attempts to create a uterovaginal canal. Following ovarian hyperstimulation, oocyte aspiration was performed and fertilization was carried out in vitro. Embryos were transferred by transtubal embryo transfer and transmyometrial transfer. A resulting pregnancy produced a 2812 g infant delivered by cesarean section. At surgery, amniotic membrane was used as an epithelial surface for a newly created tract between the vagina and the uterine cervix; 5 months later the canal remained satisfactory.

The cervical canal may also be obliterated in true hermaphrodites (Van Niekerk, 1974).

Müllerian Aplasia

Aplasia of the müllerian ducts leads to absence of the uterine corpus, uterine cervix, and upper (superior) vagina (see Fig. 8–1). The foreshortened 1-cm to 2-cm vagina is presumably derived exclusively from invagination of the urogenital sinus. Individuals with müllerian aplasia are seen because of primary amenorrhea. Secondary sexual development is normal. Traditional uterine structures do not exist, but remnants may exist in the form of bilateral cords. The appellation *Rokitansky-Küster-Hauser syndrome* is often used. At one time applied only if uterine remnants persisted, the eponoym has more recently been used synomously with müllerian aplasia. Treatment is dealt with in standard gynecologic texts. An artificially created neovagina can usually be accomplished by dilators; surgery (McIndoe procedure) is utilized for less than in the past. A recent observation is that vaginal vault prolapse may occur following an ostensibly successful procedure (Schaffer et al., 2002).

The only disorder that ordinarily needs to be considered in the differential diagnosis of müllerian aplasia is complete androgen insensitivity. Androgen insensitivity can be excluded on the basis of chromosomal studies and gonadal com-

using DNA polymorphic variants. These studies nonetheless confirmed that familial aggregates are not infrequent (Kennedy et al., 1995, 1997). The OXEGENE group recorded receipt of samples from 19 mother-daughter pairs and 56 sib pairs (Kennedy et al., 1995). In 18 families, 3 or more relatives in more than one generation were observed. All but 2 of 16 monozygotic twin pairs have been concordant for endometriosis (Hadfield et al., 1997). A similar study in Iceland yielded 15 familial aggregates (Stefansson et al., 1998). Kennedy and coworkers (1998) recommended MRI to diagnose endometriosis. Endometriosis was found on MRI in 5 of 14 (14%) first-degree relatives and 1/12 (8%) of other relatives; more equivocal findings were found even more often.

Higher concordance of endometriosis for MZ than DZ twins has been observed (Moen, 1994; Kennedy et al., 1995; Treloar et al., 1998a, b). In addition, endometriosis as a cause of surgical menopause is more highly correlated in MZ twins than in DZ twins (r = 0.52 versus 0.19) (Treloar et al., 1998a). Finally, menstrual pneumothorax was reported in two sisters with pelvic endometriosis (Hinson et al., 1981). Pneumothoraxes occurred on the right, the usual side.

GENETIC MECHANISMS

Endometriosis is clearly heritable, but the precise mechanisms remain unclear. Magnitude of the increased risk (5 to 8% of first-degree relatives) is more reminiscent of polygenic-multifactorial tendencies than of a single mutant gene. However, recurrence risk is higher than the 2 to 5% expected for polygenic inheritance. The frequency of affected relatives might be even higher if one could directly measure a gene product(s). Although mendelian mechanisms cannot be excluded, polygenic inheritance seems most likely if all endometriosis is considered a single disorder. If so, increased severity in familial cases is also consistent with predictions based on a polygenic model. Such a model (see Chapter 3) predicts that the greater the severity, the greater the underlying genetic liability and, hence, the greater the proportion of affected relatives. The finding that endometriosis was more severe in familial cases also lessens the likelihood that the presence of an affected family member led to the identification of an affected relative because of a higher index of clinical suspicion. More extensive discussion is provided in Bischoff and Simpson (2000, 2001a, b), Simpson (2001), Simpson and Bischoff (2002), and Bischoff and coworkers (2002).

The other formal explanation, and perhaps the most likely, is that not all endometriosis is the same disorder, that is, genetic heterogeneity exists. One or more forms of endometriosis might be mendelian, despite the larger proportion being nongenetic or polygenic. This has proved to be the likely explanation for peptic ulcer and other adult-onset disorders. However, the face that studies have not generally shown HLA associations with endometriosis (Moen et al., 1984; Simpson et al., 1984; Maxwell et al., 1989) is more suggestive of polygenic-multifactorial inheritance than of genetic heterogeneity. Ishii et al. (2002) found an association for the HLA-DRB1*1403 allele but not for other alleles.

MOLECULAR BASIS

Given that endometriosis is heritable and presumably polygenic-multifactorial in etiology, the task is to determine the number of genes responsible and their chromosomal location(s). This can be approached in three general ways. (1) genome-wide quantitative linkage analysis (QTL) using DNA of endometriosis and controls, (2) differences in genome-wide expression patterns between mRNA of endometriosis and controls, and (3) targeted analysis of candidate genes either identified in the former two approaches or postulated de novo as causative. The first two approaches require no knowledge of the nature of the causative genes; the third requires candidate gene hypotheses.

Quantitative Linkage Analysis (QTL)

Quantitative genetic analysis across the whole genome is being pursued by several groups who seek to localize the genes paramount to the etiology of endometriosis. These studies involve comparing DNA from individuals with or without endometriosis. Recall (see Chapter 3) that this approach is predicated on the assumption that any region could encode gene(s) of importance. The method usually used is sib-pair analysis, based on the thesis that affected relatives inherit identical copies of any given allele (identify by descent; IBD) more often than expected by chance alone (see Figs. 3–5, 3–6, 3–7). If the same locus shows allele-sharing in different families of affected individuals, a pivotal gene could be identified. The strength of sib-pair methods for QTL is that there is no dependence on identifying a specific mode of inheritance because IBD sharing at a given locus is merely compared with the random expectation of 0.5 for first-degree relatives. Excess IBD sharing can be detected irrespective of (incomplete) penetrance, phenocopy, or genetic heterogeneity. No *a priori* assumption is necessary concerning candidate genes or chromosomal regions.

Although QTL has been used successfully in the identifying genes in such complex traits as asthma or hypertension, QTL analysis in endometriosis has proved disappointing. A long-standing QTL project is being conducted in Oxford, where sib-pair analysis is being performed using polymorphic DNA markers and fluorescence-based automated analysis (Kennedy et al., 1995; Kennedy, 1998; Kennedy et al., 2001). Several regions of exclusion have been noted but no linkages published. A genome-wide linkage approach is also being pursued in Iceland. A genome-wide scan of 15 families, with a total of 33 individuals and 23 relatives affected with endometriosis, was carried out using markers 5cM apart. At one time a suggestive locus was found on 9q, although not in the region of the *GALT* gene, which is on the short arm of chromosome 9 (Stefansson et al., 1998). More recently, the same group failed to confirm with a larger sample size (Geirsson et al., 2002). A third center pursuing this approach is in Australia. Initially 289 families with 374 sib-pairs were studied; possible linkage was identified to several loci (Treloar et al., 2000). More recently, the Oxford and Australian groups have combined, including their current respective commercial partners (Oxagen and Cerylid Biosciences). A total of 557 families and 683 sib pairs have been studied. "Significant linkage" for one still undisclosed locus was reported (Treloar and Kennedy, 2002), along with four "possible" linkages.

Limits and pitfalls that abound in quantitative linkage analysis were considered in Chapter 3 but are worth repeating here. One problem is that large numbers of families need to be identified with accurate diagnoses of affected and unaffected individuals. Special difficulties exist in ascertaining sufficient numbers of extended multigenerational families and in confirming the absence of disease in ostensibly unaffected individuals. Another problem is the difficulty in demonstrating linkage using the traditional genetic criteria of a log odds ratio (LOD) score of 3.0. Given the log scale, a LOD score of 3 corresponds to 10^3 fold likelihood of accepting linkage. This high bar is considered necessary given that false assignments are a known problem in linkage analysis. Relaxing statistical requirements is genetically almost heretical. Another pitfall is disease misclassification, a problem in disorders like endometriosis that are plagued by clinical mimicry and, hence, are not always easy to detect

clinically with certainty. Misclassification (erroneous diagnosis or failure to diagnose) adversely affects statistical power, already tenuous given requirements dictated by a requisite LOD score of 3.0. Finally, another major limitation is interaction between loci (Simpson and Bischoff, 2001), which can adversely affect ability to detect an existing relationship.

Gene Expression Profiling

A second general approach for finding the genes pivotal for endometriosis involves searching for differences among gene products expressed in endometriosis and control tissue. Initial work was based on immunocytochemical studies. High protein levels were found for various proto-oncogenes compared with levels in normal endometrium: *c-myc, c-fms, c-erbB-1/2,* and *ras* (Bergqvist et al., 1991; Schenken et al., 1991). Data suggested that altered proto-oncogene expression may be involved in disregulated growth and differentiation of endometriotic cells. Monoclonal cell expansion in endometriosis has also been observed (Nibert et al., 1995; Jimbo et al., 1997). Using an established endometriosis cell line, overexpression of oncogenes *c-myc* and *c-erbB-1* and *–2* has been observed by Gogusev and coworkers (2000).

Another line of investigation involved *bcl-2* overexpression, which leads to a decreased rate of cell death (Yang and Korsmeyer, 1996). This gene plays a role in the normal endometrial cycle by regulating cellular homeostasis and apoptosis; increased expression is detected in the proliferative endometrial phase but not in the secretory phase (Lu et al., 1993). Examining the expression of *bcl-2* in endometrial carcinomas and hyperplasia has produced discrepant results (Henderson et al., 1996). In one study, *bcl-2* overexpression in ectopic endometrial lesions by immunohistochemical staining was reported, indicating that endometriotic cells fail to undergo apoptosis (Watanabe et al., 1997). Using a cell death detection enzyme-linked immunosorbent assay (ELISA), Dmowski and colleagues (1998) demonstrated that apoptosis is significantly decreased in the eutopic endometrium of women with endometriosis compared with infertile controls.

The above studies examined gene products one by one. The current approach to differential gene expression utilizes microarray technology. Large-scale simultaneous gene expression profiling involves examining expression; many and possibly all relevant genes can be tested simultaneously. High-density oligonucleotide or cDNA arrays are described elsewhere and mentioned in Chapter 2.

Briefly, many thousand 20 mer oligonucleotides of defined sequence (referred to as probes) are synthesized directly onto derivatized glass slides using photolithography and oligonucleotide chemistry (Schena et al., 1995; Lockhart et al., 1996). Surface-bound oligonucleotides or probes subsequently bind or hybridize to labeled mRNA. RNAs present at frequencies of 1:300,000 can be unambiguously detected and quantified. This use of synthetic oligonucleotides permits application of the growing body of sequence information, with thousands of genes examined concurrently. However, selection of appropriate endometriosis and control tissues and proper RNA standardization are crucial. Early work has identified many genes that were upregulated or downregulated; investigation of their significance is under way.

A general caveat of gene expression profiling is that overexpressed genes are not necessarily those involved in initiating endometriosis. The converse also holds true. Uncontaminated endometriosis tissue must be studied; admixtures encompassing contiguous (normal) endometrium or connective tissues could produce spurious results.

A few reports have been published using endometriosis tissue. Eyster et al. (2002) studied three patients (eutopic endometrium and endometriotic implants). Eight genes were overexpressed in the latter, several of which were relevent to the cytoskeleton. Studying 2 patients, Guidice et al. (2002) used Affymetric microarrays, having probe sets for 558 human genes. Upregulation was observed for several genes: cytokines, growth factors, HOX genes, cell adhesion genes, mediators of cAmp signal transduction pathways and others. A similar spectrum was found by Chen et al. (2002). At Baylor the approach is to use tissue microarrays, the converse of approaches using DNAs or oligonucleatides.

Candidate Genes and Chromosomal Regions

The third general approach to uncovering genes pivotal to endometriosis is to search systematically for DNA perturbations in selective candidate loci or chromosomal regions. There is certainly no shortage of candidates gene, as reviewed by Sharpe-Timms (2002). Especially attractive seem to be steroid-related genes, angiogenic factors (Taylor et al., 2002) matrix-metalloproteinases (Henriet et al., 2002; Osteen et al., 2002), integrins (Lessey, 2002), and many others. In contrast to gene expression profiling, an advantage to this approach is that loci need not be expressed at the time tissue is obtained, unlike requirements for the expression assays

discussed in the previous section. The obvious disadvantage is that the correct gene or region must be selected and the DNA perturbation detectable by the method chosen. Any observed changes in DNA may or may not parallel any changes found in expression patterns (messenger RNA or protein) using techniques in the previous section. Theoretically, DNA-based approaches should more closely approximate causality. However, uninformative or fruitless studies are not uncommon. Irrespective of whether a candidate gene or chromosomal region is sought, the principle usually involves searching for loss of alleles at a given locus (loss of heterozygosity) or for an entire chromosomal region (comparative genome hybridization). Gain of an allele or chromosomal region can also exist.

If it is hypothesized that endometriosis involves only a somatic mutation, one need only compare DNA derived from non-endometriosis and endometriosis tissue from the same individual. A somatic mutation would be present only in the latter. If the hypothesis is that endometriosis involves an (inherited) germline mutation, one would need to compare DNA of any source (e.g., blood) from individuals with or without endometriosis.

Initial work in this general area was disappointing. Dangel and associates (1994) failed to find cytogenetic abnormalities in any of 42 endometrial implants. Another group failed to find mutations in the *Ras* oncogene or *p53* tumor suppressor gene in ectopic and eutopic endometrial tissue from 10 women with severe endometriosis (Vercellini et al., 1994). The likely explanation for these negative studies was that normal tissue (fibrous tissue or decidua) was unwittingly analyzed rather than endometriotic tissue *per se*. Indeed, positive findings were later found in a human endometriosis-derived permanent cell line (fBEM-1) established and characterized by Bouquet de Joliniere and coworkers (1997). Chromosomal studies (R-banding) showed numerous chromosomal aberrations: monosomy X; dup(Yq or 5q); trisomy 7, 8, and 10; and tetrasomy for chromosomes 17, 18, 19, and 20. Comparative genomic hybridization (CGH) was later used to identify somatic chromosomal alterations in DNA from both this cell line and from endometriotic lesions (n = 9) (Gogusev et al., 2000). CGH revealed these chromosome abnormalities in the FbEM-1 line: 1q+, 4q-, 11p-, 13q-; loss of 9, 12, and 18; and amplification of 6p. However, these changes were not consistent with previous cytogenetic results, suggesting that the cultured cells may be unstable and, hence, genetically heterogeneous.

Chromosomal alterations were observed in only four of the nine endometriotic tissue samples, with unbalanced aberrations involving gains of 1q, 4q, 11p, 17, and 20. Failure to find genetic imbalance among the remaining five cases may have been attributable to the presence of contaminating normal DNA.

The cytogenetic findings cited above suggest a genetic basis for endometriosis but do not necessarily indicate which gene is responsible. Of course, there is no shortage of specific candidate genes. Obvious examples include genes governing immunology, cell adhesion, or steroidogenesis. In assessing putative genes that exert their action through these mechanisms, the first steps usually involve searching for an association between endometriosis and normal individuals for selected genes (or polymorphisms at these loci).

Perhaps the first candidate gene postulated was galactose 1-phosphate uridyltransferase (*GALT*), located on chromosome 9p13. The specific alteration was an adenine to guanine change (polymorphism) in exon 10 that results in substitution of aspartate for asparagine (*N314D*). This polymorphism was found to be associated with endometriosis by Cramer and coworkers (1996). However, these results were not confirmed by Morland and coworkers (1998), Hadfield and coworkers (1999) or Geirsson et al. (2002). Stefannson et al. (2001) formally disproved linkage (quantitative linkage analysis) between *GALT* and endometriosis in the Icelandic population. Hadfield et al. (1999) found frequencies of *N314D* to be 15.8% (9/57) and 14.3% (13/91) in familial and sporadic endometriosis cases, respectively, versus 11.3% (6/53) in female controls and 13.7% (13/95) in male controls. Goumenou and associates (2001) reported allelic imbalance for polymorphic markers on *9p21* in 27.3% of the 22 matched samples (endometriosis tissue and normal endometrial tissue from the same individual). Loss of a functional allele at another locus — p16[Ink4], also located at 9p13, was observed in 1 of the 22 specimens.

Another attractive candidate gene is aromatase, known to be expressed in endometriotic tissue and stimulated by prostaglandin E_2 (PGE_2). (Bulun et al., 2000). Local production of estrogen and induction of PGE_2 would establish a positive feedback cycle. 17β-hydroxysteroid dehydrogenase type II expression has also been shown to be deficient in endometriosis, further leading to impaired inactivation of estradiol (E_2) to estrone. Collectively, these molecular aberrations favor accumulation of increasing quantities of E_2 and PGE_2 in endometriosis (Bulun et al., 2000).

An estrogen receptor (ER) gene polymorphism detectable by PvuII restriction endonuclease was reported by Georgiou et al. (1999). Homozygosity or heterozygosity was found in 72% (82/114) of subjects with endometriosis versus 49% (56/114) of controls. However, in a study of 50 Chinese women Fu and Wei (2002) reported no significant differences between endometriosis subjects and controls for PvuII polymorphism of the ER genes. Goumenou and coworkers (2001) have sought loss of heterozygosity (allelic imbalance) for several other regions housing candidate genes. Negative results were found for DNA mismatch repair genes (*MSH2*, *MSH6*, *MLH1*, *PMS1*). However, the same study detected loss of heterozygosity for *APOA2*, a high-density lipoprotein.

Increased frequency for the null (deletion) allele of glutathione S transferase M1 (*GSTM1*) was reported by Baronova and coworkers (1997): 86% (43/50) in endometriosis subjects versus 46% (33/72) in controls. The pharmacogenetic significance of polymorphism for this detoxification enzyme was discussed by Bischoff and Simpson (2000). In addition to their studies on *GSTM1*, Baranova and associates (1997) reported increased frequency of the slow acetylation allele of arylamine N-acetyltransferase 2 (*NAT2*); however, neither Hadfield et al. (2001), Yoshida and coworkers (2001) nor Baxter and coworkers (2001) could confirm this finding, studying one family with four affected members (mother and three daughters). Goumenou et al. (2002) reported association of the disease with the combination of CYPIA 1 ml and GSTM1 null allele.

Bischoff et al. (2002) found on 27% of endometriosis to be homozygous, for the GSTM1 null allele, far lower than other studies. The likelihood of discrepant results based on ethnic stratification seems high for this gene. Bischoff et al. (2002) also failed to find differences between fast and slow acetylataes for *NAT2* in subjects having and not having endometroisis, albeit increased frequency for mutant allele *6A being observed in endometriosis.

Other work on detoxification enzymes has dealt with Class I detoxification. No association was found in studies involving Ah receptor and CYPIA polymorphisms (Hadfield et al., 2001; Watanabe et al., 2001).

Another attractive set of candidate genes are the cell adhesion genes. A host of in *vitro* work make clear the plausibility of a relationship. Vigano et al. (2002) studied the intecellular adhesion molecule 1 (ICAM-1) gene, finding increased frequency of the rare allele R241.

GENETIC MECHANISMS

Heritable tendencies clearly exist in "essential" PCOS, i.e., PCOS not associated with adrenal enzyme deficiencies (nonclassic adrenal hyperplasia). The mode of inheritance is not certain, but dominant tendencies are clearly more pertinent than recessive ones (Simpson, 1991). Homozygosity for an enzyme defect is an unlikely explanation for multigenerational familial aggregates because enzyme deficiencies are usually autosomal recessive. Heterozygous expression of an enzyme defect is a formal but unlikely possibility. Another formal possibility is pseudoautosomal dominant inheritance in selected kindreds, vertical transmission reflecting homozygotes mating with heterozygotes.

Heritability exclusively caused by a single dominant gene seems unlikely because far fewer than 50% of symptomatic first-degree relatives seem clinically affected. Notwithstanding results of certain studies cited above, most clinicians have the impression that perhaps 5 to 10% of first-degree relatives of PCOS cases are similarly symptomatic. Mandel and coworkers (1983) studied 23 PCOS subjects in Los Angeles and found only four to have an affected relative; all four had an affected sister, and one had an affected mother as well. Lunde and associates (1989) studied 132 Norwegian women identified on the basis of ovarian wedge resection, multicystic ovaries, or other PCOS-like symptoms. Female first-degree relatives showed hirsutism and menstrual irregularities more often than controls. Among sisters, the frequencies were 6% and 15%, respectively; among mothers, 12% and 13%. Male first-degree relatives showed early baldness.

Formal explanations for the extant genetic data include not only a single dominant gene of low penetrance and variable expressivity but also polygenic-multifactorial inheritance or genetic heterogeneity. That HLA associations exist for *DRW6* (Hague et al., 1990) and *DQA1 O501* (Ober et al., 1992) suggests genetic heterogeneity, given that HLA association is usually found to be heterogeneous in adult-onset disorders with recurrence risks of 5 to 10%.

MOLECULAR BASIS

The 5% of PCOS women who have demonstrable adrenal biosynthetic defects should have a mutation in the gene coding for the respective enzyme (namely, 21-hydroxylase, 17α-hydroxylase/17,20-lyase, or 11 β-hydroxylase). Otherwise, the enzyme deficiency would be a secondary phenomenon. The same statement applies to PCOS associated with insulin resistance. Thus, Sorbara and coworkers (1994) sequenced the entire insulin receptor (*INSR*) gene in 2 PCOS cases and found no mutations; Talbot and colleagues (1996) studied 32 PCOS cases and found no perturbations in *INSR*.

Franks and colleagues at St. Mary's Hospital have long sought linkage and associations between PCOS and the various cyproterone *P450* genes involved in the adrenal biosynthetic pathways. Originally interest centered on *CYP17*, but linkage now seems excluded. The gene of current interest is *CYP11* which was shown in association with PCOS (Gharani et al., 1997). Waterworth and coworkers (1997) reported linkage with INS VNTR polymorphism.

Polygenic-multifactorial inheritance implies several causative genes. Linkage analysis to assess candidate genes responsible for PCOS is being conducted by a multicenter consortium, a collaborative effort between Penn State University, University of Pennsylvania, and UCLA. This group envisions PCOS as a disorder in which approximately 50% of cases show insulin resistance. Whether insulin resistance, which clearly has a genetic component independent of PCOS *per se*, leads to the hyperandrogenesis characteristic of PCOS is not certain. Nonetheless, the specific biochemical defect is considered to involve insulin-mediated receptor phosphorylation. Insulin receptor mutations were found in two PCOS cases in whom all 22 exons were sequenced (Sorbara et al., 1994); however, in 32 women studied by Talbot and coworkers (1996), no mutations were found in *INSR*. These data indicate that if insulin receptor perturbation is integral to PCOS, the mechanism of action involves a more distant (downstream) effect of insulin action (e.g., translation). Legro and coworkers (1998) provide a thorough discussion of the biochemical basis of PCOS.

A total of 150 families (all but two of European origin) were studied for linkage to 37 candidate genes (Table 8–11), using affected sib pair analysis and transmission-disequilibrium methods (Urbanek et al., 1999). Diagnostic criteria consisted of oligomenorrhea (<6 menses/year) and hyperandrogenism (>58 ng/dL total testosterone or >15 ng/dL not bound to sex hormone binding globulin). Of the 134 sisters of index cases, 39 were affected, 46 unaffected, and 49 unknown. Polymorphic markers within 1 cM of each candidate were available for 28 candidate genes; for 9 candidate genes, polymorphic markers were 1–4cM distant. Included in the analysis were several regions that had previously stated to show association or linkage to PCOS:

INS, *VNTR* (insulin variable number tandem repeats), *CYP11A*, *CYP1A*, *CYP17*, and *INSR* (insulin receptor). Strongest evidence for linkage was found between PCOS and follistatin; 72% identity by descent was observed. However, a later presentation by this group reported that analysis of additional families no longer revealed significant linkage to follistatin (Franks et al., 2001; Urbanek, 2001).

The nature of any perturbation of follistatin is also uncertain but a relationship is plausible. Follistatin neutralizes activin, a member of the transforming growth factor (TGF-β) family that promotes ovarian follicular development, inhibits these cells' androgen production, and increases both pituitary FSH and pancreatic β-cell insulin secretions. Inappropriately high follistatin levels should inhibit follicular development, increase ovarian androgen production, and impair insulin release. These features are all characteristic of PCOS. As predicted, overexpression of follistatin in transgenic mice results in a PCOS-like ovarian phenotype (Guo et al., 1998). However, Calvo and coworkers (2001) found no mutations after sequencing exons 1, 2, 3, 4, and 6 of the follistatin gene in 34 Spanish PCOS cases. Liao and coworkers (2000) similarly found no follistatin perturbations in 64 Chinese cases.

Of the other candidate genes, *CYP11A* showed nominally significant linkage ($P = 0.02$ before correction but $P > 0.05$ after correction). Although Gharani and associates (1997) also showed association between *CYP11A* and PCOS, the specific allele they used (*D15S520*) was not shown to be linked to PCOS in the study of Urbanek and coworkers (1999). Among genes failing to show linkage and thus contradicting association studies were *INS*, *VNTR* (linkage shown by Waterworth et al., 1997), *CYP19*, *CYP17*, and *INSR*.

In 38 PCOS subjects Oksanen and coworkers (2000) found no abnormalities in serum leptin, leptin, or leptin receptor genes. This is consistent with failure to find linkage by Urbanek and associates (1999). Takakura and coworkers (2001) found no inactivating mutations of *FSHR* (FSH receptor) in 38 PCOS cases. The search focused on exons 6, 7, 9, and 10.

Premature Ovarian Failure (POF)

The causes of POF overlap with those responsible for complete ovarian failure and primary amenorrhea, a topic covered in detail in Chapter 10. Autosomal genes and X chromosomal abnormalities causing ovarian failure were discussed in

detail in that context. In this chapter we focus our comments on familial tendencies in POF, specifically when caused by other mechanisms.

POF can result from these general causes: (1) X-chromosomal abnormalities, (2) autosomal recessive genes resulting in the various forms of XX gonadal dysgenesis; (3) autosomal chromosomal rearrangements, and (4) autosomal dominant genes, including those whose action is restricted to POF. The latter is our focus here.

X-CHROMOSOMAL ABNORMALITIES

Premature rather than complete ovarian failure occurs to a varying extent with all X-abnormalities. At least 10 to 15% of 45,X/46,XX individuals menstruate compared with fewer than 5% of 45,X individuals (Simpson, 1975). This percentage is surely a minimum because many mosaic individuals are so mildly affected that they are never detected clinically. Spontaneous menstruation occurs in about half of all 46,X,del(X)(p11) and in most 46,X,del(X)(p21 or 22) cases, although followed often by secondary amenorrhea and premature ovarian failure (Simpson and Rajkovic, 1999). Terminal deletions or X-autosomal translocations originating at Xq21 to Xq26 are more likely to be associated with premature ovarian failure than is complete ovarian failure. This topic is explored in detail in Chapter 10.

FRAXA premutation accounts for some familial POF, as discussed in Chapter 10. A relationship between *FRAXA* premutation and POF may or may not be independent of the terminal Xq ovarian maintenance genes.

AUTOSOMAL RECESSIVE POF

In some families the proband may have gonadal dysgenesis and streak gonads, but a sib may show ovarian hypoplasia and a few oocytes. These sibships indicate that the mutant gene responsible for XX gonadal dysgenesis shows variable expressivity. The autosomal recessive mutations responsible for the various forms of XX gonadal dysgenesis may thus be manifested as less severe ovarian pathology. In Finland (Aittomaki, 1994, 1995), POF caused by an FSH receptor mutation (C566T) not infrequently coexisted in the same kindred as complete ovarian failure. XX gonadal dysgenesis genes are therefore responsible for some familial premature ovarian failure.

AUTOSOMAL CHROMOSOMAL REARRANGEMENTS

Autosomal chromosomal rearrangements can also lead to premature ovarian failure (Hens et al., 1989; Kawano et al., 1998; Bunton et al., 2000). The common mechanism for many different reciprocal translocations is presumably meiotic breakdown. One to five percent of azoospermic or oligospermic men who are otherwise clinically normal show balanced autosomal translocations; these men are candidates for intracytoplasmic sperm injection (ICSI) (Van Assche et al., 1996; Bonduelle et al., 1998). Another 10% of ICSI candidates have sex chromosomal abnormalities, but usually these men show other abnormalities (Klinefelter syndrome). A problem of similar magnitude presumably exists in women, but lack of a readily assayed end point makes studies more difficult in females than in men. Nevertheless, the pathogenesis in both sexes presumably involves meiotic breakdown secondary to failure of synapsis. Detecting individuals with a chromosomal rearrangement is important because their offspring are at risk for unbalanced chromosomal abnormalities.

AUTOSOMAL DOMINANT POF

Autosomal dominant familial tendencies *per se* have long been recognized in cytogenetically normal women with premature ovarian failure. Some samples of POF women report very high frequencies of these associated abnormalities. Kim and associates (1997) reported that 22 of 119 POF women (18.5%) had hypothyroidism and 3 had Addison disease. For many years it tended to be assumed that familial tendencies in POF reflected autoimmune phenomena. In POF women antibodies coexisted against adrenal (Rebar et al., 1982; LaBarbera et al., 1988; Karlsson et al., 1993), thyroid (Alper et al., 1985), and pancreas (LaBarbera et al., 1988; Belvisi et al., 1993). Of interest here are familial tendencies in nonautoimmune POF. Coulam and coworkers (1983) reported POF in sibs who had an affected mother and aunt. Affected individuals in more than one generation were reported by Starup and Sele (1973), Austin and coworkers (1979), and Mattison and coworkers (1984). In these families autoimmune phenomena were excluded.

Studies of interest are under way in Italy (Testa et al., 1997; Vegetti et al., 1998). Women with POF (menopause < 40 years of age) recruited from a large northern Italian population underwent pedigree studies to identify heritable POF.

After excluding 10 cases with known etiologies (5 chromosomal, 3 prior ovarian surgery, 1 prior chemotherapy, 1 galactosemia), 71 probands remained. In all, cessation of ovarian function (POF) occurred under age 40 years. Of the 71, 22 (31%) had other affected relatives. An expanded sample of 130 cases found an incidence of 28.5% familial cases (Vegetti et al., 2000). Patterns of inheritance observed were consistent with autosomal or X-linked dominant inheritance; transmission through both maternal and paternal lineage was observed. Among 30 other women experiencing early menopause (40 to 50 years old), half showed other affected relatives. There is further evidence that POF (<40 years) and early menopause (menopause 40 to 50 years) represent the same phenomena. The two different phenotypes were observed within a single kindred, transmission through either a paternal or maternal relative.

Pathogenic mechanisms for autosomal dominant premature ovarian failure might include a decreased number of primordial follicles or human homologues of mouse gene cited in Chapter 10. Harris et al. (2002) found FOXL2 mutations in 2 of 70 POF patients. (See Chapter 10 for FOXL2 and the blepharophimosis-ptosis-epicanthus syndrome.) Nongenetic etiologies (phenocopies) might include infiltrative disease (e.g., sarcoidosis), toxins, or autoimmune phenomena. Environmental causes are unlikely to explain intergenerational familial aggregates.

PREMATURE OVARIAN FAILURE AS NORMAL CONTINUOUS VARIATION

It is to be expected that oocyte number (reservoir) will be low in some women simply on statistical (stochastic) grounds. Normal distribution exists for all common anatomic traits (e.g., height), and this principle must apply to oocyte number and reservoir at birth. Different rodent strains show characteristic breeding duration, implying genetic control over either the rate of oocyte depletion or the number of oocytes initially present. That a normal distribution of germ cell number exists in ostensibly normal females is thus well established in animals but is difficult to prove in humans. Nonetheless, some ostensibly normal (menstruating) women should have decreased oocyte reservoir or increased oocyte attrition on a genetic basis, analogous to animal models.

In humans, a genetic basis for the above can also be presumed by analogy to the heritability of age at human menopause, a characteristic that clearly shows familial tendencies. (See the discus-

▼ **Table 8–11.** CANDIDATE PCOS GENES SURVEYED BY URBANEK AND COWORKERS (1999)*

Candidate gene and its chromosomal location (parenthesis)

Linkage was shown to follistatin and *CYP-11A*	Inhibin C (12q13)
Androgen receptor (Xq 11.2)	Sex hormone binding globulin (17p13.2)
CYP11A-cytochrome P450 side-chain cleavage enzyme (15q23-24)	Luteinizing hormone/choriogonadotropin receptor (2p21)
CYP17-cytochrome P450 17a-hydroxylase/17,20-desmolase (10q24.3)	Follicle-stimulating hormone receptor (2p21)
CYP19-cytochrome P450 aromatase (15q21)	Mothers against decapentaplegic homolog 4 (18q21)
17-β-hydroxysteroid dehydrogenase types (17q11-21)	Melanocortin 4 receptor (18q21.32)
17-β-hydroxysteroid dehydrogenase, type II (16q24.2)	Leptin (7q31.3-32.1)
17-β-hydroxysteroid dehydrogenase, type III (9q22)	Leptin receptor (1p31)
3-β-hydroxysteroid dehydrogenase, types I and II (1p31.1)	Pro-opiomelanocortin (2p23)
Steroidogenic acute regulatory protein (8p11.2)	Uncoupling protein 2 + 3 (11q13)
Activin receptor 1 (12q13.12)	Insulin-like growth factor I (12q22-23)
Activin receptor 2A (2q22.2)	Insulin-like growth factor I receptor (15q25-26)
Activin receptor 2B (3p22.2)	Insulin-like growth factor binding protein 1 + 3 (7p13-7p12)
Follistatin (5p14)	Insulin gene *VNTR* (11p15.5)
Inhibin A (2q33.34)	Insulin receptor (19p13.3)
Inhibin β-A (7p13-15)	Leydig insulin-like protein 3 (19p13.1)
Inhibin β-B (2cen-2q13)	Insulin receptor substrate 1 (2q36-37)
	Peroxisome proliferator-activated receptor-gamma (3p25-24.2)

*Strongest linkage was shown for follistatin. Modified from or data from Legro et al. (1998).

sion earlier in this chapter.) Other confounding factors (e.g., leiomyomas or uterine cancer) also must be taken into account.

REFERENCES

Adams J, Polson DW, Franks S: Prevalence of polycystic ovaries in women with anovulation and idiopathic hirsutism. Br Med J 293:355, 1986.

Adams J, Franks S, Polson DW, et al.: Multifollicular ovaries: Clinical and endocrine features and response to pulsatile gonadotropin releasing hormone. Lancet 2:1375, 1985.

Aittomaki K, Lucena JL, Pakarinen P, et al.: Mutation in the follicle-stimulating hormone receptor gene causes hereditary hypergonadotropic ovarian failure. Cell 82:959, 1995.

Alam NA, Bevan S, Churchman M, et al.: Localization of a gene (MCUL1) for multiple cutaneous leiomyomata and uterine fibroids to chromosome 1q42.3-q43. Am J Hum Genet 68:1264, 2001.

Algovik M, Lagercrantz J, Westgren M, et al.: No mutations found in candidate genes for dystocia. Hum Reprod 14:2451, 1999.

Alper MM, Garner PR: Premature ovarian failure: Its relationship to autoimmune disease. Obstet Gynecol 66:27, 1985.

Amesse L, Yen FF, Weisskopf B, et al.: Vaginal uterine agenesis associated with amastia in a phenotypic female with a de novo 46,XX,t(8;13)(q22.1;q32.1) translocation. Clin Genet 55:493, 1999.

Anger D, Hemet J, Ensel J: Familial form of Rokitansky-Kuster-Hauser syndrome. Bull Fed Soc Gynecol Obstet Lang Fr 18:229, 1966.

Arnold LL, Meck JM, Simon JA: Adenomyosis: Evidence for genetic cause. Am J Med Genet 55:505, 1995.

Arnold LL, Ascher SM, Simon JA: Familial adenomyosis: A case report. Fertil Steril 61(6):1165, 1994.

Ashar HR, Fejzos MS, Tkachenko A, et al.: Disruption of the architectural factor HMG1-C: DNA-binding AT hook motifs fused in lipomas to distinct transcriptional regulatory domains. Cell 82:57, 1995.

Austin GE, Coulam CB, Ryan JR: A search for antibodies to luteinizing hormone receptors in premature ovarian failure. Mayo Clin Proc 54:394, 1979.

Baird PA, Lowry RB: Absent vagina and the Klippel-Feil anomaly. Am J Obstet Gynecol 118:290, 1974.

Baranova H, Bothorishvilli R, Canis M, et al.: Glutathione S-transferase M1 gene polymorphism and susceptibility to endometriosis in a French population. Mol Hum Reprod 3:775, 1997.

Battaglia C, Regnani G, Mancini F, et al.: Polycystic ovaries in childhood: a common finding in daughters of PCOS patients. A pilot study. Hum Reprod 17:771, 2002.

Baxter SW, Thomas EJ, Campbell IG: GSTM1 null polymorphism and susceptibility to endometriosis and ovarian cancer. Carcinogenesis 22:63, 2001.

Belvisi L, Bombelli F, Sironi L, et al.: Organ-specific autoimmunity in patients with premature ovarian failure. J Endocrinol Invest 16:889, 1993.

Berg-Lekas ML, Hogberg U, Winkvist A: Familial occurrence of dystocia: Am J Obstet Gynecol 179:117, 1998.

Bergqvist A, Borg A, Ljungberg O: Proto-oncogenes in endometriotic and endometrial tissue. Ann NY Acad Sci 626:276, 1991.

Bhagavath B, Stelling JR, van Lingen BL, et al.: Congenital absence of the uterus and vagina (CAUV) is not associated with the N314D allele of the galactose-1-phosphate uridyl transferase (*GALT*) gene. J Soc Gynecol Invest 5:140, 1998.

Birrell FN, Adebajo AO, Hazleman BL, et al.: High prevalence of joint laxity in West Africans. Br J Rheumatol 33:56, 1994.

Bischoff FZ, Marquez-Do D, Dant D, et al.: Nat2 and GSMT1 DNA polymorphisms: increased GSTM1 (active) genotypes in endometriosis. Fertil Steril 77:S17, 2002.

Bischoff FZ, Heard M, Simpson JL: Somatic DNA alterations in endometriosis: Frequency of chromosome 17 and P53 loss in late-stage endometriosis. J Reprod Immunol 55:49, 2002.

Bischoff FZ, Simpson JL: Heritability and molecular genetic studies of endometriosis. Hum Reprod Update 6:37, 2000.

Mushkat Y, Bukovsky I, Langer R: Female urinary stress incontinence—does it have familial prevalence? Am J Obstet Gynecol 174:617, 1996.

Nager GT, Chen SCA, Hussels IE: A new syndrome in two unrelated females: Klippel-Feil deformity, conductive deafness, and absent vagina: Case II. Birth Defects Orig Artic Ser 7(6):312, 1971.

Naylor AF, Warburton D: Genetics of obstetrical variables: A study from the Collaborative Perinatal Project. Clin Genet 6:351, 1974.

Nibert M, Heim S: Uterine leiomyoma cytogenetics. Genes Chromosomes Cancer 2:3, 1990.

Nibert M, Pejovic, T, Mandahl N, et al.: Monoclonal origin of endometriosis cysts. Int J Gynecol Cancer 5:61, 1995

Norman RJ, Masters S, Hague W: Hyperinsulinemia is common in family members of women with polycystic ovary syndrome. Fertil Steril 66:942, 1996.

Norton PA, Baker JE, Sharp HC, et al.: Genitourinary prolapse and joint hypermobility in women. Obstet Gynecol 85:225, 1995.

Nykiforuk NE: Uterus didelphys. Can Med Assoc J 38:175, 1938.

Obata K, Morland SJ, Watson RH, et al.: Frequent PTEN/MMAC mutations in endometrioid but not serous or mucinous epithelial ovarian tumors. Cancer Res 58:2095, 1998.

Ober C, Abney M, McPeek MS: Genetic studies of age at menarche in a founder population: Estimates of heritability and genome-wide association studies. J Soc Gynecol Investig 7:180A, 2000.

Ober C, Weil S, Steck T, et al.: Increased risk for polycystic ovary syndrome associated with human leukocyte antigen DQA1*0501. Am J Obstet Gynecol 167:1803, 1992.

O'Driscoll JB, Mamtora H, Higginson J, et al.: A prospective study of the prevalence of clear-cut endocrine disorders and polycystic ovaries in 350 patients presenting with hirsutism or androgenic alopecia. Clin Endocrinol (Oxf) 41:231, 1994.

Oksanen L, Tiitinen A, Kaprio J, et al.: No evidence for mutations of the leptin or leptin receptor genes in women with polycystic ovary syndrome. Mol Hum Reprod 6:873, 2000.

Okolo S, Gentry C, Wong Te Fong L, et al.: Familial versus sporadic—a new concept in our understanding of uterine fibroids. Hum Reprod 16(P245):194, 2001.

Osteen KG, Bruner-Tran KL, Ong D, et al.: Paracrine mediators of endometrial matrix metalloprotenaise expression: potential targets for progestin-based treatment of endometriosis. Ann NY Acad Sci 955:139, 2002.

Ozisik YY, Meloni AM, Powell M, et al.: Chromosome 7 biclonality in uterine leiomyoma. Cancer Genet Cytogenet 67:59, 1993.

Pandis N, Heim S, Bardi G, et al.: Chromosome analysis of 96 uterine leiomyomas. Cancer Genet Cytogenet 55:11, 1991.

Park IJ, Jones HW Jr: A new syndrome in two unrelated females: Klippel-Feil deformity, conductive deafness and absent vagina. Birth Defects Orig Artic Ser 7(6):311, 1971.

Peacock L, Wiskind A, Wall L: Clinical features of urinary incontinence and urogenital prolapse in a black inner-city population. Am J Obstet Gynecol 171:1464, 1994.

Petri E: Untersuchungen zur Erbbedingtheit der Menarche. Z Morphol Anthropol 33:43, 1934.

Petrij F, Giles RH, Dauwerse HG, et al.: Rubinstein-Taybi syndrome caused by mutations in the transcriptional co-activator CBP. Nature 376:348, 1995.

Petrozza JC, Gray MR, Davis AJ, et al.: Congenital absence of the uterus and vagina is not commonly transmitted as a dominant genetic trait: Outcomes of surrogate pregnancies. Fertil Steril 67:387, 1997.

Phelan JT, Counseller VS, Greene LF: Deformities of the urinary tract with congenital absence of the vagina. Surg Gynecol Obstet 97:1, 1953.

Pinsky L: A community of human malformation syndromes involving the müllerian ducts, distal extremities, urinary tract, and ears. Teratology 9:65, 1974.

Polishuk WZ, Ron MA: Familial bicornuate and double uterus. Am J Obstet Gynecol 119:982, 1974.

Polson DW, Adams J, Wadsworth J, et al.: Polycystic ovaries—a common finding in normal women. Lancet 1:870, 1988.

Poznanski AK, Kuhns LR, Lapides J, et al.: A new family with the hand-foot-genital syndrome: A wider spectrum of the hand-foot-uterus syndrome. Birth Defects Orig Artic Ser 11(4):127, 1975.

Ranney B: Endometriosis: IV. Hereditary tendency. Obstet Gynecol 37:734, 1971.

Rebar RW, Erickson GF, Yen SS: Idiopathic premature ovarian failure: Clinical and endocrine characteristics. Fertil Steril 37:35, 1982.

Reed WB, Walker R, Horowitz R: Cutaneous leiomyomata with uterine leiomyomata. Acta Derm Venereol 53:409, 1973.

Rein MS, Friedman AJ, Barbieri RL, et al.: Cytogenetic abnormalities in uterine leiomyomata. Obstet Gynecol 77:923, 1991.

Resendes BL, Sohn SH, Stelling JR, et al.: Role for anti-müllerian hormone in congenital absence of the uterus and vagina. Am J Med Genet 98:129, 2001.

Rheaume E, Sanchez R, Simard J, et al.: Molecular basis of congenital adrenal hyperplasia in two siblings with classical nonsalt-losing 3 beta-hydroxysteroid dehydrogenase deficiency. J Clin Endocrinol Metab 79:1012, 1994.

Romaguera J, Moran C, Diaz-Montes TP, et al.: Prevalence of 21-hydroxylase-deficient nonclassic adrenal hyperplasia and insulin resistance among hirsute women from Puerto Rico. Fertil Steril 74:59, 2000.

Rosenblatt KA, Thomas D: Reduced risk of ovarian cancer in women with a tubal-ligation or hysterectomy. Cancer Epidemiol Biomarkers Prev 5:933, 1996.

Sait SN, Dal Cin P, Ovanessoff S, et al.: A uterine leiomyoma showing both t(12;14) and del(7) abnormalities. Cancer Genet Cytogenet 37:157, 1989.

Sakkal-Alkaddour H, Zhang L, et al.: Studies of 3 beta-hydroxysteroid dehydrogenase genes in infants and children manifesting premature pubarche and increased adrenocorticotropin-stimulated delta 5-steroid levels. J Clin Endocrinol Metab 81:3961, 1996.

Sanchez-Andres A: Genetic and environmental factors affecting menarcheal age in Spanish women. Anthropol Anz 55:69, 1997.

Sargent MS, Weremowicz S, Rein MS, et al.: Translocations in 7q22 define a critical region in uterine leiomyomata. Cancer Genet Cytogenet 77:65, 1994.

Sayer TR, Dixon JS, Hosker GL, et al.: A study of paraurethral connective tissue in women with stress incontinence of urine. Neurourol Urodyn 9:319, 1990.

Schaffer J, Fabricant C, Carr BR: Vaginal vault prolapse after nonsurgical and surgical treatment of mullerian agenesis. Obstet Gynecol 99:947, 2002.

Schena M, Shalon D, Davis RW, et al.: Quantitative monitoring of gene expression patterns with a complemtary DNA microarray. Science 270:467, 1995.

Schenken RS, Johnson JV, Riehl RM: C-myc proto-oncogene polypeptide expression in endometriosis. Am J Obstet Gynecol 164:1031, 1991.

Schinzel A, Giedion A: A syndrome of severe midface retraction, multiple skull anomalies, clubfeet, and cardiac and renal malformations in sibs. Am J Med Genet 1:361, 1978.

Schoenberg-Fejzo M, Ashar HR, Krauter KS, et al.: Translocation breakpoints upstream of the *HMGIC* gene in uterine leiomyomata suggest dysregulation of this gene by a mechanism different from that in lipomas. Genes Chromosomes Cancer 17:1, 1996.

Searle AG: The genetics and morphology of two "luxoid" mutants in the house mouse. Genet Res 5:171, 1964.

Sell SM, Altungoz O, Prowse AA, et al.: Molecular analysis of chromosome 7q21.3 in uterine leiomyoma: Analysis using markers with linkage to insulin resistance. Cancer Genet Cytogenet 100:165, 1998.

Semmens JP: Congenital anomalies of female genital tract: Functional classification based on review of 56 personal cases and 500 reported cases. Obstet Gynecol 19:328, 1962.

Sharpe-Timms KL: Endometrial anomalies in women with endometriosis. Ann NY Acad Sci 955:89, 2002.

Shin JC, Ross HL, Elias S, et al.: Detection of chromosomal aneuploidy in endometriosis by multi-color fluorescence in situ hybridization (FISH). Hum Genet 100:401, 1997.

Shokeir MH: Aplasia of the müllerian septum system: Evidence of probable sex-limited autosomal dominant inheritance. Birth Defects Orig Artic Ser 14(6c):147, 1978.

Simpson JL: Endometriosis. *In* Arici A (ed): Obstetrics and Gynecology of North America. Philadelphia: WB Saunders, in preparation, 2003.

Simpson JL: Disorders of the gonads, genital tract and genitalia. *In* Rimoin DL, Connor MJ, Pyeritz RE, et al. (eds): Emery and Rimoin's Principles and Practice of Medical Genetics, 4th Edition, London: Churchill Livingstone, 2002a, p 2315.

Simpson JL: Genetics of gynecologic disorders. *In* King RA, Motulsky AG, Rotter JI (eds): The Genetic Basis of Common Diseases, 2nd ed. San Francisco: Oxford University Press, in press, 2002b.

Simpson JL: Genetic factors in common disorders of female infertility. Reprod Med Rev 8:173, 2001.

Simpson JL: Genetic programming in ovarian development and oogenesis. *In* Lobo RA, Kelsey J, Marcus R (eds): Menopause Biology and Pathobiology. London: Academic Press, 2000, p 77.

Simpson JL: Genetics of the female reproductive ducts. Am J Med Genet 89:224, 1999.

Simpson JL: Elucidating genetics of polycystic ovarian disease (PCOD). *In* Dunaif A, Givens J, Merriam G, et al. (eds): Polycystic Ovary Syndrome. Cambridge, MA: Blackwell Scientific Publications, 1991, p 59.

Simpson JL: Disorders of Sexual Differentiation: Etiology and Clinical Delineation. (Embryological contribution by JE Jirasek.) New York: Academic Press, 1976.

Simpson JL: Gonadal dysgenesis and abnormalities of the human sex chromosomes: Current status of the phenotypic-karyotypic correlations. Birth Defects Orig Artic Ser 11(4):23, 1975.

Simpson JL: Genetic aspects of gynecologic disorders occurring in 46,XX individuals. Clin Obstet Gynecol 15:157, 1972.

Simpson JL, Bischoff FZ: Heritability and molecular genetic studies of endometriosis. Ann NY Acad Sci 955:239, 2002.

Simpson JL, Elias S, Malinak LR, et al.: Heritable aspects of endometriosis: I. Genetic studies. Am J Obstet Gynecol 137:327, 1980.

Simpson JL, Malinak LR, Elias S, et al.: HLA association in endometriosis. Am J Obstet Gynecol 148:395, 1984.

Simpson JL, Rajkovic A: Ovarian differentiation and gonadal failure. Am J Med Genet 89:186, 1999.

Slavotinek AM, Stone EM, Mykytyn K, et al.: Mutations in *MKKS* cause Bardet-Biedl syndrome. Nat Genet 26:15, 2000.

Snell GD, Dickie MM, Smith P, et al.: Linkage of loop-tail, leaden, splotch, and fuzzy in the mouse. Heredity 8:271, 1954.

Snieder H, MacGregor AJ, Spector TD: Genes control the cessation of a woman's reproductive life: A twin study of hysterectomy and age at menopause. J Clin Endocrinol Metab 83:1875, 1998.

Sorbara LR, Tang Z, Cama A, et al.: Absence of insulin receptor gene mutations in three insulin-resistant women with the polycystic ovary syndrome. Metabolism 43:1568, 1994.

Speiser PW, Dupont B, Rubinstein P, et al.: High frequency of nonclassical steroid 21-hydroxylase deficiency. Am J Hum Genet 37:650, 1985.

Sreekantaiah C, Li FP, Weidner N, Sandberg AA: An endometrial stromal sarcoma with clonal cytogenetic abnormalities. Cancer Genet Cytogenet 55:163, 1991.

Starup J, Sele V: Premature ovarian failure. Acta Obstet Gynecol Scand 52:259, 1973.

Stefansson H, Einarsdottir A, Geirsson RT: Endometriosis is not associated with or linked to the GALT gene. Fertil Steril 76:1019, 2001.

Stefansson H, Geirsson RT, Steinthorsdottir V, et al.: Genetic factors contribute to the risk of developing endometriosis. Hum Reprod 17:555, 2002.

Stefansson H, Geirsson RT, Guanason GA, et al.: A genome-wide search for endometriosis genes in Icelandic patients. Am J Hum Genet 63:A311, 1998.

Stelling JR, Bhagavath B, Gray MR, et al.: HOX13 homeodomain mutation analysis in patients with müllerian system anomalies. J Soc Gynecol Invest 5:140A, 1998b.

Stelling JR, Gray MR, Davis AJ, et al.: Familial transmission of imperforate hymen. Fertil Steril 70(Suppl) Abstracts, XVI Congress on Fertility and Sterility, San Francisco (Abstract O-125) S47, 1998a.

Stevenson AC, Dudgeon MY, McCluire HI: Observations on the results of pregnancies in women residents in Belfast: II. Abortions, hydatidiform moles, and ectopic pregnancies. Ann Hum Genet 23:395, 1959.

Stern AM, Gall JC Jr, Perry BL, et al.: The hand-foot-uterus syndrome: A new hereditary disorder characterized by hand and foot dysplasia, dermatoglyphic abnormalities, and partial duplication of the female genital tract. J Pediatr 77:109, 1970.

Stone DL, Agarwala R, Schaffer AA, et al.: Genetic and physical mapping of the McKusick-Kaufman syndrome. Hum Mol Genet 7:475, 1998.

Stone DL, Slavotinek A, Bouffard GG, et al.: Mutation of a gene encoding a putative chaperonin causes McKusick-Kaufman syndrome. Nat Genet 25:79, 2000.

Strong LC, Hollander WF: Hereditary loop-tail in the house mouse accompanied by imperforate vagina and with lethal craniorachischisis when homozygous. J Hered 40:329, 1949.

Sugimoto Y, Yamasaki A, Segi E, et al.: Failure of parturition in mice lacking the prostaglandin F receptor. Science 277:681, 1997.

Sueiro MM, Piloti R: Adrenica incomplete dos pequenos labios cam caracter familiar. Arch Anat Antrop 32:187, 1964.

Tajima T, Nishi Y, Takase A, et al.: No genetic mutation in the type II 3 beta-hydroxysteroid dehydrogenase gene in patients with biochemical evidence of enzyme deficiency. Horm Res 47:49, 1997.

Takakura K, Takebayashi K, Wang HQ, et al.: Follicle-stimulating hormone receptor gene mutations are rare in

Japanese women with premature ovarian failure and polycystic ovary syndrome. Fertil Steril 75:207, 2001.

Talbot JA, Bicknell EJ, Rajkhowa M, et al.: Molecular scanning of the insulin receptor gene in women with polycystic ovarian syndrome. J Clin Endocrinol Metab 81:1979, 1996.

Tamura M, Fukaya T, Murakami T, et al.: Analysis of clonality in human endometriotic cysts based on evaluation of X chromosome inactivation in archival formalin-fixed, paraffin-embedded tissue. Lab Invest 78:213, 1998.

Taylor RN, Lebovic DI, Mueller MD: Angiogenic factors in endometriosis. Ann NY Acad Sci 943:131, 2002.

Teebi AS: Limb/pelvis/uterus-hypoplasia/aplasia syndrome. J Med Genet 30:797, 1993.

Testa G, Vegetti W, Tibiletti MG, et al.: Pattern of inheritance in familial premature ovarian failure. Hum Reprod 12:202(P174), 1997.

Thompson JD, Wharton LR, Te Linde RW: Congenital absence of the vagina: An analysis of thirty-two cases corrected by the McIndoe operation. Am J Obstet Gynecol 74:397, 1957.

Tisserant-Perrier M: Etude comparative de certains processus de chroissance chez les jumeaux. J Genet Hum 2:87, 1953.

Tomlinson IPM, Alm A, Rowan AJ, et al.: Germline mutations in FH predispose to dominantly inherited uterine fibroids, skin leiomyomata and papillary renal cell cancer. Nat Genet 30:406, 2002.

Torgerson DJ, Thomas RE, Reid DM: Mothers and daughters menopausal ages: Is there a link? Europ J Obstet Gynecol Reprod Biol 74:63, 1997.

Treloar SA, Kennedy SH: Preliminary results from two combined genome-wide scans in endometriosis. Fertil Steril 77(Suppl 2):S19, 2002.

Treloar SA, Bahlo M, Ewen K, et al.: Suggestive linkage for endometriosis found in genome-wide scan. Am J Hum Genet 67(Suppl 2):318, 2000.

Treloar SA, Do KA, Martin NG: Genetic influences on the age at menopause. Lancet 352:1084, 1998a.

Treloar SA, Martin NG, Heath AC: Longitudinal genetic analysis of menstrual flow, pain, and limitation in a sample of Australian twins. Behav Genet 28:107, 1998b.

Treloar SA, Martin NG: Age at menarche as a fitness trait: Nonaddictive genetic variance detected in a large twin sample. Am J Hum Genet 47:137, 1990.

Treloar SA, Martin NG, Dennerstein L, et al.: Pathways to hysterectomy: Insights from longitudinal twin research. Am J Obstet Gynecol 167:82, 1992.

Turunen A, Unnerus CE: Spinal changes in patients with congenital aplasia of the vagina. Acta Obstet Gynecol Scand 46:99, 1967.

Tyler GT: Didelphys in sisters. Am J Surg 45:337, 1939.

Urbanek M: Proceedings: Polycystic Ovary Syndrome: Basic Biology and Clinical Intervention. In Dunaif AD, Chang RJ, Heindel J (eds): National Institute of Environmental Health Sciences (NIH), 2001.

Urbanek M, Legro RS, Driscoll DA, et al.: Thirty-seven candidate genes for polycystic ovary syndrome: strongest evidence for linkage is with follistatin. Proc Natl Acad Sci USA 96:8573, 1999.

Utsch B, Becker K, Brock D, et al.: A novel stable polyalanine [poly(A)] expansion in the HOXA13 gene associated with hand-foot-genital syndrome: proper function of poly(A)-harbouring transcription factors depends on a critical repeat length? Hum Genet 110:488, 2002.

Van Assche E, Bonduelle M, Tournaye H, et al.: Cytogenetics of infertile men. Hum Reprod 11(Suppl):1, 1996.

van Lingen BL, Eccles MR, Reindollar H, et al.: Molecular genetic analysis of the PAX2 gene in patients with congenital absence of the uterus and vagina. Fertil Steril 70(Suppl):S402, 1998a.

van Lingen BL, Reindollar RH, Davis AJ, et al.: Further evidence that the WT1 gene does not have a role in the development of the derivatives of the müllerian duct. Am J Obstet Gynecol 179:597, 1998b.

van Lingen BL, Reindollar RH, Davis AJ, et al.: Physical mapping of a chromosomal translocation breakpoint in a patient with congenital absence of the uterus and vagina. J Soc Gyn Invest 5:F420, 1998c.

Van Niekerk WA: True Hermaphroditism. New York: Harper & Row, 1974.

Varner MW, Fraser AM, Hunter CY, et al.: The intergenerational predisposition to operative delivery. Obstet Gynecol 87:905, 1996.

Vegetti W, Grazia Tibiletti M, Testa G, et al.: Inheritance in idiopathic premature ovarian failure: Analysis of 71 cases. Hum Reprod 13:1796, 1998.

Vegetti W, Marozzi A, Manfredini E, et al.: Premature ovarian failure. Mol Cell Endocrinol 161:53, 2000.

Vercellini P, Trecca D, Oldani S, et al.: Analysis of p53 and ras gene mutations in endometriosis. Gynecol Obstet Invest 38:70, 1994.

Verp MS: Urinary tract abnormalities in hand-foot-genital syndrome. Am J Med Genet 32:555, 1989.

Verp MS, Simpson JL, Elias S, et al.: Heritable aspects of uterine anomalies: I. Three familial aggregates with müllerian fusion anomalies. Fertil Steril 40:80, 1983.

Vigano P, Infantino M, Ponti E, et al.: Analysis of G/R241 intercellular adhesion molecule-1 (ICAM-1) gene polymorphism in a ggroup of Italian endometriosis patients. Fertil Steril 77:S20, 2002.

Vikhlyaeva EM, Khodzhaeva ZS, Fantschenko ND: Familial predisposition to uterine leiomyomas. Int J Gynaecol Obstet 51:127, 1995.

Watanabe T, Imoto I, Kosugi Y, et al.: Human arylhydrocarbon receptor repressor (AHRR) gene: genomic structure and analysis of polymorphism in endometriosis. J Hum Genet 46:342, 2001.

Watanabe H, Kanzaki H, Narukawa S, et al.: Bcl-2 and Fas expression in eutopic and ectopic human endometrium during the menstrual cycle in relation to endometrial cell apoptosis. Am J Obstet Gynecol 176:360, 1997.

Waterworth DM, Bennett ST, Gharani N, et al.: Linkage and association of insulin gene VNTR regulatory polymorphism with polycystic ovary syndrome. Lancet 349:986, 1997.

Way S: The influence of minor degrees of fusion of the müllerian ducts on pregnancy and labor. J Obstet Gynaecol Br Emp 52:325, 1945.

Werempwicz S, Somberger K, Dah Cin P, et al.: Characterization of HMGIC gene rearrangements in uterine leiomyomas by fluorescence in situ hybridization (FISH). Am Soc Hum Genetics 63:A91, 1998.

White AJ: Vaginal atresia: High transverse septum. Obstet Gynecol 27:695, 1966.

Williams AJ, Powell WL, Collins T, et al.: HMGI(Y) expression in human uterine leiomyomata: Involvement of another HMG architectural factor in a benign neoplasm. Am J Pathol 150:911, 1997.

Wilroy RS Jr, Givens JR, Wiser WL, et al.: Hyperthecosis: An inheritable form of polycystic ovarian disease. Birth Defects: Orig Artic Ser 11(4):81, 1975.

Winkler H, Hoffman W: Zur Frage der Veriebbarket des Uterusymom. Dtsch Med Wochenschr 64:253, 1938.

Winter JS, Kohn G, Mellman WJ, et al.: A familial syndrome of renal, genital and middle ear anomalies. J Pediatr 72:88, 1968.

Xiao S, Lux M, Reeves R, et al.: HMGI(Y) activation by chromosome 6p21 rearrangements in multilineage mesenchymal cells from pulmonary hamartoma. Am J Pathol 150:901, 1997.

Xing YP, Powell WL, Morton CC: The del(7q) subgroup in uterine leiomyomata: Genetic and biologic characteristics. Cancer Genet Cytogenet 98:69, 1997.

Yang E, Korsmeyer SJ: Molecular thanatopsis: A discourse on the BCL2 family and cell death. Blood 88:386, 1996.

Yoshida S, Fakis G, Lyon A, et al.: Endometriosis and N-acetyltransferase 1 (NAT1) polymorphisms. Hum Reprod 16:172(P184), 2001.

Zeng WR, Scherer SW, Koutsilieris M, et al.: Loss of heterozygosity and reduced expression of the CUTL1 gene in uterine leiomyomas. Oncogene 14:2355, 1997.

Zondervan K, Cardon L, Desrosiers R, et al.: The genetic epidemiology of spontaneous endometriosis in the rhesus monkey. Ann NY Acad Sci 955:233, 2002.

CHAPTER 9

Gynecologic Cancer

Cancer is a genetic disease. Over the past several decades insights into the genetic basis of cancer have come from diverse fields, including molecular biology, tumor virology, somatic cell genetics, genetic epidemiology, and chemical carcinogenesis. It is now widely accepted that cancer results from a multistep process involving gene mutations and clonal selection of variant progeny cells. This is followed by increasingly aggressive growth properties and uninhibited cellular proliferation, invasion of neighboring tissues, and distant metastasis. The vast majority of mutations in cancer are somatic, i.e., occur only in tumor cells. However, recently an increasing number of genes have been implicated in inherited (i.e., germ-line) susceptibility to certain cancers and their mutations have been characterized.

In this chapter we review the current understanding of the genetic basis of cancer with emphasis on gynecologic malignancies.

Clonal Origin and Multistep Progression of Cancer

Pivotal to the question of whether genetic factors play a role in neoplasia is whether a given cancer originates from a single cell (unicellular or clonal) or from many cells (multicellular). If a single neoplasia arises from many cells, clinical expression of the neoplasia could require the continuous presence of a causative agent. Conversely, unicellular or clonal origin for cancer assumes that changes have occurred in DNA and have been passed on to daughter cells. These changes in DNA could have occurred spontaneously in somatic cells during cell replication or could have been induced by oncogenic agents (e.g., radiation, viruses, chemicals, random replication errors, or faulty DNA repair processes). A relatively small

subset of these mutations may be present in the germlines of these individuals and predispose them to various types of cancer.

One of the first tumors shown to be clonal in nature (i.e., derived from a single ancestral cell) was uterine leiomyoma. The original evidence came from the study of individual leiomyomas from women who were heterozygotes for the X-linked enzyme glucose-6-phosphate dehydrogenase (G-6-PD). Because of X-inactivation, only one of the X-linked alleles is expressed in a somatic cell of a heterozygous female. Cell lines derived from leiomyomas in these women express one or the other G-6-PD allele but not both, proving that each tumor originated from a single cell (Townsend et al., 1970). Other neoplasias have also been shown to be clonal in origin. Examples include multiple myeloma, chronic myelogenous leukemia, acute lymphoblastic leukemia, Burkitt lymphoma, carcinoma of the cervix, polycythemia vera, verruca vulgaris (warts), and urinary bladder cancer.

Cancer cells possess certain characteristics that distinguish them from normal cells, including (1) they are immortal, (2) they often grow more rapidly than their benign counterparts, and (3) they fail to exhibit normal cell-cell interactions (Bale and Li, 1997). Carcinogenesis is a multistep progression involving a series of genetic changes, or "hits," which result in a transition from completely normal to frank malignancy. Early "hits" may have little apparent phenotypical effect, but ultimately alterations in growth patterns and cellular morphology become evident.

Cancer Causing Genes

Two major classes of genes cause cancer—oncogenes and tumor suppressor genes. These two classes of genes act in opposite ways in causing carcinogenesis. Oncogenes act predominantly at the level of the cell to facilitate malignant transformation; a genetic change in only one allele is required to promote carcinogenesis. Tumorigenesis by oncogenes thus represents a *gain in function*. By contrast, tumor suppressor genes act recessively to block tumor development by regulating genes involved in cell growth; both alleles need to be inactivated in the cancerous cell. Thus, development of neoplasia results from a *loss of function*.

ONCOGENES

Oncogenes are altered forms of normal cellular genes (cellular oncogenes or *c-onc*) called proto-oncogenes that can lead to cancer. Proto-oncogenes are highly conserved in evolution, and their products function as regulators of normal cell growth and differentiation. Examples of proto-oncogenes are *c-src*, which codes for a cytoplasmic protein kinase involved in phosphorylation of certain amino acids; *c-erB*, which codes for the epidermal growth factor receptor; *c-jun*, a transcription factor that regulates gene expression; and *c-ras*, a guanosine triphosphate (GTP)-binding protein that plays a key role in a signal cascade that transmits messages from cell surface receptors to the nucleus (Park, 1995; Fearon and Cho, 1996).

It had been known for many years that viruses can cause tumors in animals. In 1911, Rous showed that normal chickens could be induced to develop avian sarcoma tumors following inoculation with a cell-free filtrate obtained from an independent avian sarcoma (Rous, 1911). Nearly 70 years later, it was conclusively demonstrated that the Rous sarcoma virus is a retrovirus that induces cancers in chickens because it harbors an altered version of a cellular proto-oncogene (i.e., an oncogene) called *src* (Stehelin et al., 1976). This type of transforming gene was termed a viral oncogene, or v-oncogene (*v-onc*). Soon it became clear that oncogenes were not found solely in viruses or even in malignant human cells. Even normal human cells contained useful pre-existing cellular proto-oncogenes that could be mutated into carcinogenic oncogenes. Consistent with this notion was that alteration of just one of the two proto-oncogene alleles was sufficient to cause malignant transformation in cell cultures. Such dominant mutations result in overproduction of a normal protein or an aberrant protein that is overactive. The result is that activating mutations in such genes lead to abnormal, unrestrained stimulation of cell proliferation. Proto-oncogenes must be activated to express their oncogenic potential. Activation of a proto-oncogene can occur in a variety of ways (Cooper, 1995).

Point Mutations. A point mutation (see Chapter 2) involves a single nucleotide that now may activate a proto-oncogene. For example, the single nucleotide change that alters codon 13 in the *ras*H oncogene is responsible for the potent transforming activity of the *ras*H proto-oncogene in EJ human bladder carcinoma.

Insertional Mutagenesis. A nononcogenic nucleotide sequence could become incorporated into the genome and in so doing cause a proto-oncogene to alter its function to become an oncogene. For example, the ability of a retrovirus to transform a cell without expressing the *v-onc* sequence was first noted during analysis of the bursal lymphomas caused by the transformation of B lymphocytes with the avian leukosis virus. Although the virus itself lacks an oncogene, it contains certain DNA sequences called long terminal repeat (LTR) sequences. LTRs are one of two long sections of double-stranded DNA synthesized by reverse transcriptase from the RNA of a retrovirus. When such a retrovirus is inserted into the normal DNA of the host in close proximity to a proto-oncogene, the LTR can exert its potential to produce malignant transformation. The resulting genetic disruption is called "insertional mutagenesis."

Another interesting model of insertional mutagenesis involves the relationship between Epstein-Barr virus (EBV), a herpesvirus, and some cases of Burkitt lymphoma, a human B-cell neoplasm. This oncogenic retrovirus has been shown to be integrated into the cellular genome within or in close proximity to the *c-myc* gene, with the LTR of the virus acting as a promoter of gene expression. It has been suggested that activation of *c-myc* in this way could be a mechanism that leads to the development of Burkitt lymphoma in humans, a tumor associated with EBV infection. Alternatively, EBV might induce proliferation of a preneoplastic cell population. The increased numbers of such proliferative lymphocytes might then result in an increased probability of chromosome translocations, leading to *c-myc* activation and progression to malignancy.

Gene Amplification. An increase in the number of copies of proto-oncogenes (i.e., gene amplification) has been found in tumor cells. Gene amplification can increase the number of copies of the oncogene per cell severalfold to several hundredfold, leading to greater amounts of the oncoprotein. Small doublet acentric chromosome fragments known as "double-minute" chromosomes and homogeneous staining regions of chromosomes that contain amplified DNA are cytologic counterparts to gene amplification in cancer cells. Amplification of N-*myc* or *c-myc* appears to be associated with progression of neuroblastomas and small cell lung carcinoma cells, and the *c-erb* B gene has been found to be amplified in several squamous cell carcinomas (King et al., 1985; Libermann et al., 1985). A related phenomenon occurs when leukemia cells are exposed to methotrexate, the cells acquire resistance by making multiple copies of the gene for dihydrofolate reductase, the target enzyme for methotrexate.

Chromosomal Abnormalities. Chromosomal abnormalities are characteristic of neoplastic cells; however, there is generally no consistency in the aberrations observed in different tumors of the same type of cancer or even between different cells of the same individual tumor. Such cytogenetic abnormalities do not appear to be the primary contributors to the genesis of trans-

formation in these cases but rather secondary phenomena.

In other instances, however, reproducible tumor-specific chromosomal abnormalities have been identified and shown to induce activation of proto-oncogenes (Park, 2001). For example, in 1960, Nowell and Hungerford (1960) first indicated that human chronic myelogenous leukemia was consistently characterized by the presence of an abnormal small chromosome 22, which was called the *Philadelphia chromosome* (Ph[1]), after the city in which it was discovered. The Ph[1] chromosome was shown to be an acquired abnormality found in the blood or bone marrow but not in other tissues from these patients. Subsequent studies in the 1970s established that the Ph[1] chromosome was generated by a translocation involving chromosomes 9 and 22 (Rowley, 1973). This chromosomal structural rearrangement, designated t(9;22)(q34;q11), is seen in the leukemic cells of 90% of patients with chronic myelogenous leukemia. The translocation places the *ABL* oncogene on chromosome 9 next to the break point cluster *BCR* gene of the Ph[1] gene on chromosome 22 (Fig. 9–1). A fusion gene is formed, which in turn produces an abnormal fusion protein (*BCR-ABL*). This protein retains

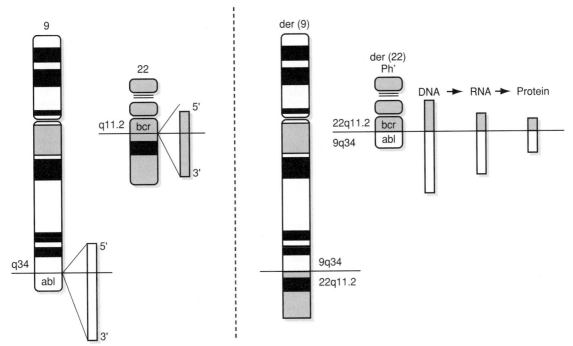

FIGURE 9–1 • Schematic representation of the chromosomes involved in the generation of the Philadelphia chromosome observed in more than 95% of patients with chronic myelogenous leukemia. The *c-ABL* proto-oncogene on the distal tip of chromosome 9q34 is translocated into the BCR locus on chromosome 22q11.2. This generates a chimeric gene that expresses a chimeric *BCR-ABL* messenger RNA and fusion protein. (From Park M: Oncogenes. *In* Scriver CR, Beaudet AL, Sly WS, et al. (eds): The Metabolic and Molecular Basis of Inherited Disease, 8th ed. New York: McGraw-Hill, 2001.)

the active protein kinase sequence from the *ABL* gene but replaces the *ABL* regulatory sequences with *BRC* sequences. The net result is generation of a protein kinase whose altered structure and function account for its transforming ability (Lugo et al., 1990). Other examples include chromosome translocations in Burkitt lymphomas that invariably involve alteration of the *c-myc* gene; this alteration occurs either as a result of the gene's moving from its normal position at 8q24 to a location distal to the immunoglobulin heavy-chain genes at 14q32 or of its fusing with immunoglobulin light-chain genes on chromosomes 2p11 and 22q11 (Kirsch et al., 1982; McBride et al., 1982). The *c-myc* protein appears to be unaltered but is now expressed in a nonregulated constitutive manner in these tumors.

Selected examples of cancers associated with chromosomal translocations that have been characterized at the molecular level are summarized in Table 9–1. The Cancer Chromosome Data Bank has registered cytogenetic studies on almost 27,000 karotypically abnormal neoplasias (Mitelman et al., 1997). These data indicated that balanced translocations, mostly translocations but also some inversions, are decidedly more disease-specific than unbalanced changes. For example, strong associations exist between t(X;1)(p11;q21) and papillary renal cell carcinoma, t(12;16)(q13;p11) and myxoid liposarcoma, and t(1;22)(q13;q13) and acute

megakaryoblastic leukemia (AML-M7). In leiomyomas, a t(7;14) translocation is associated (see Chapter 8). The reason for the difference in disease-specificity between balanced and unbalanced chromosomal abnormalities is unknown. Finally, practically all bands of the human chromosomal complement have been reported in recurrent neoplasia-associated aberrations. If we assume that all these structural chromosomal rearrangements are pathogenically important, or even essential, in the neoplastic process through structural or functional alterations of genes located in the break point regions, it follows that a large number of genes may play a role in the multistage process of tumor development.

TUMOR SUPPRESSOR GENES

Tumor suppressor genes (TSGs) are normal expressed genes that function to prevent malignant transformation. At the cellular level TSGs usually act in a recessive fashion and are defined by the effect of their absence. Thus, tumors tend to develop in cells in which both normal copies of a TSG have been inactivated or lost. One normal allele is sufficient to prevent the neoplastic transformation.

TSGs are vulnerable sites for critical DNA damage because they normally function as physiologic barriers against clonal expansion or

▼ **Table 9–1.** SELECTED CANCERS ASSOCIATED WITH CHROMOSOMAL TRANSLOCATIONS THAT
• HAVE BEEN CHARACTERIZED AT THE MOLECULAR LEVEL

Cancer	Translocation	Affected Gene	Protein Type	Reference
Chronic myelogenous leukemia and acute leukemia	t (9;22) (q34;q11)	Gene fusion: c-ABL(9q34)	Tyrosine kinase activated by BCR gene	Heisterkamp et al., 1982
Acute myleoid leukemia	t(15;17) (q21;q11-22)	Gene fusion: PML(15q21) and RAR(17q21)	Zinc finger	Borrow et al., 1990; Kakizuka et al., 1991
Burkitt lymphoma	t(8;14)(q24;q32) t(2;8)(p12;q24) t(8;22)(q24;q11)	Oncogene juxtaposed with immunoglobulin loci; C-MYC	Helix loop helix structural domain	Leder et al., 1983
Follicular lymphoma	t(14;18)(q32;q21)	Oncogene juxtaposed with immunoglobulin loci: BCL-2	Inner mitochondrial membrane	Hockenberry et al., 1990; Tsujimoto et al., 1985
Acute T-cell leukemia	t(17;19)(q35;p13)	Oncogene juxtaposed with T-cell receptor	Helix loop helix structural domain	Mellentin et al., 1989
Acute T-cell leukemia	t(7;9)(q34;34.3)	Oncogene juxtaposed with T-cell receptor	Notch homolog	Reynolds et al., 1987; Ellisen et al., 1991
B-cell chronic lymphocytic leukemia	t(8;12)(q24;q22)	BTG deregulates NYC proto-oncogene	MYC-helix loop helix structural domain	Rimokh et al., 1991
Synovial sarcoma	t(X;18)(p11;q11)	Gene fusion: SYT-SSX	Transcriptional activation domain	Kawai et al., 1998

Modified with permission from Park M: Oncogenes. *In* Scriver CR, Beaudet AL, Sly WS, et al. (eds): The Metabolic and Molecular Basis of Inherited Disease, 8th ed. New York: McGraw-Hill, 2001.

genomic mutability. They also hinder the growth, metastasis, and invasion of cells driven to uncontrolled proliferation of oncogenes (Harris and Hollstein, 1993). Loss of TSG function may occur by means of a number of mechanisms, including inactivating mutations, absent gene transcription, chromosomal rearrangement and nondisjunction, gene conversion, imprinting, or mitotic recombination. Cellular protein or viral oncoproteins can also neutralize tumor suppressor activity.

In the early 1970s, Knudson (1971) and Knudson and Strong (1972) first developed the conceptual basis for the genetic study of TSGs by constructing what is now known as the "two-hit" model. From epidemiologic studies of retinoblastoma and Wilms tumor, they predicted that two rate-limiting "hits" (i.e., mutations) are required for tumorigenesis. For example, in retinoblastoma approximately 30% of cases are hereditary (i.e., germ-line); germline tumors frequently arise in both eyes and/or multiple sites within a single eye. In these cases, one mutation is inherited in the germ-line. This is phenotypically harmless until a second "hit" occurs in a retinal cell, causing the tumor. Since there are a number of retinoblasts at risk (over 10⁷) and because they already carry one mutation, a second "hit" will occur with sufficient frequency to explain bilateral and/or multifocal tumors. This also explains why such tumors often show early age of onset as well as incomplete penetrance in individuals who inherit one mutant allele but in whom a second hit does not occur (Fig. 9–2).

In the sporadic form of retinoblastoma in which the individual does not carry a germ-line mutation, two "hits" must occur independently

Tumor Suppressor Genes
Germline Mutations

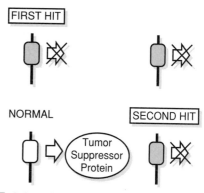

FIGURE 9–2 • Autosomal tumor recessive suppressor genes: The first "hit" is a germ-line mutation, inherited from a parent. The second is a somatic mutation. As long as some tumor suppressor protein is produced (lower row), the phenotype is normal. That is the case in the lower row, where somatic but no germ-cell mutation has occurred.

in the same retinoblast for transformation to occur (Fig. 9–3). The probability of two such events occurring in the same retinal cell is so low that it is likely to happen only once in any individual. This also explains the later age of onset in sporadic tumors and why they are virtually always unilateral and unicolar.

An important indication for the existence of TSGs within a chromosomal region is *loss of heterozygosity* (LOH) within tumor cells. The concept of LOH also can be illustrated by retinoblastomas. Comparisons of DNA sequence polymorphisms in the region of the retinoblastoma gene (*RB1*) from both sporadic and herita-

Tumor Suppressor Genes
Somatic Mutations

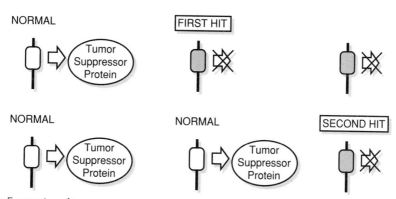

FIGURE 9–3 • Expression of tumor suppressor genes caused solely by somatic mutations. Both hits (top row) are the result of somatic mutations; in the lower row only a single mutation exists, allowing tumor suppressor protein to be expressed from the other (normal) allele.

ble retinoblastoma patients showed that peripheral blood cells exhibited heterozygosity at many loci, but tumors were hemizygous. Thus, DNA from the tumors contained alleles from only one of the two chromosome 13 homologs, revealing a loss of portion of 13q, thereby unmasking the recessive predisposing mutations at the *RB1* locus. In heritable cases, the retained chromosome 13 is the one with the abnormal *RB1* allele, i.e., the one inherited from the affected parent. Figure 9–4 shows how various mechanisms can lead to homozygosity for *RB1*.

Recently, it has been shown that at least in some cases a specific *RB1* mutation can be associated

with differential penetrance, on the basis of the sex of the transmitting parent (Klutz et al., 2002).

The *p53* tumor suppressor gene has been mapped to the short arm of chromosome 17 at band p13 (Nigro et al., 1989). Mutations in the *p53* TSG are the most common genetic abnormalities in human cancer, involving cervix, ovary, breast, bladder, and colorectal tumors (Levine et al., 1991). *p53* encodes for a sequence-specific DNA-binding phosphoprotein that acts by negatively regulating the cell cycle in the G1 phase. Figure 9–5 shows the (late) role in the clonal evolution of colorectal cancer. Loss of the ability of *p53* to bind DNA correlates with the inability to

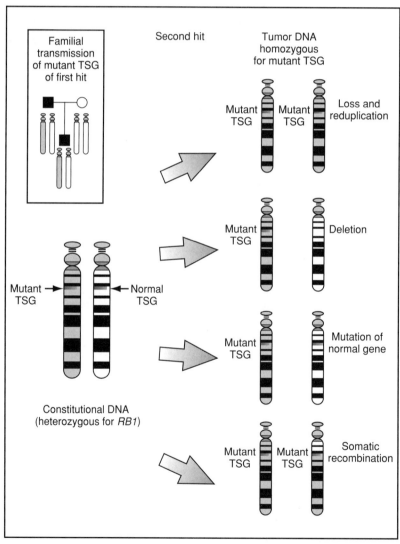

FIGURE 9–4 • Persons inheriting an *RB1* mutation are heterozygous for the mutation in all cells of their body. The second "hit" occurs during embryonic development and may consist of a point mutation, deletion, loss of the normal chromosome and duplication of the abnormal one, or somatic recombination. Each process leads to homozygosity for the mutant *RB1* allele and thus tumor development. (Modified from Cavenee WK, Dryja TP, Phillips RA, et al.: Expression of recessive alleles by chromosomal mechanisms in retinoblastoma. Nature 305:779, 1983.)

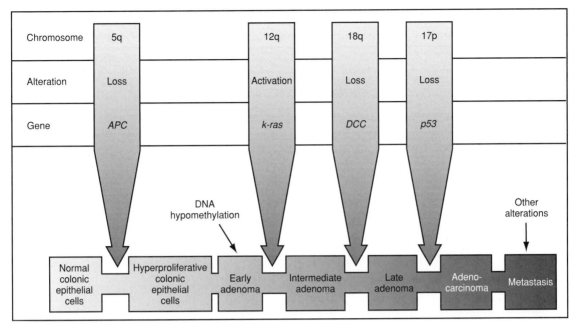

FIGURE 9–5 • Clonal evolution of colon cancer. Loss of the *APC* gene (adenomatous polyposis coli) transforms normal epithelial tissue lining the gut to hyperproliferating tissue. Hypomethlyation of DNA, activation of the *k-ras* proto-oncogene, and loss of the *DCC* (deleted in colon cancer) gene are involved in the progression to a benign adenoma. Loss of the *p53* gene and other alterations are involved in the progression to malignant carcinoma and metastasis. (Modified from Vogelstein B, Kinzler KW: The multistep nature of cancer. Trends Genet 9:138–141, 1993.)

suppress transformation. Mutant forms of *p53* may complex with normal *p53* to disrupt the structure of the normal *p53* protein. The complex consists of both normal and mutant *p53* proteins. Thus, no normal functioning *p53* alleles exists, either by loss of one allele with a mutation that inactivates the protein in the other allele, or by a dominantly acting mutation in one allele that suppresses the function of wild-type protein encoded by a normal allele. Because some mutant forms of *p53* can act in a dominant fashion to suppress wild-type *p53* and cause transformation, it was initially believed that *p53* was an oncogene. However, since the normal function of *p53* is to suppress tumorigenesis, it is more properly considered a TSG. In some families in which cancers segregate as a mendelian dominant condition (e.g., Li-Fraumeni syndrome associated with breast cancer—see further on), a mutation of the *p53* gene is transmitted through the germ-line. This is similar to transmission of the *RB1* gene in familial retinoblastoma.

Table 9–2 summarizes selected TSGs involved in the pathogenesis of human cancer.

DNA REPAIR GENES

Every cell division involves the copying of 6 billion bp of DNA. DNA polymerase has a finite error rate, and many environmental factors (e.g., ultraviolet light exposure, chemical exposures, irradiation) can damage DNA. Thus, DNA repair mechanisms are required to ensure the integrity of the genome. However, when the repair mechanisms themselves malfunction, either on the basis of an inherited or an acquired mutation, the number of mutations throughout the genome increases as cell divisions occur. The likelihood of cancer increases if the mutations involve oncogenes or tumor suppressor genes.

At least three different biochemical repair systems operate in damaged cells to safeguard DNA from permanent damage (Cleaver and Kraemer, 1995). The first system involves *nucleotide-excision repair* and *base-excision repair*. In *nucleotide-excision repair* damaged single strands of DNA are excised and replaced with a new sequence of nucleotides using the intact strand of DNA opposite the original damaged site as a template for base pairing. This type of repair is particularly important in the recovery of cells from radiation damage. In *base-excision repair*, there is removal of damaged bases, leaving the sugar-phosphate backbone of the DNA intact and creating a site lacking a purine or pyrimidine. This site is subsequently converted to a strand break and repaired. A complex second system is called postreplication repair. There are multiple mechanisms by which

▼ **Table 9–2.** SELECTED TUMOR SUPPRESSOR GENES INVOLVED IN HUMAN CANCER

Gene	Chromosomal Location	Function (Gene/Protein)	Cancer(s)
RB1	13q14	Cell cycle and transcriptional (E2F) regulation	Retinoblastoma, osteosarcoma, leukemias, rostate cancer, lung cancer
WT1	11p13	Transcriptional regulation; RNA splicing; zinc finger protein DNA binding	Wilms tumor, lung cancer
APC	5q21	Cell adhesion and signaling regulations; binds microtubules and catenins	Colorectal cancer, medulloblastoma
BRCA1	17q21	Unknown	Breast cancer, ovarian cancer, prostate cancer, colon cancer
BRCA2	13q12	Unknown	Breast cancer, male breast cancer, ovarian cancer
CDKN2A	9p21	Negative regulator of CDK4 and CDK6 cyclin-dependent kinases	Melanoma, pancreatic cancer, bladder cancer, leukemia, lung cancer
p53	17p13	Suppression of cell growth and transformation; induction of WAF1/Cip1 protein that blocks cyclin-dependent kinase enzymes, apoptosis	Ovarian cancer, brain tumors, lymphoma, breast cancer, sarcomas, Li-Fraumeni syndrome, others
NF1	17q11	RAS-mediated signal transduction regulation	Neurofibrosarcoma, colon cancer, melanoma
NF2	22q12	Cell morphology and membrane signaling regulation	Breast cancer, melanoma

disturbance of DNA replication can take place. Postreplication repair is an operational term for a particular disturbance of DNA replication by which intact new strands of DNA can be synthesized despite the presence of unexcised damage on the parental template strands (Park and Cleaver, 1979). The third repair system, called photoreactivation, reverts damaged DNA to the normal state without removing or exchanging any material from DNA. Photoreactivation is specific for one form of damage induced by ultraviolet light and involves cleavage of cyclobutane pyrimidine dimers. Although it has been identified in bacteria, yeast, fish, amphibians, and marsupials, the existence of photoreactivation in human tissue is controversial.

Cervical Cancers

Carcinoma of the cervix is one of the most common malignancies in women, accounting for 15,700 new cases (6% of all cancers) and 4900 deaths in the United States each year. Worldwide, cervical cancer is second only to breast cancer as the most common malignancy in both incidence and mortality (Cannistra and Niloff, 1996; Cervical Cancer: NIH Consensus Statement, 1996; Mohar and Frias-Mendivil, 2000).

Familial Tendencies

Almost all (95%) cervical cancer is squamous in origin. Adenocarcinoma of the cervix accounts

for the remaining 5% of cases of cervical cancer. Epidemiologic studies have not attempted to distinguish between the two histologic types. Thus, adenocarcinoma may or may not share similar causes with squamous cervical cancer. Incidence is inversely correlated with age at first intercourse and positively correlated with the number of sex partners. The disorder is relatively more common among prostitutes and extraordinarily rare among celibates. All these observations suggest an infectious cause. These striking epidemiologic features are consistent with data suggesting that heritable factors are not of paramount importance.

Earlier genetic studies have failed to detect familial tendencies in cervical cancer (Albert et al., 1977; Matlashewski et al., 1987). Other more recent studies have reached similar conclusions. The few reported familial aggregates may be more frequent than expected on the basis of either siblings sharing similar socioeconomic status or coincidental development of a relatively common neoplasia in multiple family members (Stewart et al., 1966; Munger et al., 1992; Shingleton and Thompson, 1997; Kiyono, 1998). Magnusson and colleagues (1999) used Swedish national registries of cervical cancer (126,893 relatives of 71,533 cases) and randomly selected age-matched controls (334,961 relatives of 194,810 controls) to search for genetic links to cervical cancer. For biologic mothers of cases, the relative risk (RR) was 1.83 (95% CI, 1.77–1.88), whereas for adoptive mothers the RR was 1.15 (95% CI, 0.82–1.57), which was not significantly different from unity. These results indicated an increased risk for biologic but not for nonbiologic first-degree relatives. For half-sisters of cases, the RR was 1.45 (95% CI, 1.31–1.60). Because half-sisters share, on average, 25% of their genes, this estimate was considered similar to that expected if the familial aggregation seen for first-degree relatives is caused mainly by genetic factors. The authors concluded that on the basis of epidemiologic evidence, there is a genetic predisposition for cervical cancer and its precursor forms. The magnitude of predisposition risk was believed to be similar to that of other forms of cancer, such as prostate cancer.

Human Papillomavirus

Both invasive cervical cancers and precursor lesions have been firmly associated with the presence of human papillomavirus (HPV) DNA. In humans, more than 70 molecular types of HPV have been cloned. HPV has a circular, 7900 bp, double-stranded DNA genome, a nonenveloped virion, and an icosahedral cosmid composed of 72 capsomers that measure 45 to 55 nm in diameter. Because the capsid proteins are antigenically similar, HPVs are not subdivided into serotypes based on structural antigenic features but instead are subdivided into genotypes and subtypes based on their DNA characteristics. To be classified as a distinct HPV type, a new isolate must have <50% homology with other known HPV types.

The genome HPV consists of early and late coding regions, encoding seven early and two late genetic open reading frames (ORFs). ORFs are DNA segments that are devoid of the 3-bp signals that stop protein synthesis ("stop codons") and can encode one or more exons. During DNA translation, different RNAs are produced by alternative splicing of the primary transcript, allowing more than one gene product from a single gene. Thus, all viral gene products are produced through alternative gene splicing. A noncoding "upstream regulatory region" contains the sequences regulating expression (i.e., transcriptional repressors and activators) or ORFs (Stoler, 1996). The early HPV sequence region is downstream of the upstream regulatory region and consists of six ORFs, designated E1, E2, E3, E4, E5, E6, and E7. Two of the early region ORFs, E6 and E7, encode for oncoproteins critical for viral replication as well as for host cell immortilization and transformation (Park et al., 1995). The transforming E7 protein of HPV type 16 has structural and functional

similarities to other E1A antigens of adenovirus and the large T antigen of SV40, all of which bind to the retinoblastoma protein and inactivate it (Phelps et al., 1988). Similar complexing and inactivation of the *p53* tumor suppressor gene by HPV E6 have been demonstrated (Cooper, 1995). In the rare instances in which both HPV DNA and a *p53* mutation in the cellular genome are present, the cancers are particularly aggressive (Harris and Hollstein, 1993).

Two dozen or so types of HPV have been characterized that infect the female and male anogenital tracts. Although squamous epithelium appears to be the principal site of HPV infection, it has been shown to occur in the reserve or undifferentiated epithelial cells, which give rise to both the squamous and glandular components of the cervix mucosa. Moreover, HPV DNA has been isolated from neoplasms not clearly derived from squamous-committed epithelial cells, most notably adenocarcinomas and small cell carcinomas of the cervix (Smotkin et al., 1986).

HPVs can be broadly classified into those with a low risk of lesion progression to cancer and those with a moderate to high risk. HPV types 6 and 11 primarily cause benign exophytic genital warts or condyloma acuminatum. In aggregate these viruses are present in more than 90% of condylomas, two thirds by HPV type 6 and one third by HPV type 11. HPV 6 and 11 may also be associated with low-grade squamous intraepithelial lesions. Similar associations occur with HPV types 42, 43, and 44. By contrast, HPV type 16 is the most likely virus to be associated with the entire range of intraepithelial and invasive squamous neoplasia as well as with cervical glandular neoplasia. The moderate to high risk viruses most closely related to HPV type 16 include types 31, 33, 35, 52, and 58. HPV 18 is the other cancer-associated prototype that is also most associated with nonsquamous cervical neoplasma. The viruses most related to type 18 include types 39, 45, and 59 (Stoler, 1996).

Expression of telomerase reverse transcriptase (hTERT) is required for activation of telomerase during immortalization and transformation of human cells. Zhang et al. (2002) examined hTERT amplification as a genetic event contributing to telomerase activation in cervical cancer. hTERT gene amplification was found in 21 of 88 primary tumor samples derived from patients with cervical carcinomas, and an increase in the hTERT copy number was significantly correlated with higher levels of hTERT protein expression. Moreover, the hTERT alterations were only found among those tumors with high-risk HPV infection.

Although HPV appears to be casually related to with cervical cancer, HPV screening has limited, if any, value in identifying women with abnormal Papanicolaou smear results who can be safely followed up with cytologic studies rather than colposcopically directed biopsies (Kaufman et al., 1997; ALTS Group, 2000). Recently Mandelblatt et al. (2002) has suggested that HPV screening plus Papanicolaou smears every two years may save additional years of life at reasonable costs.

Other Genetic Associations

Although no specific chromosomal numerical or structural abnormalities have been associated with cervical cancer, abnormalities of chromosome 1 have been reported most frequently (Atkin and Baker, 1979; Sreekantaiah et al., 1991). In a report using fluorescence *in situ* hybridization in cervical smears, Mian and colleagues (1999) found a relationship between trisomy 7, HPV, and cervical carcinogenesis.

In a study of 53 cervical cancers, Mitra and coworkers (1994) found that in about one fourth of informative cases, tumors had allelic losses involving chromosomes 1q, 3p, 4p, 5p, 5q, 6p, 10q, 11p, 18q, and X q, suggesting tumor-suppressor gene loci. Of particular interest is a candidate tumor suppressor gene called *FHIT* located at 3p14.2. The gene spans a fragile site called *FRA3B*, which also contains a spontaneous HPV type 16 integration site (Wilke et al., 1996). In addition to being a cervical cancer aberrant, *FHIT* transcripts have been found in cancers of the breast, colon, and gastrointestinal tract. Together these data suggest that alterations of this region at 3p (including *FHIT* mutation, chromosome deletions, chromosome translocations, and HPV integration) play an important role in cervical cancer (Cho, 1997). However, the presence of wild-type transcripts and the lack of protein-altering point mutations raise questions about the function of *FHIT* as a classic tumor suppressor gene in cervical tissue (Muller et al., 1998; Yoshino et al., 2000).

Cancer of the Uterine Corpus (Endometrial Carcinoma)

Like cancers of the cervix, uterine cancers consist of several different histologic types. By far the most common endometrial cancer involves the endometrial glands (endometrial adenocarcinoma). Rarer lesions arise from leiomyomas (leiomyosarcoma) or from the myometrium (sar-

comas, mixed müllerian type). Since >95% of endometrial cancers are adenocarcinomas, the terms endometrial cancer and endometrial carcinoma are often used interchangeably by epidemiologists. An additional problem relevant to this heterogeneity is that most epidemiologic studies naively combine cancers of the uterine cervix and uterine corpus. As a result, many potentially informative studies unfortunately must be discounted. Endometrial cancer is the most common malignancy of the female genital tract. Approximately 36,100 new cases and over 6300 deaths occur annually in the United States (Landis et al., 1998). Table 9–3 summarizes known risk factors for endometrial carcinoma. Twenty-five percent of women with endometrial cancer are premenopausal and 5% are less than 40 years of age. The majority of young women with endometrial carcinoma are obese or have high levels of endogenous unopposed estrogen due to chronic anovulation, for example as caused by polycystic ovary disease. Pregnancy confers protection from endometrial cancer by interrupting continuous estrogen stimulation of the endometrium by estrogen. In the 1960s and 1970s it was common practice to administer unopposed estrogens for menopausal symptoms; however, it was subsequently recognized that such treatment was associated with an eightfold increase in the incidence of endometrial cancer. Since the introduction of combined estrogen-progesterone regimens, the incidence of endometrial carcinoma has decreased (Rose, 1996).

Although most cases of endometrial carcinoma are considered sporadic, there is clearly a heritable component to this disease (Sandles et al., 1992). Studying 64 probands, our group found four families in which endometrial adenocarcinoma was found in at least one first-degree relative; in none of the four did relatives have colon or ovarian cancer. In none of the 34 con-

▼ Table 9–3. RISK FACTORS FOR ENDOMETRIAL
• CANCER

Characteristic	Relative Risk
Nulliparity	2–3
Late menopause	2.4
Obesity	
21-50 lbs	3
>50 lbs	10
Diabetes mellitus	2.8
Unopposed estrogen therapy	4–8
Tamoxifen	2–3
Atypical endometrial hyperplasia	8–29

Reproduced with permission from Lurain, JR: Uterine cancer. *In* Berek JS (ed): Novak's Gynecology, 12th ed. Baltimore: Williams and Wilkins, 1996, p 1057.

trols were other family members affected. Mothers and sisters of women with endometrial carcinoma have a 2.7-fold increased risk of the disease compared with controls (Schildkraut et al., 1989). These two studies suggest existence of site-specific heritable adenocarcinoma of the endometrium.

A better established form of inherited endometrial cancer is hereditary nonpolyposis colorectal cancer (HNPCC) (Boland, 1998), once called Lynch syndrome II. HNPCC is a relatively common autosomal dominant disorder characterized by an increased risk of cancers of the colon, rectum, endometrium, ovary, small intestines, hepatobiliary system, kidney, and ureters. There appears to be no increased risk for cancer of the breast, prostate, lung, bladder, larynx, bone marrow or brain (Watson and Lynch, 1993). It is estimated that 3 to 4% of all colorectal cancers occur in HNPCC families, and the prevalence of the disease is one in 200 to 1000 individuals in the general population (Mecklin, 1987; Boland, 1998). Clinically, HNPCC is defined by the following criteria (Vasen et al., 1991):

1. At least three relatives with colorectal cancer with one a first-degree relative of the other two.
2. The presence of tumors in at least two successive generations.
3. One family member affected by colorectal cancer before age 50.

The percentage of all endometrial cancers due to HNPCC is unknown. Endometrial cancer is not universally considered a criterion for HNPCC (Vasen et al., 1991). However, in four other families in the study of Sandles and coworkers (1992) other relatives had adenocarcinoma of the uterus, ovary, or colon indicative of Lynch syndrome II. Moreover, the incidence of endometrial carcinoma in women belonging to HNPCC families is 20% by age 70 compared to a 3% risk in the general population (Watson et al., 1994). The median age at diagnosis of endometrial cancer in women with HNPCC is 46 years, which is 15 to 20 years younger than the median age at diagnosis in the general population (Mecklin and Jarvinen, 1991; Watson and Lynch, 1993; Parc et al., 2000). Other selection criteria for the identification of HNPCC have been developed, including the Amsterdam Criteria I and II (Park et al., 1999) and the Japanese Criteria (Fuji et al., 1996).

HNPCC is the result of a germ-line mutation in one of at least four DNA mismatch repair genes: *hMSH2* on chromosome 2p15-16; *hML1* on chromosome 3p21; *hPMS1* on chromosome 2q31; *hPMS2* on 7p22; and *MSH6* on 2P16 (Wijnen et al., 1999). Germ-line mutations in any of these four genes appear to produce the same disease. The mutations in the genes involved in HNPCC appear to follow the tumor suppressor model. Loss of the wild-type allele in a target tissue results in a hypermutable cell that is susceptible to the accumulation of mutations at a greatly accelerated rate, which in turn leads to other mutations that are more closely responsible for the development of cancer in multistep carcinogenesis. It remains uncertain why certain organs are at selective risk of developing cancer (Boland, 1998). However, Wijnen and coworkers (1999) have found an unusually high prevalence of *MSH6* mutations, as shown by changes in the repeat numbers of simple repetitive sequences (microsatellite instability) that serve as markers for DNA mismatches. In atypical families with HNPCC, fundamentally defined as those with relatively fewer cases of colorectal cancer and relatively more of endometrial cancer, *MSH6* mutations lead to truncated proteins far more commonly than the *MSH2* and *MLH1* mutations that predominate in individuals with colorectal cancer.

In sporadic endometrial carcinoma, the most common mutated proto-oncogene is K-*ras*. It has been shown to be mutated in 10 to 30% of endometrial carcinomas (Mizuuchi et al., 1992; Enomoto et al., 1993). Other oncogenes that have been associated with endometrial carcinoma include *HER-1/neu* and *bcl-2*. Mutations in the tumor-suppressor gene *p53* have been reported in 11 to 45% of sporadic endometrial carcinomas (Hendrick, 1998). Alterations in the PTEN and *p53* genes seem to define distinct subgroups of endometrial carcinoma, the former associated with diploidy and microsatellite instability, the latter with macroscopic chromosomal instability (Koul et al., 2002).

Breast Cancer

In the United States over 180,000 women develop breast cancer annually, and about 44,000 women die of the disease (Parker et al., 1997; Landis et al., 1998). The risk of a woman's developing breast cancer between birth and age 39 is 1 in 227; between ages 40 to 59 the risk is 1 in 25; and between ages 60 to 79 the risk is 1 in 15. The lifetime risk of a woman's developing breast cancer is 1 in 8.

The best studied and most significant risk factor for breast cancer is a positive family history (Couch and Weber, 1998). Other risk factors include women who (1) experience early menarche and late menopause, (2) have few interruptions in menstrual cycling for pregnancy or breast-feeding, (3) smoke or are exposed to radiation, and (4) have atypical hyperplasia (Dupont and Page, 1985; Tokunaga et al., 1994; Pritchard, 1997; Chlebowski, 2000). Data are conflicting regarding the significance of alcohol consumption, oral contraceptive use, hormone replacement therapy, and bottle feeding as opposed to breast-feeding (Dupont and Page, 1985; Harris et al., 1992; DiSaia et al., 1996). Initial reports that induced abortion and increased fat consumption increased the risk for breast cancer have not been confirmed (Hunter et al., 1996; Melbye et al., 1997).

Whether mammographic screening actually reduces breast cancer mortality has recently been challenged and is now an area of considerable controversy (Olsen and Gøtzche, 2001; Miettinen et al., 2002).

Over the past several decades, the incidence of breast cancer has risen steadily to an average increase of about 1.2% per year (Miller et al., 1991; Chu et al., 1996; Coleman et al., 2000). Although this may reflect the increased use of mammography screening and an increased aging population, the trend probably also reflects environmental or lifestyle changes (Couch and Weber, 1998). The encouraging news is that since 1987 the mortality rate from breast cancer has declined about 25% (Beral et al., 1995; Chu et al., 1996, Ries et al., 1997; Lacey et al., 2002).

As mentioned earlier, a family history of breast cancer is the strongest risk factor. Current estimates are that 5 to 10% of all breast cancers are directly attributable to germ-line mutations in breast cancer susceptibility genes (Newman et al., 1988; Claus et al., 1991; American Cancer Society, 2000). Inherited breast cancer has several characteristic features, including earlier age at onset compared with sporadic cases, higher prevalence of bilateral disease, and the presence of other tumors in some families (e.g., ovary, colon, prostate, endometrium, sarcomas) (Anderson et al., 1993; Nelson et al., 1993; Couch and Weber, 1998). However, inherited breast cancer does not appear to be associated with any particular histologic type, pattern of metastasis, or survival time.

BRCA1

In 1990, linkage studies of early-onset breast and ovarian cancers indicated the location of a susceptibility gene on chromosome 17q21. In 1994, Miki and colleagues (1994) isolated and sequenced the gene, *BRCA1*. *BRCA1* is a novel gene that spans approximately 100 kb of genomic sequence that encodes 5592 nucleotides with a 126 bp of homology to a ring finger motif near the 5′ end. This suggests that the 1863 amino acid protein encoded by *BRCA1* may function as transcription factors (Miki et al., 1994; Couch and Weber, 1998). However, the precise biochemical function of the *BRCA1* gene product is unknown.

Germ-line mutations detected in *BRCA1* include missense mutations, nonsense mutations, insertions, deletions, and intronic mutations. Over 75% of mutations result in truncated proteins. Of the more than 100 mutations that have been identified, the eleven most common mutations in the *BRCA1* gene account for 43% of all the mutations. The *185delAG* mutation, a 2bp deletion in exon 2, has been found to be the most common overall (Simard et al., 1994; Struewing et al., 1995). Population studies have shown that 1 to 2% of the Ashkenazi Jewish population carries the *185delAG* mutation (Struewing et al., 1995; Richards et al., 1997). Approximately 2.0 to 2.5% of Ashkenazi Jewish women carry one of three founding mutations: BRCA1 (195delAG and 5382insC) and one of BRCA2 (6174delT), which is discussed below (Hartge et al., 1999; Warner et al., 1999). *185delAG* contributes to 21% of breast cancer cases among young Ashkenazi Jewish women; this mutation is associated with an increase in the risk of early-onset breast cancer by a factor of 27 (95% CI 8–89) (Krainer et al., 1997). In a few families the disease is linked to *BRCA1*, but mutations have not been detected, suggesting perturbation of mutations in regulatory sequences (Langston et al., 1996).

Gene susceptibility to breast cancer is conferred by tumor-suppressor function through inactivation of one *BRCA1* allele in the germline, followed by the loss of the remaining allele in somatic breast tissue (Futreal et al., 1994; Miki et al., 1994). Unlike mutations in other tumor suppressor genes, *BRCA1* mutations have almost always been detected in specimens of breast cancer tissue when there is a mutated germ-line allele; *BRCA1* mutations are rare in sporadic tumors. The role of *BRCA1* mutations in breast cancer is therefore essentially limited to women with genetic susceptibility to this tumor (FitzGerald et al., 1996).

Initial estimates predicted that women with *BRCA1* mutations had about an 85% lifetime risk of developing breast cancer and a 40 to 60% lifetime risk of developing ovarian cancer (Easton et al., 1993b; Easton et al., 1994). About 20% of female *BRCA1* mutation carriers were predicted to develop breast cancer by age 40 years, 50% by age 50 years, and 85% by age 70 years. It was also determined that *BRCA1* mutation carriers have an increased incidence of bilateral breast cancer. However, these penetrance figures are most certainly overestimated because of a bias of ascertainment (Collins, 1996; Hopper et al., 1999; Warner et al., 1999). Original risk estimates were based on data derived from families collected for linkage analysis, and in general only the most severely affected families were investigated. Struewing and colleagues (1997) studied 5318 persons of Ashkanazi Jews ancestry with the three most common *BRCA1* and *BRCA2* mutations and showed that the lifetime risks for breast or ovarian cancer were 56% and 16%, respectively.

Individuals with an inherited *BRCA1* mutation may also be at increased risk for other cancers. The risk of ovarian cancer by age 80 in *BRCA1* carriers is 27.8% and 1.8% in noncarriers (Whittemore et al., 1997). Again, these risks may be overestimated. Data from the Ontario Cancer Registry suggested that 16% of all fallopian tube cancers are caused by germ-line mutations in *BRCA1* or *BRCA2* (Aziz et al., 2001). The relative risk for prostate cancer is 3.3 and the relative risk for colon cancer is 4.1 in *BRCA1* carriers (Arason et al., 1993; Ford et al., 1994). Male breast cancer is only rarely associated with *BRCA1* germ-line mutations (Couch and Weber, 1998).

BRCA2

In 1994 a second breast cancer susceptibility gene called *BRCA2* was localized by linkage studies to 13q12-13 (Wooster et al., 1994). Subsequently the *BRCA2* cDNA was shown to be 11.5 kb in length and contained within 70 kb of genomic DNA (Tavtigian et al., 1996). *BRCA2* cDNA has no significant homology to any previously described gene, and the function of the protein is unknown.

Mutations in *BRCA2* are thought to account for 30 to 40% of inherited breast cancers. Lifetime breast cancer risk for *BRCA2* mutation carriers is estimated to be 85% (Ford et al., 1998); lifetime ovarian cancer risk appears to be 27%. These risks, however, may be overestimated (Thorlacius et al., 1998). In contrast to *BRCA1*, in which male breast cancer is rare, *BRCA2* mutations are associated with a 6% lifetime risk of male breast cancer (Wooster et al., 1995; Couch et al., 1996; Tavtigian et al., 1996).

More than 100 mutations have been identified in *BRCA2*, spanning the entire coding region of the gene. Most mutations involve small insertions and deletions that result in protein truncation (Couch and Weber, 1998). The single mutation 616delT was identified in 7 of 108 Ashkenazi Jewish women diagnosed with breast cancer <50 years of age and in three Ashkenazi Jewish men with breast cancer (Couch et al., 1996; Neuhausen et al., 1996). As mentioned earlier, mutations in *BRCA1* and *BRCA2* together account for a carrier frequency of about 2.0 to 2.5 present in Ashkenazi Jewish individuals (Richards et al., 1997; Hartge et al., 1999; Warner et al., 1999).

OTHER BREAST CANCER SUSCEPTIBILITY GENES

BRCA1 and *BRCA2* account for 80 to 90% of inherited breast cancers. The remaining 10 to 20% involve other rare genetic disorders, several of which have been identified. Other mutations causing heritable breast cancer doubtless exist but have not yet been elucidated.

Ataxia-Telangiectasia (AT). AT is an autosomal recessive syndrome characterized by oculocutaneous telangiectasia, cerebellar ataxia, and variable immunodeficiency. AT homozygotes develop cancers at 180 times the rate of the age-specific population (Morrell et al., 1986). Lymphoid cancers predominate in childhood; epithelial cancers, including breast cancer, are seen in adolescent and young AT patients (Swift et al., 1990). Chromosomal fragility and resulting DNA rearrangement are thought to result from the genetic defect that underlies the clinical syndrome of AT.

Swift (1997) suggested that AT heterozygotes, who do not display the typical clinical features of AT homozygotes, have a fivefold increased incidence of breast cancer. Given that 1.4% individuals in the U.S. population are AT heterozygotes, it can be calculated that approximately 6.6% of all breast cancers in the U.S. occur in AT heterozygotes. Moreover, the breast cancer risk for AT heterozygotes appears not to be limited to young women but applies at older ages as well (Athma et al., 1996). The question has been raised of whether medical diagnostic x-ray procedures, including mammography, increase the risk of breast cancer in AT heterozygotes (Morrell et al., 1990; Swift et al., 1991; Couch and Weber, 1998; Khanna, 2000).

The gene responsible for AT, called AT-mutated (*ATM*), has been mapped to chromosome 11q22 and encodes a 13 kb transcript.

ATM is a member of a large family of high-molecular-weight protein kinases. These appear to play a major role as intracellular signal transducers that give warning to the cell, via cell cycle checkpoints, of DNA damage that must be repaired before the next cell cycle division (Gatti, 1998).

The association between AT heterozygosity and increased risk for breast cancer has been challenged (Bebb et al., 1997; FitzGerald et al., 1997). However, more data from France and the Netherlands appear to confirm the increased risk (Janin et al., 1999). This issue is of great clinical importance, and further research is warranted (Swift, 1997; Werneke, 1997).

Li-Fraumeni syndrome (LFS) is an autosomal dominant condition in which family members are characterized by the occurrence of childhood bone or soft-tissue sarcomas, early-onset breast cancer, acute leukemias, brain tumors, carcinoma of the lung, carcinoma of the pancreas, adrenocortical carcinoma, melanoma, and other cancers. Affected individuals also have a significant excess of second malignancies (Varley et al., 1997). A "classic" LFS individual has been defined as a proband under age 45 years with a sarcoma who has (1) a first-degree relative under 45 years old with any cancer, and (2) an additional first- or second-degree relative under 45 years old in the same lineage with any cancer or sarcoma (Li et al., 1988).

In 1990, germ-line mutations in the *p53* tumor suppressor gene located on chromosome 17p13 were first identified (Malkin et al., 1990). This 20-kb gene encodes a 53-kD nuclear phosphoprotein composed of 393 amino acids. The *p53* protein binds specific DNA sequences and appears to be a transcription factor that may regulate the expression of other growth regulatory genes (Malkin, 1998).

Premenopausal breast cancer is common in LFS families. Patients with germ-line mutations contribute significantly to the number of breast cancer cases with a strong inherited component, particularly when breast cancer is diagnosed before age 40. Easton and coworkers (1993a) estimated that about 1% of breast cancer cases diagnosed between the ages of 30 and 40 years arise within Li-Fraumeni families. Although this is clearly lower than the proportion of early-onset cancers attributable to *BRCA1* or *BRCA2*, it is nonetheless significant. A network of regulatory proteins, called "checkpoint" kinases, has been identified. Activation of these proteins in response to DNA damage prevents cells from entering mitosis and the cascade leading to cancer. Heterozygous germ-line mutations in a known checkpoint gene (tumor suppressor gene) called *hCHK2* have been shown to cause some cases of LFS in patients who lack *p53* mutations (Bell et al., 1999). There is speculation that *p53* is directly phosphorylated by hCHK2 in an ATM-dependent manner.

Cowden Disease. Also known as multiple hamartoma syndrome, Cowden disease is an autosomal dominant disorder characterized by mucocutaneous lesions (e.g., trichilemmomas, acral keratosis, varicoid or papillomatous papules), thyroid abnormalities (e.g., goiter, cancer), breast lesions (e.g., fibroadenomas, fibrocystic disease, adenocarcinoma), hamartomatous polyps of the gastrointestinal tract, macrocephaly, and uterine leiomyomas (Eng and Parsons, 1998). The susceptibility gene for Cowden disease is a tumor-suppressor gene called *TEN* on chromosome 10q23. In one study of 25 families by Lynch and coworkers (1997) germ-line *TEN* mutations were detected in all of five families with both Cowden disease and breast cancer. Other signs of Cowden disease may be subtle when associated with breast cancer. Germ-line mutations in PTEN have also been associated with another hamartoma disorder, the Bannayan-Rile-Ruvalcaba syndrome. This syndrome is characterized by macrocephaly, cognitive and motor dysfunction, subcutaneous and visceral lipomas and hemangiomas, and intestinal juvenile polyposis (Marsh et al., 1999).

Gorlin syndrome. This rare autosomal dominant syndrome characterized by nevoid basal cell carcinomas, medulloblastoma/astrocytoma, agenesis of the corpus callosum, odontogenic keratocysts, skeletal malformations, and variable mental retardation. There is an increased frequency of breast cancer and possibly ovarian cancer (Gorlin, 1987). The gene has been mapped to 9q31 (Farndon et al., 1992).

Muir-Torre Syndrome. This syndrome is an autosomal dominant disorder that involves skin lesions (keratoacanthomas and sebaceous adenomas, and variable cancers of the gastrointestinal tract, bladder, uterus breast [postmenopausal], and ovary [Hall et al., 1994]). As various malignancies in Muir-Torre syndrome display microsatellite instability similar to that seen in colon cancer patients with hereditary nonpolyposis colorectal (HNPCC), it is postulated that mutations in one or more of the HNPCC-related genes (*MLH1, MSH2, PMS1,* and *PMS2*) may be the underlying defect (Couch and Weber, 1998). Recently, a rare case of sebaceous carcinoma of the breast has been reported in a patient with Muir-Torre syndrome (Propeck et al., 2000).

Peutz-Jeghers Syndrome. This is an autosomal dominant disorder characterized by hyperpigmented deposits in and around the mouth and hamartomatous polyposis (Kitagawa et al., 1995). Malignancies over-represented in families with this syndrome include cancers of the breast, ovary, cervix, and testes (Giardiello et al., 1987). The gene has been mapped to the telomeric region of chromosome 19p (Giardiello et al., 1987; Hemminki et al., 1997).

Partial Androgen Insensitivity (formerly Reifenstein syndrome). This is an X-linked recessive condition resulting from a germ-line mutation in the androgen receptor gene (Wooster et al., 1992). Affected males show perineoscrotal hypospadias and gynecomastia. However, the spectrum of defective virilization involves cryptorchidism and azoospermia. Affected males have an increased risk of developing breast cancer (Poujol et al., 1997). The androgen receptor gene has been localized to Xq11-Xq12 (see Chapter 11).

Genetic Counseling in Breast Cancer

Risk Assessment

In recent years, breast cancer awareness has increased considerably both on the part of the medical profession and of the general population. Assessment and counseling for persons with a family history of breast cancer with or without ovarian cancer are complex and have many ramifications. The Committee on Genetics of the American College of Obstetricians and Gynecologists has stated the following: "In selected families (multiple family members affected with breast and/or ovarian cancer or a family in which a *BRCA* mutation has been discovered), *BRCA* testing may be useful." However, "...testing of the general population is not recommended."

The Committee on Genetics of the American College of Obstetricians and Gynecologists believes that genetic testing for breast-ovarian cancer should be performed only with the individual's full informed consent. Currently, such testing continues to be best performed by investigators working under research protocols approved by an institutional review board. Individuals should be counseled before and after testing to ensure their understanding of the scope, implications, and limitations of the testing process. Counseling should include discussions of the uncertainties of applying genetic test results to the prevention and treatment of breast and ovarian cancer and the potential for genetic discrimination and loss of insurance coverage. The standard of care should emphasize genetic services, genetic information, and education and counseling rather than the testing procedures alone (American College of Obstetricians and Gynecologists, 2000).

The first step in risk assessment is to obtain a complete personal and family history with emphasis on all types of cancer. Details such as age at diagnosis and age of unaffected individuals, tumor histology, the occurrence of bilateral primary tumors, and sites of primary tumors and metastatic disease should be obtained. This should cover at least three generations and include all first-degree relatives (parents, siblings, and offspring) and second-degree relatives (grandparents, grandchildren, aunts, uncles, half-siblings, nieces, and nephews). Note should be taken of any genetic syndromes in the family, since some inherited disorders predispose affected individuals to a variety of malignancies (e.g., Fanconi anemia, xeroderma pigmentosum, Bloom syndrome, and ataxia-telagiectasia) (Hoskins et al., 1995).

Cumulative data are available to predict the prevalence of *BRCA1* and *BRCA2* mutations in women based on personal and family history (Table 9–4). Because of the higher prevalence of mutations in women of Ashkenazi Jewish ancestry, those data are reported separately (Table 9–5). Criteria defining families with the highest risk for harboring such mutations vary.

The American College of Medical Genetics (1999) has recommended the following to define families at risk:

- A positive family history of breast and/or ovarian cancer (in three or more first- or second-degree relatives on the same side of the family;
- Early age of onset (especially before age 45) of breast cancer in the patients;
- A patient or family member with ovarian cancer (at any age) in addition to one or more family members with breast cancer at any age);
- Bilateral or multifocal breast disease or multiple primary tumors (at least one involving the breast) in the patient or family member;

▶ **Table 9–4.** PREVALENCE OF MUTATIONS IN *BRCA1* AND *BRCA2* BY PERSONAL AND FAMILY HISTORY OF CANCER IN 4518 WOMEN
• (EXCLUDING WOMEN OF ASHKENAZI JEWISH ANCESTRY)

		FAMILY HISTORY				
	No Breast Cancer <50 Years or Ovarian Cancer in Anyone (%)	Breast Cancer <50 Years in One Relative; No Ovarian Cancer in Anyone (%)	Breast Cancer <50 Years in More Than One Relative; No Ovarian Cancer in Anyone (%)	Ovarian Cancer at Any Age in One Relative; No Breast Cancer <50 Years in Anyone (%)	Ovarian Cancer in More Than One Relative; No Breast Cancer <50 Years in Anyone (%)	Breast Cancer <50 Years and Ovarian Cancer at Any Age (%)
PATIENT'S HISTORY						
No breast cancer or ovarian cancer at any age	4.1	4.0	11.1	2.7	7.3	16.8
Breast cancer ≥50 years	2.4	9.6	10.7	4.8	5.6*	24.7
Breast cancer <50 years	9.7	18.9	37.6	16.3	18.4	48.2
Ovarian cancer at any age, no breast cancer	6.4	34.1	40.7	28.0	37.9	47.8
Breast cancer ≥50 years and ovarian cancer at any age	20.8	10.0*	36.4*	16.7*	33.3*	40.0*
Breast cancer <50 years and ovarian cancer at any age	18.2	46.2*	66.7*	50.0*	66.7*	78.9*

* = N<20.
From American Medical Association: Identifying and managing hereditary risk for breast and ovarian cancer. An AMA Continuing Medical Education Program, April 2001.

▶ **Table 9–5.** PREVALENCE OF MUTATIONS IN BRCA1 AND BRCA2 BY PERSONAL AND FAMILY HISTORY OF CANCER IN 2252 WOMEN OF ASHKENAZI JEWISH ANCESTRY

	FAMILY HISTORY					
	No Breast Cancer <50 Years or Ovarian Cancer in Anyone (%)	Breast Cancer <50 Years in One Relative; No Ovarian Cancer in Anyone (%)	Breast Cancer <50 Years in More Than One Relative; No Ovarian Cancer in Anyone (%)	Ovarian Cancer at Any Age in One Relative; No Breast Cancer <50 Years in Anyone (%)	Ovarian Cancer in More Than One Relative; No Breast Cancer <50 Years in Anyone (%)	Breast Cancer <50 Years and Ovarian Cancer at Any Age (%)
PATIENT'S HISTORY						
No breast cancer or ovarian cancer at any age	5.5	13.5	18.9	17.5	23.7	31.9
Breast cancer ≥50 years	4.5	9.7	12.5	13.0	37.5*	37.0
Breast cancer <50 years	12.3	26.6	43.4	44.6	66.7*	58.6
Ovarian cancer at any age, no breast cancer	22.6	15.4*	71.4*	47.4*	70.0*	82.4
Breast cancer ≥50 years and ovarian cancer at any age	33.3*	0*	100*	33.3*	None tested	50.0*
Breast cancer <50 years and ovarian cancer at any age	77.8*	83.8*	50*	0*	None tested	None tested

* = N<20.
From American Medical Association: Identifying and Managing Hereditary Risk for Breast and Ovarian Cancer, An AMA Continuing Medical Education Program, April, 2001.

- Breast cancer in a male patient or a male family member.

Women whose family history does not indicate high risk for an inherited breast-ovarian cancer susceptibility gene need to be reassured and advised that their risk is comparable to that of the general population, i.e., 1 in 8 lifetime risk of developing breast cancer. They should also be counseled about the recommendations from the American Cancer Society for the early detection of breast cancer as follows:

- Women 20 years of age and older should perform breast self-examination every month;
- Women 20 to 39 years old should have a physical examination of the breast every 3 years, performed by a health care professional such as a physician, a physician assistant, or a nurse or nurse practitioner;
- Women 40 years of age should have a physical examination of the breast every year, performed by a health care professional, such as a physician, physician assistant, nurse, or nurse practitioner;
- Women over 40 years of age and older should have a mammogram every year.

Patient or Family at Increased Risk

If the patient or family history indicates an increased risk for an inherited breast-ovarian cancer susceptibility gene, an in-depth discussion about the risks and benefits of genetic testing may be appropriate. However, pretest counseling is essential and must provide the basic elements of informed consent (Statement of the American Society of Clinical Oncology: Genetic Testing for Cancer Susceptibility, 2001):

1. Information on the specific test being performed.
2. Implications of a positive and a negative result.
3. Possibility that the test will not be informative.
4. Options for risk estimation without testing.
5. Risk of passing a mutation to children.
6. Technical accuracy of the test.
7. Fees involved in testing and counseling.
8. Risks of psychological distress.
9. Risks of insurance or employer discrimination.
10. Confidentiality risks.
11. Options and limitations of medical surveillance and screening following testing.

If after pretest counseling the patient decides to proceed with genetic testing, it should be carried out in a systematic fashion. If the patient has not had breast or ovarian cancer, a close blood relative should be tested first. A negative test result in the patient is informative only after a familial mutation has been identified. All family members who are approached about genetic testing should receive the same level of pretest counseling as the presenting patient; they must make their own independent decisions about undergoing genetic testing.

If a person is tested and no mutation is detected, she should be counseled that she nonetheless carries the same 10 to 12% lifetime risk of developing breast cancer as found in the general population and that standard early breast cancer detection measures should be taken (see earlier). In cases in which others in the family are detected to carry a susceptibility gene mutation, postcounseling of individuals who are tested and found to be unaffected is vital because they often experience serious guilt and depression. In addition, counseling must take into account psychological interfamily relationships.

If a woman is determined to be a carrier for a *BRCA1* or *BRCA2*, two options can be considered. The first is breast-ovarian cancer surveillance. This includes (Burke et al., 1997a):

1. Monthly breast self-examination beginning early in adult life (i.e., by age 18 to 21 years).
2. An annual or semiannual clinical breast examination beginning at age 25 to 35 years.
3. An annual mammogram beginning at age 25 to 35 years.
4. An annual or semiannual transvaginal ultrasound examination with color flow Doppler ultrasound and determination of carcinoembryonic (CA)-125 levels.

The second option is prophylactic surgery. A decision analysis study by Schrag and coworkers (1997) indicated that, on average, 30-year-old women who carry *BRCA1* and *BRCA2* mutations gain from 2.9 to 5.2 years of life expectancy from prophylactic mastectomy and from 0.3 to 1.7 years of life expectancy from prophylactic oophorectomy, depending on their cumulative risk of cancer. Gains in life expectancy from prophylactic surgery decline with advancing age, such that they become minimal at 60 years of age. The authors caution about limitations of their study and that calculated gains in life expectancy should be interpreted carefully. Hartmann and coworkers (1999) conducted a retrospective study of all women who underwent bilateral prophylactic mastectomy at the Mayo Clinic between 1960 and 1993. The women were divided into two groups—high risk and moderate risk—on the basis of family history. A control group of the sisters of the high-risk probands and the Gail model (Gail et al., 1989) were used to predict the number of breast cancers expected to occur in these two groups in the absence of prophylactic mastectomy. They identified 639 women (214 at high risk and 425 at moderate risk) who had undergone bilateral prophylactic mastectomy. According to the Gail model, 37.4 breast cancers were predicted in the moderate-risk group; 4 breast cancers occurred (reduction in risk, 89.5%, $P < 0.001$). The 214 high-risk probands who had undergone prophylactic mastectomies were compared with 403 sisters who had not undergone such surgeries. Of these sisters, 156 (38.7%) had been given a diagnosis of breast cancer (115 cases were diagnosed before the respective proband's prophylactic mastectomy). By contrast, breast cancer was diagnosed in 3 of 214 (1.4%) of the probands. Prophylactic mastectomy was associated with a reduction in the incidence of breast cancer of at least 90%. Moreover, there appears to be decreased emotional concern about developing breast cancer and generally favorable psychological and social outcomes among patients who have undergone prophylactic mastectomy (Frost et al., 2000).

Although data concerning prophylactic mastectomy are potentially of importance, a number of concerns have been raised about the methodologies used in the study reported by Hartmann and colleagues (1999) and the interpretation of the results (Ernster, 1999; Hamm et al., 1999; Kuerer et al., 1999; Haffty et al., 2002). Patients should be counseled that there is currently insufficient evidence to recommend for or against prophylactic mastectomy as a means of reducing breast cancer risk. However, these women should be told that this is an alternative option and that some authorities are now learning towards recommending bilateral prophylactic mastectomy (Narod, 2002). They also should be informed that the development of cancer following prophylactic surgery has been documented in case reports and observational series (Lopez and Porter, 1996). Most experts prefer simple mastectomy for prophylactic procedures; however, the optimal approach has not been tested in prospective or case-controlled studies of women with genetic breast-ovarian cancer susceptibility genes (Burke et al., 1997; Lynch and Casey, 1997).

Similar issues should be raised about prophylactic oophorectomy in women identified with BRCA1 or BRCA2 mutations. Again, there is currently insufficient evidence to absolutely recommend for or against prophylactic oophorectomy as a measure for reducing ovarian cancer risk (Rebbeck, 2000). However, recent data indicate that bilateral prophylactic salpingo-oophorectomy in carriers of BRCA1 and BRCA2 mutations can decrease the risk of coelomic epithelial cancer, breast cancer and fallopian tube cancer (Kauff et al., 2002; Rebbeck et al., 2002). Patients should be counseled that cancer has been documented to occur after the procedure. The optimal age for oophorectomy is unknown, but since the mean age for ovarian cancer in women in hereditary breast-ovarian families is in the middle forties, prophylactic oophorectomy logically might be considered after completion of childbearing or at age 35 (NIH Consensus Development Panel on Ovarian Cancer, 1995).

Walker et al. (2002) recently reported a population-based case-controlled study of 725 cases and 1303 control subjects with positive or negative family history of ovarian cancer and known duration of oral contraceptive (OC) use. They found that women with a first-degree family history of ovarian cancer are at a decreasing risk of ovarian cancer with increasing duration of OC use ($P = .014$, test of trend). Four to 8 years of OC was believed to reduce the risk of ovarian cancer by age 70 years in women with a family history of ovarian cancer, from approximately 4 women per 100 women who did not use OC to 2 women per 100 women who did use OC. Thus, in most women with a positive family history of ovarian cancer OC use may not only be recommended as a method of birth control, but also as a primary preventative measure for the development of ovarian cancer.

Women diagnosed with breast cancer who are carriers of a susceptibility gene are at increased risk for developing a second breast cancer in the contralateral breast as well as ovarian cancer (Easton et al., 1995). Thus, the option of bilateral mastectomy and/or oophorectomy should be discussed.

Narod and colleagues (2000) reported a matched case-control study comparing 209 women with bilateral breast cancer and BRCA1 or BRCA2 mutation (bilateral disease cases), with 384 women with unilateral disease and BRCA1 or BRCA2 mutation (controls). The multivariate odds ratio for contralateral breast cancer associated with tamoxifen use was 0.50 (95% CI, 0.28–0.89). Tamoxifen protected against contralateral breast cancer for BRCA1 carriers (OR 0.38; 95% CI, 0.19–0.74) and for those with BRCA2 mutations (OR 0.63; 95% CI, 0.20–1.50). Among women who used tamoxifen for 2 to 4 years, the risk of contralateral breast cancer was reduced by 75%. The authors concluded that the risk of contralateral breast cancer in women with mutations in *BRCA1* and *BRCA2* is increased, and that this drug can reasonably be offered to such women. However, they acknowledge that the effect of taxomifen on reduction of cancer-associated mortality has not yet been established. They also state that tamoxifen will reduce the occurrence of primary cancers in *BRCA1* and *BRCA2* mutation carriers and that tamoxifen chemoprevention and other preventions (discussed earlier) should be discussed with healthy women who carry *BRCA1* or *BRCA2* mutations.

Even though there is a threefold increased risk for prostate cancer in males carrying *BRCA1* mutations (Aragon et al., 1993), there are insufficient data to recommend for or against prostate cancer screening in this group (Burke et al., 1997a). The American Cancer Society recommends an annual digital rectal examination and measurement of prostate-specific antigen levels beginning at age 50 for all men, with considerations for earlier screening for men in high-risk groups, including those with a strong familial predisposition (Mettlin et al., 1993). However, controversy exists about effectiveness of screening in reducing morbidity and mortality. Many prostate cancers are not clinically evident, and most men with prostate cancer do not die from the disease (Chodak et al., 1994).

It has been recommended that male and female carriers of *BRCA1* mutations be informed of a possible increased risk of colorectal cancer, and that they be encouraged to follow screening recommendations for the general population (Burke et al., 1997a).

Ovarian Epithelial Cancer

In the United States, ovarian cancer accounts for about 25% of all malignant neoplasms of the female genital tract and over 50% of the deaths ascribed to gynecologic cancer. Ovarian cancer is the fifth leading cause of cancer-related mortality, accounting for 5% of all cancer deaths (Piver and Hempling, 1997). In 1998, approximately 25,400 new cases of ovarian cancer were diagnosed, and 14,500 women died of the disease (Landis et al., 1998).

The lifetime risk of a woman's developing ovarian cancer in the United States is about 1.8% (Whittemore et al., 1997). The combined 5-year survival rate for all patients with ovarian cancer is 40%. Although a small proportion of women are diagnosed with ovarian cancer confined to the ovary, for which cure rates are in the range of 90%, 75% of patients have advanced disease (stage III or IV), and only 12% are disease-free at 5 years (Piver and Hempling, 1997). Unfortunately, most women with early-stage disease are asymptomatic. Thus, many cases pass undetected until late stage disease is manifested by a pelvic mass, ascites, omental metastases, or bowel obstruction.

Ovarian cancer encompasses ovarian epithelial neoplasia, derived from the germinal epithelium located on the surface of the ovary; germ-cell neoplasia; and stromal neoplasia. Germ-cell tumors, especially benign lesions, are relatively more common during childhood. By the fourth decade, ovarian epithelial tumors are far more common; the median age at diagnosis is 63 years (Piver and Hempling, 1997). Approximately 90% of ovarian tumors are epithelial. Seventy-five percent of epithelial cancers are serous; 20% are mucinous: the remaining few less common histologic types include endometrial, clear cell, Brenner, and undifferential carcinomas (Berek et al., 1996).

Most ovarian cancers are sporadic epithelial tumors. However, the most significant risk factor for ovarian cancer is a positive family history; it is estimated that up to 10% of ovarian carcinomas occur in women with familial disposition to this disease (Dubeau, 1999). Other factors that have been identified as risk factors include breast cancer, talc exposure, a high-fat diet, and infertility (Piver and Hempling, 1997). Several years ago case reports and studies implicated drugs used for ovulation induction in infertility as associated with an increased risk of ovarian cancer (Rossing et al., 1994). More recent data suggest that nulliparity, especially when associated with infertility, may increase the risk rather than the infertility drugs *per se* (Mosgaard et al., 1997; Ness et al., 2002).

Most familial ovarian cancers appear to fall into three categories: (1) breast and ovarian cancer syndrome; (2) hereditary nonpolyposis colorectal cancer; and (3) site-specific familial ovarian cancer.

BREAST AND OVARIAN CANCER SYNDROME

In addition to breast cancer, mutations in *BRCA1* and *BRCA2* together have been associated with most inherited ovarian cancers (see previous discussion). To date, ovarian cancers associated with *BRCA1* and *BRCA2* mutations have been limited to epithelial carcinomas. Ford and colleagues (1995) estimated that the frequency of *BRCA1* mutations in the general population is 0.0006. On the basis of this estimate, 2.8% of all ovarian cancers diagnosed in women younger than 70 years are attributable to *BRCA1* and *BRCA2*. In a study of 374 women diagnosed with epithelial ovarian cancer before age 70 at the Royal Marsden Hospital in London, Stratton and coworkers (1997) determined that approximately 5% (95% confidence level, 3 to 8%) carried *BRCA1* mutations. By contrast, mutations in *BRCA1* and *BRCA2* appear to be responsible for a much higher proportion of ovarian cancers among Ashkenazi Jewish women. Among 38 cases diagnosed with ovarian cancer, 30 (79%) had mutations either in *BRCA1* (*185delAG*) or *BRCA2* (617delT) (Abeliovich et al., 1997).

Using data pooled from three population-based case control studies of ovarian cancer conducted in the United States, Whittemore and colleagues (1997) estimated that by age 80, the risk of ovarian cancer in carriers of *BRCA1* mutations was 27.8% compared with 1.8% in noncarriers. Table 9–6 gives the estimated cumulative ovarian cancer risks among *BRCA1* mutation carriers and noncarriers.

Rubin and coworkers (1996) studied 53 patients with ovarian cancer and germ-line mutations of *BRCA1*. Compared with matched controls, those women with *BRCA1* mutations has a significantly more favorable course with respect to survival. However, this observation has proved controversial because of methodologic problems and biases (Burk, 1997; Cannistra, 1997; Whitmore, 1997). Stettner and coworkers (1999) have suggested that a gene-conferring susceptibility to ovarian germ-cell cancers and possibly to germ-cell tumors in men as well is present in at least some families with multiple members affected with such cancers.

▼ **Table 9–6.** ESTIMATED CUMULATIVE RISK
· OF OVARIAN CANCER IN *BRCA1* MUTATION
CARRIERS AND NONCARRIERS

Age (Years)	Estimated Risk (95% CI) (%)		Risk Ratio*
	Carriers	Noncarriers	
40	4.0 (1.1–13.3)	0.1 (.0–.2)	73.9
50	9.4 (2.7–28.3)	0.3 (.1–.5)	34.7
60	14.6 (3.9–41.6)	0.5 (.3–.9)	29.8
70	21.5 (4.8–59.9)	1.1 (.7–1.8)	19.1
80	27.8 (5.2–73.0)	1.8 (1.1–2.8)	15.8

*Risk in carriers divided by risk in noncarriers.
Adapted with permission from Whittemore AS, Gong G, Itnyre J: Prevalence and contribution of BRCA1 mutations in breast cancer and ovarian cancer: Results from three U.S. population-based case-control studies of ovarion cancer. Am J Hum Genet 60:496, 1997.

HEREDITARY NONPOLYPOSIS COLORECTAL CANCER

Hereditary nonpolyposis colorectal cancer (HNPCC) has already been discussed in the section on endometrial carcinoma. Ovarian cancer risk in HNPCC families is 3.5 times higher than expected in the general population (Watson and Lynch, 1993). HNPCC accounts for approximately 10 to 15% of all hereditary ovarian cancer cases (Bewtra et al., 1992; Burke et al., 1997b). The estimated cumulative risk by age 70 is less than 10% (Aarnio et al., 1995; Marra and Boland, 1995). Mean age at diagnosis is 45 years, approximately 20 years earlier than in the general population (Vasen et al., 1990; Watson and Lynch, 1993; Watson et al., 1994). Considerable heterogeneity in histopathologic type of ovarian cancer occurs in HNPCC (Watson and Lynch, 1993; Boyd and Rubin, 1997).

SITE-SPECIFIC FAMILIAL OVARIAN CANCER

Site-specific familial ovarian cancer has been characterized by the presence of two or more first-degree relatives (mother, sister, daughter) or first- and second-degree relatives (aunt, grandmother) who have epithelial ovarian cancer. Whether this is a separate hereditary cancer is uncertain. Site-specific ovarian cancer could represent a variant of the hereditary breast-ovarian cancer syndrome, attributable to either *BRCA1* or *BRCA2* (Liede et al., 1998).

Ovarian Germ Cell Neoplasia

In females, germ-cell neoplasia most often takes the form of benign cystic teratomas (dermoids). By definition, at least two of the three germ-cell layers must be present. Well-formed ectodermal structures (e.g., teeth, hair) are not rare findings. Cystic teratomas can become malignant, but fortunately usually they are not. Other germ-cell tumors include Sertoli-Leydig cell tumors and dysgerminomas.

BENIGN CYSTIC TERATOMAS (DERMOIDS)

That benign cystic teratomas are heritable is evident on the basis of frequent bilaterality (20%) and early age at onset. Both characteristics suggest genetic tendencies. Indeed, teratomas have been reported in twins, in nontwin siblings, in triplets, and in three generations (Sippel, 1924; Feld, 1966; Hollander and Masterson, 1967; Plattner et al., 1973; Brown, 1979; Simon et al., 1985).

The pathogenesis of cystic teratomas involves parthenogenesis. That is, these tumors arise from a single germ-cell that produces itself. Studies using polymorphic chromosomal variants initially suggested that the error was restricted to meiosis II (Linder et al., 1975); however, the error may also involve meiosis I (Carritt et al., 1982). Coupled with observations of inherited tendencies toward teratomas, these data imply genetic control over meiosis.

No unusual characteristics have been uncovered in familial cases, but few data exist. Most often they are associated with normal karyotypes; however, cases with chromosomal abnormalities have been reported (Schmid-Braz et al., 2002). Neither HLA studies nor comparative frequencies of parthenogenesis are available. Too few cases of familial teratomas exist to compare ages at onset between familial and nonfamilial cases.

MALIGNANT TERATOMAS

No familial aggregates of malignant teratomas are reported, and a systematic survey by our group (Shulman et al., 1994) revealed no increased risk for first- or second-degree relatives of probands. Our study of 78 probands with various gene-cell malignancies included 23 with malignant teratomas. Not a single mother, sister, aunt, or grandmother was affected. The same held true for relatives of 14 cases of mixed germ-cell tumors and 9 cases of embryonal tumors.

DYSGERMINOMAS

Dysgerminomas have been reported in 46,XX individuals in two and perhaps three generations of a Jamaican kindred (Jackson, 1967). Familial dysgerminomas are otherwise not reported in 46,XX persons. However, the tumor is relatively common among individuals with 46,XY or 45,X/46,XY gonadal dysgenesis (see Chapter 10).

OVARIAN STROMAL NEOPLASIA

Ovarian neoplasias may arise from ovarian stromal cells: granulosa cells, Sertoli-Leydig (interstitial) cells, or fibrous elements (fibromas). All these tumors are rare, but familial aggregates of each are reported. Epidemiologic studies for stromal tumors are not available, but several lines of evidence suggest that genetic factors may be involved.

GRANULOSA CELL TUMORS

Granulosa cell tumors occur in both young girls and postmenopausal women, suggesting different pathogenetic mechanisms. Granulosa cell tumors are observed in the Peutz-Jeghers syndrome, which is an autosomal dominant disorder characterized by circumoral melanin deposits and colonic polyposis. Germ-line mutations in the LKB1 (STK11) gene (locus on chromosome 19p13.3) cause characteristic hamartomas and pigmentation to develop in patients with Peutz-Jeghers syndrome. Although ovarian sex cord tumors with annular tubules and minimal deviation adenocarcinomas of the uterine cervix are very rare in the general population, both tumor types occur with increased frequency in women with this syndrome. Connolly and colleagues (2000) have suggested that the LKB1 (STK11) gene, like other tumor suppressor genes, is affected by biallelic inactivation in the gynecologic tumors in women with Peutz-Jeghers syndrome. LBK1 (STK11) appears to play a minor role in sporadic tumorigenesis (Hemminki, 1999; Connolly et al., 2000).

In one series, 16 of 115 patients with Peutz-Jeghers syndrome had a coexisting ovarian tumor, typically a granulosa cell tumor (Dozois et al., 1970). On the other hand, familial aggregates in otherwise normal persons seem rare.

SERTOLI CELL-LEYDIG ARRHENOBLASTOMA

Reported familial aggregates of arrhenoblastoma involve siblings, a mother and daughter, and paternal cousins (Javert et al., 1951; Accardo et al., 1966; Serban et al., 1968; Goldstein et al., 1970; Murad et al., 1973). Too few cases exist to permit comparisons between familial and nonfamilial cases. A syndrome of familial arrhenoblastomas and thyroid disease has been claimed by some (Jensen et al., 1974; O'Brien and Wilansky, 1981) but doubted by others (Whitcomb et al., 1986).

ENDODERMAL SINUS TUMORS (YOLK SAC TUMORS)

These rare tumors are said to resemble the yolk sac of the rodent placenta. Secretion of alpha-fetoprotein is useful diagnostically and interesting ontologically. In our study of 30 cases, not a single relative was similarly affected.

FIBROMAS

Ovarian fibromas in the absence of other abnormalities are rare and usually not familial. An autosomal dominant gene appears to have caused ovarian fibromas in at least one family (Dumont-Herskowitz et al., 1978). Valle and coworkers (1997) reported two cases of sisters with bilateral ovarian fibromas. Ovarian fibromas are also associated with the nevoid basal cell syndrome (Gorlin syndrome), which is caused by a gene on 9q 22.3-0.31. The mutant gene is a homologue of *Drosophilia* patched (Hahn et al., 1996). Most mutations are premature stop codons due to frameshift mutations. Cases were reported by Burket and Rauh (1976), Raggio and associates (1983), and Seracchioli and coworkers (2001). If ovarian fibromas are bilateral or premenarchal at age of onset, Gorlin syndrome becomes a likely diagnosis.

Fibromas have also occurred in ataxia-telangectasia (Miller and Chatten, 1967). Ovarian fibrosarcoma has also been reported in each of dizygotic twins (Macklin, 1941).

Gestational Trophoblastic Disease

Gestational trophoblastic disease (GTD) describes a group of pathologic conditions whose antecedent is pregnancy. At the benign end of this spectrum is *placental-site plaque* or *nodule*, which is an exaggerated reaction at the placental site that regresses spontaneously. Another usually benign disease is *hydatidiform mole*, which can be complete or partial and may be complicated by persistent disease. Complete or partial moles that invade the myometrium are known as *invasive moles*. The malignant end of the spectrum includes *placental-site trophoblastic tumor* and *choriocarcinoma* (Berkowitz and Goldstein, 1996; Paradinas, 1997; Newlands et al., 1999). GTD usually arises after pregnancy, occasionally after delivery of a full-term infant, but more often after a spontaneous abortion. Hydropic avascular villi characterize benign trophoblastic disease (hydatidiform mole). Hydatidiform moles *per se* are benign but 5% develop into choriocarcinoma.

The incidence of trophoblastic disease is in the range of 110 per 100,000 pregnancies in the U.S. but in the range of 100 to 700 per 100,000 pregnancies in Taiwan, India, the Philippines, and

elsewhere in Asia (DiCintio et al., 1997; Kim, 1997). Because Asian women residing in the United States show incidences of trophoblastic disease lower than in their native lands, heritable factors have not traditionally been considered paramount. Rather, nutritional or other nongenetic factors are assumed to be more relevant; deficiencies of carotene and vitamin A have been implicated (Berkowitz et al., 1985; Parazzini et al., 1989; Berkowitz et al., 1995). Other risk factors include extremes of maternal age (teenagers and women over 40), multiple gestations, consanguinity, cigarette smoking, nulliparous women with a history of spontaneous abortions, and artificial insemination by donor (Kim, 1997).

COMPLETE HYDATIDIFORM MOLES

Complete hydatidiform moles (CHMs) lack identifiable embryonic or fetal tissues, and the chorionic villi show diffuse trophoblastic hyperplasia and generalized hydatidiform swelling (Berkowitz and Goldstein, 1996). CHMs usually have a 46,XX complement, with both haploid complements of paternal origin (androgenetic) (Kajii and Ohama, 1977). Thus, hydatidiform moles represent an extreme example of genomic imprinting (see Chapter 2) (Jacobs et al., 1982) (Fig. 9–6). Several mechanisms could produce diandric diploidy in CHMs: (1) A single haploid sperm, which subsequently duplicates its chromosomal complement and fertilizes an anucleate ("empty") ovum. Moles derived from this process of endoreplication, in which chromosomal material is doubled without associated cell division, would be 46,XX and completely homozygous. 46,YY Moles could also arise by this mechanism, but this genotype is presumably lethal and would be unable to survive implantation. (2) Two haploid sperm that fertilize an anucleate ("empty") ovum, resulting in a heterozygous mole that is either 46,XX or 46,YY. (A 46,YY constitution is possible but nonviable.) Because such moles are derived from two independent paternal haploid sets, each locus that is paternally heterozygous has a 50/50 chance of being homozygous or heterozygous in the mole. (3) A diploid sperm produced by failures of either the first or second meiotic division that fertilizes an anucleate ("empty") ovum. If nondisjunction occurred at the first meiotic division, the resulting sperm (and mole) would retain both homologues of all paternal chromosomes and thus could only be 46,XY. Unlike 46,XY complete moles of dispermic origin, these dispermic moles would retain all paternal heterozygous

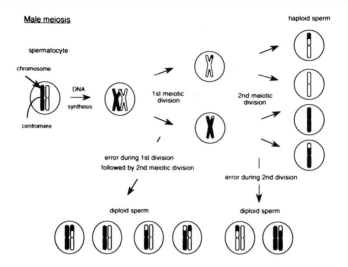

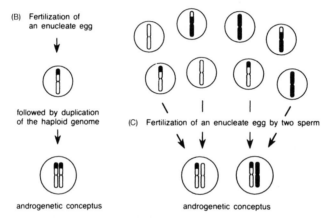

FIGURE 9–6 • Possible mechanisms of origin giving rise to two paternal chromosome complements in complete hydatidiform moles. For simplification, a single pair of chromosomes and a single recombination event has been illustrated. Fertilization of an anucleate egg by (*A*) a sperm that has failed to undergo normal meiotic division, (*B*) a haploid sperm that subsequently duplicates, or (*C*) two sperm, results in a diploid androgenic conceptus. (Reproduced with permission from Fisher RA: Genetics. *In* Hancock BW, Newlands ES, Berkowitz RS (eds): Gestational Trophoblastic Disease. London: Chapman & Hall, 1997.)

alleles. If nondisjunction occurred at the second meiotic division, the sperm would contain two copies of one paternal haploid set and would have to be 46,XX because 46,YY is apparently lethal. Most loci, particularly those near the centromeric region, would be homozygous, in which recombination is suppressed; however, heterozygosity would be expected at distal loci because of recombination before meiosis I.

Molecular genetic techniques such as analysis of restriction fragment length polymorphisms or polymerase chain reaction (PCR) amplification of various DNA sequences have revealed that approximately 75 to 85% of CHM are homozygous 46,XX resulting from a haploid sperm with endoreduplication (Kovacs et al., 1991; Lane et al., 1993). The remaining CHMs are heterozy-

gous; these are predominantly 46,XY, but some 46,XX CHMs have been reported (Wolf and Lage, 1995). Thus, a fourth possibility is dispermy fertilizing a haploid ovum, the latter then being expelled (diploid rescue), analogous to the well-established trisomic rescue. These moles could be 46,XX or 46,XY. Although chromosomes of CHMs are of paternal origin, mitochondrial DNA is of maternal origin (Azuma et al., 1991). Fisher and Newlands (1998) used molecular techniques to show that rare cases of diploid hydatidiform moles have fetal red blood cells in molar villi despite having trophoblastic hyperplasia typical of CHMs. These moles are androgenic in origin and therefore genetically CHMs. A study of similar cases in which amnion was also present showed that the amnion may also be androgenic in origin and identical to the molar vesicles, suggesting that some fetal development can occur in CHMs.

PARTIAL HYDATIDIFORM MOLES

Partial hydatidiform mole (PHM) is characterized by (1) identifiable embryonic or fetal tissues; (2) chorionic villi varying size and focal hydatidiform swelling and cavitation; (3) marked villous scalloping; and (4) prominent stromal trophoblastic inclusions (Berkowitz and Goldstein, 1996). PHMs are generally triploid with a 69,XXX, 69,XXY, or 69,XYY chromosomal complement (Jacobs et al., 1982; Szulman et al., 1984). Most triploid PHM have one maternal and two paternal contributions (diandric triploidy). Triploidy that is maternally derived (digynic triploidy) is usually not associated with molar changes in the placenta.

Several mechanisms could account for triploid conceptuses (Wolf and Lage, 1995): (1) Two haploid sperm fertilizing a haploid ovum, the resulting zygote being 69,XXX, 69,XXY, or 69,XYY. (2) Fertilization of a haploid ovum by a single haploid sperm that then replicates to produce a 69,XXX or 69,XYY zygote. (3) Fertilization of a diploid ovum by a haploid sperm, then followed by an error in the first or second meiotic division of the egg, or fertilization of an ovulated primary oocyte. The product would be either 69,XXX or 69,XXY. (4) Fertilization of a haploid ovum by a diploid sperm produced by failure of either the first or second meiotic division. Sperm produced by nondisjunction at meiosis I would yield zygotes that were either 69,XYY or 69,XXX.

Cytogenetic studies of invasive hydatidiform mole have shown the majority to be diploid, with a high proportion of cells in the tetraploid range (Makino et al., 1965). Wake and coworkers (1984) studied four invasive moles and found three to be 46,XX and one 46,XY, reflecting their origin from CHMs (Wake et al., 1984). Cytogenetic studies of choriocarcinoma cell lines have revealed numerical and structural abnormalities; however, because of possible mutation and selection, such abnormalities may not be representative of the original tumors. Although direct cytogenetic analysis and/or short-term cultures have also revealed chromosomally abnormal populations (Bettio et al., 1993), flow cytometric studies of choriocarcinomas have shown predominantly diploid cells (Hemming et al., 1988; Fukunaga and Ushigome, 1993).

In gestational trophoblastic neoplasia, patient and partner often share HLA antigens, particularly in Asian women (Ho et al., 1989). In such cases, the paternal haplotype shared with the mother almost always segregates into the mole (Couillin et al., 1985). Increased malignancy associated exclusively with paternal histocompatibility loci would be consistent with the ostensibly paradoxical observation that disparity between maternal and paternal HLA genes enhances implantation (see Chapter 5). No particular HLA antigen has been associated with gestational trophoblastic neoplasia.

In 225 Caucasian patients with trophoblastic neoplasias, Lawler (1978) found the frequencies of HLA-A and HLA-B locus antigens not to differ significantly from those of the normal control population. However, the degree of incompatibility between husband and wife, as measured by the number of antigenic incompatibilities (0, 1, or 2), indicated a trend toward patients who are more compatible with their husbands for the B locus to fall into the higher risk treatment categories.

Molecular genetic techniques may also be applied in clinical management of gestational trophoblastic tumor (GTT). Trophoblastic differentiation and human chorionic gonadotropin production, characteristic of GTT, can sometimes occur in nongestational choriocarcinoma. In contrast to women with GTT, long-term survival in patients with nongestational choriocarcinoma is uncommon. Using molecular techniques (e.g., PCR amplification of variable number tandem repeat DNA sequences, microsatellite polymorphisms, sex chromosome-specific sequences), the gestational or nongestational origin of a trophoblastic tumor can be established. Thus, using molecular techniques, it is possible to distinguish CHMs from PHMs and hydropic abortions, monospermic CHMs from dispermic CHMs, and recurrent disease from persistent disease (Newlands et al., 1999). Nongestational choriocarcinomas will have a genome that reflects the host (Fisher and Newlands, 1998).

Finally, oncogene expression in CHMs has shown an increased expression of c-fms, although neither c-fms nor c-myc has been shown to correlate with clinical course (Cheung et al., 1993). Mutations in the p53 TSG have been observed in choriocarcinoma lines (Yaginuma et al., 1995); however, no mutations have been found in the small number of CHMs studied (Cheung et al., 1994).

FAMILIAL AGGREGATES

Gestational trophoblastic disease can usually be successfully treated. Thus, the possibility of recurrence in the same person arises. Indeed, the likelihood of gestational trophoblastic disease's recurring in subsequent pregnancies in the same person is increased over the background risk (Sand et al., 1984; Berkowitz et al., 1994). Pooled data from 18 reports indicate that the frequency of recurrent trophoblastic disease is 1.3% (67/5002 subjects) (Sand et al., 1984). The actual risk is probably lower because some patients in the 18 reports were probably referred to university centers because of repetitive neoplasia. For example, only 3 of 449 (0.67%) women treated for trophoblastic neoplasia at Northwestern University manifested a subsequent tumor (Sand et al., 1984). However, after two gestational neoplastic events, the recurrence risk rises to 23% in future pregnancies (Berkowitz et al., 1998). This suggests recessive factors for a small subgroup. Most recurrences have involved complete moles, but recurrent PHM in the same subject has been reported (Honoré et al., 1987; Berkowitz et al., 1998).

Trophoblastic disease may also occur in more than one family member. Affected family members include sisters, twins, cousins, and mother-daughter pairs (Ambani et al., 1980; LaVecchia et al., 1982; Parazzini et al., 1988; Kircheisen and Ried, 1991; Seoud et al., 1995; Helwani et al., 1999).

Helwani and colleagues (1999) reported an impressive Lebanese kindred in which the offspring of two sisters, each of whom married consanguineously, produced multiple hydatidiform moles. In each case the moles were of biparental origin. The authors postulated that women with recurrent hydatidiform moles are homozygous for an autosomal recessive mutation that results in biparental pregnancies with the same phenotype (i.e., hydatidiform mole) as a uniparental paternally inherited conceptus, which suggests a defect in genomic imprinting (Moglabey et al., 1999). A genome wide-scan on two families demonstrated that the defective gene resides on chromosome 19q13.3–13.4, a region containing imprinted genes. One candidate gene, *PEG3*, which is maternally imprinted, was not mutated in the affected women (Van den Veyver et al., 2001). A global defect in imprinting was found in a hydatidiform mole of a patient with recurrent biparentally inherited molar pregnancy (Judson et al., 2002). However, in this patient there was no linkage to the candidate region on 19q13.3–13.4.

Other Gynecologic Cancers (Vagina, Vulva, Fallopian Tubes)

Other gynecologic cancers include carcinomas of the vagina, vulva, and fallopian tubes.

Carcinomas of the vagina and vulva are usually squamous in type, typically occurring in older women. Prenatal diethylstilbestrol exposure is associated with clear cell carcinomas of the vagina, a distinctly different histologic type. No familial aggregates are reported.

Carcinomas of the fallopian tube are usually adenocarcinomas and even rarer then vulvar or vaginal carcinomas. No familial aggregates have been reported, but 16% are caused by germ-line mutations in *BRCA1* or *BRCA2* (Aziz et al., 2001).

REFERENCES

Aarnio M, Mecklin J-P, Aaltonen LA, et al.: Life-time risk of different cancers in hereditary non-polyposis colorectal cancer (HNPCC) syndrome. Int J Cancer 64:430, 1995.

Abeliovich D, Kaduri L, Lerer I, et al.: The founder mutations *185delAG* and *5382insC* in *BRCA1* and *6174delT* in *BRCA2* appear in 60% of ovarian cancer and 30% of early-onset breast cancer patients among Ashkenazi women. Am J Hum Genet 60:505, 1997.

Accardo M, Condorelli BL: Arrhenoblastoma in two sisters. Riv Patol Clin Sper 7:171, 1966.

Albert S, Child M: Familial cancer in the general population. Cancer 40:1674, 1977.

ALTS Group: Human papillomavirus testing for triage of women with cytologic evidence of low-grade squamous intraepithelial lesions: Baseline data from a randomized trial. The Atypical Squamous Cells of Undetermined Significance/Low-Grade Squamous Interepithelial Lesions Triage Study (ALTS) Group. J Natl Cancer Inst 92:397, 2000.

Ambani LM, Vaidya RA, Rao CS, et al.: Familial occurrence of trophoblastic disease—report of recurrent molar pregnancies in sisters in three families. Clin Genet 18:27, 1980.

American Cancer Society, 2000: *www.cancer.org*.

American College of Medical Genetics: Genetic Susceptibility to Breast and Ovarian Cancer: Assessment, Counseling and Testing Guidelines. Web site at *http://www.faseb.rog/genetics/acmg*, 1999.

American College of Obstetricians and Gynecologists: Breast-Ovarian Cancer Screening, in Committee Opinion No. 239, August, 2000.

Anderson DE, Badzioch MD: Familial breast cancer risks: Effects of prostate and other cancers. Cancer 72:114, 1993.

Arason A, Barkardottir RB, Egilsson V: Linkage analysis of chromosome 17q markers and breast ovarian cancer in Icelandic families, and possible relationship to prostatic cancer. Am J Hum Genet 52:711, 1993.

Athma P, Rappaport R, Swift M: Molecular genotyping shows that ataxia-telangiectasia heterozygotes are predisposed to breast cancer. Cancer Genet Cytogenet 92:130, 1996.

Atkin NB, Baker MC: Chromosomal 1 in 26 carcinomas of the cervix uteri: Structural and numerical changes. Cancer 44:604, 1979.

Aziz S, Kuperstein G, Rosen B, et al. A genetic epidemiological study of carcinoma of the fallopian tube. Gynecol Oncol 80:341, 2001.

Azuma C, Saji F, Tokugawa Y, et al.: Application of gene amplification by polymerase chain reaction to genetic analysis of molar mitochondrial DNA: The detection of a nuclear empty ovum as the cause of complete mole. Gynecol Oncol 40:29, 1991.

Bale AE, Li FP: Principles of cancer management: Cancer genetics. *In* DeVita VT Jr, Hellman S, Rosenberg SA (eds): Cancer: Principles and Practice of Oncology, 5th ed. Philadelphia: Lippincott-Raven, 1997, p 285.

Bebb G, Glickman B, Gelmon K, et al.: "At risk" for breast cancer. Lancet 349:1784, 1997.

Bell DW, Varley JM, Szydlo TE, et al.: Heterozygous germ line *hCHK2* mutations in Li-Fraumeni syndrome. Science 286:2528, 1999.

Beral V, Hermon C, Reeves G, et al.: Sudden fall in breast cancer death rates in England and Wales. Lancet 345:1642, 1995.

Berek JS, Fu YS, Hacker NF: Ovarian cancer. *In* Berek JS (ed): Novak's Gynecology, 12th ed. Baltimore: Williams and Wilkins, 1996, p 1155.

Berkowitz RS, Bernstein MR, Harlow BL, et al.: Case-control study of risk factors for partial molar pregnancy. Am J Obstet Gynecol 173:788, 1995.

Berkowitz RS, Bernstein MR, Laborde O, et al.: Subsequent pregnancy experience in patients with trophoblastic disease. New England Trophoblastic Disease Center, 1965–1992. J Reprod Med 39:228, 1994.

Berkowitz RS, Cramer DW, Bernstein MR, et al.: Risk factors for complete molar pregnancy from a case-control study. Am J Obstet Gynecol 152:1016, 1985.

Berkowitz RS, Goldstein DP: Gestational trophoblastic disease. *In* Berek JS (ed): Novak's Gynecology, 12th ed. Baltimore: Williams and Wilkins, 1996, p 1261.

Berkowitz RS, Im SS, Bernstein MR, et al.: Gestational trophoblastic disease: Subsequent pregnancy outcome, including repeat molar pregnancy. J Reprod Med 43:81, 1998.

Bettio D, Giardino D, Rizzi N, et al.: Cytogenetic abnormalities detected by direct analysis in a case of choriocarcinoma. Cancer Genet Cytogenet 68:149,1993.

Bewtra C, Watson P, Conway T, et al.: Hereditary ovarian cancer: A clinicopathological study. Int J Gynecol Pathol 11:180, 1992.

Boland CR: Hereditary nonpolyposis colorectal cancer. *In* Vogelstein B, Kinzler KW (eds): The Genetic Basis of Human Cancer. New York: McGraw Hill, 1998, p 333.

Borrow J, Goddard AD, Sheer D, et al.: Molecular analysis of acute promyelocytic leukemia breakpoint cluster region on chromosome 17. Science 249:1577, 1990.

Boyd J, Rubin SC: Hereditary ovarian cancer: Molecular genetics and clinical implications. Gynecol Oncol 64:196, 1997.

Brown EH Jr: Identical twins with twisted benign cystic teratoma of the ovary. Am J Obstet Gynecol 134:879, 1979.

Burk RD: *BRCA1* mutations and survival in women with ovarian cancer. N Engl J Med 336:1255, 1997.

Burke W, Daly M, Garber J, et al.: Recommendations for follow-up care of individuals with an inherited predisposition to cancer. II. *BRCA1* and *BRCA2*. Cancer Genetics Studies Consortium. JAMA 277:997, 1997a.

Burke W, Peterson G, Lynch P, et al.: Recommendations for follow-up care of individuals with an inherited predisposition to cancer. I. Hereditary nonpolyposis colon cancer. Cancer Genetics Studies Consortium. JAMA 277:915, 1997b.

Burket R, Rauh JL: Gorlin's syndrome: Ovarian fibromas at adolescence. Obstet Gynecol 47:43S, 1976.

Cannistra SA: *BRCA1* mutations and survival in women with ovarian cancer. N Engl J Med 336:1254, 1997.

Cannistra SA, Niloff JM: Cancer of the uterine cervix. N Engl J Med 334:1030, 1996.

Carritt B, Parrington J, Welch H, et al.: Diverse origins of multiple ovarian teratomas in a single individual. Proc Nat Acad Sci USA 79:7400, 1982.

Cervical Cancer: NIH Consensus Statement 14:1, 1996.

Cheung AN, Srivastava G, Chung LP, et al.: Expression of the *p53* gene in trophoblastic cells in hydatidiform moles and normal human placentas. J Reprod Med 39:223, 1994.

Cheung AN, Srivastava G, Pittaluga S, et al.: Expression of c-myc and c-fms oncogenes in trophoblastic cells in hydatidiform mole and normal human placenta. J Clin Pathol 46:204, 1993.

Chlebowski RT: Reducing the risk of breast cancer. N Engl J Med 343:191, 2000.

Cho KR: Cervical cancer. *In* Vogelstein B, Kinzler KW (eds): The Genetic Basis of Human Cancer. New York: McGraw-Hill, 1997, p 631.

Chodak GW, Thisted RA, Gerber GS, et al.: Results of conservative management of clinically localized prostate cancer. N Engl J Med 330:242, 1994.

Chu KC, Tarone RE, Kessler LG, et al.: Recent trends in US breast cancer incidence, survival, and mortality rates. J Natl Cancer Inst 88:1571, 1996.

Claus EB, Risch N, Thompson WD: Genetic analysis of breast cancer in the Cancer and Steroid Hormone Study. Am J Hum Genet 48:232, 1991.

Cleaver JE, Kraemer KM: Xeroderma pigmentosum and Cockayne syndrome. *In* Scriver CR, Beaudet AL, Sly WS, et al. (eds): The Metabolic and Molecular Bases of Inherited Disease, 7th ed. New York: McGraw-Hill, 1995, p 4393.

Coleman MP: Trends in breast cancer incidence, survival, and mortality. Lancet 356:590, 2000.

Collins FS: BRCA1—Lots of mutations, lots of dilemmas. N Engl J Med 334:186, 1996.

Connolly DC, Katabuchi H, Cliby WA, et al.: Somatic mutations in the *STK11/LKB1* gene are uncommon in rare gynecologic tumor types associated with Peutz-Jegher's syndrome. Am J Pathol 156:339, 2000.

Cooper GM: Tumor viruses. *In* Cooper GM (ed): Oncogenes, 2nd ed. Boston: Jones and Bartlett Publishers, 1995, p 21.

Couch FJ, Farid LM, DeShano ML, et al.: BRCA2 germline mutations in male breast cancer cases and breast cancer families. Nat Genet 13:123, 1996.

Couch FJ, Weber BL: Breast cancer. *In* Vogelstein B, Kinzler KW (eds): The Genetic Basis of Human Cancer. New York: McGraw-Hill, 1998, p 537.

Couillin P, Afoutou JM, Faye O, et al.: Androgenetic origin of African complete hydatidiform moles demonstrated by HLA markers. Hum Genet 71:113, 1985.

DiCintio E, Parazzini F, Rosa C, et al.: The epidemiology of gestational trophoblastic disease. Gen Diagn Pathol 143:103, 1997.

DiSaia PJ, Grosen EA, Kurosaki T, et al.: Hormone replacement therapy in breast cancer survivors: A cohort study. Am J Obstet Gynecol 174:1494, 1996.

Dozois RR, Kempers RD, Dahlin DC, et al.: Ovarian tumors associated with the Peutz-Jeghers syndrome. Ann Surg 172:233, 1970.

Dubeau L: The cell of origin of ovarian epithelial tumors and the ovarian surface epithelium dogma: Does the emperor have no clothes? Gynecol Oncol 72:437, 1999.

Dumont-Herskowitz RA, Safaii HS, Senior B: Ovarian fibromata in four successive generations. J Pediatr 93:621, 1978.

Dupont WD, Page DL: Risk factors for breast cancer in women with proliferative breast disease. N Engl J Med 312:146, 1985.

Easton D, Ford D, Peto J: Inherited susceptibility to breast cancer. Cancer Surv 18:95, 1993a.

Easton DF, Bishop DT, Ford D, et al.: Breast and ovarian cancer incidence in BRCA1 mutation carriers. Lancet 349:962, 1994.

Easton DF, Bishop DT, Ford D, et al.: Genetic linkage analysis in familial breast and ovarian cancer. Results from 214 families. The Breast Cancer Linkage Consortium. Am J Hum Genet 52:678, 1993b.

Easton DF, Ford D, Bishop DT: Breast and ovarian cancer incidence in BRCA1 mutation carriers. Breast Cancer Linkage Consortium. Am J Hum Genet 56:265, 1995.

Ellisen LW, Bird J, West DC, et al.: TAN-1, the human homolog of the *Drosophila* notch gene, is broken by chromosomal translocations in T lymphoblastic neoplasms. Cell 66:649, 1991.

Eng C, Parsons R: Cowden syndrome. *In* Vogelstein B, Kinzler KW (eds): The Genetic Basis of Human Cancer. New York: McGraw-Hill, 1998, p 519.

Enomoto T, Fujita M, Inoue M, et al.: Alterations of the *p53* tumor suppressor gene and its association with activation of the c-K-ras-2 protooncogene in premalignant and malignant lesions of the human uterine endometrium. Cancer Res 53:1838, 1993.

Ernster VL: Prophylactic mastectomy in women with a high risk of breast cancer (Letter). N Engl J Med 340:1938, 1999.

Farndon PA, Del Mastro RG, Evans DR, et al.: Location of a gene for Gorlin syndrome. Lancet 339:581, 1992.

Fearon ER, Cho KR: The molecular biology of cancer. *In* Rimoin DL, Connor JM, Pyeritz RE (eds): Principles and Practice of Medical Genetics, 3rd ed. New York: Churchill Livingstone, 1996, p 405.

Feld D, Labes J, Nathanson M: Bilateral ovarian dermoid cysts in triplets. Obstet Gynecol 27:525, 1966.

Fisher RA, Newlands ES: Gestational trophoblastic disease. Molecular and genetic studies. J Reprod Med 43:87, 1998.

FitzGerald MG, Bean JM, Hedge SR, et al.: Heterozygous ATM mutations do not contribute to early onset of breast cancer. Nat Genet 15:307, 1997.

FitzGerald MG, MacDonald DJ, Krainer M, et al.: Germ-line BRCA1 mutations in Jewish and non-Jewish women with early-onset breast cancer. N Engl J Med 334:143, 1996.

Ford D, Easton DF, Bishop DT, et al.: Risks of cancer in BRCA1 mutation carriers. Breast Cancer Linkage Consortium. Lancet 343:692, 1994.

Ford D, Easton DF, Peto J: Estimates of the gene frequency of BRCA1 and its contribution to breast and ovarian cancer incidence. Am J Hum Genet 57:1457, 1995.

Ford D, Easton DF, Stratton M, et al.: Genetic heterogeneity and penetrance analysis of the BRCA1 and BRCA2 genes in breast cancer families. The Breast Cancer Linkage Consortium. Am J Hum Genet 62:676, 1998.

Frost MH, Schaid DJ, Sellers TA, et al.: Long-term satisfaction and psychological and social function following bilateral prophylactic mastectomy. JAMA 284:319, 2000.

Fujita S, Moriya Y, Sugihara K, et al.: Prognosis of hereditary nonpolyposis colorectal cancer (HNPec) and the role of Japanese criteria HWPCC. Jpn J Clin Oncol 26:351, 1996.

Fukunaga M, Ushigome S: Malignant trophoblastic tumors: Immunohistochemical and flow cytometric comparison of choriocarcinoma and placental site trophoblastic tumors. Hum Pathol 24:1098, 1993.

Futreal PA, Liu Q, Shattuck-Eidenens D, et al.: BRCA1 mutations in primary breast and ovarian carcinomas. Science 266:120, 1994.

Gail MH, Brinton LA, Byar DP, et al.: Projecting individualized probabilities of developing breast cancer for white females who are being examined annually. J Natl Cancer Inst 81:1879, 1989.

Gatti RA: Ataxia-telangeictasia. *In* Vogelstein B, Kinzler KW (eds): The Genetic Basis of Human Cancer. New York: McGraw-Hill, 1998, p 275.

Giardiello FM, Welsh SB, Hamilton SR, et al.: Increased risk of cancer in the Peutz-Jeghers syndrome. N Engl J Med 316:1511, 1987.

Goldstein DP, Lamb EJ: Arrhenoblastoma in first cousins: Report of two cases. Obstet Gynecol 35:444, 1970.

Gorlin RJ: Nevoid basal cell carcinoma syndrome. Medicine (Baltimore) 66:98, 1987.

Haffty BG, Harrold E, Khan AJ, et al.: Outcome of conservatively managed early-onset breast cancer by BRCA1/2 status. Lancet 359:1471, 2002.

Hahn H, Wicking C, Zaphiropoulous PG, et al.: Mutations of the human homolog of *Drosophila* patched in the nevoid basal carcinoma syndrome. Cell 85:841, 1996.

Hall NR, Williams MA, Murday VA, et al.: Muir-Torre syndrome: A variant of the cancer family syndrome. J Med Genet 31:627, 1994.

Hamm RM, Lawler F, Scheid D: Prophylactic mastectomy in women with a high risk of breast cancer (Letter). N Engl J Med 340:1837, 1999.

Harris CC, Hollstein M: Clinical implications of the *p53* tumor-suppressor gene. N Engl J Med 329:1318, 1993.

Harris JR, Lippman ME, Veronesi U, et al.: Breast cancer. N Engl J Med 327:319, 1992.

Hartge P, Struewing JP, Wacholder S, et al.: The prevalence of common BRCA1 and BRCA2 mutations among Ashkenazi Jews. Am J Hum Genet 64:963, 1999.

Hartmann LC, Schaid DJ, Woods JE, et al.: Efficacy of bilateral prophylactic mastectomy in women with a family history of breast cancer. N Engl J Med 340:77, 1999.

Heisterkamp N, Groffen L, Stephenson JR, et al.: Chromosomal localization of human cellular homologues of two viral oncogenes. Nature 299:747, 1982.

Helwani MN, Seoud M, Zahed L, et al.: A familial case of recurrent hydatidiform molar pregnancies with biparental genomic contribution. Hum Genet 105:112, 1999.

Hemming JD, Quirke P, Womack C, et al.: Flow cytometry in persistent trophoblastic disease. Placenta 9:615, 1988.

Hemminki A: The molecular basis and clinical aspects of Peutz-Jeghers syndrome. Cell Mol Life Sci 55:735, 1999.

Hemminki A, Tomlinson I, Markie D, et al.: Localization of a susceptibility locus for Peutz-Jeghers syndrome to 19p using comparative genomic hybridization and targeted linkage analysis. Nat Genet 15:87, 1997.

Hendrick L: Endometrial cancer. *In* Vogelstein B, Kinzler KW (eds): The Genetic Basis of Human Cancer. New York: McGraw-Hill, 1998, p 621.

Hockenberry D, Nuñez G, Millman C, et al.: Bcl-2, an inner mitochondrial membrane protein, blocks programme cell death. Nature 348:334, 1990.

Ho HN, Gill TJ 3rd, Kliousky B, et al.: Differences between white and Chinese populations in human leukocyte antigen sharing and gestational trophoblastic tumors. Am J Obstet Gynecol 161:942, 1989.

Hollander H, Masterson JG: Familial cystic teratoma of the ovary. Tex Rep Biol Med 25:483, 1967.

Honoré L: Recurrent partial hydatidiform mole: Report of a case. Am J Obstet Gynecol 156:922, 1987.

Hopper JL, Southey MC, Dites GS, et al.: Population-based estimate of the average age-specific cumulative risk of breast cancer for a defined set of protein-truncating mutations in BRCA1 and BRCA2. Australian Breast Cancer Family Study. Cancer Epidemiol Biomarkers Prev 8:741, 1999.

Hoskins KF, Stopfer JE, Calzone KA, et al.: Assessment and counseling for women with a family history of breast cancer: A guide for clinicians. JAMA 15:577, 1995.

Hunter DJ, Spiegelman D, Adami HO, et al.: Cohort studies of fat intake and the risk of breast cancer—a pooled analysis. N Engl J Med 334:356, 1996.

Jackson S: Ovarian dysgerminoma in three generations? J Med Genet 4:112, 1967.

Jacobs PA, Hunt PA, Matsura JS, et al.: Complete and partial hydatidiform mole in Hawaii: Cytogenetics, morphology, and epidemiology. Br J Obstet Gynaecol 89:258, 1982.

Janin N, Andrieu N, Ossian K, et al.: Breast cancer risk in ataxia-telangiectasia (AT) heterozygotes: Haplotype study in French AT families. Br J Cancer 80:1042, 1999.

Javert C, Finn WF: Arrhenoblastoma: The incidence of malignancy and the relationship to pregnancy, to sterility and to treatment. Cancer 4:69, 1951.

Jensen RD, Norris HJ, Fraumeni JF Jr: Familial arrhenoblastoma and thyroid adenoma. Cancer 33:218, 1974.

Judson H, Hayward BE, Sheridan E, Bonthron DT: A global disorder of imprinting in the human female germ line. Nature 416:539, 2002.

Kajii T, Ohama K: Androgenetic origin of hydatidiform mole. Nature 268:633, 1977.

Kakizuka A, Miller WH Jr, Umesono K, et al.: Chromosomal translocation t(15;17) in human acute promyelocytic leukemia fuses RARα (with a novel putative transcription factor, PML). Cell 66:663, 1991.

Kauff ND, Satagopan JM, Robson ME, et al. Risk-reducing salpingo-oopherectomy in women with a BRCA1 or BRCA2 mutation. N Engl J Med 346:1609, 2002.

Kaufman RH, Adam E, Icenogle J, et al.: Relevance of human papillomavirus screening in management of cervical intraepithelial neoplasia. Am J Obstet Gynecol 176:87, 1997.

Kawai A, Woodruff J, Healey JH, et al.: SYT-SSX gene fusion as a determinant of morphology and prognosis in synovial sarcoma. N Engl J Med 338:153, 1998.

Khanna KK: Carrier risk and the ATM gene: A continuing debate. J Natl Cancer Inst 92:795, 2000.

Kim SJ: Epidemiology. In Hancock BW, Newlands ES, Berkowitz RS (eds): Gestational Trophoblastic Disease. London: Chapman and Hill Medical, 1997, p 27.

King CR, Kraus MH, Aaronson SA: Amplification of a novel v-erbB-related gene in a human mammary carcinoma. Science 229:974, 1985.

Kircheisen R, Ried T: Hydatidiform moles. Hum Reprod 9:1783, 1991.

Kirsch IR, Morton CC, Nakahara K, et al.: Human immunoglobulin heavy chain genes map to a region of translocations in malignant B lymphocytes. Science 216:301, 1982.

Kitagawa S, Townsend BL, Hebert AA: Peutz-Jeghers syndrome. Dermatol Clin 13:127, 1995.

Kiyono T: Roles of HPV genes in carcinogenesis. Uirusu 48:125, 1998.

Klutz M, Brockman D, Lohman DR: A parent-of-origin effect in two families with retinoblastoma is associated with a distinct splice mutation in the RB1 gene. Am J Hum Genet 71:174, 2002.

Knudson A: Mutation and cancer: Statistical study of retinoblastoma. Proc Natl Acad Sci USA 68:820, 1971.

Knudson A, Strong L: Mutation and cancer: A model for Wilms' tumor of the kidney. J Natl Cancer Inst 48:313, 1972.

Koul A, Willen R, Bendahl PO, et al.: Distinct sets of gene alterations in endometrial carcinoma implicate alternate modes of tumorigenesis. Cancer 94:2369, 2002.

Kovacs BW, Shahbahrami B, Tast DE, et al.: Molecular genetic analysis of complete hydatidiform moles. Cancer Genet Cytogenet 54:143, 1991.

Krainer M, Silva-Arrieta S, FitzGerald MG, et al.: Differential contributions of BRCA2 and BRCA1 to early-onset breast cancer. N Engl J Med 336:1416, 1997.

Kuerer HM, Hwang ES, Esserman LJ: Prophylactic mastectomy in women with a high risk of breast cancer (Letter). N Engl J Med 340:1838, 1999.

Landis SH, Murray T, Bolden S, et al.: Cancer statistics, 1998. CA Cancer J Clin 48:6, 1998.

Lacey JV Jr, Devessa SS, Brinton LA: Recent trends in breast cancer incidence and mortality. Environ Mol Mutagen 39:82, 2002.

Lane SA, Taylor GR, Ozols B, et al.: Diagnosis of complete molar pregnancy by microsatellites in archival material. J Clin Pathol 46:346, 1993.

Langston AA, Malone KE, Thompson JD, et al.: BRCA1 mutations in a population-based sample of young women with breast cancer. N Engl J Med 334:137, 1996.

Lawler SD: HLA and trophoblastic tumours. Br Med Bull 34:305, 1978.

Leder P, Battey J, Lenoir G, et al.: Translocations among antibody genes in human cancer. Science 222:765, 1983.

LaVecchia C, Franceschi S, Fasoli M, et al.: Gestational trophoblastic neoplasms in homozygous twins. Obstet Gynecol 60:250, 1982.

Libermann TA, Nusbaum HR, Razon N, et al.: Amplification, enhanced expression and possible rearrangement of EGF receptor gene in primary human brain tumours of glial origin. Nature 313:144, 1985.

Levine AJ, Momand J, Finlay CA: The p53 tumour suppressor gene. Nature 351:453, 1991.

Li FP, Fraumeni JF, Mulvihill JJ, et al.: A cancer family syndrome in twenty-four kindreds. Cancer Res 48:5358, 1988.

Liede A, Tonin PN, Sun CC, et al.: Is hereditary site-specific ovarian cancer a distinct genetic condition? Am J Med Genet 75:55, 1998.

Linder D, McCaw BK, Hecht F: Parthenogenic origin of benign ovarian teratomas. N Engl J Med 292:63, 1975.

Lopez MJ, Porter KA: The current role of prophylactic mastectomy. Surg Clin North Am 76:231, 1996.

Lugo TG, Pendergast AM, Muller AJ, et al.: Tyrosine kinase activity and transformation potency of brc-abl oncogene products. Science 247:1079, 1990.

Lynch ED, Ostermeyer EA, Lee MK, et al.: Inherited mutations in PTEN that are associated with breast cancer, Cowden disease and juvenile polyposis. Am J Hum Genet 61:1254, 1997.

Lynch HT, Casey MJ: The role of prophylactic surgery for hereditary breast cancer and ovarian cancer. Contemp OB/GYN 42:411, 1997.

Macklin M: Tumors in monozygous and dizygous twins. Can Med Assoc J 44:604, 1941.

Magnusson PKE, Sparen P, Gyllensten UB: Genetic link to cervical tumours. Nature 400:29, 1999.

Makino S, Sasaki MS, Fukuschima T: Cytological studies of tumors. XLI. Chromosomal instability in human chorionic lesions. Okajimas Folia Anat Jpn 40:439, 1965.

Malkin D: The Li-Fraumeni syndrome. In Vogelstein B, Kinzler KW (eds): The Genetic Basis of Human Cancer. New York: McGraw-Hill, 1998, p 393.

Malkin D, Li FP, Strong LC, et al.: Germ line p53 mutations in a familial syndrome of breast cancer, sarcomas, and other neoplasms. Science 250:1233, 1990.

Marra G, Boland CR: Hereditary nonpolyposis colorectal cancer: The syndrome, the gene, and historical perspectives. J Natl Cancer Inst 87:1114, 1995.

Marsh DJ, Kum JB, Lunetta KL, et al.: PTEN mutation spectrum and genotype-phenotype correlations in Bannayan-Riley-Ruvalcaba syndrome suggests a single entity with Cowden syndrome. Hum Mol Genet 8:1461, 1999.

Matlashewski G, Schneider J, Banks L, et al.: Human papillomavirus type 16 DNA cooperates with activated ras in transforming primary cells. EMBO J 6:1741, 1987.

McBride OW, Hieter PA, Hollis GF, et al.: Chromosomal location of human kappa and lambda immunoglobulin light chain constant region genes. J Exp Med 155:1480, 1982.

Mecklin JP: Frequency of hereditary colorectal carcinoma. Gastroenterology 92:1021, 1987.

Mecklin JP, Jarvinen HJ: Tumor spectrum in cancer family syndrome (hereditary nonpolyposis colorectal cancer). Cancer 68:1109, 1991.

Melbye M, Wohlfahrt J, Olsen JH, et al.: Induced abortion and the risk of breast cancer. N Engl J Med 336:81, 1997.

Mellentin JD, Smith SD, Cleary ML: Lyl-1, a novel gene altered by chromosomal translocation in T-cell leukemia, codes for a protein with a helix-loop-helix DNA binding motif. Cell 58:77, 1989.

Mian C, Bancher D, Kohlberger P, et al.: Fluorescence in situ hybridization in cervical smears: Detection of numerical aberrations of chromosomes 7, 3 and X and relationship to HPV infection. Gynecol Oncol 75:41, 1999.

Miettinen OS, Henschke CI, Pasmantier MW, et al.: Mammographic screening: no reliable supporting evidence? Lancet 359:404, 2002.

Miki Y, Swensen J, Shattuck-Eidens D, et al.: A strong candidate for the breast and ovarian cancer susceptibility gene BRCA1. Science 266:66, 1994.

Miller BA, Feuer EJ, Hankey BF: The increasing incidence of breast cancer since 1982: Relevance of early detection. Cancer Control 2:67, 1991.

Miller ME, Chatten J: Ovarian changes in ataxia-telangectasia. Acta Paediatr Scand 56:559, 1967.

Mitelman F, Mertens F, Johansson B: A breakpoint map of recurrent chromosomal rearrangements in human neoplasia. Nat Genet 15:417, 1997.

Mitra AB, Murty VV, Li RG, et al.: Allelotype analysis of cervical carcinoma. Cancer Res 15:4481, 1994.

Mettlin C, Jones G, Averette H, et al.: Defining and updating the American Cancer Society Guidelines for the cancer-related checkup, prostate and endometrial cancers. CA Cancer J Clin 43:42, 1993.

Mizuuchi H, Nasim S, Kudo R, et al.: Clinical implications of K-ras mutations in malignant epithelial tumors of the endometrium. Cancer Res 52:2777, 1992.

Moglabey YB, Kircheisen R, Seoud M, et al.: Genetic mapping of a maternal locus responsible for familial hydatidiform moles. Hum Mol Genet 8:667, 1999.

Mohar A, Frias-Mendivil M: Epidemiology of cervical cancer. Cancer Invest 18:584, 2000.

Morrell D, Chase CL, Swift M: Cancers in 44 families with ataxia-telangiectasia. Cancer Genet Cytogenet 50:119, 1990.

Morrell D, Cromartie E, Swift M: Mortality and cancer incidence in 263 patients with ataxia-telangiectasia. J Natl Cancer Inst 77:89, 1986.

Mosgaard BJ, Lidegaard O, Kjaer SK, et al.: Infertility, fertility drugs, and invasive ovarian cancer: A case-control study. Fertil Steril 67:1005, 1997.

Muller CY, O'Boyle JD, Fong KM, et al.: Abnormalities of fragile histidine triad genomic and complementary DNAs in cervical cancer: Association with human papillomavirus type. J Natl Cancer Inst 18:433, 1998.

Munger K, Scheffner M, Huibregtse JM, et al.: Interactions of HPV E6 and E7 oncoproteins with tumour suppressor gene products. Cancer Surv 12:197, 1992.

Murad T, Mancini R, Geroge J: Ultrastructure of a virilizing ovarian Sertoli-Leydig cell. Tumor with familial incidence. Cancer 31:1440, 1973.

Narod SA, Brunet JS, Ghadiran P, et al.: Tamoxifen and risk of contralateral breast cancer in BRCA1 and BRCA2 mutation carriers: A case-control study. N Engl J Med 356:1876, 2000.

Narod S: What options for treatment of hereditary breast cancer. Lancet 359:1451, 2002.

Nelson CL, Sellers TA, Rich SS, et al.: Familial clustering of colon, breast, uterine, and ovarian cancers as assessed by family history. Genet Epidemiol 10:235, 1993.

Neuhausen S, Gilewski T, Norton L, et al.: Recurrent BRCA2 6174delT mutations in Ashkenazi Jewish women affected by breast cancer. Nat Genet 13:126, 1996.

Newlands ES, Paradinas FJ, Fisher RA: Recent advances in gestational trophoblastic disease. Hematol Oncol Clin North Am 13:225, 1999.

Ness RB, Cramer DW, Goodman MT, et al.: Infertility, fertility drugs, and ovarian cancer: a pooled analysis of case-control studies. Am J Epidemiol 155:217, 2002.

Newman B, Austin MA, Lee M, et al.: Inheritance of human breast cancer: Evidence for autosomal dominant transmission in high-risk families. Proc Natl Acad Sci USA 85:3044, 1988.

Nigro JM, Baker SJ, Preisinger AC, et al.: Mutations in the p53 gene occur in diverse human tumour types. Nature 342:705, 1989.

NIH Consensus Development Panel on Ovarian Cancer. Ovarian cancer, treatment, and follow-up. JAMA 273, 1995.

Nowell PC, Hungerford DA: A minute chromosome in human granulocytic leukemia. Science 132:1497, 1960.

O'Brien PK, Wilansky DL: Familial thyroid nodulation and arrhenoblastoma. Am J Clin Pathol 75:578, 1981.

Olsen O, Gøtzsche PC: Cochrane review of screening for breast cancer with mammography. Lancet 358:1340, 2001.

Paradinas FJ: Pathology. In Hancock BW, Newlands ES, Berkowitz RS (eds): Gestational trophoblastic disease. London: Chapman and Hall Medical, 1997, p 43.

Parazzini F, LaVecchia C, Mangili G, et al.: Dietary factors and risk of trophoblastic disease. Am J Obstet Gynecol 158:93, 1989.

Parc YR, Halling KC, Burgart LJ, et al.: Microsatellite instability and hMLH1/hMSH2 expression in young endometrial carcinoma patients: Associations with family history and histopathology. Int J Cancer 86:60, 2000.

Park JG, Vasen HF, Park KJ, et al.: Suspected hereditary nonpolyposis colorectal cancer: International Collaborative Group on Hereditary Colorectal Cancer (ICG-HNPCC) criteria and results of genetic diagnosis. Dis Color Rectum 42:710, 1999.

Park M: Oncogenes. In Scriver CR, Beaudet AL, Sly WS, et al. (eds): The Metabolic and Molecular Basis of Inherited Disease, 8th ed. New York: McGraw-Hill, 2001, p 645.

Park S, Cleaver JE: Postreplication repair: Questions of its definition and possible alteration in xeroderma pigmentosum cell strains. Proc Natl Acad Sci USA 76:3927, 1979.

Park TW, Fujiwara H, Wright TC: Molecular biology of cervical cancer and its precursors. Cancer (Suppl) 76:1902, 1995.

Parker SL, Tong T, Bolden S, et al.: Cancer statistics 1997. CA Cancer J Clin 47:5, 1997.

Phelps WC, Yee CL, Münger K, et al.: The human papillomavirus type 16 E7 gene encodes transactivation and transformation functions similar to those of adenovirus E1A. Cell 53:539, 1998.

Piver M, Hempling RE: Ovarian cancer: Etiology, screening, prophylactic oophorectomy, and surgery. In Rock JA, Thompson JD (eds): Tellinde's Operative Gynecology, 8th ed. Philadelphia: Lippincott-Raven Publishers, 1997, p 1557.

Plattner G, Oxorn H: Familial incidence of ovarian dermoid cysts. Can Med Assoc J 108:892, 1973.

Pritchard K: Breast cancer: The real challenge. Lancet 349:125, 1997.

Propeck PA, Warner T, Scanlan KA: Sebaceous carcinoma of the breast in a patient with Muir-Torre syndrome. Am J Roentgenol 174:541, 2000.

Poujol N, Lobaccaro JM, Chiche L, et al.: Functional and structural analysis of R607Q and R608K androgen receptor substitutions associated with male breast cancer. Mol Cell Endocrinol 130:43, 1997.

Raggio M, Kaplan AL, Harberg JF: Recurrent ovarian fibromas with basal cell nevus syndrome (Gorlin syndrome). Obstet Gynecol 61:95S, 1983.

Rebbeck TR, Lynch HT, Neuhausen SL, et al.: Prophylactic oophorectomy in carriers of BRCA1 or BRCA2 mutations. N Engl J Med 346:1616, 2002.

Rebbeck TR: Prophylactic oophorectomy in BRCA1 and BRCA2 mutation carriers. J Clin Oncol 18(21 Suppl):100S, 2000.

Reynolds TC, Smith SD, Sklar J: Analysis of DNA surrounding the breakpoints of chromosomal translocations involving the beta (T cell receptor) gene in human lymphoblastic neoplasms. Cell 50:107, 1987.

Richards CS, Ward PA, Roa BB, et al.: Screening for 185delAG in the Ashkenazim. Am J Hum Genet 60:1085, 1997.

Ries LAG, Kosary CL, Hankey BF, et al.: SEER Cancer Statistics Review 1973-1994: Tables and Graphs. (HIH Pub 97-2789). Bethesda, MD. National Cancer Institute, 1997.

Rimokh R, Rouault JP, Wahbi K, et al.: A chromosome 12 coding region is juxtaposed to the MYC protooncogene locus in a t(8;12)(q24;q22) translocation in a case of B-cell chronic lymphocytic leukemia. Genes Chromosomes Cancer 3:24, 1991.

Rose PG: Endometrial carcinoma. N Engl J Med 335:640, 1996.

Rossing MA, Daling JR, Weiss NS, et al.: Ovarian tumors in a cohort of infertile women. N Engl J Med 331:771, 1994.

Rous P: A sarcoma of the fowl transmissible by an agent separable from the tumor cells. J Exp Med 13:397, 1911.

Rowley JD: Letter. A new consistent chromosomal abnormality in chronic myelogenous leukemia identified by quinacrine fluorescence and Giemsa staining. Nature 243:290, 1973.

Rubin SC, Benjamin I, Behbakht K, et al.: Clinical and pathological features of ovarian cancer in women with germ-line mutations of BRCA1. N Engl J Med 335:1413, 1996.

Sand PK, Lurain JR, Brewer JI: Repeat gestational trophoblastic disease. Obstet Gynecol 63:140, 1984.

Sandles LG, Shulman LP, Elias S, et al.: Endometrial adenocarcinoma: Genetic analysis suggesting heritable site-specific uterine cancer. Gynecol Oncol 47:167, 1992.

Schildkraut JM, Risch N, Thompson WD: Evaluating genetic association among ovarian, breast, and endometrial cancer: Evidence for a breast/ovarian cancer relationship. Am J Hum Genet 45:521, 1989.

Schrag D, Kuntz KM, Garber JE, et al.: Decision analysis-effects of prophylactic mastectomy and oophorectomy on life expectancy among women with BRCA1 or BRCA2 mutations. N Engl J Med 336:1465, 1997.

Seoud M, Khalil A, Frangieh A, et al.: Recurrent molar pregnancies in a family with extensive intermarriage: Report of a family and review of the literature. Obstet Gynecol 86:692, 1995.

Seracchioli R, Bagnoli A, Colombo FM, et al.: Conservative treatment of recurrent ovarian fibromas in a young patient affected by Gorlin syndrome. Hum Reprod 16:1261, 2001.

Serban AMB, Coivirnache M, Maximillian C: Arrhenoblastoma familial. Rev Roum Embryol Cytol Ser Embryol 5:11, 1968.

Schmid-Braz AT, Cavalli LR, Cornelio DA, et al.: Comprehensive cytogenetic evaluation of a mature ovarian teratoma case. Cancer Genet Cytogenet 132:165, 2002

Shingleton HM, Thompson JD: Cancer of the cervix. In Rock JA, Thompson JD (eds): Telinde's Operative Gynecology, 8th ed. Philadelphia: Lippincott Raven, 1997, p 1413.

Shulman LP, Muram D, Marina N, et al.: Lack of heritability in ovarian germ cell malignancies. Am J Obstet Gynecol 170:6, 1994.

Simard J, Tonin P, Durocher F, et al.: Common origins of BRCA1 mutations in Canadian breast and ovarian cancer families. Nat Genet 8:392, 1994.

Simon A, Ohel G, Neri A, et al.: Familial occurrence of mature ovarian teratomas. Obstet Gynecol 66:278, 1985.

Sippel A: Dermoid of ovary in three sisters. Zentralbl Gynaekol 48:85, 1924.

Smotkin D, Berek JS, Fu YS, et al.: Human papillomavirus deoxyribonucleic acid in adenocarcinoma and adenosquamous carcinoma of the uterine cervix. Obstet Gynecol 68:241, 1986.

Sreekantaiah C, De Braekeleer M, Haas O: Cytogenetic findings in cervical carcinoma. A statistical approach. Cancer Genet Cytogenet 53:75, 1991.

Statement of the American Society of Clinical Oncology: Genetic Testing for Cancer Susceptibility, 2001, http://www.asco.org/prof/pp/html/m_ppgenetc.htm#intro

Stehelin D, Varmus HE, Bishop JM, et al.: DNA related to the transforming gene(s) of avian sarcoma viruses is present in normal avian DNA. Nature 260:170, 1976.

Stettner AR, Hartenbach EM, Schink JC: Familial ovarian germ cell cancer: Report and review. Am J Med Genet 84:43, 1999.

Stewart HL, Durham LH, Casper J, et al.: Epidemiology of cancers of uterine cervix and corpus breast and ovary in Israel and New York City. J Natl Cancer Inst 37:1, 1966.

Stoler MH: A brief synopsis of the role of human papillomaviruses in cervical carcinogenesis. Am J Obstet Gynecol 175:1091, 1996.

Stratton JF, Gayther SA, Russell P, et al.: Contribution of BRCA1 mutations to ovarian cancer. N Engl J Med 336:1125, 1997.

Struewing JP, Abeliovich D, Peretz T, et al.: The carrier frequency of the BRCA1 185delAG mutation is approximately 1% in Ashkenazi Jewish individuals. Nat Genet 11:198, 1995.

Struewing JP, Hartge P, Wacholder S, et al.: The risk of cancer associated with specific mutations of BRCA1 and BRCA2 among Ashkenazi Jews. N Engl J Med 336:1401, 1997.

Swift M: Ataxia-telangiectasia and risk of breast cancer. Lancet 350:740, 1997.

Swift M, Chase CL, Morrell D: Cancer predisposition of ataxia-telangiectasia heterozygotes. Cancer Genet Cytogenet 46:21, 1990.

Swift M, Morrell D, Massey RB, et al.: Incidence of cancer in 161 families affected by ataxia-telangiectasia. N Engl J Med 325:1831, 1991.

Szulman AE: Syndromes of hydatidiform moles: Partial vs. complete. J Reprod Med 29:788, 1984.

Tavtigian SV, Simard J, Rommens J, et al.: The complete BRCA2 gene and mutations in chromosome 13q-linked kindreds. Nat Genet 12:333, 1996.

Thorlacius S, Struewing JP, Hartge P, et al.: Population-based study of risk of breast cancer in carriers of BRCA2 mutation. Lancet 352:1337, 1998.

Tokunaga M, Land CE, Tokuoka S, et al.: Incidence of female breast cancer among atomic bomb survivors, 1950-1985. Radiat Res 138:209, 1994.

Townsend DE, Sparkes RS, Baluda MC, et al.: Unicellular histogenesis of uterine leiomyomas as determined by electrophoresis of glucose-6-phosphate dehydrogenase. Am J Obstet Gynecol 107:1168, 1970.

Tsujimoto Y, Gorham J, Cossman J, et al.: The t(14;18) chromosome translocations involved in B-cell neoplasms result from mistakes in VDJ joining. Science 229:1390, 1985.

Valle VO, Valdez B-G, Valenzuela EA: Fibroma ovarica. Informe de dos casos; incidencia familiar? Ginecol Obstet Mex 65:442, 1997.

Van den Veyver IB, Norman B, Tran CQ, et al.: The human homologue (PEG3) of the mouse paternally expressed gene 3 (Peg3) is maternally imprinted but not mutated in women with familial recurrent hydatidiform molar pregnancies. J Soc Gynecol Investig 8:305, 2001.

Varley JM, Evans DG, Birch JM: Li-Fraumeni syndrome – a molecular and clinical review. Br J Cancer 76:1, 1997.

Vasen HF, Offerhaus GJ, den Hartog Jager FC, et al.: The tumour spectrum in hereditary nonpolyposis colorectal cancer: A study of 24 kindreds in the Netherlands. Int J Cancer 46:31, 1990.

Vasen HFA, Mecklin JP, Kahn PM, et al.: The International Collaborative on hereditary nonpolyposis colorectal cancer. Dis Colon Rectum 34:425, 1991.

Walker GR, Schlesselman JJ, Ness RB: Family history of cancer, oral contraceptive use, and ovarian cancer risk. Am J Obstet Gynecol 186:8, 2002.

Wake N, Seki T, Fujita H, et al.: Malignant potential of homozygous and heterozygous complete moles. Cancer Res 44:1226, 1984.

Warner E, Foulkes W, Goodwin P, et al.: Prevalence and penetrance of BRCA1 and BRCA2 gene mutations in unselected Ashkenazi Jewish women with breast cancer. J Natl Cancer Inst 91:1241, 1999.

Watson P, Lynch HT: Extracolonic cancer in hereditary nonpolyposis colorectal cancer. Cancer 71:677, 1993.

Watson P, Vasen HF, Mecklin JP, et al.: The risk of endometrial cancer in hereditary nonpolyposis colorectal cancer. Am J Med 96:516, 1994.

Werneke U: Ataxia telangiectasia and risk of breast cancer. Lancet 350:739, 1997.

Whitcomb RW, Calkins JW, Lukert BP, et al.: Androblastomas and thyroid disease in postmenopausal sisters. Obstet Gynecol 67:89S, 1986.

Whitmore SE: BRCA1 mutations and survival in women with ovarian cancer. N Engl J Med 336:1254, 1997.

Whittemore AS, Gong G, Itnyre J: Prevalence and contribution of BRCA1 mutations in breast cancer and ovarian cancer: Results from three U.S. population-based case-control studies of ovarian cancer. Am J Hum Genet 60:496, 1997.

Wijnen J, De Leeuw W, Vasen H, et al.: Familial endometrial cancer in female carriers of MSH6 germline mutations. Nat Genet 23:142, 1999.

Wilke CM, Hall BK, Hoge A, et al.: FRA3B extends over a broad region and contains a spontaneous HPV 16 integration site—direct evidence for the coincidence of viral integration sites and fragile sites. Hum Mol Genet 5:187, 1996.

Wolf NG, Lage JM: Genetic analysis of gestational trophoblastic disease: A review. Semin Oncol 22:113, 1995.

Wooster R, Mangion J, Eeles R, et al.: A germline mutation in the androgen receptor gene in two brothers with breast cancer and Reifenstein syndrome. Nat Genet 2:132, 1992.

Wooster R, Neuhausen S, Mangion J, et al.: Localization of a breast cancer susceptibility gene, BRCA2, to chromosome 13q12-13. Science 265:2088, 1994.

Wooster R: Identification of the breast cancer susceptibility gene BRCA2. Nature 378:798, 1995.

Yaginuma Y, Yamashita T, Takuma N, et al.: Analysis of the p53 gene in human choriocarcinoma cell lines. Br J Cancer 71:9, 1995.

Yoshino K, Enomoto T, Nakamura T, et al.: FHIT alterations in cancerous and non-cancerous cervical epithelium. Int J Cancer 1:85, 2000.

Zhang A, Zheng C, Hou M, et al.: Amplification of the telomerase reverse transcriptase (hTERT) gene in cervical carcinomas. Genes Chromosomes Cancer 34:269, 2002.

CHAPTER 10

Disorders of Sex Differentiation: Gonadal Abnormalities and Hypogonadotropic Hypogonadism

The next three chapters delineate genetic aspects of sex chromosomes and sexual differentiation. Clinical management of these disorders is discussed in more detail elsewhere (Simpson and Rebar, 2001). Anomalies limited to the müllerian derivatives were discussed in Chapter 8. In this chapter we first review reproductive embryology and the genetic control of gonadal differentiation. Clinical delineation and etiologic consideration of the disorders of gonadal development follow.

Gonadal and Genital Embryology

Primordial germ cells originate in the endoderm of the yolk sac and migrate to the genital ridge to form the indifferent gonad. 46,XY and 46,XX gonads are initially indistinguishable. Indifferent gonads develop into testes if the embryo, or more specifically the gonadal stroma, is 46,XY (Fig. 10–1). This process begins about 43 days after conception. Testes become morphologically identifiable 7 to 8 weeks after conception (9 to 10 gestational or menstrual weeks).

Sertoli cells are the first cells to become recognizable in testicular differentiation. These cells organize the surrounding cells into tubules. Both Leydig cells (Patsavoudi et al., 1985) and Sertoli cells (Magre and Jost, 1984) function in dissociation from testicular morphogenesis, consistent with these cells directing gonadal development rather than the converse. These two cells secrete hormones that direct subsequent male differentiation (see Fig. 10–1).

Fetal Leydig cells produce an androgen—testosterone—that stabilizes wolffian ducts and permits differentiation of vasa deferentia, epididymides, and seminal vesicles. After conversion of testosterone by 5α-reductase to dihydrotestosterone (DHT), external genitalia are virilized. These actions can be mimicked by the administration of testosterone to female or castrated male embryos, as demonstrated clinically by the existence of teratogenic forms of female pseudohermaphroditism.

Fetal Sertoli cells produce antimüllerian hormone (AMH), also known as müllerian inhibitory substance or MIS. This glycoprotein diffuses locally to cause regression of müllerian derivatives (uterus and fallopian tubes). When AMH is chronically expressed in XX transgenic mice, oocytes fail to persist, tubule-like structures develop in gonads, and müllerian differentiation is abnormal (Behringer et al., 1990). Thus, AMH may have functions related to gonadal development as well. Steroidogenic factor I (Sf-1) appears to regulate AMH, given that lack of Sf-1 in a sex-reversed XY female is still associated with the presence of a uterus (Yu et al., 1998).

In the absence of a Y chromosome, the indifferent gonad develops into an ovary. Transformation into fetal ovaries begins at 50 to 55 days of embryonic development. Whether female (ovarian) differentiation is truly a default (constitutive) pathway or whether a yet to be determined gene product directs primary ovarian differentiation is uncertain. For many years the default hypothesis was favored (Simpson, 1987;

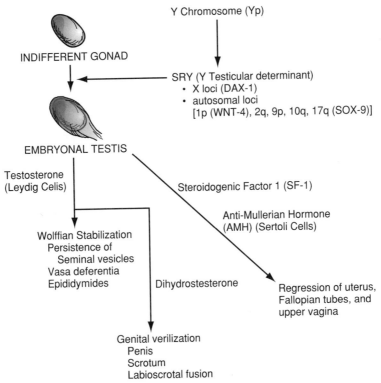

Y Chromosome (Yp)

INDIFFERENT GONAD

SRY (Y Testicular determinant)
• X loci (DAX-1)
• autosomal loci
  [1p (WNT-4), 2q, 9p, 10q, 17q (SOX-9)]

EMBRYONAL TESTIS

Testosterone
(Leydig Cells)

Steroidogenic Factor 1 (SF-1)

Anti-Mullerian Hormone
(AMH) (Sertoli Cells)

Wolffian Stabilization
Persistence of
   Seminal vesicles
   Vasa deferentia
   Epididymides

Dihydrostesterone

Regression of uterus,
Fallopian tubes, and
upper vagina

Genital verilization
Penis
Scrotum
Labioscrotal fusion

FIGURE 10–1 • Male embryology.

German, 1988). More recently, a primary directive role in ovarian differentiation has been proposed, involving DAX1 (also known as AHC) (see further on). However, it now seems unlikely that DAX1 (or at least its mouse homolog, Ahch) plays a role as a primary ovarian determinant. Nevertheless, germ cells are present in 45,X embryos (Jirásek, 1976), only to undergo atresia at a rate more rapid than that occurring in normal 46,XX embryos. Pathogenesis involves not only failure of germ cell formation but also increased atresia.

Internal ductal and external genital development are secondary to but independent of gonadal differentiation. In the absence of testosterone and AMH, external genitalia develop in female fashion (Fig. 10–2). Müllerian ducts form the uterus and fallopian tubes, and wolffian ducts regress. This scenario occurs in normal XX embryos as well as in XY embryos (animals) castrated before testicular differentiation.

Genetic Basis of Testicular Differentiation

Over 20 years ago, individuals with 46,X,i(Xq) were recognized as female in appearance. The assumption was made that the major testicular determinants (now called testis-determining factor or TDF) were located on the Y short arm (Y).

The key gene is now known to be SRY (sex determining region Y) (Fig. 10–3). Pivotal to this elucidation was its location in the Xp/Yp pseudoautosomal region (PAR), one of three regions of X-Y homology (Fig. 10–4). Crossing-over proximal in the PAR is expected. Crossing over beyond PAR and distal to SRY results in an X containing SRY and a Y lacking SRY (Fig. 10–5). Nested hierarchal analysis thus could lead to identification of SRY as TDF (Table 10–1). Several earlier candidate genes (e.g., ZFY) are closer to the centromere. Like SRY, these genes may often be interchanged in XY or XX sex reversal, but cases exist in which only SRY and not ZFY is disturbed.

The SRY gene consists of two open reading frames, 99 and 273 amino acids in length. The key sequence involves an HMG (High Mobility Group) box encompassing codons 13–82. This domain box shares characteristics in common with other DNA-binding sequences. The HMG box is the pivotal region. Approximately 10 to 15% of sporadic XY gonadal dysgenesis cases (XY females) show point mutations involving

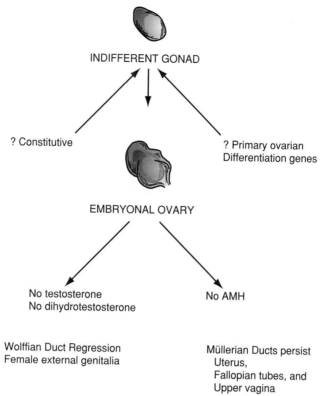

FIGURE 10–2 • Female embryology.

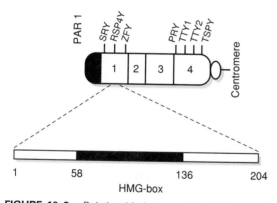

FIGURE 10–3 • Relationship between the *SRY* gene, the pseudoautosomal dominant region (PAR1), and other Yp genes. *SRY* and in particular the HMG box contains mutations responsible for 10 to 15% of cases of XY gonadal dysgensis. (From McElreavey K, Fellous M: Sex determination and the Y chromosome. *In* Seminars in Medical Genetics. Am J Med Genet 89:176, 1999.)

SRY (Pivnick et al., 1992; Cameron and Sinclair, 1997; McElreavey and Fellous, 1999). When this occurs, perturbation almost always occurs within the HMG box (see Fig. 10–3). Rarely, mutations are recognized in other regions of *SRY* (Tajima et al., 1994; Veitia et al., 1997; Brown et

al., 1998), upstream to *SRY* (McElreavey et al., 1992), or downstream to *SRY* (McElreavey et al., 1996).

SRY fulfills the key requirements for testes differentiation. Expression occurs before testicular differentiation is manifested (Gubbay et al., 1991). Transgenic XX mice with *SRY* predictably show testicular differentiation (Koopman et al., 1991). The exact function of *SRY* remains unclear at the cellular level (McElreavey and Fellous, 1999; Ostrer, 2000), but *SRY* binds DNA at a consensus sequence (AATAAC) in all species. The role of *SRY* in testes differentiation could involve DNA bending (Giese et al., 1994), presumably to juxtapose more than one testicular-determining gene and, hence, to facilitate transcription or interaction of certain gene products. The full answer may not be forthcoming until simultaneous analysis of multiple expressed proteins is undertaken in single cells (expression profiling, perhaps using cDNA microarrays).

It is fashionable to propose unifying hypotheses explaining interrelationships between *SRY* and the various autosomal and X loci that seem to play roles in testicular differentiation. For example, plausible scenarios are offered by Ostrer (2000) and by McElreavey and Fellous

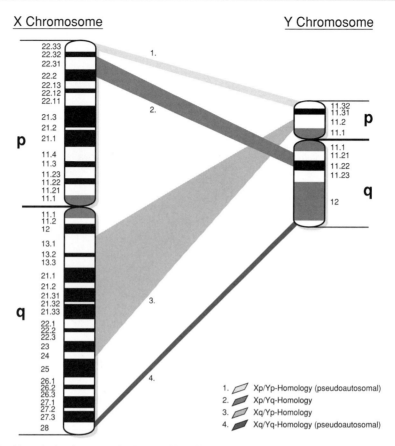

FIGURE 10–4 • Homologies between the human X and Y chromosomes. (From Vogel F, Motulsky AG: Human Genetics—Problems and Approaches, 3rd ed. Berlin: Springer-Verlag, 1997.)

(1999). In one attractive scenario *SRY* directly represses *DAX1*, an X locus, otherwise presumed capable of directing ovarian development. The underlying rationale is that in XY humans duplication of Xp and, hence, *DAX1* may be associated with ovaries. If *DAX1* is duplicated, perhaps *SRY* cannot fully exert its normal action of inducing testicular differentiation. *DAX1* could act as a result of regulation by WNT-4, a locally acting growth factor located on 1p53. Duplication of 1p and overexpression of WNT-4 resulted in upregulation of *DAX1* in a sex-reversed XY female (Jordan et al., 2001).

In another scenario the pivotal gene is near or consonant with *SOX9* and the campomelic dysplasia (CD) locus. *SOX9* has two activation domains, suggesting the ability to upregulate other genes (McDowall et al., 1999). Deletion of *SOX9* is responsible for campomelic dysplasia and XY gonadal dysgenesis (sex reversal). Conversely, duplication of 17q23.1 → q24.3, where *SOX9* is localized, results in a 46,XX individual's having bilateral scrotal gonads (pre-

sumptive testes), a small male phallus, and a perineal urethral orifice (i.e., an incompletely sex-reversed XX male) (Huang et al., 1999). Similarly, insertional mutagenesis (deletion) involving *SOX9* leads to XX mice having testes (Bishop et al., 2000). A logical deduction is that *SRY* normally derepresses a locus, which then will permit testicular differentiation (Fig. 10–6). The insertional mutation uncovered by Bishop and coworkers (2000) was presumed to lead to unscheduled derepression, thus resulting in XX mice differentiating testes. Vidal and colleagues (2001) created XX transgenic mice that ectopically expressed *SOX9*. Testes resulted despite absence of *Sry*, leading the authors to propose *SRY* as merely a molecular switch to initiate *SOX9* (the primary testes determinant).

Still other autosomal regions are important for testicular differentiation. The relationship of these genes or regions to *SRY* is even less clear, and in some cases only circumstantial reasons point to these genes as necessary for the indifferent gonad to differentiate into the testes. Autosomal regions that preclude testicular development when *deleted*

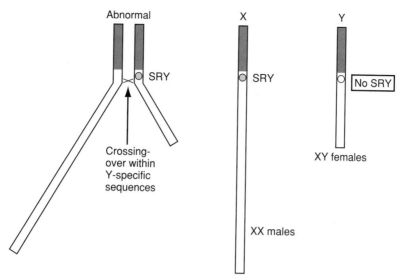

FIGURE 10–5 • X-Y interchange restricted to the Yp/Yp pseudoautosomal region (PAR) (shaded) would not perturb sexual differentiation, whereas more proximal crossing-over would involve Y-specific sequences that yield XX males with *SRY* and XY females without *SRY*. Pseudoautosomal regions also exist between Yp and Xq as well as between Yq and Xq. (From Passarge E: Color Atlas of Genetics. New York: Thieme Medical Publishers, Inc., 1995.)

include 9p24.3 (a region that encodes DMRT) (Ottolenghi and McElreavey, 2000), 10q26 (a region that encompasses *SF-1*) (Veitia et al., 1998; Waggoner et al., 1999), and 11p (a region that encodes *WT-1*) (Slavotinek et al., 1999), and 2q33. Duplication of 1p is also associated with

▼ **Table 10–1.** AN ILLUSTRATIVE EARLY (1986)
• STUDY ILLUSTRATING THE PRINCIPLE OF LOCALIZING THE TESTIS DETERMINING FACTOR BY HIERARCHICAL ANALYSIS FOR THE PRESENCE OR ABSENCE OF CLONED DNA SEQUENCES IN XX AND XY MALES

		DNA Sequences (Probe)			
		DXYS5 (47)	DXYS7 (13d)	DXYS8 (118)	DXYS1 (DP34)	Interval
Diagnosis	N					
XX Male	7	–	–	–	–	
XX Male	1	+	–	–	–	1
XX Male	6	+	+	–	–	2
XX Male	5	+	+	+	–	3
XY Male (Control)	5	+	+	+	+	4

Interpretation: Interval 3 is never present without interval 2, nor is 2 present without 1. Thus, testis-determining factor lies closer to interval 1 than to other intervals. None of these clones corresponded to the testis determinant, however, because some XX males lack (N = 7) interval 1. Later testis-determining factor was localized to a small (140 kb) portion of interval 1 (interval 1B) and proved to be *SRY*.

+, present; –, absent
Data from Vergnaud G, Page DC, Simmler MC, et al.: A deletion map of the human Y based on DNA hybridization. Am J Hum Genet 38:109, 1986.

XY sex reversal (Wieacker et al., 1996), as is 17q, as noted above.

In mice additional gene knockouts produce other gonadal perturbations, pointing to potential roles for homologous human genes: *Emx2* (Miyamoto et al., 1997) and *M33* (Duggan et al., 1999). Microarrays showing differential expression of cDNAs between male and female embryos point to the importance of other genes, like *Nexia-1* and *Vamia-I* (Grimmond et al., 2000).

Less specific but no less compelling evidence for autosomal control over testicular development is the occurrence of testicular differentiation in 46,XX true hermaphrodites, and in other heritable syndromes that deleteriously affect testicular differentiation: agonadism (de Grouchy et al., 1985), rudimentary testes syndrome (Najjar et al., 1974), and the occurrence of germ cell hypoplasia in both males (germinal cell aplasia) and female sibs (streak gonads) (Hamet et al., 1973, Smith et al., 1979; Granat et al., 1983; Al-Awadi et al., 1985; Mikati et al., 1985). Genes responsible for these disorders have not been identified.

In summary, *SOX9*, *DAX1*, and perhaps other autosomal genes interact with *SRY* to orchestrate testicular differentiation. *SRY* may represses *DAX1* and derepress *SOX9*. Other genes connoted by syndromes or chromosomal deletions or duplications could act downstream of SRY; their perturbation may lead to XY females, but the action of the gene need not be primary for testicular differentiation. A key autosomal gene

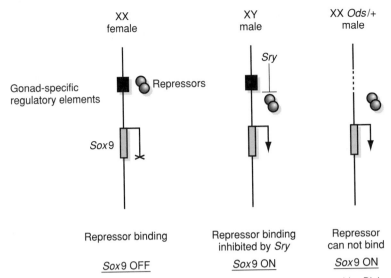

XX
female

XY
male

XX *Ods*/+
male

Sry

Gonad-specific
regulatory elements

Repressors

*Sox*9

Repressor binding

Repressor binding
inhibited by *Sry*

Repressor
can not bind

*Sox*9 OFF

*Sox*9 ON

*Sox*9 ON

FIGURE 10–6 • A double-repressor model of mammalian sex determination proposed by Bishop and colleagues (2000), based on an insertional mutation that resulted in XX mice expressing testes. Initially *Sox9* is expressed in the genital ridges of both male and female embryos. Expression is proposed to be mediated by a genital ridge–specific enhancer located upstream or downstream of *Sox9* (not shown). In wild-type XX gonads (left), *Sox9* expression is downregulated (*Sox9* OFF) by the binding of a repressor or repressor complex to gonad-specific regulatory elements (filled box) located –1.3 Mb (upstream) of *SOX9*. In the middle figure, one repressor binding is predicted to be antagonized by *Sry* protein, leading normally to upregulation of *Sox9* expression, Sertoli-cell differentiation, and testis formation (*Sox9* ON). In the XX odd sex/ods+ gonads (right), *Sox9* cannot be repressed because the gonad-specific elements for repressor binding have been deleted. As a result, *Sox9* is expressed and testes are induced despite lack of a Y. (From Bishop CE, Whitworth DJ, Qin Yi, et al.: A transgenic upstream of *SOX9* is associated with dominant XX sex reversal in the mouse. Nat Genet 26:490, 2000.)

may be perturbed in XX true hermaphrodites, and once elucidated could also be pivotal.

Yq and Spermatogenesis

Genes on the Y long arm are important for spermatogenesis. About 15% of azoospermic men have minute deletions, and about 5 to 10% of oligospermic men have such deletions. These genes are important in the evaluation of male infertility.

The most popular model assumes at least three Yq *AZF* loci (Fig. 10–7). Deletion of AZFa is the rarest, associated with absence of spermatogene-

sis and stem cells. Deletion of AZFb shows maturational arrest and corresponds to the locus RNA-Binding Motif (*RBM*). If AZFc is deleted, azoospermia and oligospermia occur. AZFc contains the locus *DAZ* (Deleted in Azoospermia). Despite severe oligospermia, males with DAZ deletions can achieve pregnancy through intracytoplasmic sperm injection (ICSI). In these pregnancies, the Yq deletion is transmitted to all males but none of the females (Page et al., 1999); phenotypical aberrations other than spermatogenesis have not been observed. However, the size of the deletion may differ between generations (expansion or deletion).

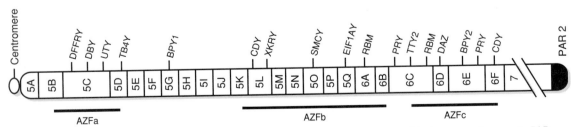

FIGURE 10–7 • Diagram showing location of Yq genes (*AZFa, AZFb, AZFc*) responsible for spermatogenesis. PAR = pseudoautosomal region (see Figure 10–4). (Modified from McElreavey K, Fellous M: Sex determination and the Y chromosome. AZFc corresponds to DAZ. Am J Med Genet 89:176, 1999.)

Other Yq Genes

Loss of the fluorescent and presumably contiguous nonfluorescent portion of Yq was first reported by Lukusa and coworkers (1986) to protect against the anticipated germ cell neoplasia in XY females. XY females with deletion of Yq failed to develop neoplasia as predicted (see below), whereas those with an intact Y did. Page (1987) proposed that the protective locus in this region be termed gonadoblastoma Y (GBY); its wild type function was postulated to affect spermatogenesis. A relationship (or identity) between the locus described by Lukusa and associates (1986) and that claimed responsible for cell growth (CGY or TSY) was proposed by Simpson (1988).

Lau (1999) noted that the exact location of GBY on the Y short arm or proximal Yq (intervals 4-6) has remained elusive. This has led to speculation that more than one GBY locus exists (Tsuchiya et al., 1995). Perhaps the most attractive candidate gene is *TSPY*, a multicopy gene located in interval 3 (Vogt et al., 1997). This gene is upregulated in gonadoblastoma tissue (Tsuchiya et al., 1995) and normally expressed in spermatogenia cells in normal testes (Schnieders et al., 1996).

The cytologic origin probably involves interchange between Xq and Yq (McElreavey and Cortes, 2001) (see Fig. 10–4).

Genetic Basis of Ovarian Differentiation

In the absence of a Y chromosome, the indifferent gonad develops into an ovary (see Fig. 10–2). Given that germ cells exist in 45,X human fetuses (Jirasék, 1976) and 39,X mice, the pathogenesis of germ cell failure clearly involves increased germ cell attrition. That is, germ cells form in monosomy X but fail to persist. If two intact X chromosomes are not present, 45,X ovarian follicles usually degenerate by birth. The second X chromosome is therefore accepted as responsible for ovarian *maintenance* as opposed to primary ovarian *differentiation*.

A topic of longstanding interest is whether primary ovarian differentiation requires a specific gene or merely occurs as the default pathway (constitutive) in the absence of *SRY* and its accompanying testicular determinants (downstream and upstream). *DAX1* has been proposed as a primary ovarian differentiation gene. When duplicated, a region of Xp(21) redirects 46,XY embryos into female differentiation (Bardoni et al., 1994). This region contains the locus AHC (Adrenal Hypoplasia Congenital), which encompasses or is identical to *DAX1* (Dosage Sensitive Sex Reversal/Adrenal hypoplasia critical region X); the mouse homolog is *Ahch*. Could this region play a primary role in ovarian differentiation in 46,XX individuals? As predicted, if *Ahch* (*DAX1*) were to play a pivotal role in primary ovarian differentiation, *Ahch* is upregulated in the XX mouse ovary. Transgenic XY mice overexpressing *Ahch* develop as females, at least in the presence of a relatively weak *Sry*. However, in XX mice lacking *Ahch* (knockout), ovarian differentiation is surprisingly not impaired, nor is ovulation or fertility (Yu et al., 1998). Further, XY mice mutant for *Ahch* unexpectedly show testicular germ cell defects. Thus, *Ahch* cannot be responsible for primary ovarian differentiation in mice, nor presumably is *DAX1* (AHC) in humans.

In conclusion, no evidence remains that primary ovarian differentiations occurs other than passively (constitutive). Loci on the X chromosome might serve to maintain germ cells, preventing premature attrition. Ovarian maintenance genes must exist on several locations on both Xp and Xq, as is detailed later in this chapter. In addition, various autosomal genes must remain intact for normal ovarian development. Some of these genes have been identified, and others can be deduced by the many disorders characterized by ovarian failure in 46,XX individuals.

Ovarian Failure Due to Monosomy X (Turner Syndrome)

The term historically applied to women with ovarian failure is gonadal dysgenesis or Turner syndrome. Unfortunately, Turner syndrome connotes different features to different physicians and investigators. In this chapter, the term gonadal dysgenesis is applied to women with streak gonads; Turner stigmata are reserved for those with short stature and certain somatic anomalies (Table 10–2). By themselves, Turner stigmata would not imply the presence of streak gonads. The term *Turner syndrome* is limited to those individuals with streak gonads, Turner stigmata, and a 45,X or X-deletion complement.

In 80% of 45,X cases the X is maternal (Xm), and in 20% the remaining X is paternal (Xp) in origin (Cockwell et al., 1991; Mathur et al., 1991).

▼ **Table 10–2.** SOMATIC FEATURES
• ASSOCIATED WITH THE 45,X
  CHROMOSOMAL COMPLEMENT

Growth
  Decreased birth weight
  Decreased adult height (141 to 146 cm)
Intellectual function
  Verbal IQ > performance IQ
  Cognitive deficits (space-form blindness)
  Immature personality, probably secondary to short
    stature
Cranofacial
  Premature fusion of spheno-occipital and other sutures,
    producing brachycephaly
  Abnormal pinnae
  Retruded mandible
  Epicanthal folds (25%)
  High-arched palate (36%)
  Abnormal dentition
  Visual anomalies, usually strabismus (22%)
  Auditory deficits; sensorineural or secondary to middle
    ear infection
Neck
  Pterygium colli (46%)
  Short, broad neck (74%)
  Low nuchal hair (71%)
Chest
  Rectangular contour (shield chest) (35%)
  Widely spaced nipples
  Tapered lateral ends of clavicle
Cardiovascular
  Coarctation of aorta or ventricular septal defect
    (10 to 16%)
Renal (38%)
  Horseshoe kidneys
  Unilateral renal aplasia
  Duplication ureters
Gastrointestinal
  Telangiectasias
Skin and lymphatics
  Pigmented nevi (63%)
  Lymphadema (38%) due to hypoplastic superficial
    vessels
Nails
  Hypoplasia and malformation (66%)
Skeletal
  Cubitus valgus (54%)
  Radial tilt of articular surface of trochlear surface
  Clinodactyly V
  Short metacarpals, usually IV (48%)
  Decreased carpal arch (mean angle 117 degrees)
  Deformities of medial tibial condyle
Dermatoglyphics
  Increased total digital ridge count
  Increased distance between palmar triradii a and b
  Distal axial triradius in position t'

MONOSOMY X

Gonads

In most 45,X adults with gonadal dysgenesis, the normal gonad is replaced by a white fibrous streak, 2 to 3 cm long and about 0.5 cm wide, located in the position ordinarily occupied by the ovary (Fig. 10–8). A streak gonad is characterized histologically by interfacing waves of dense fibrous stroma that are indistinguishable from normal ovarian stroma (Fig. 10–9). As already stated, germ cells are usually absent in 45,X adults yet present in 45,X embryos (Jirasék, 1976). Thus, the pathogenesis of germ cell failure is increased atresia, not failure of germ cell formation. This is relevant to clinical management.

That adult 45,X individuals develop streak gonads is not so obvious as might be expected given that relatively normal ovarian development occurs in many other mammals (e.g., mice) with monosomy X. Likely explanations for why normal 46,XX females do not develop streak gonads include the idea that pivotal genes on the normal heterochromatic (inactive) X are not inactivated. Alternatively, pivotal loci could be reactivated in oocytes, or oocytes alone could be spared X-inactivation (Gartler et al., 1972).

Lack of normal ovarian development predictably leads to deficient secretion of sex steroids. Estrogen and androgen levels are decreased; follicle-stimulating hormone (FSH) and luteinizing hormone (LH) levels are increased. Estrogen-dependent processes show effects predictable for hormonal deficiency. At puberty, pubic and axillary hair fail to develop (Fig. 10–10). Breasts contain little parenchymal tissue; areolar tissue is only slightly darker than the surrounding skin; external genitalia, vagina, and müllerian derivates are well differentiated but remain small (unstimulated).

Although streak gonads are usually present in 45,X individuals, about 3% of adult patients menstruate spontaneously (at least twice), and 5% show breast development (Table 10–2). Occasionally the interval between menstrual periods is almost normal in 45,X patients, and a few fertile patients have been reported. Undetected 46,XX cells (i.e., 45,X/46,XX mosaicism) should be suspected in menstruating 45,X patients; however, it is plausible that a few 45,X individuals could be fertile, inasmuch as germ cells are present in 45,X embryos. In addition, pregnancy can occasionally be achieved in hypergonadotropic women by sequential gonadotropin suppression followed by ovulation induction. Check and coworkers (1990) induced ovulation in 5% of 361 cycles in 100 hypergonadotropic women; the chromosomal complements of the women were not stated.

Infertility therapy for 45,X women usually involves hormone therapy (estrogen and cyclic progestogens) to produce normal uterine size, followed by assisted reproductive technology (ART). The process involves a partner's sperm being

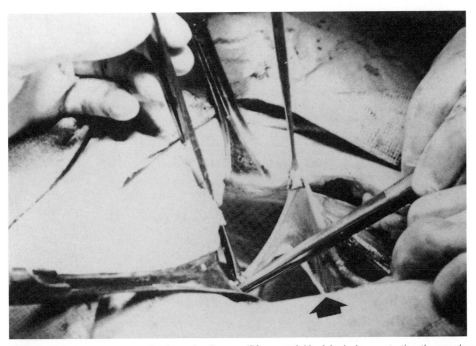

FIGURE 10–8 • Photograph taken at the time of celiotomy (Pfannenstiel incision), demonstrating the usual appearance of a streak gonad (arrow). The clamp is elevating a fallopian tube. This particular individual had XY gonadal dysgenesis, but the appearance of a streak gonad would have been almost identical in most 45,X individuals. (From Simpson JL: Disorders of Sexual Differentiation: Etiology and Clinical Delineation. New York: Academic Press, 1976.)

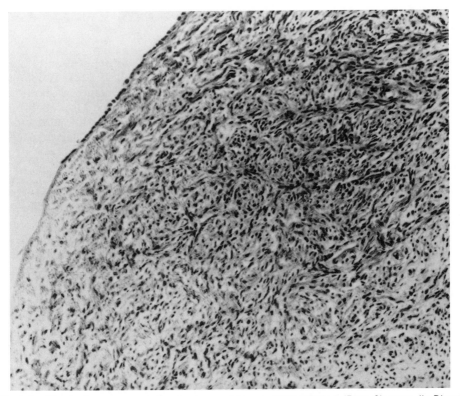

FIGURE 10–9 • Histologic appearance of a streak gonad from a 45,X individual. (From Simpson JL: Disorders of Sexual Differentiation: Etiology and Clinical Delineation. New York: Academic Press, 1976.)

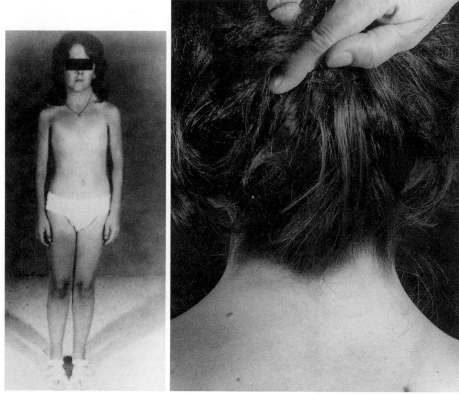

A　　　　　　　　　　　　　　　　　　　　　　　　　　　　　B

FIGURE 10–10 • Photograph of a 45,X individual (*A*). This 140-cm patient had no secondary sexual development and several somatic anomalies consisting of the Turner stigmata: webbing of the neck, low nuchal hair line, and pigmented nevi (*B*). (From Simpson JL: Disorders of Sexual Differentiation: Etiology and Clinical Delineation. New York: Academic Press, 1976.)

mixed with ova donated from another woman, fertilization *in vitro*, and transfer of the embryo to the uterus of the hormonally synchronized 45,X patient. This technique is well established, and the overall success rate (clinical pregnancies) is over 20% per cycle. Foudila and colleagues (1999) reported 20 clinical pregnancies among 18 women with Turner syndrome; the exact chromosomal complements were not stated. Clinical pregnancy rate per fresh embryo transferred was 46% (13/28); however, 7 of the 13 (54%) pregnancies resulted in spontaneous abortions. Among transferred frozen embryos, the respective rates were 28% (7/25) and 14% (1/7). Consistent results, although with lower pregnancy rates, were reported by Khastgir and coworkers (1997) and Tarani and coworkers (1998). Before embarking on such a clinical regime, the ability of a given 45,X woman to carry her pregnancy successfully must be addressed. Specifically, women with coarctation of the aorta (see next section) may be unsuitable candidates.

Offspring of 45,X women are probably at little, if any, increased risk for chromosomal abnormalities (Dewhurst, 1978; Simpson, 1981),

intuitive deductions and claims notwithstanding (Chen and Woolley, 1971; Brook et al., 1973). The increased spontaneous abortion rate noted after donor oocyte ART probably reflects hormonal dysfunction or uterine factors (hypoplasia) rather than transmission of aneuploid (monosomic) gametes.

SOMATIC ANOMALIES

45,X individuals are not only short (less than 4 feet, 10 inches) but often exhibit various somatic anomalies (Turner stigmata) (see Table 10–2). No single feature or features of the Turner stigmata are pathognomonic, although in aggregate a characteristic spectrum exists that is more likely to occur in 45,X individuals than in individuals with most other sex chromosomal abnormalities. Assessing renal, vertebral, cardiac, and auditory functions is therefore obligatory.

The region of the X responsible for protecting against these anomalies is unclear, but it is not necessarily the same as that for ovarian maintenance. The distal X short arm has in particular been implicated in somatic development. Another pseudoautosomal gene implicated in somatic development and short stature (Turner stigmata) is *SHOX*, like *RPS4X* a pseudoautosomal locus not subject to inactivation. Zinn and colleagues (1998) and Zinn and Ross (2001) correlated somatic anomalies with Xp perturbations, using molecular markers to characterize deletions and X/autosomal translocation. High-arched palate, short stature, and autoimmune thyroid disease were associated with terminal deletions of Xp11.2-22.1, the same large region noted to contain ovarian determinants. Especially informative was an interstitial deletion in the above region, observed in a 31-year-old woman with premature ovarian failure (POF) and short stature (Zinn et al., 1998). Bioné and Toniolo (2000) have also discussed candidate genes on Xp and Xq that could be important for ovarian and somatic differentiation.

GROWTH

45,X neonates have decreased birth weight (Chen and Woolley, 1971). Total body length at birth is less than normal but often close to the 50th percentile. Height velocity before puberty generally is in the 10th to 15th percentile (Brook et al., 1973), and the mean height of 45,X adults (≥ 16 years old) is between 141 and 146 cm (Simpson, 1975; Ranke et al., 1983), perhaps 20 cm less than normal. Normally, the predicted adult height in females can be estimated by taking the sum of the heights of both parents, dividing by 2, and subtracting 13 cm (for females) (Tanner et al., 1970). After taking into account decreased expected height for 45,X individuals, correlation of an offspring's height with midparental height holds for Turner syndrome as it does for 46,XX females (Brook et al., 1977). That is, the absolute predicted height in Turner syndrome is less but the midparental height correlation still holds.

Various treatments for short stature in 45,X patients have been proposed: growth hormone, anabolic steroids, low-dose estrogens (Ranke et al., 1987). All these treatment regimens show ostensible benefit, especially immediately after onset of therapy. Effect on ultimate height is less certain, but the consensus has evolved that final height can be increased by 6 to 8 cm (Rosenfeld and Grumbach, 1990). Pediatric endocrinologists favor use of human recombinant DNA-derived human growth hormone. Growth hormone therapy in a heterogeneous group (various karyotypes) of clinical Turner syndrome patients resulted in a 8.4 ± 4.5 cm increase in height over that predicted; final height was 150.4 ± 5.5 cm (Rosenfeld et al., 1998). With growth hormone and oxandrolone, the increase was 10.3 ± 4.7 cm. Early initiation of therapy at a recommended dose of 0.375 mg/kg/week is believed to produce the best outcome (Rosenfeld et al., 1998). Details on treatment regimes are discussed in standard pediatric endocrinologic treatises (e.g., Grumbach and Conte, 1998).

One reason for limited efficacy of growth hormone treatment may be that epiphyses in 45,X individuals are structurally abnormal. Not only long bones but teeth and skulls are abnormal as well (Filippson et al., 1965; Lindstein et al., 1969). Thus, patients with a 45,X chromosomal complement could be said to have a skeletal dysplasia.

INTELLIGENCE

Most 45,X patients are normal in intelligence, but any given 45,X patient has a higher probability of being retarded than a 46,XX person (Simpson, 1975). Performance IQ is lower than verbal IQ, the latter being similar to that of 46,XX matched controls. 45,X individuals often have a cognitive defect characterized by poor spatial processing skills (space-form blindness). Ross and coworkers (2000) believe that only loss of distal Xp (Xp 22.33) produces this phenotype; neurocognitive deficits were believed to be independent of statural or ovarian abnormalities.

Psychosocial deficits primarily involve behavorial immaturity and difficulties in social relationships. These are probably secondary to delayed sexual development and statural growth (McCauley et al., 1986, 1987).

ADULT-ONSET DISEASES

Many adult-onset disorders occur in 45,X cases, more so than expected in the general population. Hypertension deserves special comment, for this is present in about one third of adult 45,X individuals. Hypertension need not alter hormonal therapy, but close monitoring is required and exogenous estrogen therapy may need to be reduced. Frequencies of diabetes mellitus and autoimmune thyroiditis are increased.

45,X/46,XX AND 45,X/47,XXX MOSAICISM

If nondisjunction or anaphase lag occurs in the zygote or embryo, two or more cell lines may result; this phenomenon of mosaicism was discussed in Chapter 1 (see Fig. 1–15). The final chromosomal complement depends on the stage at which abnormal cell division occurs and the types of daughter cells that survive after the abnormal cell division (nondisjunction). Ability to recognize mosaicism depends on the number of cells analyzed per tissue and the number of tissues analyzed (Simpson, 1976). Counting 50 cells without detecting one nonmodal cell excludes ($P<0.005$) mosaicism for a minority line of 10% or more (Ford, 1969). The common practice of counting 20 cells carries a probability of 0.122 for failing to detect at least one cell representing a minority cell line of 10% frequency. With 50 cells, probability would be only 0.005 for failing to detect a 10% minority line. If the minority cell line were 30% in frequency, the probability would be 0.001 counting 20 cells are counted (Ford, 1969).

The most common form of mosaicism associated with gonadal dysgenesis is 45,X/46,XX. 45,X/46,XX individuals show fewer anomalies than 45,X individuals. Twelve percent of 45,X/46,XX individuals menstruate compared with only 3% of 45,X individuals (Simpson, 1975). Of 45,X/46,XX individuals, 18% undergo breast development compared with 5% of 45,X individuals. Mean adult height is greater in 45,X/46,XX than in 45,X individuals; more mosaic (25%) than nonmosaic (5%) patients reach adult heights greater than 162 cm (Simpson, 1975). Somatic anomalies are less likely to exist in 45,X/46,XX than in 45,X individuals. Huang et al. (2002) followed up 17 45,X/46,XX cases ascertained at amniocentesis; 5 were terminated and 3 lost to follow-up. Of the 8 liveborns, 2 had features of "Turner syndrome" at birth. Sybert (2002) followed cases of 45,X/46,XX in their own clinic and cases published by others. The author concluded that 34% had spontaneous menses, 61% short stature (< 3rd percentile).

In Sybert's review and analysis (Sybert, 2002) spontaneous menstruation occurred in 34–57% (depending on whether mode of ascertainment was in her clinic or from published reports, respectively); frequency of short stature (< 3rd percentile) was 45% (5/11) and 87% (7/8); fertility occured in 14% (1/7) and 69% (9/13). Less common but phenotypically similar to 45,X/46,XX individuals is 45,X/47,XXX. 45,X/46,XY individuals may also show bilateral streak gonads; however, they often show a unilateral streak gonad and a contralateral dysgenetic testis (mixed gonadal dysgenesis); this is discussed further under male pseudohermaphroditism (see Chapter 11).

X Short Arm Deletions and Ovarian Failure

46,X,DEL(Xp) OR 45,X/46,X, DEL(Xp) DELETIONS

Deletions of the short arm of the X chromosome show variable phenotype, depending upon the amount of Xp persisting (Fig. 10–11). The most common break point for terminal deletions is Xp 11.2→11.4 (see Fig. 10–10). In 46,X, del(X)(p11) only proximal Xp remains; the del(Xp) chromosome appears acrocentric or telocentric. Chromosomes characterized by progressively more distal (telomeric) break points have been reported: Xp21, 22.1, 22.2, 22.3. Sequencing and analysis with polymorphic DNA markers should allow precise determinations of break points in X-deletions, but relatively few molecular studies have

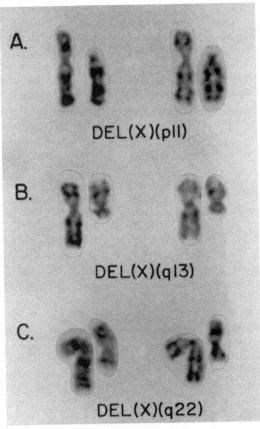

FIGURE 10–11 • A normal X chromosome and deletions of the X chromosome derived from three different persons. (From Simpson JL, LeBeau MM: Gonadal and statural determinants on the X chromosome and their relationship to in vitro studies showing prolonged cell cycles in 45,X;46,Xdel(X)(p11); 46,X,del(X)(q13) and (q22) fibroblasts. Am J Obstet Gynecol 141:930, 1981.)

▼ **Table 10–3.** OVARIAN FUNCTION AS TABULATED ON THE BASIS OF CASES REVIEWED BY
• OGATO AND MATSUO (1995)

	Percentage Complete Ovarian Failure	Percentage Partial Ovarian Failure	Percentage Normal Ovarian Failure
	(Primary Amenorrhea or Streak Gonads)	(Secondary Amenorrhea or Abnormal Menses)	(Presumed)
X Monosomy (45,X)	88	12	0
X Short-Arm Deficiency (Xp)			
del (X)(p11)	50	45	5
del (X)(p21–22.2)	13	25	62
del (X)(p22.3)	0	0	100
i(Xq)	91	9	0
idic(Xq)	80	20	0
X Long-Arm Deficiency (Xq)			
del(X)(q13–21)	69	31	0
del(X)(q22–25)	31	56	13
del(X)(q26–28)	8	67	25
idic(Xp)	73	27	0

The data of Ogato and Matsuo constitute the first two columns. The last column presumes that the remainder of cases had normal ovarian function [e.g., 5% in del(X)(p11)].

been reported (Tharapel et al., 1993; Zinn et al., 1998; Davison et al., 2000; Zinn and Ross, 2001).

Approximately half the reported 46,X,del(Xp) (p11) individuals show primary amenorrhea and gonadal dysgenesis. Others menstruate and show breast development. In a tabulation made 15 years ago, 12 of 27 reported del(X) (p11.2→11.4) individuals menstruated spontaneously; however, menstruation was rarely normal (Simpson, 1987). Similar analysis was later performed by Ogata and Matsuo (1995),

Zinn and coworkers (1998), and by one of the authors (Simpson 1998, 2000; Simpson and Rajkovic, 1999). None of these compilations has materially altered the fundamental conclusions made over a decade ago concerning location of key determinants (Simpson, 1997; Zinn et al., 1998; Zinn and Ross, 2001). Ogata and Matsuo (1995) estimate that 50% of del(Xp11) cases display primary amenorrhea and 45% show secondary amenorrhea (Table 10–3). Figure 10–12 shows our updated compilation of reported cases.

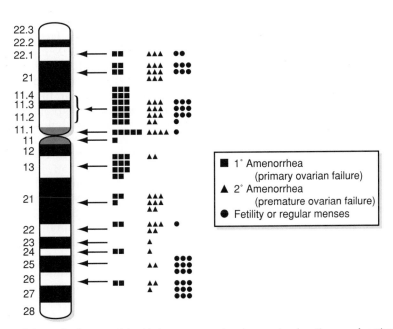

FIGURE 10–12 • Schematic diagram of the X chromosome showing ovarian function as a function of nonmosaic terminal deletions. (From Simpson JL, Rajkovic A: Ovarian differentiation and gonadal failure. Am J Med Genet 89:186, 1999.)

Ovarian development occurs more often in 46,X, del(Xp11) than in 45,X. Women with more distal deletions [del(X)(p21.1 to p22.1.22)] menstruate more often, but still many are infertile or show secondary amenorrhea. That is, ovarian failure (menopause) is often premature (<35 or <40 years of age, depending upon definition). Xp21,22.1 or 22.2 X play a lesser but still important role in ovarian development (Simpson 1998, 2000). Deletion of only the most telomeric portion of Xp (Xp22.3 → Xpter) does not result in amenorrhea (Thomas et al., 1999). Zinn and coworkers (1998) and Zinn and Ross (2001) are applying molecular approaches to better characterize the pivotal region, but to date the only conclusion has been that the still large region Xp11.3→22.1 is paramount; however, an affected patient with an interstitial deletion raises the possibility of narrowing the region of interest (Zinn et al., 1998; Zinn and Ross, 2001).

Most women with deletions of Xp are short in stature. Thus, statural determinants must exist on Xp. Given that del(Xp) women may menstruate but still be short, regions on Xp responsible for ovarian and statural determinants must be distinct (Fraccaro et al., 1977; Simpson, 1981, 1997, 1998; Soyke et al., 1998). Statural determinants are more telomeric. Zinn and coworkers (1998) concluded that a high arched palate, short stature, and autoimmune thyroid disease were controlled by a region on Xp11.2→22.1, but no other structural anomalies have been localized. Thomas and coworkers (1999) reported autism in three of eight cases involving perturbation of Xp 22.31→.33. Impaired "visual spatial/perceptual abilities" (space-form blindness) seemed to be localized to distal Xp 22.33 by Ross and colleagues (2000).

Both mother and daughter may show the same Xp deletions not only in association with X/autosome translocation but also in association with terminal deletions. In 1977 Fraccaro and associates (1977) highlighted familial distal Xp deletions. Among 10 del(Xp) cases studied by James and coworkers (1997) were two mother-daughter pairs. Familial cases have involved deletions at Xp11 as well as at Xp22-12 (Massa et al., 1992; Zinn et al., 1998). Xp interstitial deletions involving Xp11-22 and Xp11.4-22.3 (Herva et al., 1979; Wilson et al., 1983) have been reported.

ISOCHROMOSOME FOR THE X LONG ARM

Division of the centromere in the transverse rather than the longitudinal plane results in an isochromosome, a metacentric chromosome consisting of isologous arms (see Chapter 1). Both arms are structurally identical and contain the same genes. Isochromosome for the X long arm [i(Xq)] differs from terminal deletion of Xp in that not just the terminal portion but all of the Xp is deleted. An isochromosome for the X long arm is the most common X structural abnormality, but coexisting 45,X cells (mosaicism) are common.

Almost all reported 46,i(Xq) patients show streak gonads. Short stature and Turner stigmata have long been accepted as frequent (Simpson, 1975). Occasional 46,X,i(Xq) patients have menstruated, but surveys verify rarity of menstruation. The almost complete lack of gonadal development in 46,X,i(Xq) individuals contrasts with that in 46,X,del(Xp11) individuals, about half of whom menstruate or develop breasts. This could indicate that gonadal determinants exist at several different locations on Xp, one locus near the centromere deleted in i(Xq) yet retained in del(X) (p11).

CANDIDATE GENES ON Xp

A few plausible candidate genes on Xp have been proposed. Zinn and colleagues (1998) proposed *ZFX*, a DNA binding protein. Jones and coworkers (1996) proposed *DFRX*, located on Xp11.4 and homologous to a locus on Yq11.2. *DFRX* (or *USP9X*) targets proteins for degradation by the ubiquitan pathway. *USP9X* is homologous to the gene fat facets (faf) in *Drosophila*. Both *DFRX* and *ZFX* escaped inactivation in two de novo (X)(p11.2) deletions. James and colleagues (1998) considered *DFRX* an unlikely candidate after ovarian function was observed in two cases despite haploinsufficiency; however, neither case reported was completely normal, and for this reason a role for *DFRX* in gonadal development is not categorically excluded. An instructive case of an interstitial deletion of Xp11.2–11.4 (Zinn et al., 1998) led to the hypothesis of several candidate genes in that region: *DFRX* (USP9X) as discussed above, *UBE1* (another ubiquitan pathway enzyme) and *BMP15*. *BMP* is a member of the TGF-β family of signaling compounds and is structurally similar to *GDF-9*, knockout of which causes germ cell failure in mice (Dong et al., 1996; Simpson and Rajkovic, 1999).

Bione and Toniolo (2000), Zinn (2001), and Zinn and Ross (2001) reviewed several candidate X-ovarian genes on Xp; other candidates can be deduced from homologes in the mouse

▼ **Table 10–4.** SELECTED MOUSE MODELS OF OVARIAN FAILURE.

Mutant Mouse/Transgene	Human Locus	Function	Mouse Phenotype
Prenatal ovarian failure defects			
Zinc finger X (*zfx*) knockout	Xp22.1–p21.3	Transcription factor	Reduced number of oocytes, infertility, short stature (Luoh et al., 1997)
Germ-cell deficient (gcd) unknown	Unknown	Unknown gene, generated by transgene insertion	Lack of germ cells as early as day 11.5 of embryonic development (Pellas et al., 1991)
White spotting (*W*)	4p11–q12	Tyrosine kinase receptor	Reduced pigmentation, anemia, lack of germ cells (Manové et al., 1991)
Steel (*Sl*)	12q22	Mast cell growth factor	Reduced pigmentation, anemia, lack of germ cells (Matsui et al., 1990)
Steroidogenic factor 1 (*SF-1*) knockout	9q33	Nuclear receptor factor	Ovarian agenesis, XY sex reversal, adrenal agenesis (Luo et al., 1994)
*mut*S (*E. coli*) homolog 5 (*MSH 5*)	6p21.3	DNA mismatch repair	Absence of ovarian structure, normal oviducts and uteri (Edelmann et al., 1999)
Beta-cell leukemia/lymphoma 2 (*Bcl-2*) knockout	18q21.3	Cell death repressor protein	Accelerated atresia of primordial follicles (Ratts et al., 1995)
Factor in germ-line alpha (*Figα*)	Unknown	Transcription factor	Females lack primordial follicles, males are normal (Soyal et al., 1999)
Postnatal ovarian failure defects			
Growth differentiation factor 9 (*GDF9*)	5	Oocyte secreted growth factor	Block in prenatal follicle development, infertility (Dong et al., 1996)
Follicle-stimulating hormone β	11p13	Glycoprotein hormone	Female infertility, block of folliculogenesis before antral stage subunit ββ knockout (*FSHβ*) (Kumar et al., 1997)
Follicle-stimulating hormone receptor (*FSHR*) knockout	2p21-p16	Hormone receptor	Female infertility, block in folliculogenesis before antral stage (Dierich et al., 1998)
Estrogen receptor α (*Erα*) knockout	11q12	Hormone receptor	Absent corpora lutea, arrest of preovulatory follicle maturation (Lubahn et al., 1993)
Connexin 37 knockout	1p35.1	Gap junction	Lack of graafian follicles, failure to ovulate (Simon et al., 1997)
*mut*L (*E. coli*) homolog 1 (*MLH1*) knockout	3p21.3	DNA repair enzyme	Failure to complete meiosis II, normal estrous cycle (Edelmann et al., 1996)
Zona matrix protein 3 (*mZP3*) knockout	7q11.23	Zona pellucida	Infertility, oocytes lack zona pellucida (Rankin et al., 1996)
Nerve growth factor-induced gene NGFI-A knockout	2q32.3–q33	Transcription factor	Lack of corpora lutea, suppressed luteinizing hormone levels (Topilko et al., 1998)

From Simpson JL, Rajkovic A: Ovarian differentiation and gonadal failure. Am J Med Genet 89:186, 1999.

(Table 10–4) (Simpson and Rajkovic, 1999), but the location of their human homolog is often not known.

X Long Arm Deletions

46,X,DEL(Xq) AND 45,X/46,X,DEL(Xq) DELETIONS

Deletions of the X long arm vary in composition (see Figs. 10–11 and 10–12). Terminal deletions originating at Xq13 have long been shown to be associated with primary amenorrhea, lack of breast development, and complete ovarian failure (Ogata and Matsuo, 1995; James et al., 1998; Simpson, 1998, 2000; Simpson and Rajkovic, 1999). Xq13 is thus the most pivotal region for ovarian maintenance. The key loci

could lie no more distal than proximal Xq21, given that menstruation occurs in deletions of break points Xq21 or beyond (see Fig. 10–12). Menstruating del(X)(q21) women might have retained a region containing an ovarian maintenance gene, whereas del(X)(q13 or 21) women with primary amenorrhea might have lost such a locus. Figure 10–12 shows phenotypes associated with various terminal deletions of Xq.

In more distal Xq deletions, the phenotype is usually not primary amenorrhea but premature ovarian failure (Bione et al., 1998; Simpson, 1998; Simpson and Rajkovic, 1999; Susca et al., 1999; Bione and Toniolo, 2000). Distal Xq is less important for ovarian maintenance than proximal Xq, but there is evidence that the former still contains regions important for ovarian maintenance. There is no clear demarcation into discrete regions, but it is heuristically useful to stratify terminal deletions in this fashion: Xq13→21, Xq22–25, and Xq26–28. In 1995, Ogato and Matsuo correlated ovarian function using such stratification (see Table 10–3). Our most recent tabulations (see Fig. 10–12) are generally consistent.

Molecular attempts at more precisely mapping the regions of Xq integral for ovarian development have begun (Bione et al., 1998). Sala and coworkers (1997) studied seven X/autosome translocations involving Xq21–22; five of the seven had primary amenorrhea. A region of Xq spanning 15 mb encompassed break points in all seven cases. Break points in four other X-autosome translocations studied by Philippe and coworkers (1995) were also localized to the same region. The YAC contig encompassing these break points spanned most of Xq21, extending between DXS233 and DXS1171 (Willard et al., 1994). That the break points associated with ovarian failure spanned the entire Xq21 region makes it unlikely that a single gene causes ovarian failure. Alternatively, in these translocations ovarian failure is not the result of perturbation of any specific gene but rather is reflective of generalized cytologic (meiotic) instability.

Analogous to del(Xp) deletions, distal Xq deletions may be familial. Some familial aggregates are derivative of Xq/autosome translocations, but del(X)(q26) and other terminal Xq deletions may also be familial (Fitch et al., 1982; Schwartz et al., 1987; Veneman et al., 1991; Massa et al., 1992; Tharapel et al., 1993). The degree of persistent ovarian function may vary among different family members having the same deletion.

Some families have been ascertained for reasons other than premature ovarian failure. Our group ascertained one Xq interstitial deletion following detection in a fetus through amniotic fluid analysis (Tharapel et al., 1993). This suggests that heretofore unrecognized families might be ascertained if prometaphase analysis or molecular studies of polymorphic loci were performed more often in POF. Vegetti and colleagues (1998) detected one del(Xq) case among 82 Italian women with POF, and Susca and coworkers (1999) found two del(Xq) cases among 20 Italian women with POF.

Distal Xq deletions seem to have a less severe effect on stature than proximal deletions, analogous to the effect on gonadal development. Somatic anomalies of the Turner stigmata are uncommon, arguably no more common than in the general population.

An unusual case of Xp21–22 duplication and Xq21→qter deletions [46,X,der(X)/pter→ q21::pp21→pter] was reported by Nakamura

and coworkers (2001). The 20-year-old woman had streak gonads, tall stature 174 cm (>2 SD over age-matched Japanese women) multiple fractures, and endometriosis. It is tempting to postulate that the Xp duplication resulted in overexpression of SHOX, whereas Xq21→qter deletion was responsible for the gonadal failure (Nakamura et al., 2001).

DIA AND OTHER Xq CANDIDATE GENES

A popular candidate gene on the X long arm is the human homolog of the *Drosophila melanogaster* gene *diaphanous* (*dia*). This gene causes sterility in male and female flies (Castrillon and Wasserman, 1994). Sequence comparisons between *dia* and the human EST (expressed sequence tag) *DRE25* reveal significant homology. *DRE25* also maps to human Xq21–22 (Castrillon and Wasserman, 1994), a region important for ovarian maintenance. *Drosophila dia* is a member of a family of proteins that help establish cell polarity, govern cytokinesis, and reorganize the acton cytoskeleton. Studying familial POF, an Xq21/autosome translocation (Phillipe et al., 1993) was found by Sala and coworkers (1997) to be associated with disruption of *DRE25* (Bione et al., 1998).

XPNPEP2 encodes an Xaa-Pro aminopeptidase (metalloprotease) that hydrolyzes proline bonds. XPNPSP2 was disrupted in a Xq translocation reported by Prueitt and colleagues (2000). The region involved Xq25. Zinn (2001) and Bione and Toniolo (2000) considered other Xq candidate genes; Simpson and Rajkovic (1999) reviewed mouse models (see Table 10–4) pointing to possible homologous genes (X and autosomes) in the human.

Other X Chromosome Abnormalities

Many other X abnormalities have been reported. Of particular note are those women once said to have a 46,X,i(Xp) complement. Initially, several women seemed to have such a complement. They showed primary amenorrhea, but stature was usually normal. However, the consensus later arose that i(Xp) does not exist, the karyotype in these individuals instead being del(X)(q22 or 24). Centric fragments and ring X[r(X)] chromosome are mitotically unstable, frequently associated with secondarily derived monosomic (45,X) lines.

Autosomal Causes of Ovarian Failure (46,XX)

Many different autosomal genes are known to cause ovarian failure, and it can confidentially be predicted that many more will be elucidated based on genes already identified in mice (see Table 10–4). Table 10–5 lists disorders that are encountered in the differential diagnosis of 46,XX ovarian failure (gonadal dysgenesis) characterized by primary amenorrhea. We will discuss these disorders next.

XX GONADAL DYSGENESIS

Gonadal dysgenesis histologically similar to that occurring in individuals with an abnormal sex chromosomal complement may be present in 46,XX individuals, as shown over 25 years ago (Simpson et al., 1971a). Mosaicism has been reasonably excluded in many affected individuals. The general term *XX gonadal dysgenesis* can be applied to those individuals, particularly those with no somatic anomalies.

▼ **Table 10–5.** THE SPECTRUM OF XX
• GONADAL DYSGENESIS

XX gonadal dysgenesis without somatic anomalies
XX gonadal dysgenesis with neurosensory deafness
  (Perrault syndrome)
XX gonadal dysgenesis with cerebellar ataxia (heterogeneous)
XX gonadal dysgenesis and other malformation syndromes
  (see Table 10–6)
XX gonadal dysgenesis as one component of pleiotropic
  mendelian disorders (see Table 10–7)
FSH receptor mutations (*FSHR*)
LH receptor mutations (*LHR*)
Blepharophimosis-ptosis-epicanthus (*FOXL2*)
Germ cell absence in both sexes (46,XX)
  No somatic anomalies
  Hypertension and deafness (Hamet et al., 1973)
  Alopecia (Al-Awadi et al., 1985)
  Microcephaly and short stature (Mikati et al., 1985)
  Agonadia (46,XX cases)
Adrenal and ovarian biosynthetic defects
  17α-Hydroxylase (*CYP17*)
  Aromatase
Inborn errors of metabolism
  Galactosemia
  Carbohydrate-deficient glycoprotein
  (Phosphomannomutase deficiency, *PMM2*)
Dynamic mutations (triplet repeat)
  Fragile X (*FRAXA*)
  Myotonic dystrophy (uncommon cause)
Ovarian-specific autoimmunity
Polyglandular autoimmune syndrome
  (Premature ovarian failure)
Autosomal trisomies
  Trisomy 13
  Trisomy 18

Many different forms of 46,XX gonadal dysgenesis exist, but that form of XX gonadal dysgenesis *not* associated with somatic anomalies is most obviously inherited in autosomal recessive fashion. Affected individuals are normal in stature (mean height 165 cm) (Simpson et al., 1979); Turner stigmata are usually absent. Frequent reports of consanguinity have long made it clear that autosomal recessive genes are responsible. In segregation analysis by the author, Simpson and colleagues revealed segregation ratio to be 0.16 for female sibs. Thus, two thirds of gonadal dysgenesis in 46,XX individuals is genetic (Meyers et al., 1996). Nongenetic phenocopies could be caused by infection, infarction, or infiltrative or autoimmune phenomena.

The mechanism underlying failure of germ cell persistence in XX gonadal dysgenesis is unknown, but many plausible hypotheses exist. Abnormalities of meiosis would be manifested as ovarian failure and infertility in otherwise normal women. Other explanations include interference with germ cell migration, abnormal connective tissue milieu, or gonadotropin receptor abnormalities.

Of clinical relevance is variable expressivity. In some families one sib had streak gonads, whereas another had primary amenorrhea and extreme ovarian hypoplasia (presence of a few oocytes) (Boczkowski, 1970; Simpson et al., 1971b; Simpson, 1979; Portuondo et al., 1987; Aittomaki, 1994; Meyers et al., 1996). If the mutant gene responsible for XX gonadal dysgenesis were capable of variable expression, that gene may be responsible for some sporadic cases of premature ovarian failure.

Identifying autosomal genes responsible for the various forms of XX gonadal dysgenesis is difficult. A fortuitous family might arise in which an autosomal translocation cosegregates with XX gonadal dysgenesis. Sporadic cases of gonadal dysgenesis have long been associated with reciprocal autosomal translocations, but there seems to be little consistency among chromosomes involved. An alternate approach is genome-wide sib-pair analysis using polymorphic DNA markers (dinucleotide repeats; single nucleotide poly) readily available throughout the genome. Using sib-pair analysis, as few as 50 to 100 families should identify chromosomal region(s) worthy of sequencing. This method was applied successfully in Finland to elucidate the form of XX gonadal dysgenesis due to FSH receptor mutation (Aittomaki, 1994; Aittomaki et al., 1995). A host of mouse genes are also potentially relevant (see Table 10–4), and perturbations in their human homologs can be sought. The mode of action is often surprisingly disparate from that predicted. Systematic identification and analysis of cDNA libraries of ovarian specific genes represent the more omnibus approach, utilizing gene knockout technology in the mouse and sequencing in the human.

PERRAULT SYNDROME (XX GONADAL DYSGENESIS WITH NEUROSENSORY DEAFNESS)

The variant of XX gonadal dysgenesis associated with neurosensory deafness is called Perrault syndrome (Perrault et al., 1951). Like XX gonadal dysgenesis without deafness, Perrault syndrome is inherited in autosomal recessive fashion (Josso et al., 1963; Christakos et al., 1969; Pallister and Opitz, 1979; Simpson, 1979; McCarthy and Opitz, 1985; Nishi et al., 1988). Endocrine features seem identical to those of XX gonadal dysgenesis without deafness.

Of note is existence of an attractive gene knock out model. Mice null for connexin 37 show

gonadal failure due to arrest at the antral stage of *oogenesis* (Simon et al., 1997). The connexin family of genes in humans is responsible for many forms of congenital deafness, hence being of obvious relevance to Perrault syndrome.

XX GONADAL DYSGENESIS CAUSED BY FSH RECEPTOR MUTATION (*FSHR*: VAL566ALA)

This condition has been found predominantly in Finland, where Aittomaki and colleagues (Aittomaki, 1994; Aittomaki et al., 1995) searched hospitals and cytogenetic laboratories to identify 75 patients country-wide having the XX gonadal dysgenesis phenotype. Diagnostic criteria were 46,XX women with primary or secondary amenorrhea having serum FSH > 40 mIU/ml. These 75 included 57 sporadic cases and 18 cases having an affected relative (7 different families). Most cases resided in north central Finland, a more sparsely populated part of the country (Fig. 10–13). The frequency was 1

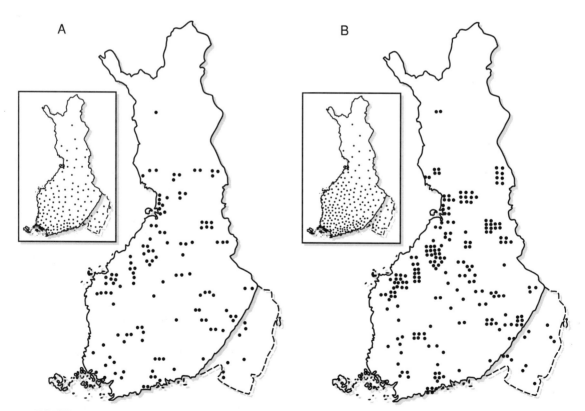

FIGURE 10–13 • Birthplaces of the parents (*A*) and grandparents (*B*) of XX gonadal dysgenesis patients in Finland. If more than one individual was affected in a family, only one symbol is present. The small reference maps show the distribution of the respective number of dots arranged according to the population density of Finland in 1940 (*A*) and 1910 (*B*). (From Aittomaki K: The genetics of XX gonadal dysgenesis. Am J Hum Genet 58:844, 1994.)

per 8300 liveborn Finnish females, a relatively high incidence attributed to a founder effect. Segregation ratio of 0.23 for female sibs was consistent with autosomal recessive inheritance, as was the high consanguinity rate (12%).

Sib pair analysis using polymorphic DNA markers first localized the gene to chromosome 2p, a region that had previously been known to contain genes for both the FSH receptor (*FSHR*) and the LH receptor (*LHR*). A specific mutation in exon 7 (Val566Ala) of the *FSHR* gene was observed in six families (Aittomaki et al., 1994, 1995) (Fig. 10–14). This cytosine-thymidine transition (C566T) was later observed in an additional six families (Aittomaki et al., 1995, 1996).

The *FSHR*:C566T mutation was not found in all Finnish XX gonadal dysgenesis cases. Could the C566T-negative cases in Finland represent XX gonadal dysgenesis with no somatic anomalies as found elsewhere? This would be consistent with the C566T mutation only rarely being detected in women with 46,XX ovarian failure who reside outside Finland. Layman and

coworkers (1998) found no mutation in the *FSHR* gene in 35 46,XX women having hypergonadotropic hypogonadism (15 with primary amenorrhea; 20 with secondary amenorrhea). Liu and coworkers (1998) found no *FSHR* abnormalities in one multigenerational POF family, four sporadic POF cases, and two other hypergonadotropic hypogonadism cases.

Similarly negative findings were reported in 46,XX POF or primary amenorrhea cases from Germany (Simoni et al., 1997), Brazil (da Fonte Kohek et al., 1998), and Mexico (de la Chesnaye et al., 2001). The last report analyzed all exons of *FSHR*. Similarily, Jiang et al. (1998) did not find C566T in 1100 normal Danish or 540 normal Singaporean individuals (v 1% in the general Finnish population); 1 in 1200 in Switzerland showed C566T heterozygosity.

When Aittomaki and colleagues (1996) compared the phenotype of C566T XX gonadal dysgenesis (Val566Ala) with non-Val566Ala XX gonadal dysgenesis, the former proved more likely to have ovarian follicles on ultrasound examination. C566T XX gonadal dysgenesis

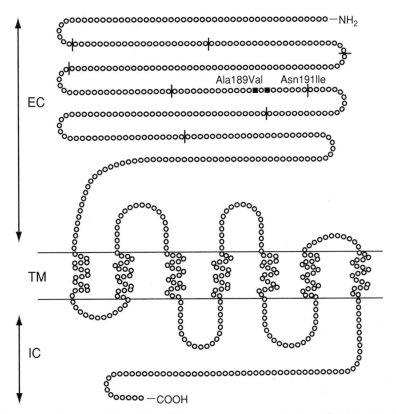

FIGURE 10–14 • Schematic presentation of the FSH receptor and gene structure. The locations of two known inactivating mutations are designated by closed symbols. Exons are separated with a short line. EC = extracellular domain; TM = transmembrane domain; IC = intracellular domain. (Modified from Aittomaki K: FSH receptor defects and reproduction. *In* Kempers RD, Cohen J, Haney AF, et al. (eds): Fertility and Reproductive Medicine. New York: Elsevier, 1998.)

showed some of the features gynecologists have long predicted for a gonadotropin resistance disorder (Savage syndrome), even if in general the phenotype found by Aittomaki (1994) was not expected. It was still a suprise to many that FSH was markedly elevated in C566T XX gonadal dysgenesis and that gonads were more reminiscent of bilateral streak gonads. However, *FSHR* (knockout) mice similarly show failure of oogenesis; thus, the necessity of FSH for progression of oogenesis is clear (Simpson and Rajkovic, 1999). Interestingly, FSH is not as pivotal for spermatogenesis (Tapanainen et al., 1997).

INACTIVATING LH RECEPTOR (LHR OR LHCGR) MUTATION (46,XX)

Another trophic hormone receptor gene in which a mutation causes gonadal dysgenesis is the LH receptor (*LHR*). (The same receptor binds to both luteinizing hormone [LH] or chorionic gonadotropin [CG], hence LHCGR.) LH receptor mutations have been reported predominantly in 46,XY cases, where phenotype may extend to complete LH resistance and XY sex-reversed female. A milder form (partial LH resistance) is associated with hypospadias or small penis (Sultan and Lumbroso, 1998). 46,XX cases have occurred in sibships in which an affected 46,XY male had Leydig cell hypoplasia.

Analogous to the FSH receptor gene, the *LHR* (LHCGR) gene is relatively large, 75 kD in length, and consists of 17 exons. Located on 2p near *FSHR*, the first 10 exons in *LHR* are extracellular; the last six are intracellular, with the 11th transmembrane. The transmembrane domain (exon) has harbored most recognized mutations. Latronico and coworkers (1996) reported primary amenorrhea in a 22-year-old woman whose family also included three males, like herself homozygous for nonsense mutation at codon 554 (Arg554 ter). The resulting stop codon produced a truncated protein. The affected female showed breast development but only a single episode of menstrual bleeding at age 20 years; LH was 37 mIU/ml, FSH 9 mIU/ml. The mutation reduced signal transduction activity of the LH receptor gene.

In another 46,XX case, Toledo and colleagues (1996) studied the female sib of the two 46,XY affected males reported by Cramer and coworkers (1995). The sister showed elevated gonadotropins but anatomically normal ovaries. The mutation was Ala593Pro. Laue and associates (1995) described two sisters with a nonsense mutation (Cys545→ter) in exon 11; LH receptor

function was lost. The father but not the mother had the mutation, suggesting a dominant negative effect. Other possibilities include the mutation's being coincidental or the mutant allele inherited from the mother simply not being detected.

Overall, females affected with *LHR* (LHCGR) mutations show oligomenorrhea or, less often, primary amenorrhea. Ovulation does not occur. Gametogenesis proceeds up until the preovulatory stage but not beyond. This is consistent with findings in the mouse knockout (see Simpson and Rajkovic, 1999).

Of interest, *activating* LH receptor mutations have little effect in females. Yet in males these mutations cause precocious puberty (Sultan and Lumbroso, 1998).

CEREBELLAR ATAXIA AND XX GONADAL DYSGENESIS

XX gonadal dysgenesis cases (hypergonadotropic hypergonadism) encompass a heterogeneous mixture of disorders associated with cerebellar ataxia. The hereditary ataxias alone are heterogeneous and confusing nosologically, principally because of ill-defined diagnostic criteria and lack of direct access to the cerebellum. Forms of ataxia characterized by hypogonadotropic *hypo*gonadism also exist but are not considered here.

The association between hypergonadotropic hypogonadism and ataxia was first reported by Skre and associates (1976), who described cases in two families. In one family a 16-year-old girl was affected, whereas in the other family three sisters were affected. In the sporadic case and in one of the three sibs, age of onset for ataxia was shortly after birth; in the two other sibs, age of onset was later during childhood. Cataracts were present in all individuals described by Skre and coworkers (1976).

Hypergonadotropic hypogonadism and ataxia were subsequently reported by De Michele and colleagues (1993), Linssen and coworkers (1994), Gottschalk and coworkers (1996), Fryns and colleagues (1998), Nishi and colleagues (1988), and Amor and coworkers (2001). The nature of ataxia has differed. Clinical findings similar to those of Skre and coworkers (1976) were reported by De Michele and coworkers (1993), Nishi and associates (1988) and Amor and associates (2001); ataxia was usually not progressive in these cases. Mitochondrial enzymopathy was evident in one case reported by De Michele and coworkers (1993), but mitochondrial studies have not been otherwise performed. Cataracts were observed only by Skre and colleagues (1976); amelogenesis was reported only by Linssen and coworkers (1994). Neurosensory deafness reminiscent of Perrault syndrome was reported by Amor and coworkers (2001). Mental retardation is variable (Amor et al., 2001).

Overall, it is difficult to determine the extent of genetic heterogeneity in cerebellar ataxia and the hypergonadotropic hypogonadism disorders. A single mutant gene is unlikely to explain every single case, but not every family need be unique.

XX GONADAL DYSGENESIS AND MULTIPLE MALFORMATION SYNDROME

The pleiotropic gene causing XX gonadal dysgenesis and neurosensory deafness (Perrault syndrome) has already received comment. Table 10–6 summarizes several such syndromes: XX gonadal dysgenesis, microcephaly, and arachnodactyly (Maximilian et al., 1970); XX gonadal dysgenesis, cardiomyopathy leading to dilation, blepharoptosis, and broad nasal bridge (Malouf et al., 1985; Narahara et al., 1992); XX gonadal dysgenesis and epibulbar dermoid (Quayle and Copeland, 1991); and XX gonadal dysgenesis, short stature and metabolic acidosis (Pober et al., 1998). These disorders are presumably distinct. If mendelian, they are presumably autosomal recessive. In Malouf syndrome, affected males have been reported. In these families subtle chromosomal rearrangements cannot be confidentially excluded.

In each of the syndromes listed in Table 10–6, an underlying biologic questions is whether the ostensibly pleiotropic gene(s) cause both somatic anomalies and ovarian failure? Or, do the somatic and gonadal phenotypes merely involve only closely linked genes, i.e., a contiguous gene syndrome? Do unrecognized parental chromosomal rearrangements exist? In turn, do any of these genes play pivotal roles in normal ovarian differentiation and maintenance upstream or downstream? Alternatively, does their perturbation merely cause ovarian failure secondarily, perhaps through generalized disturbance of connective tissue?

Primary ovarian failure is also observed infrequently in other conditions, often mendelian in etiology (Table 10–7). Of special note given potential nosologic confusion are Denys-Drash syndrome and Frasier syndrome, related syndromes both caused by mutations in *WT-1*. *WT-1* mutations are discussed in greater detail later in this chapter in the context of 46,XY sex reversal (XY females or ambiguous external). However, a 46,XX individual with Frasier syndrome has been reported (Bailey et al., 1992). This woman manifested primary amenorrhea and ovarian failure in addition to the renal parenchymal disease characteristic of Frasier syndrome. Gonadal failure in 46,XX Frasier syndrome may go unappreciated if the primary amenorrhea is assumed to be secondary to azotemia.

BLEPHAROPHIMOSIS-PTOSIS-EPICANTHUS (*FOXL2*)

Blepharophimosis-ptosis-epicanthus (BPE) is an autosomal dominant multiple malformation syndrome long known to be associated with ovarian failure (Zlotogora et al., 1983; Panidis et al., 1994). In Type I ovarian abnormalities exist, usually premature ovarian failure and not complete ovarian failure exists. In one puzzling case Fraser and coworkers (1988) reported that ovaries of an affected individual were unresponsive to gonadotropins. In Type II ovarian abnormalities do not exist but eyelid abnormalities do.

Sib-pair analysis using polymorphic DNA variants (Harrar et al., 1995) localized the gene to chromosome 3 (3q22→24), a region that facilitated positional cloning to reveal that a winged

▼ **Table 10–6.** MALFORMATION SYNDROMES WITH 46,XX GONADAL DYSGENESIS

Somatic Features	References	Etiology
Cerebellar ataxia, sensorineural deafness	Skre et al., 1976; Amor et al., 2001	Autosomal recessive
Microcephaly, arachnodactyly	Maximilian et al., 1970	Autosomal recessive
Epibulbar dermoids	Quayle and Copeland, 1991	Autosomal recessive
Short stature and metabolic acidosis	Pober et al., 1998; Hisama et al., 2001	Autosomal recessive
Blepharophimosis-ptosis-epicanthus	Zlotogora et al., 1983; Crisponi et al., 2001	Autosomal dominant (*FOXL2*)
Denys-Drash/Frasier syndrome	Bailey et al., 1992	Autosomal dominant
Dilated cardiomyopathy, mental retardation, bleparoptosis (Malouf syndrome)	Malouf et al., 1985; Narahara et al., 1992	Autosomal recessive

▼ **Table 10–7.** SELECTED MENDELIAN DISORDERS IN WHICH OVARIAN FAILURE IS FREQUENTLY
• OBSERVED

	Somatic Features	Ovarian Anomalies	Etiology
Cockayne syndrome (Nance and Berry, 1992)	Dwarfism, microcephaly, mental retardation, pigmentary retinopathy and photosensitivity, premature senility, sensitivity to ultraviolet light	Ovarian atrophy and fibrosis (Sugarman et al., 1977)	Autosomal recessive
Martsolf syndrome (Martsolf et al., 1978)	Short stature, microbrachycephaly, cataracts, abnormal facies with relative prognathism due to maxillary hypoplasia	Primary hypogonadism (Hennekam et al., 1988; Harbord et al., 1989)	Autosomal recessive
Nijmegen syndrome (Weemaes et al., 1981)	Chromosomal instability, immunodeficiency, hypersensity to ionizing radiation, malignancy	Ovarian failure (primary) (Conley et al., 1986; Chrzanowska et al., 1995)	Autosomal recessive (7;14 rearrangement)
Werner syndrome (Goto et al., 1981)	Short stature, premature senility, skin changes (scleroderma)	Ovarian failure (Goto et al., 1981)	Autosomal recessive
Rothmund-Thompson syndrome (Hall et al., 1980)	Skin abnormalities (telangiectasia, erythema, irregular pigmentation), short stature, cataracts, sparse hair, small hands and feet, mental retardation, osteosarcoma	Ovarian failure (primary hypogonadism or delayed puberty) (Starr et al., 1985)	Autosomal recessive
Carbohydrate-deficient glycoprotein syndrome, type 1 (phosphomannomutase deficiency) (Matthijs et al., 1997)	Neurologic abnormalities (e.g., unscheduled eye movements), ataxia, hypotonial/hyporeflexia strokes, joint contractures	Ovarian failure (hypogonadism) (Kristiansson et al., 1995)	Autosomal recessive
Ataxia-telangiectasia	Cerebellar ataxia, multiple telangiectasias (eyes, ears, flexor surface of extremities), immunodeficiency, chromosomal breakage, malignancy, x-ray hypersensitivity	"Complete absence of ovaries," "absence of primary follicles" (Zadik et al., 1978; Waldmann et al., 1983)	Autosomal recessive
Bloom syndrome (German, 1969; German et al., 1984; German, 1993)	Dolichocephaly, growth deficiency, sun-sensitive facial erythema, chromosomal instability (increased sister chromatical exchange), increased malignancy	Ovarian failure (German, 1993)	Autosomal recessive

helix/forkhead transcription factor gene (*FOXL2*) was mutated, yielding a truncated protein (Crisponi et al., 2001). The gene, a winged helix/forkhead transcription faetal, is expressed in mesenchyma of mouse eyelids and in adult ovarian follicles. *FOXL2* cosegregated with the form of BPE associated with ovarian failure in four families and in one patient having a de novo mutation. Mutations observed included stop codons and a 17 bp duplication causing a frameshift and, hence, truncated gene product.

Although De Baere et al. (2001) found no FOXL2 mutations in 30 premature ovarian failure patients without eyelid abnormalities, Harris et al. (2002) found mutations in 2 of 70.

Germ Cell Failure in Both Males and Females

In several sibships, male and female sibs each show germinal cell failure. Affected females show streak gonads, whereas males show germ cell aplasia (Sertoli-cell only syndrome or Del Castillo phenotype) (see below). In two families, parents were consanguineous, and in each no somatic anomalies were associated (Smith et al., 1979; Granat et al., 1983). In three other families, characteristic somatic anomalies coexisted, suggesting distinct entities. Hamet and colleagues (1973) reported germ cell failure, hypertension, and deafness; Al-Awadi and coworkers (1985) reported germ cell failure and an unusual form of alopecia ("mane-like" head hair persisted in the midline with no hair present of sides of the face and head); Mikati and coworkers (1985) reported germ cell failure, microcephaly, short stature, mental retardation, and unusual facies (synophyrs, abnormal pinnae, micrognathia, loss of teeth). The sibs reported by Al-Awadi et al. (1985) were Jordanian; those reported by Mikati et al. (1985) were Lebanese. Both families were consanguineous unions.

These families demonstrate in aggregate that a single autosomal gene can deleteriously affect germ cell development in both sexes. Presumably the gene(s) acts either at a specific site common to early germ cell development or through a non-specific mechanism producing meiotic breakdown. Elucidating any such genes could have profound implications for understanding normal developmental processes. A variety of attractive candidate genes exist in mouse and *Drosophila* (see Table 10–4). Particularly attractive is *gcd*, a mouse mutant in which germ cells are deficient in both males and females. Null mutants for *WT-1* fail to develop in mice having gonads in either sex, but kidneys are also absent (Kreidberg et al., 1993).

Gonadal Dysgenesis in 46,XY Females

Gonadal dysgenesis may occur in individuals with apparently normal male (46,XY) chromosomal complements. The phenotype is embryologically predictable because loss of testicular tissue before 7 to 8 weeks of embryogenesis would be expected to produce such a phenotype, as originally shown by Jost (1953) in rabbits. Table 10–8 lists the spectrum of these disorders.

GONADAL DYSGENESIS IN 46,XY FEMALES

The prototypic examples of XY females with gonadal dysgenesis show structurally normal female external genitalia, vagina, uterus, and fallopian tubes. In at least some cases of this condition the gonads of human XY females were embryologically ovaries (Cussen and MacMahon, 1979). At puberty, secondary sexual development fails to occur. Height is normal, and somatic anomalies are usually not present. This external appearance may be identical clinically to that of 46,XX gonadal dysgenesis without somatic anomalies. Gonadotropins (FSH, LH) are elevated and estrogens are decreased.

The risk of dysgerminoma or gonadoblastoma is approximately 20 to 30% if no medical intervention occurs (Simpson and Photopulos, 1976). Neoplasia may arise in the first or second decade. Irrespective, the relatively high likelihood of undergoing neoplastic transformation necessitates gonads being extirpated in XY gonadal dysgenesis. Laparoscopic removal of gonads or sometimes even a gonadoblastoma is possible (Wilson et al., 1992; Pisarska et al., 1998) (Fig. 10–15). Uterus and fallopian tubes should *not* be removed because the uterus may be necessary if the patient desires pregnancy through donor oocytes or donor embryos. Successful pregnancies have been

▼ Table 10–8. THE SPECTRUM OF 46,XY SEX REVERSAL (XY FEMALES)

XY gonadal dysgenesis without somatic anomalies
  Perturbations of *SRY* (HMG-box)
  Duplication Xp (*DAX1*)
  X-linked recessive form
  Forms without detectable molecular perturbation or heritability
XY gonadal dysgenesis and Wilms' tumor oncogene (WT-1)
  Denys-Drash syndrome
  Frasier syndrome
XY gonadal dysgenesis and campomelic dysplasia (SOX9)
XY gonadal dysgenesis/α-thalassemia X chromosome (ATX)
XY gonadal dysgenesis in other malformation syndromes
  Ectodermal anomalies (Brosnan)
  Genital-palato-cardiac (Gardner-Silengo-Wachtel)
  Spastic paraplegia-optic atrophy-microcephaly (Teebi)
XY gonadal dysgenesis with autosomal deletions
  Del (2p)
  Del (9p) (*DMRT*)
  Del (10q)
XY gonadal dysgenesis with autosomal duplications (1p+)
Germ cell failure in both sexes (46,XY cases)
  No somatic anomalies
  Hypertension and deafness (Hamet et al., 1973)
  Alopecia (Al-Awadi et al., 1985)
  Microcephaly and short stature (Mikati et al., 1985)
Leydig cell hypoplasia
Steroid biosynthetic defects
  Steroidogenic factor 1 (LH Receptor Deficiency) (SF1)
  17α hydroxylase/17,20 desmolase deficiency
  3β-ol dehydrogenase/3β-hydroxysteroid dehydrogenase deficiency
Agonadia (46,XY)

carried by 46,XY sex-reversed females (Kan et al., 1997).

Isolated XY gonadal dysgenesis as defined can be the result of several different etiologies. In this section we allude to four subtypes in which somatic anomalies are uncommon (see Table 10–8). One explanation is mutation or deletion of *SRY*, usually but not always involving the *SRY* HMG box (Jäger et al., 1990; Hawkins et al., 1992). As discussed, about 10 to 15% of sporadic XY gonadal dysgenesis cases show perturbations of *SRY* (Pivnick et al., 1992; McElreavey, 1996). A second form of XY gonadal dysgenesis segregates in the fashion expected of an X-linked recessive (Sternberg et al., 1968; Espiner et al., 1970; Simpson et al., 1971a; German et al., 1978; Simpson, 1979; Simpson et al., 1981; Mann et al., 1983). Third, XY sex reversal may involve the X-linked gene Dose Sensitive Sex reversal region. Duplication of this region or pertubations) of the *DAX1* gene is associated with XY sex reversal. However, only 1 of 27 "46,XY sex-reversal females"

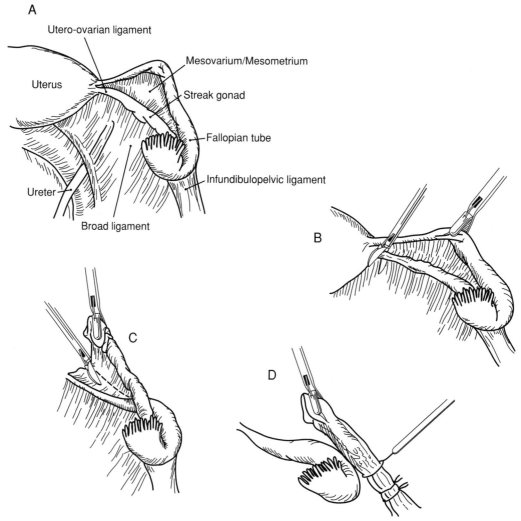

FIGURE 10–15 • Technique used for laparoscopic gonadectomy, the procedure of choice when the peritoneal reflection between fallopian tube and gonad (mesovarium/mesosalpinx) has sufficient width to allow the streak gonad to be separated from the parallel aligned fallopian tube (as indicated in *A*). (*A*) The fallopian tube is retracted laterally with grasping forceps, exposing the utero-ovarian ligament and mesovarium/mesosalpinx. (*B*) After cauterization, the utero-ovarian ligament is cut with scissors. (*C*) The mesovarium/mesosalpinx is first cauterized and then cut at 1-cm increments beginning at the utero-ovarian ligament and extending to the infundibulopelvic ligament. (*D*) Ovarian vessels entering the infundibulopelvic ligament are ligated with endoloops. (From Pisarska MD, Simpson JL, Zepeda DE, et al.: Laparoscopic removal of streak gonads in 46,XY or 45,X/46,XY gonadal dysgenesis. J Gynecol Tech 4:95, 1998.)

studied by Bardoni and coworkers (1994) showed duplication of Xp21.2→22.1. Fourth, segregation analysis long ago supported the existence of an (idiopathic) autosomal recessive form(s) (Simpson et al., 1981).

XY GONADAL DYSGENESIS AND *WT-1*

Sex reversal in 46,XY individuals occurs as part of several different multiple malformation syndromes (see Table 10–8). Several of these syndromes deserve special comment.

Alluded to already, mutations of *WT-1* (Wilms *t*umor oncogene) produce a variety of genital abnormalities. The exact mechanism is not well understood. A complex gene, *WT-1* is located on chromosome 11p. It is ten (10) exons in length, and at least 32 isoforms exist (McElreavey and Fellous, 1999). Other peculiarities include alternate translation initiation sites, alternate differential splicing in exon 5, and alternate donor acceptor sites at the exon 9 boundary. The latter results in differential splicing of the three amino acids—lysine (K), threonine (T), and serine (S) (Barbaux et al., 1997; Scharnhorst et al., 1999).

The ratio of KTS (+) and non KTS (−) transcripts differs in testes and ovary (Nachtigal et al., 1998), and could be perturbed in Frasier syndrome (see below).

Prior to recognition of the significance of *WT-1* perturbations, the association of nephropathy, genital ambiguity, and Wilms tumor was recognized in a male child. This constellation became known as Denys-Drash syndrome (Drash et al., 1970). Gessler and colleagues (1989) next observed mental retardation, aniridia, and Wilms tumor in deletions of 11p13. The *WT-1* gene is in that region. Most cases of Denys-Drash syndrome are males with genital ambiguity, but some are female. Gonadal development thus ranges from streak gonads through dysgenetic testes to true hermaphroditism (Edidin, 1985). Müeller (1994) noted that half the phenotypic females were 46,XY.

Related to Denys-Drash syndrome is Frasier syndrome, a condition in which renal parenchymal disease and XY sex reversal occurs (Fraiser et al., 1964). A case of XY gonadal dysgenesis gonadoblastoma, and renal parenchymal failure described by Simpson and colleagues (1982) represented what is now usually called Frasier syndrome. Frasier syndrome and Denys-Drash syndrome are caused by different types of perturbations involving *WT-1* (Barbaux et al., 1997).

The *WT-1* null mutation in mice results in failure of either sex to develop gonads (and kidneys) (Kreidberg et al., 1993). Given that both *SRY* and *WT-1* are found in the testes, with the latter evident earlier, it has been proposed that *WT-1* is required *upstream* of *SRY* (i.e., before *SRY* is expressed (McElreavey and Fellous, 1999).

XY GONADAL DYSGENESIS AND CAMPTOMELIC DYSPLASIA (*SOX 9*)

Camptomelic dysplasia is characterized by bowing of long bones, abnormal facies, and other skeletal anomalies (Fig. 10–16). The locus for this disorder is on 17q24.3–q25.1, and its perturbation involves the DNA binding protein *SOX9* (Kwok et al., 1995; Sudbeck et al., 1996). However, *SOX9* mutations do not always manifest as XY sex-reversal, nor do mutations in *SOX9* produce 46,XY gonadal dysgenesis in the absence of skeletal anomalies (Kwok et al., 1996). This may reflect modifying genes or mutations in the very long (1 mb) *SOX9* promoter region (Pfeifer et al., 1999), length making mutations difficult to detect. However,

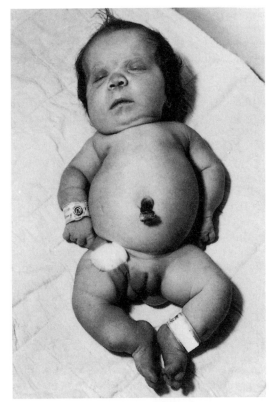

FIGURE 10–16 • Camptomelic dysplasia, often caused by perturbation of the *SOX9* gene on 17q. (From Jones KL: Smith's Recognizable Patterns of Human Malformation, 5th ed. Philadelphia: WB Saunders, 1997.)

other observations point to 17q being a pivotal autosomal region for control of sexual differentiation. Olney and colleagues (1999) reported interstitial deletion of 17q23.3q–24.3 in complete absence of *SOX9*, and campomelic dysplasia, suggesting haploinsufficiency as the molecular mechanism. Huang and colleagues (1999) reported duplication of 17p associated with presumptive bilateral testes and incomplete malelike external genitalia.

Insertional mutagenesis of a gene (odd sex, or ods) upstream of *SOX9* results in testicular development in XX mice (Bishop et al., 2000). *SRY* might normally derepress this region in order to permit testicular development in XY embryos; mutation resulting in derepression could result in the same phenotype in XX embryos.

XY GONADAL DYSGENESIS AND *ATX*

An X-linked gene (*ATX*) causes mental retardation, α-thalassemia, abnormal facies (upturned nose, carp-shaped mouth), and male pseudo-hermaphrodites. The phenotype may extend to genetic males having female external genitalia (sex reversal) (Gibbons et al., 1992, 1995a; McPherson et al., 1995; Reardon et al., 1995). Labeled *ATX* (*Alpha Thalassemia X Chromosome*), this gene is located on Xq12-q21.31. It is a member of the DNA helicase family, and over 25 mutations are reported (Gibbons et al., 1995b, 1997).

XY GONADAL DYSGENESIS IN MULTIPLE MALFORMATION SYNDROMES

Multiple malformation syndromes characterized by XY sex reversal include (1) XY gonadal dysgenesis and ectodermal anomalies (Brosnan et al., 1980); (2) XY gonadal dysgenesis in genital-palato-cardiac (Gardner-Silengo-Wachtel) syndrome (Greenberg et al., 1987); and (3) XY gonadal dysgenesis, spastic paraplegia, optic atrophy, and microcephaly (Teebi et al., 1998) (see Table 10–8). XY sex reversal also occurs with holoprosoncephaly (Witters et al., 2001). Many other multiple malformations are syndromes characterized by hypospadias without genital ambiguity (Pinsky et al., 1999) or very rarely, even genital ambiguity (male pseudohermaphroditism); however, complete XY sex reversal into female phenotype is not associated with these syndromes.

XY GONADAL DYSGENESIS AND OTHER AUTOSOMAL DELETIONS (2q, 9p, 10q)

It has been noted that perturbation of autosomal genes may cause sex reversal (XY gonadal dysgenesis). Direct molecular proof exists for campomelic dwarfism /SOX9 (17q) and for the Denys-Drash/Frasier syndromes/ *WT-1* (11p). Existence of other autosomal genes influencing sex differentiation can be deduced on the basis of malformation syndromes showing multiple affected sibs. Several autosomal deletions are associated with 46,XY sex reversal.

The association between 9p deletions and XY gonadal dysgenesis is especially well accepted (Bennett et al., 1993; McDonald et al., 1997; Veitia et al., 1997; Flejter et al., 1998; Guioli et al., 1998; Veitia et al., 1998). Interest has been piqued by reports suggesting that deletions of 9p24.3 are a major cause of *SRY*-positive XY gonadal dysgenesis (Flejter et al., 1998; Guioli et al., 1998; Veitia et al., 1998). This region

contains a domain homologous to key sex-determining genes in *Caenorhabitis elegans* (*mab3*) and *Drosophila* (double sex or *dsx*). The putative human locus was initially termed DMT, but it is now called *DMRT1* (*Doublesex and mab3 related transcription factor 1*). Ferguson-Smith and colleagues (1998) concluded that del(9p24.3) was a common cause of 46,XY gonadal dysgenesis in *SRY*-positive cases. Of 11 46,XY females with *SRY*, 3 showed complete deletion of one "*DMT1*" allele. Raymond and colleagues (1999) found that 9p24.3 actually contains two relevant domains: *DMRT1* and *DMRT2*. Sequencing 87 unexplained XY sex reversal cases revealed only one potential mutation in *DMRT1* and none in *DMRT2*. A later study by the same group found no deletions as determined by a *DMRT1* FISH probe (Mengelt et al., 1999). That the smallest reported 9p region capable of producing sex-reversal showed neither *DMRT1* nor *DMRT2* suggests that both genes must be deleted for sex reversal. Necessity for deletion of two genes implies a quantitative threshold for *DMRT* gene activity, below which testicular differentiation is impeded. With such a mechanism, phenotype might thus be expected to vary, as indeed it does in del(9) (Veitia et al., 1998).

Slavotinek and colleagues (1999) reported sex reversal with deletions of 2q33, and Waggoner and coworkers (1999) summarized sex reversal associated with deletion of 10q26. SF–1 is located on 10q but not 10q26.

XY GONADAL DYSGENESIS AND 1P DUPLICATION

Wieacker and colleagues (1996) reported XY sex reversal associated with *duplication* 1p of (p22.3 → p32.2). Jonday et al. (2001) described that duplication of 1p resulted in overexpression of WNT-4 and upregulation of DAX-1. O'Holenghi et al. (2001) reported no perturbation in Lim Hameobry Dannese 9 (LH × 9) in severed cases. This gene is located human chromosome 1.

Leydig Cell Hypoplasia (LHR Mutations)

With bilateral testes devoid of Leydig cells, 46,XY individuals have female external genitalia and no uterus. Epididymides and vasa deferentia are present, and serum LH is elevated. Affected siblings have been reported and parental consanguinity observed. Thus, autosomal recessive inheritance has long been accepted. The molecular basis was not elucidated until the last decade, shown to be a mutation in the *LHR* gene located on chromosome 2 (Sultan and Lumbroso, 1998). Leydig cells presumably fail to develop because LH cannot exert its normal effect during embryogenesis, leading to inadequate virilization and gonadal differentiation. Embryonic testes presumably secrete AMH, predictably accounting for absence of a uterus as expected in 46,XY individuals.

The *LHR* gene consists of 11 exons and 699 amino acids. These exons comprise intracellular domains, intracellular and extracellular loops, transmembrane domains, and extracellular domains. Complete resistance to LH produces XY females, whereas partial resistance leads to males with a small penis or hypospadias. Approximately one dozen different *LHR* mutations have been found in 46,XY "females" with Leydig cell hypoplasia and sometimes, as noted earlier in the chapter, their 46,XX sibs (Sultan and Lumbroso, 1998). 46,XX cases presented with primary amenorrhea. Kremer and colleagues (1995) reported two siblings of consanguineous parents; homozygosity for a missense mutation (C593R) existed. In other cases deletions, different point mutations, and stop codons have been recognized (Latronico et al., 1996; Laue et al., 1996; Latronico et al., 1998).

Deficiency of Steroidogenic Factor-1 sf-1 (46,XY Females)

Steroidogenic factor–1 (SF-1) plays a pivotal but still poorly defined role in the hypothalamic-pituitary gonadal axis. The SF-1 gene product is encoded by the gene *FTZ1*, located on human 9q33. *FTZ1* is a zinc finger protein. An orphan nuclear receptor closely related to steroid receptors, SF-1, has no known ligand (hence the designation "orphan"). Disruption of *FTZ1* in mice (knockouts) results in perturbation of adrenal *and* gonadal development as well as abnormalities of the hypothalamus and pituitary gonadotrophs (Luo et al., 1994; Parker and Schimmer, 1997). The role of SF-1 in these interactions is not clear. Irrespective, mutations in human *FTZ1* perturbing SF-1 receptors would be expected to cause significance abnormalities of sexual development.

The first human case involved an SF-1 mutation reported by Achermann and colleagues (1999). A 46,XY individual showed primary adrenal failure, female external genitalia, streak gonads, and normal müllerian derivatives. Congenital adrenal lipoid hyperplasia was initially entertained. *SRY*, *StAR*, and *DAX1* were normal. DNA sequencing revealed heterozygosity for a 2 bp substitution at codon 35 (G35E) in *FTZ1*. The mutated glycine is the last amino acid of the first zinc finger of SF–1, suggesting perturbation of a crucial site for DNA binding. A second mutation is presumably necessary to explain the phenotype, but this was not detected. In mice G35E does not exert a dominant negative effect.

Presence of a uterus is consistent with the hypothesis that SF-1 regulates repression of AMH.

Deficiency of 17α-Hydroxylase/ 17, 20-Desmolase Deficiency (CYP17)

Sex steroid synthesis requires intact adrenal and gonadal biosynthetic pathways. Various gene products (enzymes) are necessary to convert cholesterol to testosterone and androstenedione and, hence, estrogens. The various enzyme blocks have varying but predictable consequences, depending on site. The most common adrenal biosynthetic problem is female pseudohermaphroditism (see Chapter 11) caused by deficiency of 21- or 11β-hydroxylase. Ovarian development is normal in both these defects, but other adrenal enzyme deficiencies may be associated with ovarian or testicular failure. These will then need to be considered in the differential diagnosis of XX and XY gonadal dysgenesis (see Table 10–8).

Deficiency of the bifunctional enzyme 17α-hydroxylase/17,20 desmolase (Fig. 10–17) may result in primary amenorrhea and hypergonadotropic hypogonadism. Deficiency of the enzyme means that neither androgens nor estrogens are synthesized. Thus, primary amenorrhea occurs in 46,XX individuals. In 46,XY cases lack of androgen results in lack of virilization (male pseudohermaphroditism). Enzymology is complex because both 17α-hydroxylase and 17,20 desmolase(lyase) activities are governed by a single gene. This gene (CYP17) is located on 10q and codes for a cytochrome p450 enzyme. Most of the perhaps 150 cases of 17α-hydroxylase deficiency are male (46,XY) and show male genital ambiguity. Females deficient for 17α-hydroxylase/17–20 desmolase (CYP17) show hypoplastic ovaries that are sometimes streak-like in appearance; oocytes appear incapable of reaching diameters larger than 2.5 mm (Araki et al., 1987). However, stimulation with exogenous gonadotropins can produce oocytes

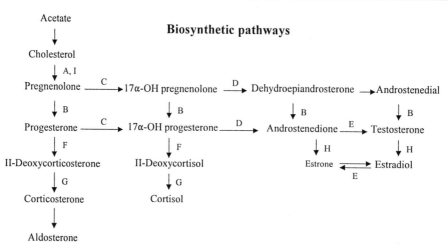

Biosynthetic pathways

FIGURE 10–17 • Pivotal adrenal and gonadal biosynthetic pathways. Letters designate enzymes or activities required for the appropriate conversions. A, 20α-hydroxylase, and 20,22-desmolase; B, 3β-ol-dehydrogenase; C, 17α-hydroxylase; D, 17,20-desmolase; E, 17-ketosteroid reductase; F, 21-hydroxylase; G, 11β-hydroxylase; H, aromatase. In addition to these enzymes, *Steroid Acute Regulatory* protein (StAR), designated I, is responsible for transporting cholesterol to the site of steroid biosynthesis. 17α-Hydroxylase (C) and 17,20-desmolase (D) activities are actually governed by a single gene.

capable of being used for fertilization *in vitro* (Rabinovici et al., 1989).

An important diagnostic clue to 17α-hydroxylase deficiency is hypertension, the pathogenesis of which is hypervolemia due to mineralocorticoid excess. If hypertension is not present, the clinical presentation is indistinguishable from XX gonadal dysgenesis without somatic anomalies. Diagnosis is based on *elevated* progesterone, deoxycorticosterone, and corticosterone levels coupled with *decreased* testosterone and estrogen levels.

In both affected males and few affected females, the molecular basis is usually point mutations rather than deletions or gene conversions.

Autosomal Trisomy

Except for trisomy 21, the liveborn autosomal trisomies are characterized by severe ovarian dysgenesis. Oocytes are usually not observed in trisomy 13, trisomy 18, and triploidy. This applies even in midtrimester abortuses (Kennedy et al., 1977; Cunniff et al., 1991), unlike 45,X. It is presumed that pathogenesis involves nonspecific meiotic perturbations, reflecting geometric impediments posed by three homologous chromosomes attempting to pair. This would be consistent with animal studies that show meiotic breakdown with translocations, insertions, and other rearrangements (Burgoyne and Baker, 1984). The same conclusion applies to other rearrangements. However, chromosomes 13 and 18 could also contain specific genes that control oogenesis. Ovarian function is more nearly normal in trisomy 21, and fertility is not uncommon.

Premature Ovarian Failure Associated with Expansion of Triplet Nucleotide Repeats

FRAGILE X (CGG REPEATS)

A molecular mechanism seemingly relevant to ovarian development is expansion of triplet nucleotide repeats. The prototype is the fragile X syndrome, caused by mutation of the *FMR-1* gene on Xq27. "Fragile" refers to a tendency toward chromosomal breakage when affected cells are cultured in folic acid–deficient media. Various fragile sites exist in humans, but only FRAXA and FRAXE in particular are relevant to the present discussion.

In FRAXA, males show mental retardation, characteristic facial features, and large testes (see Chapter 6). The molecular basis involves repetition of the triplet repeat CGG $(CGG)^n$ 230 times or more. Ordinarily, the normal number of repeats in males is only between 6 and 50. When heterozygous females show 50 to 200 repeats, a *premutation* is said to be present. During female (but not male) meiosis, the number of triplet repeats may increase (expand). A woman with a FRAXA premutation may have an affected son *if* the number of CGG repeats on the X transmitted to her offspring were to expand during meiosis to more than 230 repeats; her son would then inherit that expanded X and, hence, be affected. Females may also be affected if expansion occurs, but they show a less severe phenotype than males.

Females with the FRAXA premutation may show POF. Schwartz and colleagues (1994) reported that fragile X carrier females more often showed oligomenorrhea than noncarrier female relatives (38 versus 6%). Murray and coworkers (1998) analyzed 1268 controls, 50 familial POF cases, and 244 sporadic POF cases. Of familial cases, 16% showed FRAXA premutation; among sporadic cases, only 1.6% showed POF. In the same sample POF was not increased in FRAXE. An international collaborative survey (Allingham-Hawkins et al., 1999) of 395 premutation carriers revealed that 63 (16%) underwent menopause under 40 years of age; only 0.4% of controls did. Surprisingly, frequency of POF was not increased in 128 FRAXA cases having a full mutation. Consistent with the above observations that heterozygous FRAXA women respond poorly to ovulation-inducing agents, producing fewer oocytes and fewer embryos in ART (Black et al., 1995).

The consensus seems to be that FRAXA is associated with POF. However, Kennerson and coworkers (1997) do not agree. They argue that data are best explained by a contiguous gene syndrome. That is, they postulate two separate but closely linked loci. Both may or may not be deleted in a given individual. That Xq27–28 contains both *FMR-1* (FRAXA) and a region important for ovarian maintenance is consistent with but does not prove this hypothesis.

MYOTONIC DYSTROPHY (CTG REPEATS)

Myotonic dystrophy is an autosomal dominant disorder characterized by muscle wasting (head, neck, extremities), frontal balding, cataracts, and male hypogonadism (80%) attributable to testicular atrophy. Female hypogonadism is very much less common, if increased at all. Despite frequent textual citations, ovarian failure is actually not well documented.

Pathogenesis of myotonic dystrophy involves nucleotide expansion of CTG in the 3' untranslated region of a protein located on chromosome 19. Normally, 5–27 CTG repeats are present. Heterozygotes usually have at least 50 repeats; severely affected individuals show 600 or more. As in FRAXA, poor response to ovulation induction regions is observed. Sermon and colleagues (1998) report fewer embryos per cycle than in standard ART; thus, pregnancy rates in preimplantation genetic diagnosis are decreased.

Neither fragile X nor myotonic dystrophy need ordinarily be considered in the differential diagnosis of primary ovarian failure. However, these disorders are occasionally the explanation for POF.

Galactosemia

In the galactosemias, enzyme deficiencies prevent synthesis of glucose from galactose. All these enzyme deficiencies are inherited in autosomal recessive fashion.

Of special relevance is the form of galactosemia caused by deficiency of galactose-1-phosphate-uridyl transferase (GALT), coded by a gene on 9p. In addition to early onset renal damage to the hepatic and ocular systems, ovarian failure may occur. In 1981 Kaufman and colleagues (1981) reported POF in 12 of 18 galactosemic women. Waggoner and coworkers (1990) observed ovarian failure in 8 of 47 (17%) females with galactosemia. Pathogenesis presumably involves galactose toxicity after birth; elevated fetal levels of toxic metabolites should be cleared rapidly *in utero* by maternal enzymes. Consistent with this concept is that a neonate with galactosemia showed normal ovarian histologic appearance (Levy et al., 1984).

Given the clinical severity of galactosemia and the absolute necessity for childhood dietary treatment to prevent mental retardation, it seems highly unlikely that previously undiagnosed galactosemia would prove to be the cause of ovarian failure in women presenting solely with primary amenorrhea or POF. Of greater interest, therefore, was the report in 1989 by Cramer and coworkers that GALT heterozygotes were at increased risk for POF (Cramer et al., 1989). The same author later failed to observe GALT abnormalities in another sample of women with early menopause (Cramer et al., 1995), and Kaufman and colleagues (1993) likewise failed to confirm the observation. Moreover, not all homozygotes for human galactosemia are abnormal, nor are all transgenic mice in which GALT is inactivated (Leslie et al., 1995).

In conclusion, homozygous but probably not heterozygous GALT deficiency is associated with ovarian failure.

Carbohydrate-Deficient Glycoprotein (Phosphomannomutase Deficiency, PMM2)

In type 1 carbohydrate-deficient-glycoprotein (CDG) deficiency, mannose 6 phosphate cannot be converted to mannose 1 phosphate. As result, the lipid-linked mannose-containing oligosaccharides necessary for secretory glycoproteins is lacking. The CDG gene is located on 16p13. The usual molecular pathogenesis is a missense mutation (Bjursell et al., 1997).

The wide spectrum of neurologic abnormalities include hypotonia and hyper-reflexia, unprovoked eye movements, ataxia, joint contractions, epilepsy, and strokelike episodes (Matthijs et al., 1997). Later in life subcutaneous fat deposits, hepatomegaly, cardiomyopathy, pericardial effusion, and factor XI (clotting) deficiency develop. Ovarian failure is characterized by elevated FSH, lack of secondary sexual development, and ovaries that lack follicular activity (de Zegher and Jaeken, 1995; Kristiansson et al., 1995).

Aromatase Mutations (CYP19) in Females (46,XX)

Conversion of androgens (Δ 4-androstenedione) to estrogens (estrone) requires cytochrome P–450 aromatase, an enzyme that is the gene product of a 40-kb gene located on chromosome 15q21.1 (ER Simpson, 1998). The gene consists of 10 exons. Mutation of the gene and, hence, deficiency of the aromatase enzyme in 46,XX individuals are most often associated with genital ambiguity. For this reason, aromatase deficiency is also discussed in Chapter 11 in the context of female pseudohermaphroditism.

In addition to genital ambiguity, however, 46,XX aromatase deficiency may present as primary amenorrhea in phenotypical females. Ito and coworkers (1993) reported aromatase mutation (CYP19) in a 46,XX 18-year-old Japanese woman having primary amenorrhea and cystic ovaries. The patient was a compound heterozygote, having two different point mutations in exon 10. The mutant protein had no activity. Conte and coworkers (1994) reported aromatase deficiency in a 46,XX woman presenting with primary amenorrhea, elevated gonadatropins, and ovarian cysts. Compound heterozygosity for two different mutations in exon 10 was found. One was a C1303T transition leading to cysteine rather than arginine, whereas the other was a G1310A transition resulting in tyrosine rather than cysteine.

The above phenotype is different from that reported by Mullis and coworkers (1997). They observed clitoral enlargement at puberty but no breast development. Multiple ovarian follicular cysts were evident. FSH was elevated; estrone and estradiol were decreased. Estrogen and progesterone therapy resulted in a growth spurt, decreased FSH, decreased androstenedione and testosterone, breast development, menarche, and decreased follicular cysts. Compound heterozygosity existed at the CYP19 locus.

Premature Ovarian Failure and Polyglandular Autoimmune Syndrome

Type 1 polyglandular autoimmune syndrome is an autosomal recessive disorder especially common in Finland and in the Iranian Jewish population (Ahonen et al., 1990). Deficiencies of the parathyroids, adrenals, and gonad occur. Moniliasis as result of immune deficiencies is common. Hypergonadotropic ovarian failure is common (60%.) Localized on 2q22.3 (Aaltonen et al., 1994), the human gene has a murine homologue: *AutoImmune Regulation* gene (AIRE). Type 1 polyglandular autoimmune syndrome is uncommon outside the Finnish and Iranian Jewish populations.

Type II polyglandular autoimmune syndrome, also called Schmidt syndrome, is a heterogeneous disorder inherited in autosomal *dominant* fashion. Failure or hypofunction occurs in gonads, adrenals, thyroid, and pancreas. Other defects involve the hematologic, gastrointestinal, ocular, and integumental (hair) systems. Immunologic dysfunction is often pronounced. As in type 1 autoimmune syndrome, moniliasis is common. An association exists with HLA-B8 and to a lesser extent DR3 and DR4 (Butler et al., 1984).

Premature Ovarian Failure and Antiovarian Antibodies

A relationship between POF and antiovarian antibodies has been proposed. Antiovarian antibodies may be either generalized in nature or directed against a specific cellular component (e.g., gonadotropin receptor, stromal cells, zona pellucida). The role of anti-ovarian antibodies in ovarian failure was reviewed by Anasti (1998). In our opinion, a casual relationship seems less likely than a secondary effect (epiphenomenon), antibodies arising only after ovarian damage has occurred for unrelated but primary reasons. If causative, POF rather than primary amenorrhea would be expected.

Similar reasoning applies as well to the relationship of oophoritis to ovarian failure.

46,XY and 46,XX Agonadia

Agonadia usually occurs in 46,XY individuals. Gonads are absent rather then just being present in the form of streaks. External genitalia are abnormal but female-like; no more than rudimentary müllerian *or* wolffian derivatives are present. External genitalia usually consist of a phallus about the size of a clitoris, underdeveloped labia majora, and nearly complete fusion of labioscrotal folds. Sometimes external genitalia are nearly female in appearance. In about one half of cases, somatic anomalies coexist – craniofacial anomalies vertebral anomalies, and mental retardation. Because almost all cases are 46,XY, pathogenic explanations have always focused on loss of testes early in embryogenesis. The pathogenesis of agonadia in 46,XY individuals must take into account not only the absence of gonads (presumably testes), but also abnormal external genitalia and lack of internal genital ducts. One possibility is the transient presence of fetal testes, sufficiently long to initiate male differentiation and suppress müllerian differentiation but not long enough to complete male differentiation. Another possibility is defective connective tissue. Given the existence of both heritable tendencies (de Grouchy et al., 1985) and frequent coexistence of somatic anomalies, defective connective tissue has seemed an especially plausible explanation for certain cases. No mutations have been reported in *SRY* (Pivnick et al., 1992; Mendonca et al., 1994b; Zenteno et al., 2001).

46,XX agonadia is rare but reported (Duck et al., 1975; Levinson et al., 1976); thus, agonadia may need to be considered in the differential diagnosis of 46,XX primary amenorrhea. In addition to the sporadic cases cited above, Mendonca and coworkers (1994b) reported agonadia without somatic anomalies in phenotypic sibs having unlike chromosomal complements (46,XY and 46,XX). The family was later studied for pertubation in LHX9, with none found (Ottolenghi et al., 2001). Kennerknecht and colleagues (1993a) reported agonadism, hypoplasia of the pulmonary artery and lung, and dextrocardia in XX and XY sibs.

46,XY agonadia has been observed in the CHARGE association (Kushnick et al., 1992).

True Hermaphroditism

True hermaphrodites have both ovarian and testicular tissue. They may have a separate ovary and a separate testis, or, more often, one or more ovotestes. Most true hermaphrodites (60%) have a 46,XX chromosomal complement; however, 46,XX/46,XY, 46/XY, 46,XX/47,XXY and other complements may exist (Simpson, 1978). Phenotype probably reflects specific chromosomal constitution (Simpson, 1978), but clinically

it suffices to generalize about the overall phenotype of true hermaphrodites.

If medical intervention were not to occur (obviously now a rarity in most venues), two thirds of true hermaphrodites would be raised as males (Simpson, 1976). By contrast, external genitalia are usually ambiguous or predominantly female. Breast development occurs at puberty, even with predominantly male external genitalia. Gonadal tissue may be located in the ovarian, inguinal, or labioscrotal regions. A testis or an ovotestis is more likely to be present on the right than on the left. Spermatozoa are rarely present (Wachtel, 1983); however, ostensibly normal oocytes are often present, even in ovotestes (Fig. 10–18).

The greater the proportion of testicular tissue in an ovotestis, the greater the likelihood of gonadal descent. In 80% of ovotestes, testicular and ovarian components are juxtaposed end-to-end (Sternberg et al., 1968). An ovotestis may thus be detectable by inspection or palpation; testicular tissue is softer and darker than ovarian tissue. Accurate identification by ultrasound or magnetic resonance imaging is particularly necessary if the inappropriate portion of the ovotestis is to be extirpated. Both gonadal neoplasia and breast carcinoma have been reported in these individuals (Simpson, 1978; Verp and Simpson, 1987). The former may reflect risks associated with the intra-abdominal location of testicular tissue.

True hermaphrodites have become pregnant (Tegenkamp et al., 1979; Minowada et al., 1984), usually but not always after removal of testicular tissue. A single 46,XX/46,XY true hermaphrodite has become pregnant (Verp et al., 1992), but the other dozen pregnancies were 46,XX. Offspring seem no more likely to be abnormal than in the general population.

A uterus is usually present, although sometimes it is bicornuate or unicornuate. Absence of a uterine horn usually indicates ipsilateral testes or ovotestes. The fimbriated end of the fallopian tube is not infrequently occluded ipsilateral to an ovotestis. Squamous metaplasia of the endocervix may occur (van Niekerk, 1974). Menstruation is not uncommon and may be manifested as cyclic hematuria.

Presence of a uterus is diagnostically useful in true hermaphroditism and particularly invaluable in the rare 46,XY cases. Of individuals with genital ambiguity having a Y chromosome, only 46,XY hermaphrodites and 45,X/46,XY mosaics have a uterus. A uterus is absent in only 10 to 20% of XX true hermaphrodites, but the frequency is much higher in the families in which XX males and XX true hermaphrodites coexist (Simpson, 1978, 2000) (see below).

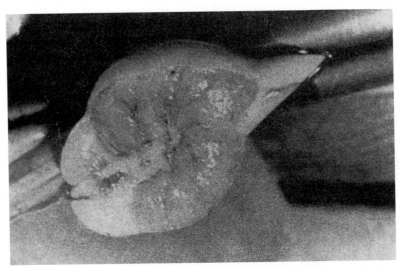

FIGURE 10–18 • A bisected ovotestis from a patient of Van Niekerk. The patient had a 46,XX complement. The ratio of ovarian to testicular tissue is about 1:4; ovarian tissue is present at the lower left. The testicular portion appeared yellowish brown, whereas the ovarian portion was white, although, in this photograph, color differentiation cannot be appreciated. The ovarian portion was firmer than the testicular portion. In 80% of ovotestes, just as in this patient, ovarian and testicular tissues are arranged end-to-end. (From Van Niekerk WA: True Hermaphroditism. New York: Harper & Row, 1974.)

Diagnosis is usually made only after excluding male and female pseudohermaphroditism. If rearing the child in the female sex is chosen, extensive surgery may or may not be necessary. If a male sex of rearing is chosen, genital reconstruction and selective gonadal extirpation are invariably indicated.

46,XX/46,XY AND 46,XY

46,XX/46,XY true hermaphroditism is usually caused by chimerism, the presence in a single individual of two or more cell lines, each derived from different zygotes. 46,XY cases may be unrecognized chimeras (Simpson, 1978).

46,XX/47,XXY and other mosaic or chimeric states are probably more likely to have resulted from nondisjunction on analysis lag.

46,XX

Chimerism is not the likely explanation for 46,XX true hermaphrodites. Explanations for the presence of testes in individuals who ostensibly lack a Y include (1) translocation during paternal meiosis of *SRY* from the Y to an X, (2) translocation of *SRY* from the Y to an autosome, (3) undetected mosaicism or chimerism, and (4) autosomal sex-reversal genes.

46,XX true hermaphrodites usually do not show DNA sequences from their father's Y (Ramsay et al., 1988), in contrast with 46,XX males in whom 80% show *SRY*. Still unexplained is why H-Y antigen was reported present in almost all 46,XX true hermaphrodites (Aaronson, 1985). However, a few 46,XX true hermaphrodites have shown *SRY* (Berkovitz et al., 1992; McElreavey et al., 1992). In the latter report, *SRY* was found in both 46,XX true hermaphrodites and 46,XX phenotypic male sibs. This suggests that Yp/Xp translocation *can* be involved. However, when *SRY* is present in true hermaphrodites, why, one wonders, is the phenotype not that of a 46,XX male (see Chapter 12)? One possibility is that a mutation was concomitantly present within the *SRY* HMG box. Another hypothesis is stochastic nonrandom inactivation of the X chromosome containing *SRY* (Fechner et al., 1994). Third, complete sex reversal (XX males) could occur when the more common Xp/Yp interchange occurs, but XX true hermaphroditism could occur with other interchanges. Recall that there are actually several regions of X-Y homology: Xp/Yp; Xq/Yp;Xp/Yq (McElreavey and Cortes, 2001). If *SRY* is translocated to Xq, where the X-inactivation gene (*XIST*) is located, spending of inactivation could mitigate against complete sex reversal and result in XX true hermaphroditism. Margarit and colleagues (2000) describe such a case. Kusz and coworkers (1999) also reported incomplete masculinization of XX individuals having *SRY* on the inactive X; however, those cases were not true hermaphrodites.

Somatic mutations of embryonic postzygotic origin are another explanation for XX true hermaphroditism (Braun et al., 1993). Braun described a sporadic case in which perturbation of *SRY* (two point mutations) was restricted to gonadal tissue (ovotestes). Peripheral blood revealed that the subject and his father had the same DNA perturbation. However, Somenice et al. (2001) similarly sought SRY in gonadal tissue, and failed to find it.

Finally, mendelian mutations could also cause true hermaphroditism. This is presumably the explanation for reported sibships with XX true hermaphroditism (Clayton et al., 1958; Rosenberg et al., 1963; Berger et al., 1970; Armendares et al., 1975; Fraccaro et al., 1979). Familial XX true hermaphroditism is more likely to be characterized by bilateral ovotestes and uterine absence than is nonfamilial true hermaphroditism (Simpson, 1978). It is probable that these families reflect autosomal recessive sex-determining genes, although subtle cytogenetic abnormalities could also exist. Both gonads are morphologically similar (Salameh et al., 1995), which favors a central basis for gonadal perturbation as opposed to chimerism (46,XX/46,XY). Occurrence of 46,XX males and 46,XX true hermaphrodities in the same kindred also has been observed (Berger et al., 1970; Kasdan et al., 1973; Skordis et al. 1987; Ramos et al., 1996; Ostrer, 2001; McElreavey et al., 2002). The 46,XX male in these kindreds usually show genital ambiguity, in contrast to the typical 46,XX male. In the family studied by Ramos et al. (1996) affected individuals were SRY negative as were two XX male sibs reported by Zenteno et al. (1997). It is likely that the phenomenon being observed in these families, which show dominant transmission, is not the same as that responsible for the families in which multiple affected sib showed XX true hermaphroditism but no other disorder of sex differentiation.

It could be postulated that perturbation (derepression) of normally dormant autosomal gene(s) induces inappropriate (testicular) gonadal development in 46,XX individuals. This argument was offered over a decade ago (Simpson, 1987a, b; Simpson et al., 1988), and it seems even more plausibile given the many autosomal genes since shown to influence testicular differentiation. Autosomal regions that have piqued interest include 2q, 9p (*DMT1*), 10p (*PAX2*), 11p (*WT-1*), and 17q (*SOX9*). Deletions of all are associated with XY sex reversal, and if duplicated any one could play a role in producing true hermaphroditism.

The converse holds for 1p, which if duplicated shows XY sex reversal.

Other Disorders Affecting Gonads

GERMINAL CELL APLASIA (SERTOLI CELL-ONLY SYNDROME; DEL CASTILLO SYNDROME)

Del Castillo and colleagues (1947) described several normally virilized but sterile males. Their seminiferous tubules lacked spermatogonia and their testes were slightly smaller than average. Leydig cells appeared normal, explaining normal secondary sexual development. FSH levels predictably proved elevated; LH levels were normal. In contrast to Klinefelter syndrome (Chapter 12), tubular hyalinization and sclerosis rarely occur in germinal cell aplasia. Occasionally a few spermatozoa are present, but affected males should be considered sterile. Androgen therapy is unnecessary because secondary sexual development is normal.

Occasionally reported as familial in the older literature (Edwards and Bannerman, 1971), germinal cell aplasia is probably more often nongenetic. The phenotype could be the end result of a variety of prenatal or postnatal testicular insults. When the phenotype coexists with somatic anomalies, a genetic cause is more likely.

RUDIMENTARY TESTES

Bergada and colleagues (1962) were the first to report males who, despite well-formed testes less than 1 cm in greatest diameter, had small penises. Testes show a few Leydig cells, small tubules containing Sertoli cells, and occasional spermatogonium. Wolffian derivatives were present; müllerian derivatives were absent. The phenotype is clearly heterogeneous – cytogenetic, mendelian, and nongenetic. Najjar and coworkers (1974) described five affected sibs of consanguineous parents, suggesting that at least one form of this entity is caused by a single mutant gene.

Pathogenesis is unclear. Testes could have initially been normal during embryogenesis, only later decreasing in size. This would be analogous to what occurs in anorchia (see below).

ANORCHIA

Males (46,XY) with unilateral or bilateral anorchia have unambiguous male external genitalia, normal wolffian derivatives, no müllerian derivatives, and no detectable testes (Simpson, 1976; Kogan et al., 1986). Unilateral anorchia is asymptomatic and not extraordinarily rare. Bilateral anorchia is relatively rare. Somatic abnormalities are not ordinarily present.

Despite the absence of testes, the phallus is well differentiated. Pathogenesis presumably involves atrophy of fetal testes after 12 to 16 weeks' gestation, by which time genital virilization has been completed. Vasa deferentia terminate blindly, often in association with spermatic vessels. The diagnosis should be applied only if testicular tissue is not detected in the scrotum, the inguinal canal, or the entire path along which the testes descend during embryogenesis. Splenic-gonadal fusion can occur, mimicking the disorder. Laparoscopy (Boddy et al., 1985), ultrasound, and magnetic resonance imaging are helpful in confirming the diagnosis.

Heritable tendencies clearly exist (Hall et al., 1975), but the occurrence of monozygotic twins discordant for bilateral anorchia (Simpson et al., 1971c) indicates that genetic factors are not paramount in all cases. Pathogenesis could involve *in utero* torsion of the testicular artery, a heritable tendency (Castilla et al., 1975; Collins et al., 1989). However, this explanation does not account for a potential relationship between agonadism and anorchia observed by the report of Josso and Briard (1980) of two sibs having these different disorders.

Testes are absent in several malformation syndromes in which external genitalia are unequivocally male (Table 10–9). These include Cross syndrome (Cross et al., 1967); the OEIS syndrome (omphalocele, extrophy, imperforate anus, spine deformity) (Stevenson et al., 1989; Keppler-Noreuil, 2001), Saldino syndrome (anorchia with cone-shaped epiphyses) (Saldino et al., 1972) and sirenomelia (Simpson, 1976; Stevenson et al., 1986).

ACCESSORY OR MALPOSITIONED GONADS

Reports exist of more than two ovaries or more than two testes (Wharton, 1959; Case, 1985). Gonadal malposition or fusion with other organs also occurs, for example to the kidney (Levy et al., 1997) or, as already noted, toward the spleen (Walther et al., 1988). Familial aggregates have not been reported. Polyorchidism is far more common than polyovaries, with over 100 cases of the former reported (Shabtai, 1991). Half have scrotal testes; others do not descend properly, sometimes locating in an intra-abdominal location.

RUDIMENTARY OVARY SYNDROME AND UNILATERAL STREAK OVARY SYNDROME

The rudimentary ovary syndrome is a poorly defined if not anachronistic term. It was traditionally applied to ovaries characterized by decreased numbers of follicles. Cases have been associated with sex chromosomal abnormalities, particularly 45,X/46,XX mosaicism. Similar statements also apply to individuals said to have the unilateral streak ovary syndrome.

Hypogonadotropic Hypogonadism

In hypogonadotropic hyprogonadism, FSH and LH are not produced. Thus, gonads cannot produce sex steroids or complete gametogenesis. The phenotype reflects inadequate pubertal development (primary amenorrhea in females) and infertility. In females external genitalia are well differentiated and a uterus is present. Etiology is disparate, reflecting abnormalities in the hypothalamus or anterior pituitary gland. The

▼ **Table 10–9.** MALFORMATION SYNDROMES ASSOCIATED WITH ABSENCE OF TESTES

Disorders	Major Features	Etiology
Cross (Cross et al., 1967)	Microphthalmia, corneal opacity, deficient pigmentation, extrapyramidal movements, mental retardation	Autosomal recessive
OEIS (Keppler-Noreuil, 2001)	Omphalocele, exstrophy, imperforate anus, spine deficiency	Sporadic; distinctiveness from exstrophy cloaca uncertain (Carey, 2001)
Sirenomelia (Simpson, 1976; Stevenson, 1986)	Fused lower limbs, absent genitalia and anus, renal agenesis	Sporadic
Saldino (Saldino et al., 1972)	Cone-shaped epiphyses (distal phalanges)	Sporadic

Modified from McGillivray BC: Male genital system. *In* Stevenson RE, Hall JG, Goodman RM (eds): Human Malformations and Related Anomalies, vol 11. New York: Oxford University Press, 1993, p 551.

▼ **Table 10–10.** MUTATIONS CAUSING HYPOGONADOTROPIC HYPOGONADISM (HH)

Gene	Chromosomal Location	Clinical Features other than HH	CNS Defect	Inheritance
KAL1	Xp22.3	Anosmia	Hypothalamic	X-linked recessive
AHC	Xp21	Congenital adrenal hypoplasia	Hypothalamus, pituitary	X-linkaged recessive
GNRHR	4q21.2	–	Pituitary	Autosomal recessive
Leptin	7q31.3	Obesity	Hypothalamic	Autosomal recessive
Leptin receptor	1p31	Obesity	Hypothalamic	Autosomal recessive
HESX1	3p21.1-21.2	Septo-optic dysplasia	Pituitary	Autosomal recessive
LH-β	19q13.3	Isolated LH deficiency	Pituitary	Autosomal recessive
FSH-β	11p13	Isolated FSH deficiency	Pituitary	Autosomal recessive
PROP-1	5q	Short stature, hypothryoidism, hypoprolactinemia	Pituitary	

CNS, central nervous system; LH, luteinizing hormone; FSH, follicle-stimulating hormone; XLR, X-linked recessive; AR, autosomal recessive.
From Layman L: Genetics of human hypogonadotropic hypogonadism. Am J Med Genet 89:242, 1999.

former would encompass abnormalities of gonadotropin-releasing hormone (GnRH), the latter FSH, LH, or both. Table 10–10 lists key genes that if mutant can cause some of the disorders discussed below.

KALLMANN SYNDROME (KAL1)

In Kallmann syndrome hypogonadotropic hypogonadism (HH) exists in conjunction with characteristic somatic features. The most prominent somatic finding is decreased or absent olfaction (anosmia or hyposmia). The anatomic basis is

aplasia of the olfactory bulbs. Pathogenesis involves perturbation of the KAL1 protein, called anosmin KAL1. KAL1 is localized on distal Xp and not subject to X-inactivation. A pseudogene exist on Yq. Anosmin forms a lattice on which GnRH neurons and olfactory nerves migrate. Failure of lattice formation deleteriously affects migration of GnRH neurons, which during embryogenesis normally migrate along with the olfactory nerves from the olfactory placode to their eventual destination in the hypothalamus (Fig. 10–19). Absence of the olfactory bulb thus impedes GnRH neuronal migration. Unilateral renal agenesis, cleft palate, and occasionally other

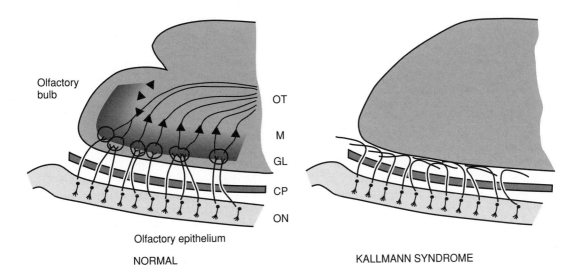

FIGURE 10–19 • The hypothalamic-pituitary-gonadal axis is shown, as are key regulators of reproductive function. Genes in which there are known mutations are enclosed in boxes, and their suggested sites of involvement are shown with arrows. LEP, leptin; LEPR, leptin receptor; *Kal*, Kallmann syndrome gene; *AHC*, congenital adrenal hypoplasia gene; GnRHR, GnRH receptor; FSH, follicle-stimulating hormone; LH, luteinizing hormone. (From Layman L: Genetics of human hypogonadotropic hypogonadism. Am J Med Genet 89:240, 1999.)

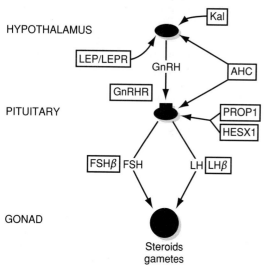

HYPOTHALAMUS

Kal

LEP/LEPR

GnRH

AHC

GnRHR

PITUITARY

PROP1

HESX1

FSHβ FSH

LH LHβ

GONAD

Steroids
gametes

FIGURE 10–20 • Model for pathogenesis of Kallman syndrome (KS) involving mutation of the *KAL* gene. In normal individuals axons of olfactory neurons (ON) transverse the cribriform plate (GL) and make snyapses with dendrites of mitral cells (M), whose axons form the olfactory tracts (OT). The KAL protein (shaded area) is secreted by the mitral cells and is required in the glomerular layer for the establishment and maintenance of proper interactions with olfactory axons. In KS, KAL protein is absent; therefore, olfactory axons cannot interact properly with their target, ending their migration between the cribriform plate and the forebrain. The migration defect of GnRH neurons in KS would be a secondary effect caused by lack of contact "migration route." (From Ballabio A, Rugarli EI: Kallmann Syndrome. *In* Scriver CR, Beaudet AL, Sly WS, et al. (eds): The Metabolic and Molecular Bases of Inherited Disease, 8th ed Vol IV. New York: McGraw-Hill, 2001. Used by permission of the Journal of the American Medical Association.)

somatic anomalies may exist. Figure 10–20 shows the relationship of KAL to other elements of the hypothalamic-pituitary-gonadal axis.

This disorder has long been recognized as the most common cause of HH (Santen and Paulsen, 1973a, b). Encoded at Xp22.3, KAL consists of 14 exons and is approximately 210 kb in length (del Castillo et al., 1992; Incerti et al., 1992). Thus, Kallman syndrome is X-linked recessive. Heterozygous females show HH, but hyposomia is far more pronounced in males. Molecular perturbations include deletions (Legouis et al., 1991; Bick et al., 1992) and point mutations (Hardelin et al., 1993). Of all Kallman syndrome aggregates demonstrating X-linked inheritance, approximately half show KAL gene mutations (Hardelin et al., 1993).

Molecular heterogeneity is usually observed, although a 514 G → A substitution (Glu → Lys) was reported in six unrelated subjects of Mexican origin (Maya-Nunez et al., 1998). Other perturbations include stop codons, frameshift mutation,

splice junction mutations, and, rarely, point mutation (Ballabio and Rugarli, 2001). Molecular diagnosis has been hindered by the existence of a nonfunctional KAL homolog on the Y (KAL-Y). Several exons are deleted in KAL-Y. X-Y interchange leading to an X/Y fusion gene is reported (Guioli et al., 1992).

Given that no KAL mutations have been found in females with idiopathic HH and anosmia, an autosomal recessive gene has been invoked to explain affected females. The same gene might explain males with Kallmann syndrome who fail to show KAL mutations.

ISOLATED HYPOGONADOTROPIC HYPOGONADISM

In isolated hypogonadotropic hypogonadism (IHH), FSH and LH deficiencies exist without deficiencies of other pituitary tropic hormones and without associated somatic anomalies. IHH is less common than Kallmann syndrome. Affected females show primary amenorrhea and lack secondary sexual development. Ovaries are characterized by numerous primordial follicles but no oocytes. Affected males fail to undergo normal secondary sexual development. They usually consult a physician because of a small penis, small testes, high-pitched voice, and scanty beard growth. Sense of smell is by definition intact. External genitalia are small yet well differentiated. Testes are characterized by decreased Leydig cells and maturational arrest in spermatogenesis. If major somatic anomalies exist, a disorder other than IHH should by definition be considered. Autosomal recessive inheritance (Betend et al., 1977; Toledo et al., 1985) is presumed to exist, distinguishing idiopathic HH from those forms of Kallmann syndrome caused by KAL mutations.

Pathogenesis of isolated hypogonadotropic hypogonadism could theoretically involve abnormalities of either the hypothalamus or the pituitary (see Fig. 10–20) and be caused by perturbation of any of the genes listed in Table 10–10. Because both FSH and LH are deficient, it has long been assumed that pathogenesis of idiopathic hypogonadotropic hypogonadism involves GnRH deficiency. A mouse model exists in which absence of GnRH is caused by the deletion of the GnRH gene (Krieger et al., 1982; Mason et al., 1986). This trait is autosomal recessive, identical to the mode of inheritance in humans. Given this attractive model, it has been a surprise that to date no human GnRH deletions have been identified. Negative studies were reported by

Weiss and coworkers (1989, 1991), Nakayama and coworkers (1990), and Layman (1999) and Layman and coworkers (1992, 1993).

Mutations have been found in the GnRH *receptor* gene located on 4q21.2. Deletions have been found both in affected males and in affected females. De Roux (1997) studied a 22-year-old male who had idiopathic HH but no evidence of anosmia. He experienced puberty at age 18 but developed neither facial nor pubic hair. Penis and testes were small, and testosterone levels were low. Sperm count was normal, although with diminished sperm mobility. Gonadotropin levels were low but nonetheless responsive to GnRH. The proband's sister experienced thelarche at age 24 years and had only a single menstrual period at age 18. Both sibs showed compound heterozygosity for missense mutations Gln106Arg and Arg262Gln in the GnRH receptor gene. Layman and colleageus (1998, 2001) studied a family with one affected male and three affected females. All three women lacked secondary sexual development, failing to undergo puberty by ages 30, 21, and 17, respectively; their 29-year-old brother also showed pubertal delay. In this family compound heterozygosity also existed: Arg262Gln and Tyr284Cys. One sib had bilateral seromucinous cystadenomas (Layman et al., 2001). De Roux and colleagues (1999) described one male and two additional females, both of whom had breast development despite primary amenorrhea; compound heterozygosity consisted of Arg262Gln on one chromosome and two mutations (Gln106Arg/Ser217Arg) on the other. Caron and colleagues (1999) reported pubertal failure and primary amenorrhea in a woman whose two brothers had small penises and bilateral cryptorchidism; compound heterozygosity existed (Arg262Gln/Ala129Asp). Costa et al. (2001) studied 17 Brazilian cases from 14 families. The inactivating Gln106Arg mutation was found in several cases in homozygous or compound heterozygous form.

The cases cited above notwithstanding, mutations in the GnRH receptor gene remain uncommon explanations for idiopathic HH. Layman and colleagues (1998) studied 46 probands, none of whom had hyposmia or anosmia. The sole mutation found was the case previously described, the proband in the family with four affected individuals.

Other candidate genes have thus been screened in idiopathic HH but without evidence of perturbation. For example, Taylor and associates (1999) found no mutations in the homeobox gene *EMX2* in 120 patients.

ISOLATED FSH DEFICIENCY AND FSH-β MUTATION

Rabin and coworkers (1972) and later Bell and colleagues (1975) reported primary amenorrhea and lack of secondary sex characteristics due to isolated FSH deficiency. The affected female had small ovaries with numerous primordial follicles but no mature oocytes. FSH was undetectable (less than 3 mIU/mL), whereas LH was markedly elevated (40 to 90 mIU/mL). Given that GnRH governs both FSH and LH secretion, pathogenesis would seem more likely to involve the pituitary than the hypothalamus.

Mutations in *FSH*-β have been observed by Matthews and coworkers (1993) and Layman and coworkers (1997). The case of Matthews involved a 13-year-old girl with no secondary sexual development, undetectable FSH, and elevated LH; other pituitary hormones were normal. GnRH stimulation resulted in increased LH but no increase in FSH levels. Molecular analysis of the *FSH*-β gene, located on 11p13, demonstrated a two-base deletion that produced a frameshift altering amino acids 61–86 and resulting in a premature stop codon at position 61 (Val 61X); amino acids 87–11 were thus not transcribed. Layman and associates (1997) found the same mutation in compound heterozygous form in a 16-year-old girl with no breast development, undetectable FSH and elevated LH; the other mutant allele was Cys51Gly, a missense mutation in exon 3. In addition to these two affected females, *FSH*-β gene mutations were reported in two FSH-deficient males (Lindstedt et al., 1998; Phillip et al., 1998). In the first case a Cys82Arg missense mutation was detected, whereas in the second Val61X (stop codon). In both cases another dysfunctional allele presumably exists.

ISOLATED LH DEFICIENCY ("FERTILE EUNUCH SYNDROME")

Males who show normal or nearly normal spermatogenesis despite failure to undergo normal sexual development have been termed "fertile eunuchs." These males have high-pitched voices, poor muscle development, and scanty beard growth. Their testes have normal numbers of germ cells but practically no Leydig cells. The phenotype could be explained by deficient LH secretion or partial LH receptor defect. Sperm counts are usually normal, and administration of hCG and testosterone has resulted in well-documented cases of paternity. Females with an analogous condition have not been reported.

Located on 19q13.3, the LH gene governs both LH and CG functions. Molecular perturbation has been noted in one male (Weiss et al., 1992). This 17-year-old boy had pubertal delay, small testes, and low testosterone levels; homozygosity existed for Gln54Arg.

The phenotype is less pronounced than that of LH receptor (LHR) mutation (see above), presumably reflecting the presence of some LH, at least embryologically. Fetal or Leydig cells could also respond *in utero* to hCG.

LEPTIN AND LEPTIN-RECEPTOR DEFICIENCIES

HH may also be caused by abnormalities of leptin or the leptin receptor. This was anticipated in humans once it became known that several mouse models (ob/ob and db/db) long used to study diabetes mellitus were actually caused by deficiencies of leptin and leptin resistance, respectively (Montague et al., 1997). Searches were thus undertaken to detect mutations in families having markedly obese children. Few mutations were found, although Montague and colleagues (1997) detected a leptin mutation in two obese prepubertal children, and Strobel and associates (1998) found a leptin mutation in three sibs of consanguineous parents. In the latter, a 14-year-old girl had primary amenorrhea; her 22-year-old brother had pubertal delay and low testosterone levels. Both sibs were homozygous for Arg105Trp. Similar to the ob/ob mouse, the two sibs showed extreme obesity, hyperinsulinemia, and idiopathic hypogonadism; however, hyperglycemia was not observed in the humans.

Mutations in the leptin receptor produce a similar phenotype. Clement and coworkers (1998) found a homozygous point mutation at the splice donor site 3′ to exon 16. Affected individuals in the family showed obesity, idiopathic hypogonadism, and elevated leptin. Mild abnormalities of growth hormones (GH) and thyroxine (T_4) were observed but not diabetes mellitus.

HYPOGONADOTROPIC HYPOPITUITARISM IN MULTIPLE MALFORMATION SYNDROMES

HH can occur as part of deficiencies involving two or more pituitary tropic hormones. For example, hypopituitary dwarfism may result in deficiencies of growth hormone, gonadotropins (FSH, LH), thyroid-stimulating hormone and adrenocortico-tropic hormone. Discussed elsewhere in detail (Pinsky et al., 1999), these heterogeneous group of disorders can result from mutant autosomal recessive genes or X-linked recessive genes or from phenocopies (infection, neoplasia).

Pituitary HH can also be one component of a variety of multiple malformation syndromes. One example is *PROP1* deficiency (Wu et al., 1995). Affected individuals have an autosomal recessive form of pituitary HH showing deficiencies of growth hormone, thyrotropin, prolactin, and gonadotropins. Missense and nonesense deletions mutations are reported (Cogan et al., 1998; Fluck et al., 1998; Fofanova et al., 1998). Mutations in *Prop1*, the mouse equivalent of human *PROP1*, constitute the basis of the mouse model Ames dwarfism (Wu et al., 1998). Another multiple malformation syndrome in which HH occurs is that involving the *AHC* gene (adrenal hyperplasia congenital). *AHC* codes for the 470 amino acid protein *DAX1*, an orphan receptor that if duplicated can cause sex reversal (XY → XX mammals) and has been alluded to several times already. Nonduplicative perturbations in *AHC* are associated with idiopathic HH. Missense mutations have been reported (Zhang et al., 1998) in the C terminal region; mutations in the amino acid terminal region have not been reported. Given that the latter should confer a less severe phenotype, it has been postulated that individuals with such mutations in this region of *DAX1* might present solely with idiopathic HH. However, Achermann and colleagues (1999) screened 100 cases with idiopathic HH and found no *DAX1* mutations.

A third disorder in which a multiple malformation pattern is associated with HH is septo-optic dysplasia, caused by the homeobox gene *HESX1*, located on 3p21. This autosomal recessive disorder is characterized by panhypopituitarism, optic nerve atrophy, agenesis of the corpus callosum, and agenesis of the septum pellucidum (Dattani et al., 1998). A mouse gene (*Hesx1*) homologous to human *HESX1* is expressed in the early forebrain, specifically in the region of Rathke's pouch that ultimately becomes the anterior pituitary gland. Not surprisingly then, molecular perturbations of *HESX1* have been detected in idiopathic HH (Arg53Cys) (Dattani et al., 1998).

Additional discussion of HH syndromes are tabulated by Pinsky and coworkers (1999).

REFERENCES

Aaltonen J, Bjorses P, Sandkuiji L, et al.: An autosomal locus causing autoimmune disease: Autoimmune polyglandular disease type I assigned to chromosome 21. Nature Genet 8:83, 1994.

Aaronsen IA: True hermaphroditism. A review of 41 cases with observations on testicular history and function. Br J Urol 57:775, 1985.

Achermann JC, Ito M, Ito M, et al.: A mutation in the gene encoding steroidogenic factor-1 causes XY sex reversal and adrenal failure in humans. Nat Genet 22:125, 1999.

Ahonen P, Myllarniemi S, Sipila I, et al.: Clinical variation of autoimmune polyendocrinopathy-candidiasis-ectodermal dystrophy (APECED) in a series of 68 patients. N Engl J Med 322:1829, 1990.

Aittomaki K: The genetics of XX gonadal dysgenesis. Am J Hum Genet 54:844, 1994.

Aittomaki K, Dieguez Luccena JL, Pakarinen P, et al.: Mutation in the follicle-stimulating hormone receptor gene causes hereditary hypergonadotropic ovarian failure. Cell 82:959, 1995.

Aittomaki K, Herva R, Stenman UH, et al.: Clinical features of primary ovarian failure caused by a point mutation in the follicle-stimulating hormone receptor gene. J Clin Endocrinol Metab 81:3722, 1996.

Al-Awadi SA, Farag TI, Teeb AS, et al.: Primary hypergonadism and partial alopecia in three sibs with müllerian hypoplasia in the affected females. Am J Med Genet 22:619, 1985.

Allingham-Hawkins DJ, Babul-Hirji R, Chitayat D, et al.: Fragile X premutation is a significant risk factor for premature ovarian failure: The International Collaborative POF in Fragile X study—preliminary data. Am J Med Genet 83:322, 1999.

Amati P, Gasparini P, Zlotogora J, et al.: A gene for premature ovarian failure associated with eyelid malformation maps to chromosome 3q22-q23. Am J Hum Genet 58:1089, 1996.

Amor DJ, Martin B, Delatycki RJ, et al.: New variant of familial cerebellar ataxia with hypergonadotropic hypogonadism and sensorineural deafness. Am J Med Genet 99:29, 2001.

Araki S, Chikazawa K, Sekiguchi I, et al.: Arrest of follicular development in a patient with 17 alpha-hydroxylase deficiency: Folliculogenesis in association with a lack of estrogen synthesis in the ovaries. Fertil Steril 47:169, 1987.

Armendares S, Salamanca F, Canty SD, et al.: Familial true hermaphroditism in three siblings. Humangenetik 29:99, 1975.

Bailey WA, Zwingman TA, Reznik VM, et al.: End-stage renal disease and primary hypogonadism associated with a 46,XX karyotype. Am J Dis Child 146:1218, 1992.

Ballabio A, Rugarli EI: Kallmann syndrome. In Scriver CR, Beaudet AL, Sly WS, et al. (eds): The Metabolic and Molecular Bases of Inherited Disease. New York: McGraw Hill, 2001, p 5729.

Barbaux S, Niaudet P, Gubler M-C, et al.: Donor splice-site mutations in WT1 are responsible for Frasier syndrome. Nat Genet 17:467, 1997.

Bardoni B, Xanaria E, Guioli S, et al.: A dose sensitive locus at chromosome Xp21 is involved in male to female sex reversal. Nat Genet 7:497, 1994.

Behringer RR, Cate RL, Froelick GJ, et al.: Abnormal sexual development in transgenetic mice chronically expressing müllerian inhibiting substance. Nature 345:16, 1990.

Bell J, Benveniste R, Spitz I, Rabinowitz DJ: Isolated deficiency of follicle-stimulating hormone: Further studies. Clin Endocrinol Metab 40:790, 1975.

Bennett CP, Docherty Z, Robb SA, et al.: Deletion 9p and sex reversal. J Med Genet 30:518, 1993.

Bergada C, Cleveland WW, Jones HW, et al.: Variants of embryonic testicular dysgenesis: Bilateral anorchia and the syndrome of rudimentary testes. Acta Endocrinol (Copenh) 40:521, 1962.

Berger R, Abonyi D, Nodot A: Hermaphroditism vrai et "garcon XX" dans une fratrie. Revue Europeenne de Etudes Clinique Biologie 15:330, 1970.

Berkovitz GD, Fechner PY, Marcantonio SM, et al.: The role of the sex-determining region of the Y chromosome (SRY) in the etiology of 46,XX true hermaphroditism. Hum Genet 88:411, 1992.

Betend B, Lebacq E, David L, et al.: Familial idiopathic hypogonadotrophic hypogonadism. Acta Endocrinol (Copenh) 84:246, 1977.

Bick D, Franco B, Sherins RJ, et al.: Brief report: Introgenic deletion of the KALIG-1 gene in Kallmann's syndrome. N Engl J Med 326:1752, 1992.

Bione S, Sala C, Manzini C, et al.: A human homologue of the Drosophilia melanogaster diaphanous gene is disrupted in a patient with premature ovarian failure: Evidence for conserved function in oogenesis and implications for human sterility. Am J Hum Genet 62:533, 1998.

Bione S, Toniolo D: X chromosome genes and premature ovarian failure. Semin Reprod Med 18:51, 2000.

Bishop CE, Whitworth DJ, Qin Y, et al.: A transgenic insertion upstream of SOX9 is associated with dominant XX sex reversal in the mouse. Nat Genet 26:490, 2000.

Bjursell C, Stibler H, Wahlstrom J, et al.: Fine mapping of the gene for carbohydrate-deficient glycoprotein syndrome, Type I (CDG1): Linkage disequilibrium and founder effect in Scandinavian families. Genomics 39:247, 1997.

Black SH, Levinson G, Harton GL, et al.: Preimplantation genetic testing (PGT) for fragile X (fraX). Am J Hum Genet 57:A31, 1995.

Boddy SA, Corkery JJ, Gornall P: The place of laparoscopy in the management of the impalpable testis. Br J Surg 72:918, 1985.

Boczkowski K: Pure gonadal dysgenesis and ovarian dysplasia in sisters. Am J Obstet Gynecol 106:626, 1970.

Braun A, Kammerer S, Cleve H et al.: True hermaphtoditism in a 46,XY individual, caused by a postzygotic somatic point mutation in the male gonadal sex-determining locus (SRY): Molecular genetics and histological findings in a sporadic case. Am J Hum Genet 52:578, 1993.

Brook CG, Gasser T, Werder EA, et al.: Height correlations between parents and mature offspring in normal subjects and in subjects with Turner's and Klinefelter's and other syndromes. Ann Hum Biol 4:17, 1977.

Brook CGD, Wagner H, Zachman M, et al.: Familial occurrence of persistent müllerian structures in otherwise normal males. Br Med J 1:771, 1973.

Brosnan PC, Lewandowski RC, Toguri AG, et al.: A new familial syndrome of the 46,XY gonadal dysgenesis with anomalies of ectodermal and mesodermal structures. J Pediatr 97:586, 1980.

Brown S, Yu C, Lanzano P, et al.: De novo mutation (Gln2Stop) at the 5' end of the SRY gene leads to sex reversal with partial ovarian function. Am J Hum Genet 62:189, 1998.

Burgoyne PS, Baker TG: Meiotic pairing and gametogenic failure. Symp Soc Exp Biol 38:349, 1984.

Butler MG, Hodes, ME, Conneally PM, et al.: Linkage analysis in a large kindred with autosomal dominant transmission of polyglandular autoimmune disease type II (Schmidt syndrome). Am J Med Genet 18:61, 1984.

Cameron F, Sinclair AH: Mutations in SRY and SOX9: Testis-determining genes. Hum Mutat 9:388, 1997.

Carey JC: Exstrophy of the cloaca and the OEIS complex: One and the same. Am J Med Genet 99:270, 2001.

Caron P, Chauvin S, Christin-Maitre S, et al.: Resistance of hypogonadotropic patients with mutated GnRH receptor genes to pulsatile GnRH administration. J Clin Endocrinol Metab 84:990, 1999.

Case WG: Triorchidism. Eur Urol 11:433, 1985.

Castilla EE, Sod R, Anzorena O, et al.: Neonatal testicular torsion in two brothers. J Med Genet 12:112, 1975.

Castrillon DH, Wasserman SA: *Diaphanous* is required for cytokinesis in *Drosophila* and shares domains of similarity with the products of the limb deformity gene. Development 120:3367, 1994.

Chen YC, Woolley PV: Genetic studies on hypospadias in males. J Med Genet 8:153, 1971.

Check JH, Nowroozi K, Chase JS, et al.: Ovulation induction and pregnancies in 100 consecutive women with hypergonadotropic amenorrhea. Fertil Steril 53:811, 1990.

Christakos AC, Simpson JL, Younger JB, et al.: Gonadal dysgenesis as an autosomal recessive condition. Am J Obstet Gynecol 104:1027, 1969.

Chrzanowska KH, Kleijer WJ, Krajewska-Walasek M, et al.: Eleven Polish patients with microcephaly, immunodeficiency, and chromosomal instability: The Nijmegen breakage syndrome. Am J Med Genet 57:462, 1995.

Clayton GW, Smith JD, Rosenberg HS: Familial true hermaphroditism in pre- and postpubertal genetic females. Hormonal and morphologic studies. J Clin Endocrinol Metab 18:1349, 1958.

Clement K, Vaisse C, Lahlou N, et al.: A mutation in the human leptin receptor gene causes obesity and pituitary dysfunction. Nature 392:398, 1998.

Cockwell A, MacKenzie M, Youings S, et al.: A cytogenetic and molecular study of a series of 45,X fetuses and their parents. J Med Genet 28:152, 1991.

Cogan JD, Wu W, Phillips JAI, et al.: The PROP1 2 base pair deletion is a common cause of combined pituitary hormone deficiency. J Clin Endocrinol Metab 83:3346, 1998.

Collins K, Broecker BH: Familial torsion of the spermatic cord. J Urol 141:128, 1989.

Conley ME, Spinner NB, Emanuel BS, et al.: A chromosomal breakage syndrome with profound immunodeficiency. Blood 67:1251, 1986.

Conte FA, Grumbach MM, Ito Y, et al.: A syndrome of female pseudohermaphrodism, hypergonadotropic hypogonadism, and multicystic ovaries associated with missense mutations in the gene encoding aromatase (*P450*arom). J Clin Endocrinol Metab 78:1287, 1994.

Costa EMF, Bedecarrats GY, Mendonca BB, et al.: Two novel mutations in the gonadotropin-releasing hormone receptor gene in Brazilian patients with hypogonadotropic hypogonadism and normal olfaction. J Clin Endocrinol Metab 86:2680, 2001.

Cramer DW, Harlow BL, Barbieri RL, et al.: Galactose-1-phosphate uridyl transferase activity associated with age at menopause and reproductive history. Fertil Steril 51:609, 1989.

Cramer DW, Xu H, Harlow BL: Family history as a predictor of early menopause. Fertil Steril 64:740, 1995.

Crisponi L, Deiana M, Loi A, et al.: The putative forkhead transcription factor FOXL2 is mutated in blepharophimosis/ptosis/epicanthus inversus syndrome. Nat Genet 27:132, 2001.

Cross HE, McKusick VA, Breen W: A new oculocerebral syndrome with hypopigmentation. J Pediatr 70:398, 1967.

Cunniff C, Jones KL, Benirschke K: Ovarian dysgenesis in individuals with chromosomal abnormalities. Hum Genet 86:552, 1991.

Cussen LJ, MacMahon RA: Germ cells and ova in dysgenetic gonads of a 46,XY female dizygote twin. Am J Dis Child 133:373, 1979.

da Fonte Kohek MB, Batista MC, Russell AJ, et al.: No evidence of the inactivating mutation (C566T) in the follicle-stimulating hormone receptor gene in Brazilian women with premature ovarian failure. Fertil Steril 70:565, 1998.

Dattani T, Martinez-Barbera JP, Thomas PQ, et al.: Mutations in the homeobox gene HESX1/Hesx1 associated with septo-optic dysplasia in human and mouse. Nat Genet 19:125, 1998.

Davison RM, Fox M, Conway GS: Mapping of the POF1 locus and identification of putative genes for premature ovarian failure. Mol Hum Reprod 6:314, 2000.

De Baere E, Dixon MJ, Small KW, et al.: Spectrum of FOXL2 gene mutations in blepharophimosis-ptosis-epicanthus inversus (BPES) families demonstrates a genotype-phenotype correlation. Hum Mol Genet 10:1591, 2001.

De Grouchy J, Gompel A, Salomon-Bernard Y: Embryonic testicular regression syndrome and severe mental retardation in sibs. Ann Genet De Genetique 28:154, 1985.

de la Chesnaye E, Canto P, Ulloa-Aguirre A, et al.: No evidence of mutations in the follicle-stimulating hormone receptor gene in Mexican women with 46,XX pure gonadal dysgenesis. Am J Med Genet 98:125, 2001.

De Michele G, Filla A, Striano S, et al.: Heterogeneous findings in four cases of cerebellar ataxia associated with hypogonadism (Holmes' type ataxia). Clin Neurol Neursurg 95:23, 1993.

de Roux N, Young J, Brailly-Tabard S, et al.: The same molecular defects of the gonadotropin-releasing hormone determine a variable degree of hypogonadism in affected kindred. J Clin Endocrinol Metab 84:567, 1999.

de Roux N, Young J, Misrahi M, et al.: A family with hypogonadotropic hypogonadism and mutations in the gonadotropin-releasing hormone receptor. N Engl J Med 337:1597, 1997.

Dewhurst J: Fertility in 47,XXX and 45,X patients. J Med Genet 15:132, 1978.

de Zegher F, Jaeken J: Endocrinology of the carbohydrate-deficient glycoprotein syndrome type 1 from birth through adolescence. Pediatr Res 37:395, 1995.

del Castillo EB, Trabucco A, De La Balze FA: Syndrome produced by absence of the germinal epithelium without impairment of the Sertoli or Leydig cells. J Clin Endocrinol 7:493, 1947.

del Castillo I, Cohen-Salmon M, Blanchard S, et al.: Structure of the X-linked Kallmann syndrome gene and its homologous pseudogene on the Y chromosome. Nat Genet 2:305, 1992.

Dierich A, Sairam MR, Monaco L, et al.: Impairing follicle-stimulating hormone (FSH) signaling in vivo: Targeted disruption of the FSH receptor leads to aberrant gametogenesis and hormonal imbalance. Proc Natl Acad Sci USA 95:13612, 1998.

Domenice S, Nishi MY, Billerbeck AE, et al.: Molecular analysis of SRY gene in Brazilian 46,XX sex reversed patients: absence of SRY sequence in gonadal tissue. Med Sci Monit 7:238, 2001.

Dong J, Albertini DF, Nishimori K, et al.: Growth differentiation factor-9 is required during early ovarian folliculogenesis. Nature 383:531, 1996.

Drash A, Sherman F, Hartmann WH, et al.: A syndrome of pseudohermaphroditism, Wilms' tumor, hypertension, and degenerative renal disease. J Pediatr 76:585, 1970.

Duck SC, Sekkan GS, Wilbois R, et al.: Pseudohermaphroditism with testes and 46,XX karyotypes. J Pediatr 87:58, 1975.

Duggan DJ, Bittner M, Chen Y, et al.: Expression profiling using cDNA microarrays. Nat Genet 21:10, 1999.

Edelmann W, Cohen PE, Kane M, et al.: Meiotic pachytene arrest in MLH1-deficient mice. Cell 85:1125, 1996.

Edelmann W, Cohen PE, Kneitz B, et al.: Mammalian MutS homologue 5 is required for chromosome pairing in meiosis. Nat Genet 21:123, 1999.

Edidin DV: Pseudohermaphroditism, glomerulopathy, and Wilms' tumor (Drash syndrome). J Pediatr 107:988, 1985.

Edwards JA, Bannerman RM: Familial gynecomastia. Birth Defects Orig Artic Ser 7(6):193, 1971.

Espiner EA, Veale AMO, Sands VE, et al.: Familial syndrome of streak gonads and normal make karyotype in five phenotypic females. N Engl J Med 238:6, 1970.

Fechner PY, Rosenberg C, Stetten G, et al.: Nonrandom inactivation of the Y-bearing X chromosome in a 46,XX individual: Evidence for the etiology of 46,XX true hermaphroditism. Cytogenet Cell Genet 66:22, 1994.

Ferguson-Smith MA, Sanoudou D, Lee C: Microdeletion of DMT1 at 9p24.3 is the commonest cause of 46,XY females. Am J Hum Genet 63:A162, 1998.

Filippson R, Lindsten J, Almqvist S: Time of eruption of the permanent teeth, cephalometric and tooth measurement and sulphation factor activity in 45 patients with Turner's syndrome with different types of X chromosome aberration. Acta Endocrinol (Copenh) 48:91, 1965.

Fitch N, de Saint, VJ, Richer CL, et al.: Premature menopause due to small deletion in long arm of the X chromosome: A report of three cases and a review. Am J Obstet Gynecol 142:968, 1982.

Flejter WL, Fergestad J, Gorski J, et al.: A gene involved in XY sex reversal is located on chromosome 9, distal to marker D9S1779. Am J Hum Genet 63:794, 1998.

Fluck C, Deladoey J, Rutishauser K, et al.: Phenotypic variability in familial combined pituitary hormone deficiency caused by a PROP 1 gene mutation resulting in the substitution of Arg to Cys at codon 120 (R120C). J Clin Endocrinol Metab 83:3727, 1998.

Fofanova O, Takamura N, Kinoshita E, et al.: Compound heterozygous deletion of the PROP-1 gene in children with combined pituitary hormone deficiency. J Clin Endocrinol Metab 83:2601, 1998.

Ford CE: Mosaics and chimaeras. Br Med Bull 25:104, 1969.

Foudila T, Soderstrom-Anttila V, Hovatta O: Turner's syndrome and pregnancies after oocyte donation. Hum Reprod 14:532, 1999.

Fraccaro M, Maraschio P, Pasquali F, et al.: Women heterozygous for deficiency of the (Xpter—➜ X21) region of the chromosome are fertile. Hum Genet 39:283,1977.

Fraccaro M, Tiepolo L, Zuffardio-Chiumello G, et al.: Familial XX true hermaphroditism and H-Y antigen. Hum Genet 48:45, 1979.

Fraiser JE, Andres GA, Cooney DR, et al.: A syndrome of pure gonadal dysgenesis: Gonadoblastoma, Wilms' tumour and nephron disease. Lab Invest 48:4P, 1964.

Fraser IS, Shearman RP, Smith A, et al.: An association among blepharophimosis, resistant ovary syndrome, and true premature menopause. Fertil Steril 50:747, 1988.

Fryns JP, Van Lingen C, Devriendt K, et al.: Two adult females with a distinct familial mental retardation syndrome: Nonprogressive neurological symptoms with ataxia and hypotonia, similar facial appearance, hypergonadotrophic hypogonadism, and retinal dystrophy. J Med Genet 35:333, 1998.

Gartler SM, Liskay RM, Campbell BK, et al.: Evidence of two functional X chromosomes in human oocytes. Cell Differ 1:215, 1972.

German J: Bloom syndrome: A mendelian prototype of somatic mutational disease. Medicine (Balt) 72:393, 1993.

German J: Gonadal dimorphism explained as a dosage effect of a locus on the sex chromosomes, the gonad-differentiation locus (GDL). Am J Hum Genet 42:414, 1988.

German J, Bloom D, Passarge E: Bloom's syndrome XI. Progress report for 1983. Clin Genet 25:166, 1984.

German J, Simpson JL, Chaganti RSK, et al.: Genetically determined sex reversal in 46,XY humans. Science 202:53, 1978.

Gessler M, Thomas GH, Couillin P, et al.: A deletion map of the WAGR region on chromosome 11. Am J Hum Genet 44:486, 1989.

Gibbons RJ, Bachoo S, Pickett DJ, et al.: Mutations in transcriptional regulator ATRX establish the functional significance of PHD-like domain. Nat Genet 17:146, 1997.

Gibbons RJ, Brueton I, Buckle VJ, et al.: Clinical and hematologic aspects of the X-linked α-thalassemia/mental retardation syndrome (ATR-X). Am J Med Genet 55:288, 1995b.

Gibbons RJ, Picketts DJ, Villard L, et al.: Mutations in a putative global transcriptional regulator cause X-linked mental retardation with α-thalassemia (ATR-X syndrome). Cell 80:837, 1995a.

Gibbons RJ, Suthers GK, Wilkie AOM, et al.: X-linked α-thalassemia/mental retardation (ART-X) syndrome: Localization to Xq12-q21.31 by X inactivation and linkage analysis. Am J Hum Genet 51:1136, 1992.

Giese K, Pagel J, Grosschedl R: Distinct DNA-binding properties of the high mobility group domain of murine and human SRY sex-determining factors. Proc Natl Acad Sci USA 91:3368, 1994.

Goto M, Tanimoto K, Horiuchi Y, et al.: Family analysis of Werner's syndrome: A survey of 42 Japanese families with a review of the literature. Clin Genet 19:8, 1981.

Gottschalk ME, Coker SB, Fox LA: Neurologic anomalies of Perrault syndrome. Am J Med Genet 65:274, 1996.

Granat M, Amar A, Mor-Yosef S, et al.: Familial gonadal germinative failure: Endocrine and human leukocyte antigen studies. Fertil Steril 40:215, 1983.

Greenberg F, Gresik MW, Carpenter RJ, et al.: The Gardner-Silengo-Wachtel or Genito-Palato-Cardiac syndrome: Male pseudohermaphroditism with micrognathia, cleft palate, and conotruncal cardiac defects. Am J Med Genet 26:59, 1987.

Grimmond S, Van Heteren N, Siggers P, et al.: Sexually dimorphic expression of protease nexin-1 and vanin-1 in the developing mouse gonad prior to overt differentiation suggests a role in mammalian sexual development. Hum Mol Genet 9:1553, 2000.

Grumbach MM , Conte FA: Disorders of sex differentiation. In Wilson JD, Foster DW, Kronenberg HM, et al. (eds): Williams Textbook of Endocrinology, 9th ed. Philadelphia: WB Saunders Co. 1998, p 1303.

Gubbay J, Collignon J, Koopman P, et al.: A gene mapping to the sex-determining region of the mouse Y chromosome is a member of a novel family embryonically expressed genes. Nature 346:245, 1991.

Guioli S, Incerti B, Zanaria E, et al.: Kallmann syndrome due to a translocation resulting in an X/Y fusion gene. Nat Genet 1:337, 1992.

Guioli S, Schmitt K, Critcher R, et al.: Molecular analysis of 9p deletions associated with XY sex reversal: Refining the localization of a sex-determining gene to the tip of the chromosome. Am J Hum Genet 63:905, 1998.

Hall JG, Morgan A, Blizzard RM: Familial congenital anorchia. Birth Defects Orig Artic Ser 11:115, 1975.

Hall JG, Pallister PD, Clarren SK, et al.: Congenital hypothalamic hamartoblastoma, hypopituitarism, imperforate anus and postaxial polydactyly—a new syndrome? Part I: Clinical, causal, and pathogenetic considerations. Am J Med Genet 7:47, 1980.

Hamet P, Kuchel O, Nowacynski JM, et al.: Hypertension with adrenal, genital, renal defects, and deafness. Arch Intern Med 131:563, 1973.

Harbord MG, Baraitser M, Wilson J: Microcephaly, mental retardation, cataracts, and hypogonadism in sibs: Martsolf's syndrome. J Med Genet 26:397, 1989.

Hardelin JP, Levilliers J, Blanchard S, et al.: Heterogeneity in the mutations responsible for X chromosome-linked Kallmann syndrome. Hum Mol Genet 2:373, 1993.

Harrar HS, Jeffrey S, Patton MA: Linkage analysis in blepharophimosis-ptosis syndrome confirms localization to 3q21-24. J Med Genet 32:774, 1995.

Harris SE, Chand AL, Winship IM, et al.: Idenfication of novel mutations in FOXL2 associated with premature ovarian failure. Mol Hum Reprod 8:729, 2002.

Hawkins JR, Taylor A, Berta P, et al.: Mutational analysis of SRY; nonsense and missense mutations in XY sex reversal. Hum Genet 88:471, 1992.

Hennekam RC, van de Meeberg AG, van Doorne JM, et al.: Martsolf syndrome in a brother and sister: Clinical features and pattern of inheritance. Eur J Pediatr 47:539, 1988.

Herva RB, Kaluzewski B, de la Chapelle A: Inherited interstitial del(Xp) with minimal clinical consequences: with a note on the location of genes controlling phenotypic features. Am J Med Genet 3:43, 1979.

Hisama FM, Zemel S, Cherniske EM, et al.: 46,XX gonadal dysgenesis, short stature, and recurrent metabolic acidosis in two sisters. Am J Med Genet 98:121, 2001.

Huang B, Thangavelu M, Bhatt S, et al.: Prenatal diagnosis of 45,X and 45,X mosaicism: the need for thorough cytogenetic and clinical evaluations. Prenat Diagn 22:105, 2002.

Huang B, Wang S, Ning Y, et al.: Autosomal XX sex reversal caused by duplication of SOX9. Am J Med Genet 87:349, 1999.

Incerti B, Guioli S, Pragliola A, et al.: Kallmann syndrome gene on the X and Y chromosomes: Implications for evolutionary divergence of human sex chromosomes. Nat Genet 2:311, 1992.

Ito Y, Fisher CR, Conte FA, et al.: Molecular basis of aromatase deficiency in an adult female with sexual infantilism and polycystic ovaries. Proc Natl Acad Sci USA 90:11673, 1993.

Jäger RJ, Anvret M, Hall K, et al.: A human XY female with a frame shift mutation in the candidate testis-determining gene SRY. Nature 348:452, 1990.

James RS, Coppin B, Dalton P, et al.: A study of females with deletions of the short arm of the X chromosome. Hum Genet 102:507, 1998.

James RS, Dalton P, Gustashaw K, et al.: Molecular characterization of isochromosomes of Xq. Ann Hum Genet 61:485, 1997.

Jiang M, Aittomaki K, Nilsson C, et al.: The frequency of an inactivating point mutation (566C → T) of the human follicle-stimulating hormone receptor gene in four populations using allele-specific hybridization and time-resolved fluorometry. J Clin Endocrinol Metab 83:4338, 1998.

Jirasék J: Principles of reproductive embryology. In Simpson JL (ed): Disorders of Sexual Differentiation: Etiology and Clinical Delineation. San Diego: Academic Press, 1976, p 51.

Jones MH, Furlong RA, Burkin H, et al.: The Drosophila developmental gene fat facets has a human homologue in Xp11.4 which escapes X-inactivation and has related sequences on Yp11.2. Hum Mol Genet 5:1695, 1996.

Jordan BK, Mohammed M, Ching ST, et al.: Up-regulation of WNT-4 signaling and dosage-sensitive sex reversal in humans. Am J Hum Genet 68:1102, 2001.

Josso N, De Grouchy J, Frezal J, et al.: Le syndrome de Turner familial etude de deux familles avec caryotypes XO et XX. Ann Pediatr 39:775, 1963.

Josso N, Briard ML: Embryonic testicular regression syndrome: Variable phenotypic expression in siblings. J Pediatr 97:200, 1980.

Jost A: Problems of fetal endocrinology. The gonadal and hypophyseal hormones. Recent Prog Horm Res 8:379, 1953.

Kan AK, Abdalla HI, Oskarsson T: Two successful pregnancies in a 46,XY patient. Hum Reprod 12:1434, 1997.

Kasdan R, Nankin HP, Troen P, et al.: Paternal transmission of maleness in XX human beings. N Engl J Med 288:539, 1973.

Kaufman FR, Devgan S, Donnell GN: Results of a survey of carrier women for the galactosemia gene. Fertil Steril 60:727, 1993.

Kaufman FR, Kogut MD, Donnell GN, et al.: Hypergonadotropic hypogonadism in female patients with galactosemia. N Engl J Med 304:994, 1981.

Kennedy JF, Freeman MG, Benirschke K: Ovarian dysgenesis and chromosome abnormalities. Obstet Gynecol 50:13, 1977.

Kennerknecht I, Sorgo W, Oberhoffer R, et al.: Familial occurrence of agonadism and multiple internal malformations in phenotypically normal girls with 46,XY and 46,XX karyotypes, respectively: A new autosomal recessive syndrome. Am J Med Genet 47:1166, 1993.

Kennerson A, Cramer, DW, Warren ST: Fragile X premutations are not a major cause of early menopause. Am J Hum Genet 61:1362, 1997.

Keppler-Noreuil KM: OEIS complex (omphalocele-exstrophy-imperforate anus-spinal defects): A review of 14 cases. Am J Med Genet 99:271, 2001.

Khastgir G, Abdalla H, Thomas A, et al.: Oocyte donation in Turner's syndrome: An analysis of the factors affecting the outcome. Hum Reprod 12:279, 1997.

Kogan SJ, Gill B, Bennett B, et al.: Human monorchism: A clinicopathological study of unilateral absent testes in 65 boys. J Urol 135:758, 1986.

Koopman P, Gubbay J, Vivian N, et al.: Male development of chromosomally female mice transgenic for Sry. Nature 351:117, 1991.

Kreidberg JA, Sariola H, Loring JM, et al.: WT-1 is required for early kidney development. Cell 74:679, 1993.

Kremer H, Kraaij R, Toledo SP, et al.: Male pseudohermaphroditism due to a homozygous missense mutation of the luteinizing hormone receptor gene. Nat Genet 9:160, 1995.

Krieger DT, Perlow MJ, Gibson MJ, et al.: Brain grafts reverse hypogonadism of gonadotropin releasing hormone deficiency. Nature 298:468, 1982.

Kristiansson B, Stibler H, Wide L: Gonadal function and glycoprotein hormones in the carbohydrate-deficient glycoprotein (CDG) syndrome. Acta Paediatr 84:655, 1995.

Kumar TR, Wang Y, Lu N, et al.: Follicle stimulating hormone is required for ovarian follicle maturation but not male fertility. Nat Genet 15:201, 1997.

Kushnick T, Wiley JE, Palmer SM: Agonadism in a 46,XY patient with CHARGE association. Am J Med Genet 42:96, 1992.

Kusz K, Kotecki M, Wojda A, et al.: Incomplete masculinisation of XX subjects carrying the SRY gene on an inactive X chromosome. J Med Genet 36:452, 1999.

Kwok C, Tyler-Smith C, Mendonca BB, et al.: Mutation analysis of the 2 kb 5' to SRY in XX females and Y intersex subjects. J Med Genet 33:465, 1996.

Kwok C, Weller PA, Guioli S, et al.: Mutations in SOX9, the gene responsible for campomelic dysplasia and autodomal sex reversal. Am J Hum Genet 57:1028, 1995.

Latronico AC, Anasti J, Arnhold IJ, et al.: Brief report: Testicular and ovarian resistance to luteinizing hormone caused by inactivating mutations of the luteinizing hormone-receptor gene. N Engl J Med 334:507, 1996.

Latronico AC, Chai Y, Arnhold IJ, et al.: A homozygous microdeletion in helix 7 of the luteinizing hormone receptor associated with familial testicular and ovarian resistance is due to both decreased cell surface expression and impaired effector activation by the cell surface receptor. Mol Endocrinol 12:442, 1998.

Lau YF: Gonadoblastoma, testicular and prostate cancers, and the TSPY gene. Am J Hum Genet 64:921, 1999.

Laue LL, Wu SM, Kudo M, et al.: Compound heterozygous mutations of the luteinizing hormone receptor gene in Leydig cell hypoplasia. Mol Endocrinol 10:987, 1996.

Laue L, Wu SM, Kudo M, et al.: A nonsense mutation of the human luteinizing hormone receptor gene in Leydig cell hypoplasia. Hum Mol Genet 4:1429, 1995.

Layman LC: Genetics of human hypogonadotropic hypogonadism. Am J Med Genet 89:240, 1999.

Layman LC: Human gene mutations causing infertility. J Med Genet 39:153, 2002.

Layman LC, Amde S, Cohen DP, et al.: The Finnish follicle-stimulating hormone receptor gene mutation is rare in North American women with 46,XX ovarian failure. Fertil Steril 69:300, 1998.

Layman LC, Lanclos KD, Tho SPT, et al.: Patients with idiopathic hypogonadotropic hypogonadism have normal gonadotropin-releasing hormone gene structure. Adolesc Pediatr Gynecol 6:214, 1993.

Layman LC, Lee EJ, Peak DB, et al.: Delayed puberty and hypogonadism caused by a mutation in the follicle stimulating hormone β-subunit gene. N Engl J Med 337:607, 1997.

Layman LC, McDonough PG, Cohen DP, et al.: Familial gonadotropin-releasing hormone resistance and hypogonadotropic hypogonadism in a family with multiple affected individuals. Fertil Steril 75:1148, 2001.

Layman LC, Wilson JT, Huey LO, et al.: Gonadotropin-releasing hormone, follicle-stimulating hormone beta, and luteinizing hormone beta gene structure in idiopathic hypogonadotropic hypogonadism. Fertil Steril 57:42, 1992.

Legouis R, Hardelin JP, Levilliers J, et al.: The candidate gene for the X-linked Kallmann syndrome encodes a protein related to adhesion molecules. Cell 67:423, 1991.

Leslie ND, Yager K, Bai S: A mouse model for transferase deficiency galactosemia. Am J Hum Genet 57:191: A38, 1995.

Levinson G, Zarate A, Guzman-Toledano R, et al.: An XX female with sexual infantilism, absent gonads, and lack of müllerian ducts. J Med Genet 13:68, 1976.

Levy B, DeFranco J, Parra R, et al.: Intrarenal supernumerary ovary. Urology 157:2240, 1997.

Levy HL, Driscoll SG, Porensky RS, et al.: Ovarian failure in galactosemia. N Engl J Med 310:50, 1984.

Lindstedt G, Nystrom E, Matthews C, et al.: Follitropin (FSH) deficiency in an infertile male due to FSHbeta gene mutation: A syndrome of normal puberty and virilization but underdeveloped testicles with azoospermia, low FSH but high lutropin and normal serum testosterone concentrations. Clin Chem Lab Med 36:663, 1998.

Lindstein J, Fraccaro M: Turner's syndrome. In Rashad MN, Morton WRM (eds): Genital Anomalies. Springfield IL: Charles C Thomas Publishers, 1969, p 396.

Linssen WH, Van den Bent MJ, Brunner HG, et al.: Deafness, sensory neuropathy, and ovarian dysgenesis: A new syndrome or a broader spectrum of Perrault syndrome? Am J Med Genet 51:81, 1994.

Liu JY, Gromoll J, Cedars MI, et al.: Identification of allelic variants in the follicle-stimulating hormone receptor genes of females with or without hypergonadotropic amenorrhea. Fertil Steril 70:326, 1998.

Lubahn DB, Moyer JS, Golding TS, et al.: Alteration of reproductive function but not prenatal sexual development after insertional disruption of the mouse estrogen receptor gene. Proc Natl Acad Sci USA 90:11162, 1993.

Lukusa T, Fryns JP, Van den Berge H: Gonadoblastoma and Y-chromosome fluorescence. Clin Genet 29:311, 1986.

Luo X, Ikeda Y, Parker KL: A cell-specific nuclear receptor is essential for adrenal and gonadal development and sexual differentiation. Cytogenet Cell Genet 80:128, 1994.

Luoh SW, Bain PA, Polakiewicz RD, et al.: Zfx mutation results in small animal size and reduced germ cell number in male and female mice. Development 124:2275, 1997.

Magre S, Jost A: Dissociation between testicular morphogenesis and endocrine cytodifferentiation of Sertoli cells. Proc Natl Acad Sci USA 81:783, 1984.

Malouf J, Alam S, Kanj H, et al.: Hypergonadotropic hypogonadism with congenital cardiomyopathy: An autosomal-recessive disorder? Am J Med Genet 20:483, 1985.

Mann JR, Corkery JJ, Fisher HJW, et al.: The X-linked recessive form of XY gonadal dysgenesis with high incidence of gonadal cell tumours: Clinical and genetic studies. J Med Genet 20:264, 1983.

Manová K, Bachvárová RF: Expression of c-kit encoded at the W locus of mice in developing embryonic germ cells and presumptive melanoblasts. Dev Biol 146:312, 1991.

Margarit E, Coll MD, Oliva R, Gomez D: SRY gene transferred to the long arm of the X chromosome in a Y-positive XX true hermaphrodite. Am J Med Genet 90:25, 2000.

Martsolf JT, Hunter AG, Haworth JC: Severe mental retardation, cataracts, short stature, and primary hypogonadism in two brothers. Am J Med Genet 1:291, 1978.

Massa G, Vanderschueren-Lodeweyckx M, Fryns JP: Deletion of the short arm of the X chromosome: A hereditary form of Turner syndrome. Eur J Pediatr 151:893, 1992.

Mason AJ, Hayflick JS, Zoeller T, et al.: A deletion truncating the gonadotropin-releasing hormone gene is responsible for hypogonadism in the hpg mouse. Science 234:1366, 1986.

Mathur A, Stekol L, Schatz D, et al.: The parental origin of the single X chromosome in Turner syndrome: Lack of correlation with parental age or clinical phenotype. Am J Hum Genet 48:682, 1991.

Matsui Y, Zsebo KM, Hogan BL: Embryonic expression of a haematopoietic growth factor encoded by the Sl locus and the ligand for c-kit. Nature 347:667, 1990.

Matthews CH, Borgato S, Beck-Peccoz P, et al.: Primary amenorrhea and infertility due to a mutation in the β-subunit of follicle-stimulating hormone. Nat Genet 5:83, 1993.

Matthijs G, Schollen E, Pardon E, et al.: Mutations in PMM2, a phosphomannomutase gene on chromosome 16p13, in carbohydrate-deficient glycoprotein type I syndrome (Jaeken syndrome). Nat Genet 16:88, 1997.

Maximilian C, Ionescu B, Bucur A: Deux soeurs avec dysgenesie gonadique majeure, hypotrophic staturale, microcephalie, arachnodactylie et caryotype 46,XX. J Genet Hum 10:26, 1970.

Maya-Nunez G, Zenteno JC, Ulloa-Aguirre A, et al.: A recurrent missense mutation in the KAL gene in patients with X-linked Kallmann's syndrome. J Clin Endocrinol Metab 83:1650, 1998.

McCarthy DJ, Opitz JM: Perrault syndrome in sisters. Am J Med Genet 22:629, 1985.

McCauley E, Kay T, Ito I, et al.: The Turner's syndrome: Cognitive defects, affective discrimination and behavioral problems. Child Dev 58:464, 1987.

McCauley E, Sybert VP, Ehrhardt A: Psychological adjustments of adult women with Turner syndrome. Clin Genet 29:284, 1986.

McDonald MT, Flejter W, Sheldon S, et al.: XY sex reversal and gonadal dysgenesis due to 9p24 monosomy. Am J Med Genet 73:321, 1997.

McDowall S, Argentaro A, Ranganathan S, et al.: Functional and structural studies of wild type SOX9 and mutations causing campomelic dysplasia. J Biol Chem 274:24023, 1999.

McElreavey K, Cortes LS: X-Y translocations and sex differentiation. Semin Reprod Med 19:133, 2001.

McElreavey K, Fellous M: Sex determination and the Y chromosome. *In* Seminars in Medical Genetics. Am J Med Genet 89:176, 1999.

McElreavey K, Jawaheer D, Le Caignec C, et al.: A gene for human testis determination maps to chromosome 5. Hum Reprod 17:40 (Abstract O-116), 2002.

McElreavey K, Rappaport R, Vilain E, et al.: A minority of 46,XX true hermaphrodites are positive for the Y-DNA sequence including *SRY*. Hum Genet 90:121, 1992.

McElreavey K, Vilain E, Barbaux S, et al.: Loss of sequences 3' to the testis-determining gene, *SRY* including the Y pseudoautosomal boundary associated with partial testicular determination. Proc Natl Acad Sci USA 93:8590, 1996.

McGillivray BC: Male genital System. *In* Stevenson RE, Hall JG, Goodman RM (eds): Human Malformations and Related Anomalies, vol 11. New York: Oxford University Press, 1993, p 551.

McPherson EW, Clemens MM, Gibbons RJ, et al.: X-linked alpha-thalassemia/mental retardation (ART-X) syndrome: A new kindred with severe genital anomalies and mild hematologic expression. Am J Med Genet 55:302, 1995.

Mendonca BB, Barbosa AS, Arnhold IJP, et al.: Gonadal agenesis in XX and XY sisters: Evidence for the involvement of an autosomal gene. Am J Med Genet 52:39, 1994.

Mengelt AM, Raymond CS, Brown LG, et al.: FISH screening for microdeletions of DMRT1 in 46,XY sex reversed individuals. Am J Hum Genet 65(Suppl A):351, 1999.

Meyers CM, Boughman JA, Rivas M, et al.: Gonadal dysgenesis in 46,XX individuals: Frequency of the automosal recessive form. Am J Med Genet 63:518, 1996.

Mikati MA, Samir SN, Sahil IF: Microcephaly, hypergonadotropic hypogonadism, short stature and minor anomalies: A new syndrome. Am J Med Genet 22:599, 1985.

Minowada S, Fukutani K, Hara M, et al.: Childbirth in true hermaphrodite. Eur Urol 10:414, 1984.

Miyamoto N, Yoshida M, Kuratani S, et al.: Defects of urogenital development in mice lacking Emx2. Development 124:1653, 1997.

Montague CT, Farooqi S, Whitehead FP, et al.: Congenital leptin deficiency is associated with severe early-onset obesity in humans. Nature 387:903, 1997.

Müeller RF: Syndrome of the month: The Denys-Drash syndrome. J Med Genet 31:471, 1994.

Mullis PE, Yoshimura N, Kuhlmann B, et al.: Aromatase deficiency in a female who is compund heterozygote for two new point mutations in the P450 arom gene: Impact of estrogens on hypergonadotropic hypogonadism, multicystic ovaries, and bone densitometry in childhood. Clin Endocrinol Metab 82:1739, 1997.

Murray A, Webb J, Grimley S, et al.: Studies of FRAXA and FRAXE in women with premature ovarian failure. J Med Genet 35:637, 1998.

Nachtigal MW, Hirokawa Y, Enyeart-Van-houten DL, et al.: Wilms' tumor 1 and *Dax-1* modulate the orphan nuclear receptor SF-1 in sex-specific gene expression. Cell 93:445, 1998.

Najjar SS, Takla RJ, Nassar VH: The syndrome of rudimentary testes: Occurrence in five siblings. J Pediatr 84:119, 1974.

Nakamura Y, Suehiro Y, Sugino N, et al.: A case of 46,X,der(X) (pter→q21::p21→pter) with gonadal dysgenesis, tall stature, and endometriosis. Fertil Steril 75:1224, 2001.

Nakayama Y, Wondisford FE, Lash RW, et al.: Analysis of gonadotropin-releasing hormone gene structure in families with familial central precocious puberty and idiopathic hypogonadotropic hypogonadism. J Clin Endocrin Metab 70:1233, 1990.

Nance MA, Berry SA: Cockayne syndrome: Review of 140 cases. Am J Med Genet 42:68, 1992.

Narahara K, Kamada M, Takahashi Y, et al.: Case of ovarian dysgenesis and dilated cardiomyopathy supports existence of Malouf syndrome. Am J Med Genet 44:369, 1992.

Nishi Y, Hamamoto K, Kajiyama M, et al.: The Perrault syndrome: Clinical report and review. Am J Med Genet 31:623, 1988.

Ogata T, Matsuo N: Turner syndrome and female sex chromosome aberrations: Deductions of the principal factors involved in the development of clinical features. Hum Genet 95:607, 1995.

Olney PN, Kean LS, Graham D, et al.: Campomelic syndrome and deletion of *SOX9*. Am J Med Genet 84:20, 1999.

Ostrer H: Sexual differentiation. Semin Reprod Med 18:41, 2000.

Ostrer H, Jawaheer D, Juo S-H, et al.: A gene for human testis determination maps to chromosome 5. Am J Hum Genet 69:A188, 2001.

Ottolenghi C, Moreira-filho C, Mendonca BB, et al.: Absence of mutations involving the lim homeobox domain gene LHX9 in 46,XY gonadal agenesis and dysgenesis. J Clin Endocrinol Metab 86:2465, 2001.

Ottolenghi C, McElreavey K: Deletions of 9p and the quest for a conserved mechanism of sex determination. Mol Genet Metabol 71:397, 2000.

Page DC: Hypothesis: A Y-chromosome gene causes gonadoblastoma in poorly differentiated gonads. Development 101(suppl):151, 1987.

Page DC, Silber S, Brown LG: Men with infertility caused by AZFc deletion can produce sons by intracytoplasmic sperm injection, but are likely to transmit the deletion and infertility. Hum Reprod 14:1722, 1999.

Pallister PD, Opitz JM: The Perrault syndrome: Autosomal recessive ovarian dysgenesis with facultative, non-sex-limited sensorineural deafness. Am J Med Genet 4:239,1979.

Panidis D, Rousso D, Vavilis D, et al.: Familial blepharophimosis with ovarian failure. Hum Reprod 9:2034, 1994.

Parker KL, Schimmer BP: Steroidogenic factor 1: A key determinant of endocrine development and function. Endocr Rev 18:361, 1997.

Patsavoudi E, Magre S, Castinior M, et al.: Dissociation between testicular morphogenesis and functional differentiation of Leydig cells. J Endocrinol 28:235, 1985.

Pellas TC, Ramachandran B, Duncan M, et al.: Germ-cell deficient (gcd), an insertional mutation manifested as infertility in transgenic mice. Proc Natl Acad Sci USA 88:8787, 1991.

Perrault M, Klotz P, Housset E: Deux cas de syndrome de Turner avec surdi-mutité dans une même fratrie. Bull Soc Med Hop Paris 67:79, 1951.

Pfeifer D, Kist R, Dewar K, et al.: Campomelic dysplasia translocation breakpoints are scattered over 1mb proximal to *SOX9*: Evidence for an extended control region. Am J Hum Genet 55:111, 1999.

Phillip M, Arbelle JE, Segev Y, et al.: Male hypogonadism due to a mutation in the gene for the β-subunit of follicle stimulating hormone. New Engl J Med 338:1729, 1998.

Philippe C, Arnould C, Sloan F, et al.: A high-resolution interval map of the q21 region of the human X chromosome. Genomics 27:539, 1995.

Philippe C, Cremers FPM, Chery M, et al: Physical mapping of DNA markers in the q13-q22 region of the human X chromosome. Genomics 17:147,1993.

Pinsky L, Erickson RP, Schimke RN: Genetic Disorders of Human Sexual Development. New York: Oxford University Press, 1999.

Pisarska MD, Simpson JL, Zepeda DE, et al.: Laparoscopic removal of streak gonads in 46,XY or 45,X/46,XY gonadal dysgenesis. J Gynecol Tech 4:95, 1998.

Pivnick EK, Wachtel S, Woods D, et al.: Mutations in the conserved domain of SRY are uncommon in XY gonadal dysgenesis. Hum Genet 90:308, 1992.

Pober BR, Zemel S, Hisama FM: 46,XX gonadal dysgenesis, short stature and recurrent metabolic acidosis in two sisters. 48th Annual Meeting, The American Society of Human Genetics. Am J Hum Genet 63:652, A117, 1998.

Prueitt RL, Ross JL, Zinn AR: Physical mapping of nine Xq translocation breakpoints and identification of XPNPEP2 as a premature ovarian failure candidate gene. Cytogenet Cell Genet 89:44, 2000.

Portuondo JA, Neyro JL, Benito JA, et al.: Familial 46,XX gonadal dysgenesis. Int J Fertil 32:56, 1987.

Quayle SA, Copeland KC: 46,XX gonadal dysgenesis with epibulbar dermoid. Am J Med Genet 40:75, 1991.

Rabin D, Spitz I, Bercovici B, et al.: Isolated deficiency of follicle-stimulating hormone. Clinical and laboratory features. N Engl J Med 287:1313, 1972.

Rabinovici J, Blankstein J, Goldman B, et al.: In vitro fertilization and primary embryonic cleavage are possible in 17α-hydroxylase deficiency despite extremely low intrafollicular 17β-estradiol. J Clin Endocrinol Metab 68:693, 1989.

Ramos ES, Moreira-Filho CA, Vicente YA, et al.: SRY-negative true hermaphrodites and an XX male in two generations of the same family. Hum Genet 97:596, 1996.

Ramsay M, Bernstein R, Zwane E, et al.: XX true hermaphroditism in South African blacks: An enigma of primary sexual differentiation. Am J Hum Genet 43:4, 1988.

Ranke MB, Blum WF, Hang F, et al.: Growth hormone, somatomedin in levels and growth regulation in Turner's syndrome. Acta Endocrinol 116:305, 1987.

Ranke MB, Pfluger H, Rosendahl W, et al.: Turner's syndrome: Spontaneous growth in 150 cases and review of the literature. Eur J Pediatr 141:81, 1983.

Rankin T, Familari M, Lee E, et al.: Mice homozygous for an insertional mutation in the Zp3 gene lack a zona pellucida and are infertile. Development 122:2903, 1996.

Ratts VS, Flaws JA, Kolp R, et al.: Ablation of bcl-2 gene expression decreases the numbers of oocytes and primordial follicles established in the post-natal female mouse gonad. Endocrinology 136:3665, 1995.

Raymond CS, Parker ED, Kettlewell JR, et al.: A region of human chromosome 9p required for testis development contains two genes related to known sexual regulators. Hum Mol Genet 8:989, 1999.

Reardon W, Gibbons RJ, Winter RM, et al.: Male pseudohermaphroditism in sibs with the alpha-thalassemia/mental retardation (ATR-X) syndrome. Am J Med Genet 55:285, 1995.

Rosenberg HS, Clayton GW, Hsu TC: Familial true hermaphroditism. J Clin Endocrinol Metabol 23:203, 1963.

Rosenfeld RG, Attie KM, Frane J, et al.: Growth hormone therapy of Turner's syndrome: Beneficial effect on adult height. J Pediatr 132:319, 1998.

Rosenfeld RG, Grumbach MM (eds): Turner Syndrome. New York: Marcel Dekker, 1990.

Ross JL, Roeltgen D, Kushner H, et al.: The Turner syndrome-associated neurocognitive phenotype maps to distal Xp. Am J Hum Genet 67:672, 2000.

Sala C, Arrigo G, Torri G, et al.: Eleven X chromosome breakpoints associated with premature ovarian failure (POF) map to a 15-Mb YAC contig spanning Xq21. Genomics 40:123, 1997.

Salameh W, Shoukair M, Keswani A, et al.: Evidence for a deletion in the LH receptor gene in a case of Leydig cell aplasia. In 77th Annual Meeting of Endocrine Society, June 14-17, Washington, DC, Abstract P2-150:328, 1995.

Saldino RM, Marshall S, Taybi H: Cone-shaped epiphyses in the distal phalanges. Case report of a child with anorchia. Radiol Clin Biol 41:449, 1972.

Santen RJ, Paulsen CA: Hypogonadotropic eunuchoidism. I. Clinical study of the mode of inheritance. J Clin Endocrinol Metab 36:47, 1973a.

Santen RJ, Paulsen CA: Hypogonadotropic eunuchoidism. II. Gonadal responsiveness to exogenous gonadotropins. Clin Endocrinol Metab 36:55, 1973b.

Scharnhorst V, Dekker P, van der Eb AJ, et al.: Internal translation initiation generates novel WT1 protein isoforms with distinct biological properties. J Biol Chem 27:23456, 1999.

Schnieders F, Dork T, Arnemann J, et al.: Testis-specific protein. Y-encoded (TSPY) expression in testicular tissues. Hum Mol Genet 5:1801, 1996.

Schwartz C, Fitch N, Phelan MC, et al.: Two sisters with a distal deletion at the Xq26/Xq27 interface. DNA studies indicate that the gene locus for factor IX is present. Hum Genet 76:54, 1987.

Schwartz CE, Howard-Peebles PN, Bugge M: Obstetricial and gynecological complications in fragile X carriers: multicenter study. Am J Med Genet 51:400, 1994.

Sermon K, De Vos A, Van de Velde H, et al.: Fluorescent PCR and automated fragment analysis for the clinical application of preimplantation genetic diagnosis of myotonic dystrophy. Mol Hum Reprod 4:791, 1998.

Shabtai F, Schwartz A, Hart J, et al.: Chromosomal anomaly and malformation syndrome with abdominal polyorchidism. J Urol 146:833,1991.

Simon AM, Goodenough DA, Li E, et al.: Female infertility in mice lacking connexin 37. Nature 385:525, 1997.

Simoni M, Gromoll J, Nieschlag E: The follicle-stimulating hormone receptor: Biochemistry, molecular biology, physiology, and pathophysiology. Endocr Rev 18:739, 1997.

Simpson ER: Genetic mutations resulting in estrogen insufficiency in the male. Mol Cell Endocrinol 145:55, 1998.

Simpson JL: Genetic programming in ovarian development and oogenesis. In Lobo RA, Kelsey J, Marcus R (eds): Menopause Biology and Pathobiology. London: Academic Press, 2000, p 77.

Simpson JL: Genetics of female infertility. In Filicori M, Flamigni C (eds): Proceedings of the Conference, Treatment of Infertility: The New Frontiers. Boca Raton, Florida: Communications Media for Education, Inc, 1998, p 37.

Simpson JL: Genetics of oocyte depletion. In Lobo RA (ed): Perimenopause. Serono Symosia USA Norwell. Massachusetts, New York, Springer, 1997, p 36.

Simpson JL: Ovarian maintenance determinants on the X chromosome and on autosomes. In Coutifaris C, Mastroianni L (eds): New Horizons in Reproductive Medicine—Proceedings of the IXth World Congress on Human Reproduction. Philadelphia: 1996; 1997, p 439.

Simpson JL: Phenotypic-karyotypic correlations of gonadal determinants: Current status and relationship to molecular studies. In Sperling K, Vogel F (eds): Human Genetics Proceedings of the Seventh International Congress, Berlin, 1986. Heidelberg, Berlin: Springer-Verlag, 1987.

Simpson JL: Pregnancies in women with chromosomal abnormalities. In Schulman JD, Simpson JL (eds): Genetic Diseases in Pregnancy. New York: Academic Press, 1981, p 439.

Simpson JL: Gonadal dysgenesis and sex chromosome abnormalities. Phenotypic/karyotypic correlayions. In Valllet

HL, Perter IH (eds): Genetic mechanisms of sexual development. New York: Academic Press, 1979, p 365.

Simpson JL: True hermaphroditism. Etiology and phenotypic considerations. Birth Defects 14(6C):9, 1978.

Simpson JL: Disorders of Sexual Differentiation: Etiology and Clinical Delineation. New York: Academic Press, 1976.

Simpson JL: Gonadal dysgenesis and abnormalities of the human sex chromosomes: Current status of phenotypic-karyotypic correlations. Birth Defects 11:113, 1975.

Simpson JL, Baum LD, Depp R, et al.: Low maternal serum alpha-fetoprotein and perinatal outcome. Am J Obstet Gynecol 156:852, 1987a.

Simpson JL, Chaganti RSK, Mouradian J, et al.: Chronic renal disease, myotonic dystrophy, and gonadoblastoma in an individual with XY gonadal dysgenesis. J Med Genet 19:73, 1982.

Simpson JL, Christakos AC, Horwith M, et al.: Gonadal dysgenesis associated with apparently chromosomal complements. Birth Defects 7(6):215, 1971a.

Simpson JL, Horwith M, Morillo-Cucci G, et al.: Bilateral anorchia: Discordance in monozygotic twins. Birth Defects 7(6):196, 1971c.

Simpson JL, Gray RH, Queenan JT, et al.: Pregnancy outcome associated with natural family (NFP): Scientific basis and experimental design for an international cohort study. Adv Contracept 4:247, 1988.

Simpson JL, Mills JL, Holmes LB, et al.: Low fetal loss rates after ultrasound-proved viability in early pregnancy. JAMA 258:2555, 1987b.

Simpson JL, New M, Peterson RE, et al.: Pseudovaginal perineoscrotal hypospadias (PPSH) in sibs. Birth Defects 7(6):140, 1971b.

Simpson JL, Photopulos G: The relationship of neoplasia to disorders of abnormal sexual differentiation. Birth Defects 12(1):15, 1976.

Simpson JL, Rajkovic A: Ovarian differentiation and gonadal failure. Am J Med Genet 89:186, 1999.

Simpson JL, Rebar R: Normal and abnormal sexual differentiation and development. In Becker KL (ed): Principles and Practice of Endocrinology and Metabolism, 3rd ed. Philadelphia: Lippincott Williams and Wilkins, 2001, p 852.

Skordis NA, Stetka DG, MacGillivray MH, et al.: Familial 46,XX coexisting with familial 46,XX true hermaphrodites in same pedigree. J Pediatr 110:244, 1978.

Skre H, Bassoe HH, Berg K, et al.: Cerebellar ataxia and hypergonadotropic hypogonadism in two kindreds. Chance concurrence, pleiotropism or linkage? Clin Genet 9:234, 1976.

Slavotinek A, Schwarz C, Getty JF, et al.: Two cases with interstitial deletions of chromosome 2 and sex reversal in one. Am J Med Genet 86:75, 1999.

Smith A, Fraser IS, Noel M: Three siblings with premature gonadal failure. Fertil Steril 32:528, 1979.

Soyke A, Stumm M, Krebs P, et al.: Familial occurrence of a del(Xp-) chromosome: Pitfall in karyotype/phenotype correlation. Am J Med Genet 80:436, 1998.

Soyal S, Rankin T, Dean J: International Workshop on Early Folliculogenesis and Oocytes Development: Basic and clinical aspects. London, UK: Abstract Presentation, 1999.

Starr DG, McClure JP, Connor JM: Non-dermatological complications and genetic aspects of the Rothmund-Thomson syndrome. Clin Genet 27:102, 1985.

Sternberg WH, Barclay DL, Kloepfer HW: Familial XY gonadal dysgenesis. N Engl J Med 278:695, 1968.

Stevenson RE, Jones KL, Phelan MC, et al.: Vascular steal: The pathogenetic mechanism producing sirenomelia and associated defects of the viscera and soft tissues. Pediatrics 78:451, 1986.

Stevenson RE, Phelan MC, Saul RA: Defects of the abdominal wall: Association with vascular steal. Proc Greenwood Genet Center 8:15, 1989.

Strobel A, Issad T, Camoin L, et al.: A leptin missense mutation associated with hypogonadism and morbid obesity. Nat Genet 18:213, 1998.

Sudbeck P, Schmitz ML, Baeuerle PA: Sex reversal by loss of the C-terminal transactivation domain of human SOX9. Nat Genet 13:230, 1996.

Sugarman GI, Landing BH, Reed WB: Cockayne syndrome: Clinical study of two patients and neuropathologic findings in one. Clin Pediatr (Phila) 16:225, 1977.

Sultan LH, Lumbroso S: LH receptor defects. In Kempers RD, Cohen J, Haney AF, Younger JB (eds): Fertility and Reproductive Medicine—Proceedings of the XVI World Congress on Fertility and Sterility. Amsterdam: Elsevier Science, 1998, p 769.

Susca F, Apa R, Vicino M, et al.: Xq deletion and premature ovarian failure. Hum Reprod 14 (abstract):236, 1999.

Sybert VP: Phenotypic effects of mosaicism for a 47,XXX cell line in turner syndrome. J Med Genet 39:217, 2002.

Tajima T, Nakae J, Shinohara N, et al.: A novel mutation localized in the 3' non-HMG box region of the SRY gene in 46,XY gonadal dysgenesis. Hum Mol Genet 3:1187, 1994.

Tanner JM, Goldstein H, Whitehouse RH: Standards for children's height at ages 2-9 years allowing for heights of parents. Arch Dis Child 45:755, 1970.

Tapanainen JS, Aittomaki K, Min J, et al.: Men homozygous for an inactivating mutation of the follicle-stimulating hormone (FSH) receptor gene present variable suppression of spermatogenesis and fertility. Nat Genet 15:205, 1997.

Tarani L, Lampariello S, Raguso G, et al.: Pregnancy in patients with Turner's syndrome: Six new cases and review of literature. Gynecol Endocrinol 12:83, 1998.

Taylor HS, Block K, Bick DP, et al.: Mutation analysis of the EMX2 gene in Kallmann's syndrome. Fertil Steril 72:910, 1999.

Teebi AS, Miller S, Ostrer H, et al.: Spastic paraplegia, optic atrophy, microcephaly with normal intelligence, and XY sex reversal: A new autosomal recessive syndrome? J Med Genet 35:759, 1998.

Tegenkamp TR, Brazzell JW, Tegenkamp I, et al.: Pregnancy without benefit of reconstructive surgery in a bisexually active true hermaphrodite. Am J Obstet Gynecol 135:427, 1979.

Tharapel AT, Anderson KP, Simpson JL, et al.: Deletion (X) (q26.1 → q28) in a proband and her mother: Molecular characterization and phenotypic-karyotypic deductions. Am J Hum Genet 52:463, 1993.

Thomas NS, Sharp AJ, Browne CE, et al.: Xp deletions associated with autism in three females. Hum Genet 104:43, 1999.

Toledo SP, Arnhold IJ, Luthold W, et al.: Leydig cell hypoplasia determining familial hypergonadotropic hypogonadism. Prog Clin Biol Res 200:311, 1985.

Toledo SP, Brunner HG, Kraaij R, et al.: An inactivating mutation of the luteinizing hormone receptor causes amenorrhea in a 46,XX female. J Clin Endocrinol Metab 81:3850, 1996.

Topilko P, Schneider-Maunoury S, Levi G, et al.: Multiple pituitary and ovarian defects in Krox-24 (NGFI-A, Egr-1)-targeted mice. Mol Endocrinol 12:107, 1998.

Tsuchiya K, Reijo R, Page, DC, et al.: Gonadoblastoma: Molecular definition of the susceptibility region on the Y chromosome. Am J Hum Genet 57:1400, 1995.

van Niekerk WA: True Hermaphroditism. New York: Harper & Row, 1974.

Vegetti W, Grazia Tibiletti M, Testa G, et al.: Inheritance in idiopathic premature ovarian failure: Analysis of 71 cases. Hum Reprod 13:1796, 1998.

Veitia R, Ion A, Barbaux S, et al.: Mutations and sequence variants in the testis-determining region of the Y chromosome in individuals with a 46,XY female phenotype. Hum Genet 99:648, 1997.

Veitia R, Nunes M, Brauner R, et al.: Deletions of distal 9p associated with 46,XY male to female sex reversal: Definition of the breakpoints at 9p23.3-p24.1. Genomics 41:271, 1997.

Veitia RA, Nunes M, Quintana-Murci L, et al.: Swyer syndrome and 46,XY partial gonadal dysgenesis associated with 9p deletions in the absence of monosomy-9p syndrome. Am J Hum Genet 63:901, 1998.

Veitia R, Nunes M, Rapport R, et al.: Sywer syndrome and 46,XY partial gonadal dysgenesis associated with 9p deletions and the absence of monosomy 9p syndrome. Am J Hum Genet 63:901, 1998.

Veneman TF, Beverstock GC, Exalto N, et al.: Premature menopause because of an inherited deletion in the long arm of the X-chromosome. Fertil Steril 55:631, 1991.

Vergnaud G, Page DC, Simmler MC, et al.: A deletion map of the human Y chromosome based on DNA hybridization. Am J Hum Genet 38:109, 1986.

Verp MS, Harrison HH, Ober C, et al.: Chimerism as the etiology of a 46,XX/46,XY fertile true hermaphrodite. Fertil Steril 57:346, 1992.

Verp MS, Simpson JL: Abnormal sexual differentiation and neoplasia. Cancer Genet Cytogenet 25:191, 1987.

Vidal V, Chaboissier M-C, deRooij DG, et al.: *SOX9* induces testis development in XX transgenic mice. Nat Genet 28:216, 2001.

Vogt PH, Affara N, Davey P, et al.: Report of the Third International Workshop on Y Chromosome Mapping 1997. Heidelberg, Germany, April 13-16, 1997. Cytogenet Cell Genet 79:1, 1997.

Wachtel SS: H-Y Antigen and the Biology of Sex Determination. New York: Grune & Stratton, 1983.

Waggoner DD, Buist NR, Donnell GN: Long-term prognosis in galactosaemia: Results of a survey of 350 cases, J Inherit Metab Dis 13:802, 1990.

Waggoner DJ, Chow CK, Dowton SB, et al.: Partial monosomy of distal 10q: Three new cases and a review. Am J Med Genet 86:1, 1999.

Waldmann TA, Misiti J, Nelson DL, et al.: Ataxia-telangiectasia: A multisystem hereditary disease with immunodeficiency, impaired organ maturation, x-ray hypersensitivity, and a high incidence of neoplasia [clinical conference]. Ann Intern Med 99:367, 1983.

Walther MM, Trulock TS, Finnerty DP, et al.: Splenic gonadal fusion. Urology 32:521, 1988.

Weemaes CM, Hustinx TW, Scheres JM, et al.: A new chromosomal instability disorder: The Nijmegen breakage syndrome. Acta Paediatr Scand 70:557, 1981.

Weiss J, Adams E, Whitcomb RW, et al.: Normal sequence of the gonadotropin-releasing hormone gene in patients with idiopathic hypgonadotropic hypogonadism. Biol Reprod 45:743, 1991.

Weiss J, Axelrod L, Whitcomb RW, et al.: Hypogonadism caused by a single amino acid substitution in the β-subunit of luteinizing hormone. N Engl J Med 326:179, 1992.

Weiss J, Crowley WF, Jameson JL: Normal structure of the gonadotropin-releasing hormone (GnRH) gene in patients with GnRH deficiency and idiopathic hypogonadotropic hypogonadism. J Clin Endocrinol Metab 69:299, 1989.

Wharton LR: Two cases of supernumerary ovary and one of accessory ovary, with an analysis of previously reported cases. Am J Obstet Gynecol 78:1101, 1959.

Wieacker P, Missbach D, Jakubiczka S, et al.: Sex reversal in a child with the karyotype 46,XY, dup (1) (p22.3p32.3). Clin Genet 49:271, 1996.

Willard HF, Cremers FP, Mandel JL, et al.: Report of the fifth international workshop on human X chromosome mapping. Cytogenet Cell Genet 67:295, 1994.

Wilson EE, Vuitch F, Carr BR: Laparoscopic removal of dysgenetic gonads containing a gonadoblastoma in a patient with Swyer syndrome. Obstet Gynecol 79:842, 1992.

Wilson MG, Modebe O, Towner JW, et al.: Ullrich-Turner syndrome associated with interstitial deletion of Xp11.4 leads to p22.31. Am J Med Genet 14:567, 1983.

Witters I, Moerman P, Muenke M, et al.: Semilobar holoprosencephaly in a 46,XY female fetus. Prenat Diagn 21:839, 2001.

Wu E, Jiang H, Simon MI: Different 1-adrenergic receptor sequences required for activating G subunits of Gq class of G proteins. J Biol Chem 270:9829, 1995.

Wu W, Cogan JD, Pfaffle RW, et al.: Mutations in PROP1 cause familial combined pituitary hormone deficiency. Nat Genet 18L147, 1998.

Yu RN, Ito M, Saunders TL, et al.: Role of *Ahch* in gonadal development and gametogenesis. Nat Genet 20:353, 1998.

Zadik Z, Levin S, Prager-Lewin R, et al.: Gonadal dysfunction in patients with ataxia-telangiectasia. Acta Paediatr Scand 67:477, 1978.

Zenteno JC, Jimenez AL, Canto P, et al.: Clinical expression and *SRY* gene analysis in XY subjects lacking gonadal tissue. Am J Med Genet 99:244, 2001.

Zenteno JC, Lopez M, Vera C, et al.: Two SRY-negative XX male brothers without genital ambiguity. Hum Genet 100:606, 1997.

Zhang YH, Guo W, Wagner RL, et al.: DAX1 mutations map to putative structural domains in a deduced-dimensional model. Am J Hum Genet 62:855, 1998.

Zinn AR: The X chromosome and the ovary. J Soc Gynecol Investig 8:S34, 2001.

Zinn AR, Ross JL: Molecular analysis of genes on Xp controlling Turner syndrome and premature ovarian failure (POF). Semin Reprod Med 19:141, 2001.

Zinn AR, Tonk VS, Chen Z, et al.: Evidence for a Turner syndrome locus or loci Xp11.2-p22.1. Am J Hum Genet 63:1757, 1998.

Zlotogora J, Sagi M, Cohen, T: The blepharophimosis-ptosis and epicanthus inversus syndrome: Delineation of two types. Am J Hum Genet 33:1020, 1983.

CHAPTER **1 1**

Abnormal Genital Development (Male and Female Pseudohermaphroditism)

External genitalia are normally distinctly male or distinctly female. Gonads are appropriate for genetic sex (46,XY or 46,XX). Normal male differentiation occurs if testes in 46,XY individuals provide sufficient androgens to virilize the undifferentiated fetus along male lines. If external genitalia in individuals with a Y chromosome are not virilized to the extent expected of a normal male, *male pseudohermaphroditism* is said to exist. If excess androgens are present, female fetuses virilize inappropriately. If external genitalia in 46, XX individuals is not that expected of normal females, *female pseudohermaphroditism* is said to exist.

This chapter discusses the major forms of *male* and *female pseudohermaphroditism*, both of which may lead to genital ambiguity. A third general category of individuals with genital ambiguity are those with *true hermaphroditism*, which was discussed in Chapter 10 as a primary disorder of gonadal development.

Female Pseudohermaphroditism

In female pseudohermaphrodite 46,XX individuals the external genitalia fail to develop as expected for normal females. By far the most common cause is congenital adrenal hyperplasia, resulting from deficiencies of the various enzymes required for steroid biosynthesis (Fig. 11–1): 21-hydroxylase, 11β-hydroxylase, and 3β-ol-dehydrogenase. The common pathogenesis involves decreased production of adrenal cortisol, which regulates secretion of adrenocorticotropic

hormone (ACTH) through a negative feedback inhibition mechanism. If cortisol production is decreased, ACTH secretion is not inhibited. Elevated ACTH levels lead to increased quantities of steroid precursors, from which androgens can be synthesized.

Syndromes of adrenal hyperplasia must be excluded rapidly when assessing an infant with genital ambiguity because cortisol and corticosterone deficiencies result in sodium wasting that may be life-threatening. If salt wasting does not exist and cortisol is not administered, affected individuals initially experience increased growth during early childhood; however, premature epiphyseal closure leads to decreased final adult height. Even if cortisol administration is begun immediately following birth, patients with adrenal hyperplasia historically have attained heights only between the third and fifteenth percentiles (Riddick et al., 1975). However, with long-term routine use of dexamethasone, predicted adult heights can often be obtained if bone age is not already advanced when treatment is begun (Rivkees and Crawford, 2000). This holds for both 21- and 11β-hydroxylase deficiencies.

DEFICIENCY OF 21-HYDROXYLASE (*CYP21*)

Clinical

Deficiency of 21-hydroxylase, inherited in autosomal recessive fashion, is the most common cause of genital ambiguity. The incidence in Europe and

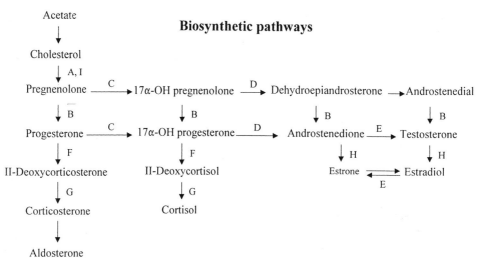

FIGURE 11–1. • Pivotal adrenal and gonadal biosynthetic pathways. Letters designate enzymes or activities required for the appropriate conversions. A, 20α-hydroxylase, and 20,22-desmolase; B, 3β-ol-dehydrogenase; C, 17α-hydroxylase; D, 17,20-desmolase; E, 17-ketosteroid reductase; F, 21-hydroxylase; G, 11β-hydroxylase; H, aromatase. In addition to these enzymes, *St*eroid *A*cute *R*egulatory protein (StAR), designated I, is responsible for transporting cholesterol to the site of steroid biosynthesis. 17α-hydroxylase (C) and 17,20-desmolase (D) activities are actually governed by a single gene.

North America overall is about 1/12,000 to 1/18,000 (Pang and Clark, 1993). Much higher incidences are observed in Yupik Eskimoes (Alaska) and in Reunion (South Pacific). 21-Hydroxylase deficiency is the result of deficiency of a cytochrome P-450 enzyme that converts 17α-hydroxyprogesterone to 11-deoxycortisol (see Fig. 11–1). Serum cortisol and deoxycortisol are decreased; 17α-hydroxyprogesterone (17α-OHP), androstenedione, estrone, and testosterone are increased. Increased 17α-OHP in either serum (affected neonate) or amniotic fluid (affected fetus) provides the basis for diagnosis.

Females deficient for 21- or 11β-hydroxylase show clitoral hypertrophy, labioscrotal fusion, and displacement of the urethral orifice to a location more nearly approximating that expected for a male. Extent of virilization may vary among individuals having the same enzyme deficiency. Wolffian derivatives (vasa deferentia, seminal vesicles, epididymides) are rarely present, probably because fetal adrenal function begins too late in embryogenesis to stabilize the wolffian ducts. Müllerian derivatives develop normally, as would be expected in the absence of antimüllerian hormone AMH (MIS). Ovaries develop normally. Scrotal and areolar hyperpigmentation may occur, presumably because ACTH has melanocyte-stimulating properties. Increased synthesis of pro-piomelanocortin (POMC), the parent hormone of both melanocyte-stimulating hormone (MSH) and ACTH, also occurs. In fact, hyperpigmentation

suggests the diagnosis of 21- or 11β-hydroxylase deficiencies in males whose external genitalia are normal at birth. If not ascertained by birth, 21- or 11 β-hydroxylase deficiencies may pass undetected in males until the child is 2 years of age or older. At that time genital enlargement, pubic hair, and prematurely increased height are manifested.

Sodium wasting occurs in 75% of 21-hydroxylase deficiency cases showing virilization. In the form of 21-hydroxylase deficiency not associated with sodium wasting (non–sodium-wasting 21-hydroxylase deficiency), it is assumed that increased ACTH secretion results in aldosterone and cortisol levels sufficient to prevent sodium wasting. Mineralocorticoid and sodium chloride must be administered to correct hyperkalemia and restore fluid-electrolyte balance. If sodium wasting is untreated, hyponatremia, hyperkalemia, dehydration, and death may occur. Cortisol administration must be continued into adulthood, although after infancy requirements per unit weight may diminish. Long-term replacement with sodium-retaining hormone (e.g., fluorinated hydrocortisone) may also be necessary.

Molecular

21-Hydroxylase is a P450 enzyme and thus located in mitochondria. Its gene (*CYP21*) is located on chromosome 6p21, closely linked to human leukocyte antigen (HLA). This linkage can

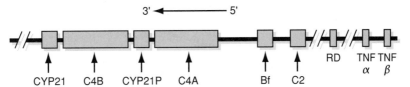

FIGURE 11–2 • Relationship among *CYP21, CYP21P,* complement (C4B, C4A) genes. This complex is located between HLA-B and HLA-DR.

be exploited for heterozygote identification and antenatal genetic diagnosis. *CYP21* is tandemly arranged with the gene(s) encoding the C4 component of complement (Fig. 11–2). This entire arrangement is then repeated. Both complement genes (C4A and C4B) are active, but only a single *CYP21* gene is active. The other *CYP21* is a pseudogene, called *CYP21P.* Although *CYP21* and *CYP21P* are 98% homologous, the latter contains a number of deletion sequences that result in a truncated gene product. Particularly common is an 8 bp deletion in exon 3 that is produced as result of an altered reading frame; the protein (gene) product is thus truncated and nonfunctional. The actual order is C4A-*CYP21P*-C4B-*CYP21,* oriented with the sense strand left to right. It is presumed that this *CYP21*/C4 tandem configuration arose by gene duplication through recombination. The *CYP21*/C4 tandem arrangement predisposes toward unequal crossing over as a result of chromosomal misalignment (Fig. 11–3). This may lead to molecular perturbations, in which one chromosome has a duplication whereas its homolog has a deficiency for the same sequence. The result could be an allele consisting only of *CYP21*P sequences (large gene conversion) or an allele lacking *CYP21* (deletion). The phenomenon of gene conversion is characteristic of 21-hydroxylase deficiency.

Various perturbations in the *CYP21* gene are found in 21-hydroxylase deficiency (Table 11–1). Homozygous deletions and large gene conversions leading to persistence of only *CYP21P* alleles predictably result in severe salt-wasting 21-hydroxylase deficiency (Wedell, 1998). This accounts for one third of cases overall. Point mutations and splice junction mutations account for perhaps 50%, with nine mutations in various combinations accounting for the great majority of Swedish cases (Table 11–1). Point mutations causing dysfunctional *CYP21* genes are usually found in the pseudogene (*CYP21P*), and thus can be presumed to have arisen by recombination. Deletions, large conversions, and *CYP21P*-derived point mutations account for 90 to 95% of all mutated *CYP21* alleles in French, American, Italian, and Swedish populations

(Morel et al., 1992; Speiser et al., 1992; Wedell, 1998; Bobba et al., 1999). All but 5% of point mutations in *CYP21* are derived from the accompanying pseudogene (*CYP21P*) through unequal cross-over.

Simple virilizing 21-hydroxylase deficiency is more likely to be associated with missense nucleotide substitution, whereas salt-wasting 21-hydroxylase deficiency is naturally more likely to be associated with large deletions or gene conversion frame shifts and nonsense mutations (see Table 11–1). The phenotype cannot always be

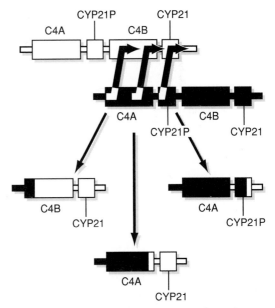

FIGURE 11–3 • Schematic representation of crossing-over events involving genes for the C4 complement and 21-hydroxylase. Depending on the extent of unequal crossing over, one can obtain one complement gene made mainly of CB4 sequences in its 3′ area with one *CYP21*; or one complement gene made mainly of C4A in its 5′ area with one *CYP21*; or one C4A and a 21-hydroxylase gene that includes mainly the 5′ part of *CYP12P*. In the third type of crossing over, the 21-hydroxylase gene, although it contains some sequences of the 3′ part of *CYP21*, is made mainly of the 5′ part of *CYP21P*, including deleterious mutations characteristic of *CYP21P*. (From Miegon CJ, Donohoue PA: Congenital adrenal hyperplasia caused by 21-hydroxylase deficiency. Its molecular basis and its remaining therapeutic problems. Endocrinol Metab Clin North Am 20:277, 1991.)

▼ **Table 11–1.** *CYP21* MUTATION FOUND IN SWEDEN BY WEDELL (1998)

Mutation		Perturbation	Nucleotide Position	Exon	Frequency (%)
A. Deletion/Apparent large gene conversion (*CYP21P* but not *CYP21* present)					32.2%
B. Pseudogene-derived mutations:					
1	I2 splice	AA/AC → AG	656	Intron 2	26.6
2	Ile172Asn	ATC → AAC	1001	Exon 4	19.8
3	Val281Leu	GTG → TTG	1685	Exon 7	5.7
4	Arg356Trp	CGG → TGG	2110	Exon 8	3.0
5	Gln318stop	CAG → TAG	1996	Exon 8	2.4
6	Pro30Leu	CCG → CTG	89	Exon 1	1.6
7	E3 del 8bp		del 708-715	Exon 3	1.1
8	Cluster E6:				
	Ile236Asn	ATC → AAC	1382	Exon 6	
	Val237Glu	GTG → GAG	1385	Exon 6	1.1
	Met239Lys	ATG → AAG	1391	Exon 6	
9	Leu307insT	ins T	1765	Exon 7	<1
C. Combinations of mutations in B:					
	I2 splice + Gln318stop		(two *CYP21*/ chromosome)		<1
	I2 splice + Val281Leu		(two mutations/ *CYP21* allele)		<1
	I2 splice + IleI72Asn		"		<1
	Leu307insT + Gln318stop		"		<1
	Gln318stop + Arg356Trp		"		<1
	Cluster E6 + Val281Leu		"		<1
	Val281Leu + L307insT		"		<1
	Ile172Asn–Arg356Trp		(six mutations/ *CYP21* allele)		<1
D. Rare mutations (but present more than once):					
10	Pro453Ser	CCC → TCC	2581	Exon 10	<1
11	Arg483Pro	CGG → CCG	2672	Exon 10	<1
12	Arg483GGtoC	GG → C	2672-73	Exon 10	<1
E. Unique mutations (single families):10 different mutations					
					<2.5%

Approximately 400 mutations constituted the data base. Gene conversions, gene deletions, and nine mutations were responsible for 95% of cases. From Wedell A: Molecular genetics of congenital adrenal hyperplasia (21-hydroxylase deficiency): implications for diagnosis, prognosis and treatment. Acta Paediatr 87:159, 1998.

predicted precisely from the mutation, but some predictions are possible (Fig. 11–4). The most common gene conversion involves nucleotide 656, either an adenine or cytosine being replaced by a guanine, nucleotide (nt) 656A/C→G. The nt656A/C→G mutation results in a premature splice of intron 2 and, hence, a frame shift. This mutation usually causes virilization without salt wasting (Tusie-Luna et al., 1990; Speiser et al., 1992; New and White, 1995). A major diagnostic difficulty in diagnosing of nt656A/C→G is poor amplification (allele dropout) of the normal allele in heterozygotes (Day et al., 1996; Van de Velde et al., 1999). The next most common mutation is a 172→A transition (Ile172Asn). This causes the same phenotype and shows 3 to

7% of normal enzyme activity (Tusie-Luna et al., 1990; New and White, 1995).

Late-onset 21-hydroxylase may produce hirsutism and a polycystic ovary-type phenotype. This is especially common in individuals of Ashkenazi Jewish descent, who may show Val281Leu. This mutation decreases enzyme activity to 20 to 50% of normal. Heterozygote frequencies for late onset 21-hydroxylase deficiency as high as one in three have been reported in Ashkenazi Jews, an astonishingly high frequency derived from a presumptive homozygote frequency (q^2) of 1 in 30 (see Chapter 2 for Hardy-Weinberg equilibrium). The phenotype is hirsutism, acne, and polycystic ovarian disease. If compound heterozygosity

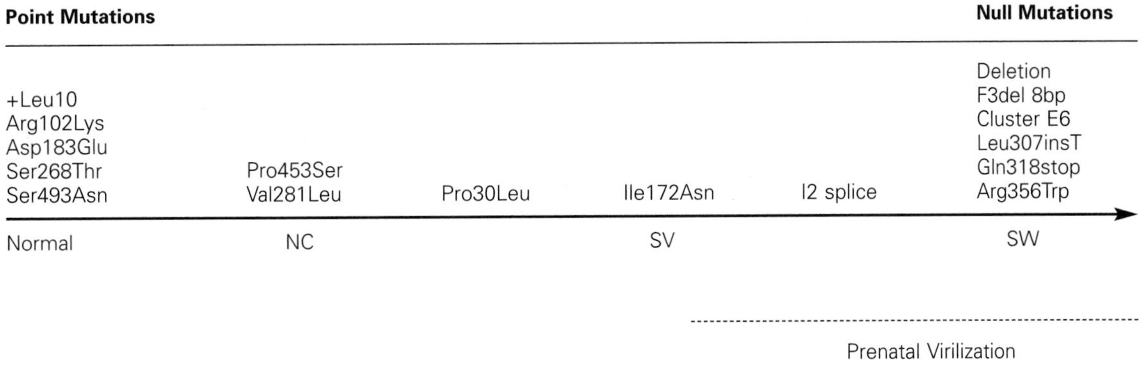

Point Mutations
Null Mutations
+Leu10
Arg102Lys
Asp183Glu
Ser268Thr
Ser493Asn
Pro453Ser
Val281Leu
Pro30Leu
Ile172Asn
I2 splice
Deletion
F3del 8bp
Cluster E6
Leu307insT
Gln318stop
Arg356Trp
Normal
NC
SV
SW
Prenatal Virilization

FIGURE 11–4 • Steroid 21-hydroxylase mutations, graded according to severity. Slight variation may occur between mutations, but they generally fall into four major clinical groups: normal, nonclassic (NC), simple virilizing (SV), and salt-wasting (SW) congenital adrenal hyperplasia. (From Wedell A: Molecular genetics of congenital adrenal hyperplasia [21-hydroxylase deficiency]: Implications for diagnosis, prognosis and treatment. Acta Paediatr 87:159, 1998.)

exists for the Val281Leu allele and one causing classic 21-hydroxylase deficiency, the phenotype is that of late-onset 21-hydroxylase. This is consistent with the principle that phenotype reflects the less severe genotype in compound heterozygosity. This scenario was illustrated earlier with respect to cystic fibrosis (see Chapter 4).

DEFICIENCY OF 11β-HYDROXYLASE (CYB11B1)

Less common than 21-hydroxylase deficiency, 11β-hydroxylase deficiency is also inherited in autosomal recessive fashion. In this disorder there is decreased conversion of 11-deoxycortisol to cortisol and 11-deoxycorticosterone to corticosterone (see Fig. 11–1). The predominant metabolite of 11-deoxycortisol is tetrahydrocortisol, which is increased. Because deoxycortisol and deoxycorticosterone are potent sodium-retaining hormones, increased levels may lead to hypervolemia and, hence, hypertension. In 11β-hydroxylase deficiency infants thus manifest not only the genital virilization characteristic of 21-hydroxylase deficiency but also hypertension.

The gene responsible for this form of female pseudohermaphroditism is *CYP11B1*, located on 8q22 (Mornet and White, 1989). There are two 11β-hydroxylase genes, coding for the mitochondrial cytochrome P450 enzymes *CYP11B1* and *CYP11B2*. The latter gene is expressed only in the zona glomerulosa and is important for aldosterone synthesis.

The most common molecular perturbations in *CYP11B1* are point mutations (White et al., 1991; Naiki et al., 1993; Skinner and Rumsby, 1994). Over two dozen different mutations have been associated with 11β-hydroxylase deficiency (Fig. 11–5). These include nonsense mutations, missense mutations, and frameship mutations and insertions (White et al., 1994; Nakagawa et al., 1995; Geley et al., 1996). Mutations tend to cluster in exons 6 to 8, which could indicate a "hot spot" for mutation. Alternatively, mutations in proximal exons, i.e., closer to the DNA binding region, could be lethal. In support of the hotspot hypothesis, Arg448His is a common

356
Q-Ter
356
Q-Ter
374
R-Q
394*
448
R-H
441
V-G
32*
116
W-Ter
174
K-Ter
318
T-M
384
R-Q
CYS
1
2
3
4
5
6
7
8
9

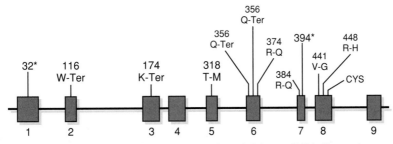

FIGURE 11–5 • Locations of mutations causing 11β-hydroxylase deficiency. CYS indicates the conserved cysteine that coordinates the heme group. Asterisks indicate the position of frameshift mutations. (From Donohoue PA, Parker KL, Migeon CJ: Congenital adrenal hyperplasia. *In* Scriver CR, Beaudet AL, Sly WS, et al. (eds): The Metabolic and Molecular Bases of Inherited Disease, 8th ed, vol. III. New York: McGraw-Hill, 2001.)

mutation in Ashkenazi Jews (White et al., 1991), whereas Arg448Cys is observed in other ethnic groups (Geley et al., 1996).

Although *CYP11B1* has a homologous gene on the same chromosome (*CYP11B2*), gene conversion is uncommon in 11β-hydroxylase deficiency because both genes are functional. This contrasts with a 21-hydroxylase deficiency (*CYP21* and *CYP21P*).

DEFICIENCY OF 3β-HYDROXYSTEROID-DEHYDROGENASE (3β-HSD)

In 3β-ol-dehydrogenase deficiency (see Fig. 11–1), the principal synthesized androgen is dehydroepiandrosterone (DHEA). This relatively weak androgen cannot be converted to either androstenedione or testosterone. Females with 3β-ol-dehydrogenase deficiency are thus less virilized than females with 21- or 11β-hydroxylase deficiencies. On the other hand, DHEA is such a weak androgen that males with 3β-ol-dehydrogenase deficiency fail to masculinize completely (male pseudohermaphroditism). 3β-ol-Dehydrogenase deficiency is therefore the only form of adrenal hyperplasia in which both males and females show genital ambiguity. During embryogenesis, 3β-ol-dehydrogenase activity reaches its maximum capacity earlier in testes (third month) than in adrenals and ovaries (fourth month). Otherwise, external genitalia might be identical in affected males and affected females.

Complete deficiency of 3β-ol-dehydrogenase results in severe sodium wasting secondary to deficiency of sodium-retaining hormones. Sodium wasting is often so pronounced that affected infants die precipitously. Less severe deficiencies are compatible with long-term survival, many cases having been detected in older infants (Bongiovanni, 1979).

3β-ol-Dehydrogenase deficiency is inherited in autosomal recessive fashion and can be diagnosed on the basis of serum steroids measured before and after ACTH stimulation. Located on chromosome 1, the gene is not mitochondrial like *CYP21* and *CYP11B* but microsomal. Thus, 3βol-dehydrogenase is *not* a cytochrome P450 enzyme.

Molecular

There are two 3β-HSD genes (I and II), both located on chromosome 1 (p11-13) and both consisting of 4 exons. Type II is expressed in gonads and adrenals. Mutations causing both virilization and salt-wasting have almost completely abolished enzyme activity; mutations causing only virilization are missense mutations characterized by 1 to 10% enzyme activity (Simard et al., 1995a). Mutations causing the two phenotypes are scattered among all exons (Fig. 11–6). In each of 11 families with severe salt-wasting 3β-HSD, different mutations were found (Simard et al., 1995a, b; Taijma et al., 1997). In six non-salt-wasting 3β-HSD deficiency families, different

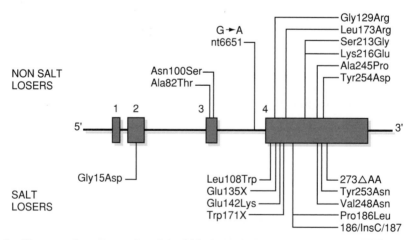

FIGURE 11–6 • Diagrammatic representation of the *3b*-hydroxysteroid dehydrogenase type 2 (*HSD3B2*) gene with the mutations that result in 3β-HSD deficiency. The numbered solid boxes indicate the exons. Missense mutations causing amino acid substitutions in the enzyme are indicated by the three letter abbreviation for the wild-type amino acid, followed by the amino acid number in the enzyme and then the three-letter abbreviation for the substituted amino acid. Mutations with less than 1% 3β-HSD activity are indicated below the gene and cause salt loss. Missense and splicing mutations, indicated above the gene, result in 2 to 4.7% enzymatic activity and are associated with the non–salt losing phenotype. (From Grumbach MM, Conte FA: Disorders of sex differentiation. *In* Wilson JD, Foster DW, Kronenberg HM, et al. (eds): Williams Textbook of Endocrinology, 9th ed. Philadelphia: WB Saunders, 1998.)

mutations were also usual (Simard et al., 1995b); however, Ala 82 Thr was observed in two Brazilian families. Moisan and coworkers (1999) found 8 mutations in 11 patients from 7 families.

DEFICIENCY OF 17α-HYDROXYLASE/ 17,20-LYASE (CYP17)

If the cytochrome P450 enzyme 17α-hydroxylase/17-20-lyase is deficient, pregnenolone cannot be converted to 17α-hydroxy-pregnenolone. If the enzyme defect were complete, cortisol, androstenedione, testosterone, and estrogens could not be synthesized; however, 11-deoxycorticosterone and corticosterone could be. With a compensatory increase in ACTH secretion, 11-deoxycorticosterone and corticosterone increase to result in hypernatremia, hypokalemia, and hypervolemia. Hypertension occurs. Aldosterone is decreased, presumably because hypervolemia suppresses the renin-angiotensin system. Affected males usually have genital ambiguity (male pseudohermaphroditism).

Females with 17α-hydroxylase deficiency have normal external genitalia but at puberty fail to undergo normal secondary sexual development (primary amenorrhea). Affected females are ordinarily encountered in differential diagnosis of XX gonadal dysgenesis. Hypertension is the major diagnostic clue. Oocytes appear incapable of spontaneously exceeding a diameter greater than 2.5 mm (Araki et al., 1987), but ovaries nonetheless respond to exogenous gonadotropins (Rabinovici et al., 1989).

17α-Hydroxylase deficiency is inherited in autosomal recessive fashion. The gene (CYP17) is located on 10q24-25, and the gene product is a cytochrome P450 enzyme. This single gene (and enzyme) is responsible for both 17α-hydroxylase and 17,20-desmolase (lyase) actions (see Fig. 11–1).

Molecular

Over 20 different mutations have been identified in CYP17, scattered among the 8 exons. Mutations include missense mutations, duplications, deletions, and premature protein truncation (Yanase, 1995). Most mutations have been observed in only a single family, yet another example of molecular heterogeneity. An exception exists in Mennonites of Dutch origin, in whom a 4-base duplication in exon 8 accounts for most cases (Imai et al., 1992). This founder mutation originated in Friesland.

Few patients having deficiency of both 17α-hydroxylase *and* 17,20 lyase activities have been

analyzed, but mutations different from those only showing deficient 17α-hydroxylase activity have been found (Kaneko et al., 1994; Miura et al., 1996). Transfection experiments show that only 5% of 17α-hydroxylase activity is sufficient for the estrogen production necessary for normal secondary sexual characteristics in a 46,XX individual; however, 25% of enzyme activity is necessary to virilize external genitalia in males (Yanase, 1995; Miura et al., 1996). Targeted mutagenesis in the rat gene indicates that mutations closer to the 5′ end are more deleterious (Fig. 11–7).

For further discussion of molecular aspects of CYP17α, see the section on Male Pseudohermaphroditism (below).

AROMATASE MUTATIONS (CYP19)

Conversion of androgens (Δ4-androstenedione) to estrogens (estrone) requires cytochrome P-450 aromatase, an enzyme that is the gene product of a single 40-kb gene located on chromosome 15q21.1 (ER Simpson et al., 1997). The CYP19 gene consists of 10 exons (Fig. 11–8). A dysfunctional enzyme leads to excess androstenedione, an androgen capable of virilizing female fetuses. Thus, aromatase deficiency can cause female pseudohermaphroditism.

CYP19 mutation has been associated with either primary amenorrhea or genital ambiguity in 46,XX individuals. The former was considered in Chapter 10. Here we consider aromatase deficiency causing 46,XX genital ambiguity, for these cases are encountered in the differential diagnosis of female pseudohermaphroditism.

Shozu and colleagues (1991) were the first to recognize *placental* aromatase deficiency, manifested as maternal virilization during the third trimester and confirmed in studies of placental tissue. The 46,XX infant had genital ambiguity (female pseudohermaphroditism), but no adrenal enzyme defects were evident. Instead, the molecular basis of the mutation was a 87-bp insert in exon 6 of the aromatase gene, altering a splice junction site to produce a novel protein with 29 additional amino acids (Harada et al., 1992). The mutation resulted in less than 0.3% normal enzyme activity (Harada et al., 1992).

Aromatase mutations in 46,XX female infants have also produced clitoromegaly (Mullis et al., 1997). Clitoral enlargement occurred at puberty, but breast development did not. Multiple ovarian follicular cysts were evident. Follicle-stimulating hormone (FSH) was elevated, estrone and estradiol levels low. Estrogen and progesterone therapy resulted in a growth spurt, decreased

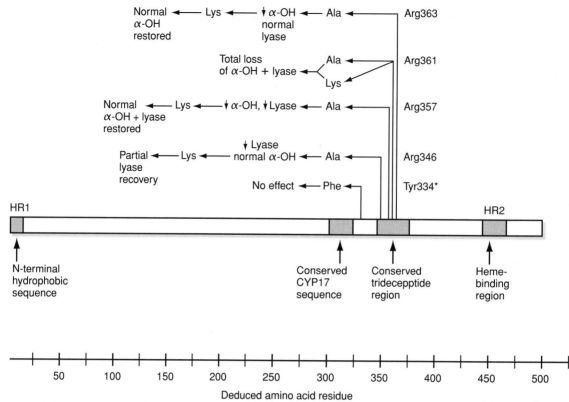

FIGURE 11–7 • Results of site-directed mutations in the rat *CYP17* gene. *CYP17* cDNA underwent site-directed mutagenesis to produce the codon changes shown. The mutants were expressed in COS-1 cells, and 17*a*-hydroxylase (*α*-OH) and 17,20-layse (lyase) activities were measured. The mutations at arginine 346,357 and 363 were corrected by a second mutation replacing the mutant alanine with lysine. The only residue tested that is not conserved between the rat and the human: is that of HR1 and HR2- homologous regions 1 and 2; both contain highly conserved critical cysteine residues. (From Donohoue PA, Parker KL, Migeon CJ: Congenital adrenal hyperplasia. *In* Scriver CR, Beaudet AL, Sly WS, et al. (eds): The Metabolic and Molecular Bases of Inherited Disease, 8th ed, vol III. New York: McGraw-Hill, 2001.)

FSH, decreased levels of androstenedione and testosterone, breast development, menarche, and decreased numbers of follicular cysts.

A sibship has been reported with affected female (46,XX) and male (46,XY). The former had genital ambiguity; the latter was tall (Morishima et al., 1995). Homozygosity existed for a missense mutation (R375C) (Mulaikal et al., 1987).

TERATOGENIC FEMALE PSEUDOHERMAPHRODITISM

To interfere with genital differentiation, a teratogen must exert its action during organogenesis. Before that time, no organ-specific structure can be affected. In humans the genital tubercle first becomes evident around 5 weeks of embryogenesis (7 weeks' gestation). If an androgenic teratogen is administered prior to 12 weeks of gestation, labioscrotal fusion may occur. After 12 weeks, an androgenic teratogen may cause clitoral enlargement but not labioscrotal fusion.

Female pseudohermaphroditism can result from administration of androgens or certain (19-nortestosterone) progestins during early pregnancy (Carson and Simpson, 1984). When testosterone and other androgens masculinize the female offspring of pregnant women, phallic enlargement, labioscrotal fusion, and displacement of the urogenital sinus invagination result. Excessive androgen production does not affect müllerian differentiation or ovarian differentiation.

Androgen-induced female pseudohermaphroditism was not uncommon decades ago, when women were more frequently treated during pregnancy with high doses of synthetic progestins. Not infrequently, virilized female offspring resulted (Grumbach et al., 1959; Carson and Simpson, 1984). Administration of progestins during pregnancy, especially at high doses, is now rarely indicated. Female pseudohermaph-

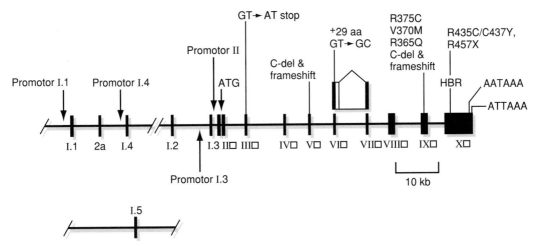

FIGURE 11–8 • Structure of the human *CYP19* gene showing the known mutations. Five of the mutations are single base pair changes giving rise to single amino acid substitutes. Of these, two are in the heme binding region (HBR) of exon X (R435C and C437Y) in compound heterozygosity. Three are in exon IX (R375C, V370M, R365Q). Another single base pair change resulted in a stop codon (R457X) in exon X. A Japanese infant showed a splice junction terminating mutation in exon VI, giving rise to a read-through of 87 bp before a cryptic splice junction is recognized; the net result is an insertion of 29 amino acids. A 4-year-old Swiss girl was found to be a compound heterozygote. On one chromosome was a frameshift that led to a nonsense codon; on the other chromosome was a splice junction mutation leading a premature stop codon. A Swiss newborn boy carried a homozygous 1-bp deletion in exon V, resulting in a frameshift. (From Bulun SE: Aromatase deficiency and estrogen resistance: from molecular genetics to clinic. Semin Reprod Med 18:31, 2000.)

roditism from this cause is now rare but nonetheless still important because it is preventable.

Teratogens most likely to be relevant at present include testosterone, ethinyl testosterone, norethindrone acetate, norethindrone, and danocrine. In doses administered therapeutically for conditions such as endometriosis, female pseudohermaphroditism (Simpson, 1976; Carson and Simpson, 1984) may result. Acetoxyprogesterones (norethynodrel, medroxyprogesterone, and 17α-OH-progesterone caproate) are rarely implicated. 19-Nortestosterones (e.g., norethindrone) can produce virilization but only at very high doses (10–20 mg daily); thus, a single oral contraceptive pill (1 mg daily) should not produce a teratogenic female pseudohermaphrodite. Danazol is capable of producing teratogenic female pseudohermaphroditism in clinically administered doses (Duck et al., 1981; Brunskill et al., 1992). Older reports of female virilization following administration of maternal diethyl-stilbestrol remain unexplained (Bongiovanni et al., 1959). Perhaps there was contamination with androgens in the preparations administered.

MATERNAL VIRILIZING TUMORS

Fetal masculinization has been reported in pregnancies associated with Sertoli cell tumors (arrhenoblastoma), Leydig cell tumors, luteomas of pregnancy, and adenocarcinomas that metastasize to the ovary (e.g., Krukenberg tumor). Frequently cited in texts as a cause of masculinizing female fetuses, androgen-secreting tumors during pregnancy are actually very rare causes of female pseudohermaphroditism. Moreover, patients with pre-existing androgen-secreting tumors rarely become pregnant. In 1973 Verhoeven and colleagues (1973) collected 45 reports in which virilizing tumors were associated with pregnancy. Among the offspring were 18 females whose external genitalia were described; nine had clitoral or labial hypertrophy and only one had labioscrotal fusion. Luteomas are non-neoplastic but hormone-dependent ovarian lesions that occurs during pregnancy and regress thereafter. Some fetal virilization is not uncommon and complete masculinization in a 46,XX female fetus is reported (Mazza et al., 2002)

IDIOPATHIC CLITORAL HYPERTROPHY

Marked clitoral enlargement of unexplained origin sometimes exists. Hemangiomas, neurofibromas, or tumors should be considered, and a computed tomographic scan or magnetic resonance imaging study ordered. Some reported cases could have been the result of unrecognized aromatase deficiency, as illustrated by Mullis and coworkers (1997). In other cases the enlargement truly seems idiopathic and may reflect end-organ hyper-responsiveness.

Table 11–2 lists some multiple malformation syndromes in which clitoral hypertrophy exists.

AUTOSOMAL XX SEX REVERSAL CAUSED BY *SOX9* DUPLICATION

Huang and coworkers (1999) reported a highly informative, and, to date, unique case of 46,XX sex reversal. Alluded to in Chapter 10, external genitalia in this 46,XX newborn were ambiguous but predominantly male. The phallus was 1.2 cm in length; the urethral orifice opened at the base of the phallus. The scrotum was bifid with palpable gonads; however, no histologic information was provided. Cytogenetic studies revealed duplication of 17q23.1→924.3 in one cell line; the other cell was 46,XX.

Microsatellite analysis revealed that the duplication was maternal in origin, defined by a region beginning 12cM proximal and extending 2cM distal to the *SOX9* gene. This region of 17q encodes the *SOX9* gene. In Chapter 10, we noted that perturbations of *SOX9* in 46,XY are associated with sex reversal and campomelic dysplasia. *SOX9* duplication causes sex reversal in 46,XX, further indicating that *SOX9* is crucial for normal sexual differentiation. In the case above there might have been unexpected derepression of a locus ordinarily derepressed by *SRY*. This would be consistent with insertional mutagenesis near *SOX9* causing testes development in XX mice (Bishop et al., 2000).

FEMALE PSEUDOHERMAPHRODITISM WITH SKELETAL ABNORMALITIES (JONES-PARK SYNDROME)

A distinct syndrome was observed in two sibs having clitoral hypertrophy, a single perineal

▼ **Table 11–2.** SYNDROMES ASSOCIATED WITH CLITOROMEGALY

Syndrome	Prominent Features	Causation
Beckwith-Wiedemann	Macrosomia, macroglossia, omphalocele	Autosomal dominant
Bowen (Bowen et al., 1964)	Failure to grow, absent or weak sucking and swallowing, flexion of fingers, congenital glaucoma, malformed ears, small mandible, heart malformations, hypospadias, agenesis of the corpus callosum, death at an early age	Unknown
Fraser (Greenberg et al., 1986; Gafusso et al., 1987)	Cryptophthalmia, defect of auricle, hair growth on lateral forehead to lateral eyebrow, hypoplastic nares, mental deficiency, partial cutaneous syndactyly, urogenital malformations	Autosomal recessive
Leiomyoma of vulva and esophagus (Wahlen and Astedt, 1965; Schapiro and Sandrock, 1973)	Lower esophageal leiomyoma with obstruction; leiomyoma at base of clitoris causes enlargement of clitoris	Autosomal dominant
LEOPARD (Peixoto et al., 1981)	*L*entigines (multiple), *E*CG abnormalities, *o*cular hypertelorism, *p*ulmonic stenosis, *a*bnormalities of genitalia, *r*etardation of growth, *d*eafness, macroglossia, multiple dental anomalies, basilar impression and platybasia, megacolon, anal ectopy.	Autosomal dominant
Leprechaunism (Donohue) (Donohue and Uchida, 1954; Elsas et al., 1985)	Elfin facies, low-set ears, growth retardation, acanthosis nigricans, pachyderma, insulin resistance, hyperinsulinemia, hypertrophy of pancreatic β cells	Autosomal recessive
Neurofibromatosis, type I (Diekmann et al., 1967)	Café-au-lait spots, neurofibromas, enlargement of clitoris with significant firmness, compatible with neurofibroma; usually appears during adolescence or later	Autosomal dominant
Silver-Russell (Angehrn et al., 1979)	Short stature of prenatal onset; skeletal asymmetry; small, incurved fifth finger; small, triangular facies; bluish sclerae; café au lait spots	Unknown
Rutledge (Rutledge et al., 1984)	Joint contractures, cerebellar hypoplasia, renal hypoplasia, other urogenital anomalies, tongue cysts, shortness of limbs, eye abnormalities, defects of the heart, gallbladder agenesis, ear malformations	Autosomal recessive

Modified from Simpson JL, Verp MS, Plouffe L: Female genital system. *In* Stevenson RE, Hall JG, Goodman RM (eds): Human Malformations and Related Anomalies, vol 2. London: Oxford Press, 1993.

orifice leading anteriorly to a urethra and posteriorly to a vagina, and numerous skeletal anomalies (hypoplasia of the mandible and maxilla, brachycephaly, narrow vertebral bodies, relatively long slender bones, dislocation and fusion of the radial heads leading to abnormal-appearing elbows, coxa valga, and phalangeal fusion of several toes) (Jones and Park, 1971; Park et al., 1992). Müllerian derivatives and ovaries were normal. Both sibs developed breasts and pubic hair but failed to menstruate. Their parents were consanguineous; thus, autosomal recessive inheritance seems probable.

FEMALE PSEUDOHERMAPHRODITISM, RENAL AND GASTROINTESTINAL ANOMALIES

Female pseudohermaphroditism may be associated with one or more of the following anomalies: absence or duplication of the uterus; renal absence, duplication, or hydronephrosis; and imperforate anus (Perloff, 1953; Lubinsky, 1980;

Seaver et al., 1994). Short stature, mental retardation, deafness, ear and nasal malformations, and a blindly ending colon are less often associated. Ovaries are usually normal. This condition appears to be distinct from that in which disturbances of external genitalia are associated with exstrophy of the bladder or cloaca (see below).

DUPLICATION OF THE CLITORIS DUE TO EXSTROPHY OF THE BLADDER

Two separate clitori or a single clitoris that is bifid are usually associated with urethral anomalies like female epispadias, urethral duplication, and/or bladder anomalies (Jones, 1973). These patients typically have exstrophy of the bladder (Fig. 11–9). Feins and Cranley (1986) demonstrated how the bladder exstrophy causes the clitoris to separate and become bifid. In a review by Schey and coworkers (1980), female epispadias have been considered a mild form of bladder exstrophy.

The underlying mechanism reflects disruptions of the lower abdomen and pelvis, secondarily

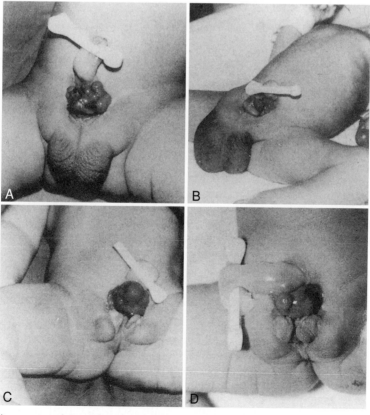

FIGURE 11–9 • Appearance of the abdomen and external genitalia in two male (A and B) and two female (C and D) newborn infants. (From Martinez-Frias ML, Bermejo E, Rodriguez-Pinilla E, et al.: Exstrophy of the cloaca and exstrophy of the bladder: Two different expressions of a primary developmental field defect. Am J Med Genet 99:261, 2001.)

altering development of the clitoris. The end result is a bifid clitoris, which may be rudimentary. Cloacal exstrophy can produce a similar condition. Current opinion is that exstrophy of the cloaca and exstrophy of the bladder are two different expressions of the same developmental field defect (Martinez-Frias et al., 2001).

Primary attention must be devoted to repair of the associated exstrophy. Females with epispadias may have incontinence, and corrective surgery can be very difficult. Severe cases may be diagnosed in utero by ultrasonography.

DUPLICATION OF THE EXTERNAL GENITALIA

Complete duplication of the external genitalia, including the clitoris, was reported by Kapoor and Saha (1987). Complete duplication of the bladder, urethra, and external genitalia was observed. Other anomalies included ventriculoseptal defect, malrotation of the gut, ectopic anal opening, maldescended left kidney, rachischisis of the lumbar spine and sacrum, and umbilical hernia.

ABSENCE OF THE EXTERNAL GENITALIA

Hypoplasia or absence of any evidence of development of external genitalia can occur. Hypoplasia of the clitoris is one component.

In this relatively rare defect the external genitalia of the newborn female may assume a relatively hypoplastic appearance. The obese child may display only a genital fold because of the thick fat pad underlying the labia majora. Chronic inflammatory processes can lead to fusion of the labia majora and minora, imparting to the perineum a flat, cleftlike appearance. It is sometimes difficult to exclude this explanation for cases described in the literature.

The normal appearance of the external female genitalia does not depend on any hormonal input until the pubertal phase. Androgen action is key for normal male sexual development *in utero*, but no hormonal counterpart is necessary for the female. As an isolated defect, genital hypoplasia is purely cosmetic and should resolve on its own at puberty. When genital hypoplasia occurs as one feature of a syndrome, other anomalies invariably prove of greater importance.

Hypoplasia of the external genitalia is less often an isolated defect than observed in multiple malformation syndromes (Robinow et al., 1969; Chen et al., 1980; Duncan et al., 1988; Ayme et al.,

1989; Aughton and Cassidy, 1990; Litwin et al., 1991) (Table 11–3). Some of these syndromes may be diagnosed prenatally using ultrasonography (Ayme et al., 1989). A positive family history is of great assistance. Hypoplasia of the external genitalia is also commonly seen with cloacal anomalies.

ABSENCE OF THE CLITORIS (AGENESIS)

The clitoris may be absent in females with otherwise normal or near-normal external genitalia. Diagnostic criteria assume clitoral agenesis is not secondary to exstrophy or cloacal defects. Cases without associated anomalies were reported by Russu (1938) and by Falk and Hyman (1971). There were not even such minor midline fusion failure defects as absence of midline pubic hair or a patulous urethra.

Del Giudice and Nydorf (1986) described agenesis of the clitoris in a patient with cutis marmorata telangiectatica congenita (CMTC). This rare disorder is characterized by persistent livedo reticularis, telangiectases, and superficial ulceration.

EXSTROPHY OF THE CLOACAL AND RELATED CAUDAL ABNORMALITIES

Genital abnormalities may also result from maldevelopment of the genital tubercle, cloacal membrane, urogenital membrane, or the entire hind end of the embryo (i.e., caudal regression syndrome). The protypical example is exstrophy of the cloaca, whose incidence is perhaps 1:200,000. This is much rarer than exstrophy of the bladder, whose incidence is 1:30,000–1:50,000 (Martinez-Frias et al., 2001). In some cloacal malformations the external genitalia are so abnormal that the sex of rearing is in doubt (Dougherty and Spencer, 1972; Martinez-Frias et al., 2001). Disorders of reproductive tracts are commonly associated. Anomalies of the cardiac, gestational renal, skeletal (limb) and brain (Arnold-Chiari malformation) are not uncommon.

Expressivity probably encompasses not only exstrophy of the cloaca, as defined by caudal dysplasia (sacral agenesis) (Passarge and Lenz, 1966; Fullana et al., 1986) but also caudal duplication and sirenomelia. Both males and females may be affected. In particular, consensus seems to exist that the complex of exstrophy of the cloaca, body wall abnormalities (omphalopagus, spinal defects), and imperforate arms constitutes a single entity (Carey, 2001; Keppler-Noreuil, 2001).

▼ **Table 11–3.** MULTIPLE MALFORMATION SYNDROMES ASSOCIATED WITH ABSENCE OF
• EXTERNAL GENITALIA

Syndrome	Prominent Features	Causation
CHARGE association	Coloboma, *h*eart disease, *a*tresia choanae, *r*etarded growth, *g*enital hypoplasia, *e*ar defects	Unknown (heterogenous occasionally familial)
Fryns	Diaphragmatic defects, lung hypoplasia, cleft lip and palate (often bilateral), cardiac defects, renal cysts, urinary tract malformation, distal limb hypoplasia, hypoplastic external genitalia, duodenal atresia, pyloric hyperplasia, malrotation and common mesentery, Dandy-Walker anomaly and agenesis of corpus callosum; almost always lethal	Autosomal recessive
Limb-body wall complex	Body wall defect, neural tube defect, limb abnormalities, complete absence of external genitalia	Unknown
Prader-Willi	Hypotonia, genital hypoplasia, obesity, acromicria, large head circumference, large anterior fontanelle, mild micrognathia, mild anomalies of the gingivae or alveolar ridges, skin changes	15q Deletion, uniparental (maternal) disomy 15
Pterygium	Normal intelligence; short stature; pterygia of neck, axillary, antecubital, popliteal, digital, and intercrural areas; multiple joint contractures, unusual facies; cleft palate; bilateral pulmonary hypoplasia; small heart; absent appendix; attenuation of the ascending and transverse colon; cervical vertebral fusion; aplasia of labia majora; small clitoris	Heterogeneous, (autosomal dominant, autosomal recessive, or X-linked recessive)
Robinow (Robinow et al., 1969)	Short stature, macrocephaly, prominent eyes, short forearms, hemivertebrae, hypoplastic genitalia	Autosomal dominant or recessive
Sirenomelia (Stevenson et al., 1986)	Single fused lower limb, renal aplasia, imperforate anus, absence of genitalia	Unknown, perhaps vascular in basis

Modified from Simpson JL, Verp MS, Plouffe L: Female genital system. *In* Stevenson RE, Hall JG, Goodman RM (eds): Human Malformations and Related Anomalies, vol 2. London: Oxford Press, 1993.

Genital ambiguity can also occur with prune belly syndrome (Rabinowitz and Schillinger, 1977).

Male Pseudohermaphroditism

In male pseudohermaphroditism, individuals with a Y chromosome have external genitalia that fail to develop as expected for normal males. External genitalia are sufficiently ambiguous to confuse the sex of rearing. Cytogenetic forms of male pseudohermaphroditism (45,X/46,XY and variants) are also discussed here to contrast their phenotype with the spectrum of male pseudohermaphroditism attributable to genetic (mendelian) causes (Table 11–4).

TERATOGENIC MALE PSEUDOHERMAPHRODITES

If administered in sufficiently high doses in the first trimester to a woman pregnant with a male fetus, several agents would be expected to produce female external genitalia. The mode of action of cyproterone involves blocking the androgen receptor. Finasteride inhibits 5α-reductase. Con-

sequences of perturbing these functions are clarified below. Both agents are approved in the U.S. for treatment of hirsutism; thus, the risk for teratogenic male pseudohermaphroditism exists. Fortunately, no cases of human teratogenicity appear to have been reported.

There is some controversy concerning whether administration of progestins or progesterones during pregnancy can produce hypospadias. However, the weight of evidence is that these agents do not adversely affect male genital development (Simpson and Kaufman, 1998; Phillips and Simpson, 2001).

CYTOGENETIC FORMS

45,X/46,XY Individuals have both a 45,X cell line and at least one cell line containing a Y chromosome. Based on cohort studies of 45,X/46,XY cases detected *in utero* (prenatal genetic diagnosis), well over 90% of cases are normal males (Chang et al., 1990). The phenotype of cases ascertained postnatally differs, manifesting a variety of phenotypes extending from almost normal males with cryptorchidism or penile hypospadias through genital ambiguity to phenotypically normal females (Simpson, 1976;

▼ **Table 11–4.** SPECTRUM OF DISORDERS CAUSING MALE PSEUDOHERMAPHRODITISM

A. Teratogenic
   Cyproterone acetate (no reported cases)
   Finasteride (no reported cases)
   Flutamide (no reported cases)
   Progestins (alleged but unproved)
B. Cytogenetic (45,X/46,XY) Mosaicism
   Female external genitalia
   Ambiguous external genitalia
C. Male Pseudohermaphroditism (Genital Ambiguity or Sex Reversal) in Multiple Malformation Syndromes
   Smith-Lemli-Opitz (SLO)
   Genito-palato-cardiac
   Meckel-Gruber
   Other (see Table 11–5)
D. Testosterone Biosynthetic Defects (Adrenal or Testis)
   Congenital adrenal lipoid hyperplasia (*StAR* deficiency) (*CYP11A*)
   3β-ol-Dehydrogenase/3β-hydroxysteroid dehydrogenase deficiency (3β-HSD)
   17α-Hydroxylase/17, 20-desmolase (lyase) deficiency (*CYP17*)
   17β-Hydroxysteroid dehydrogenase/17-ketosteroid reductase (17-HSD-3)
E. Steroidogenic Factor-1 (SF-1) deficiency (*FTZ1*)
F. Androgen Receptor Insensitivity (*ARG*)
   Complete (CAI)
   Partial (PAI)
   Mild
G. 5α-Reductase Deficiency (*SRD5A2*)
H. Agonadia (Testicular Regression)
I. Leydig Cell Hypoplasia (LH Receptor Defect) (LHR)

McDonough and Tho, 1983; Rosenberg et al., 1987). Different phenotypes presumably reflect different tissue distributions of the various cell lines. A structurally abnormal Y chromosome may be present. Given that structurally abnormal chromosomes (e.g., dicentric) are often unstable, it is likely that the 45,X line arises secondarily following loss of the structurally abnormal Y.

45,X/46,XY Unambiguous Female External Genitalia

45,X/46,XY Individuals may have Turner stigmata and thus would be clinically indistinguishable from 45,X individuals. However, such individuals usually are normal in stature and show no somatic anomalies. As in other types of gonadal dysgenesis, the external genitalia, vagina, and müllerian derivatives remain unstimulated because of the lack of sex steroids. Breasts fail to develop, and little pubic or axillary hair develops. If breast development occurs in a 45,X/46,XY individual, an estrogen-secreting tumor like gonadoblastoma or dysgerminoma should be suspected (Verp and Simpson, 1987). Virilization has also been claimed to result from gonadotropin stimulation of streak gonads (Bosze et al., 1986); modern studies of such cases could be informative.

Although streak gonads of 45,X/46,XY individuals may be histologically indistinguishable

from streak gonads of 45,X individuals, gonadoblastomas or dysgerminomas develop in about 15 to 20% of 45,X/46,XY individuals (Simpson and Photopulos, 1976). A locus on Yq termed GBY (gonado*b*lastoma Y chromosome) is believed to predispose to neoplasia if retained in a phenotypical XY female. If GBY is deleted, as in deletions of Yq, the risk of neoplasia is diminished in sex-reversal females (Lukusa et al., 1986).

Neoplasia may develop in the first or second decade of life. Even if the presumptive GBY locus were absent, gonadal extirpation is recommended for all 45,X/46,XY individuals having female external genitalia. The uterus should be retained, given that pregnancy may be achievable through donor oocytes or donor embryos. Gonadectomy can usually be accomplished by laparoscopy (Pisarska et al., 1998) (see Fig. 10–15). Although it is preferable to remove only gonads in such cases, technically it may be necessary to remove the adnexa as well. Only rarely should laparotomy prove necessary.

45,X/46,XY Ambiguous External Genitalia

Asymmetric or mixed gonadal dysgenesis is applied to individuals with one streak gonad and one dysgenetic testis. These individuals usually have ambiguous external genitalia and a 45,X/46,XY complement and usually a uterus. Many investigators believe that the phenotype is invari-

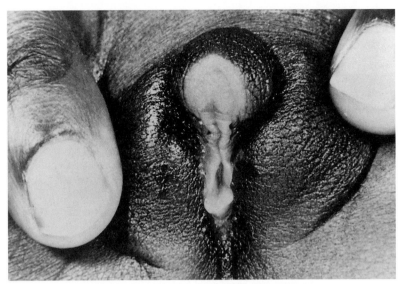

FIGURE 11–10 • External genitalia of an infant with 45,X/46, Y, dup (Yq) mosaicism. (From Morillo-Cucci G, German J: Abnormal Y chromosomes and monosomy 45,X: A concept derived from the study of three patients. Birth Defects Orig Artic Ser 7(6): 210, 1971.)

ably associated with 45,X/46,XY mosaicism. Occasionally only 45,X or only 46,XY cells are demonstratable. These ostensibly nonmosaic cases may merely reflect inability to sample enough tissues or cells.

45,X/46,XY Individuals with ambiguous external genitalia usually have müllerian derivatives (e.g., a uterus) (Fig. 11–10). Presence of a uterus is an important diagnostic sign because that organ is absent in almost all genetic (mendelian) forms of male pseudohermaphroditism, as discussed below. If an individual has ambiguous external genitalia, bilateral testes, and a uterus, it is reasonable to infer that individual actually has 45,X/46,XY mosaicism. This holds regardless of whether both lines can be demonstrated cytogenetically. Occasionally the uterus may be rudimentary, or a fallopian tube may fail to develop ipsilateral to a testis.

45,X/46,XY with Nearly Normal Male External Genitalia

45,X/46,XY Mosaicism may be detected in individuals with nearly normal male external genitalia. In fact, this is the most common phenotype, based on the liveborn follow-up of 45,X/46,XY fetuses ascertained at amniocentesis; 90% on more have a normal male phenotype (Hsu, 1986, 1998; Huang et al., 2002). The fact that 45,X/46,XY neonates far more commonly show genital ambiguity merely reflects biases of ascertainment. Those with male phenotypes pass unrecognized.

45,X/46,XY Individuals having almost normal male external genitalia seem not to develop neoplasia as often as 45,X/46,XY individuals with female or frankly ambiguous genitalia (Simpson and Photopulos, 1976). Gonadal extirpation may not be necessary if a male sex of rearing is chosen, provided gonads can be assessed periodically within the scrotum by ultrasound or palpation (Simpson and Photopulos, 1976).

MALE PSEUDOHERMAPHRODITISM IN MULTIPLE MALFORMATION SYNDROMES

Genital ambiguity may occur in individuals with various multiple malformation syndromes. Genital ambiguity may exist with the Meckel-Gruber syndrome, Smith-Lemli-Opitz type I syndrome, brachioskeletal-genital syndrome (el-Sahy and Waters, 1971), esophageal-facial-genital syndrome (Opitz and Howe, 1969), and several other disorders. These disorders are usually inherited in either autosomal recessive or X-linked recessive fashion, as shown in Table 11–5. Many additional syndromes are associated with cryptorchidism or simple hypospadias (Pinsky et al., 1999).

Syndromes associated with XY sex reversal are discussed in Chapter 10 and listed in Table 10–8. Examples include campomelic dysplasia (*SOX9*), Denys/Drash and Frasier syndromes (*WT-1*) and autosomal perturbations involving 1q, 2q, 9p, 10q. In each condition the phenotype in affected 46,XY individuals is usually complete sex reversal

▼ **Table 11–5.** MULTIPLE MALFORMATION SYNDROMES ASSOCIATED WITH AMBIGUOUS GENITALIA

Syndrome	Prominent Features	Etiology
Ablepharon-macrostomia (Hornblass and Reifler, 1985)	Absent eyelids, eyebrows, eyelashes, external ears; fusion defects of the mouth; ambiguous genitalia; absent or rudimentary nipples; parchment skin, delayed development of expressive language	Autosomal recessive
Aniridia-Wilms tumor association (Riccardi et al., 1978, 1987)	Moderate to severe mental deficiency, growth deficiency, microcephaly, aniridia, nystagmus, ptosis, blindness, Wilms tumor, ambiguous genitalia, gonadoblastoma	Chromosomal or autosomal dominant (*WT-1*)
Antley-Bixler (Antley and Bixler, 1975; Kelley et al., 2002)	Traphezoidocephaly due to premature fusion of calvarial sutures, midface hypoplasia, choanal atresia, nadioulnar synostoses, bowed femurs, longbone fractures	Autosomal recessive; heterogeneous may be caused by lanosterol 14-alpha demethylase deficiency
Asplenia-cardiovascular anomalies-caudal deficiency (Rodriguez et al., 1991)	Hypoplasia or aplasia of the spleen complex, cardiac malformations, abnormal lung lobulation, anomalous position and development of the abdominal organs, agenesis of corpus callosum, imperforate anus, ambiguous genitalia, contractures of the lower limb	Autosomal recessive
Beemer (Beemer and Ertbruggen, 1984)	Hydrocephalus, dense bones, cardiac malformation, bulbous nose, broad nasal bridge, ambiguous genitalia	Autosomal recessive
Brachio-skeletal-genital (el-Sahy and Waters, 1971)	Maxillary hypoplasia, prognathism, fusional cervical vertebrae, bifid uvula	Autosomal recessive
Deletion 11q (Sirota et al., 1984)	Trigonocephaly, flat and broad nasal bridge, micrognathia, carp mouth, hypertelorism, low-set ears, severe congenital heart disease, anomalies of limbs, external genitalia	Chromosomal
Drash (Habib et al., 1985; Turleau et al., 1987)	Wilms tumor, nephropathy, ambiguous genitalia with 46,XY karyotype	Unknown
Esophogeal-facial-genital (Opitz et al., 1969)	Hypertelorism, slanting palpebral fissures, swallowing difficulties	? Autosomal dominant
Fraser (Greenberg et al., 1986; Gattuso et al., 1987)	Cryptophthalmia, defect of auricle, hair growth on lateral forehead to lateral eyebrow, hypoplastic nares, mental deficiency, partial cutaneous syndactyly, urogenital malformation	Autosomal recessive
Lethal acrodysgenital dysplasia (Merrer et al., 1988)	Failure to thrive, facial dysmorphism, ambiguous genitalia, syndactyly, postaxial polydactyly, Hirschprung disease, cardiac and renal malformations	Autosomal recessive
Meckel-Gruber (Mecke and Passenge, 1971)	Polycystic kidneys, occipital encephalocele, polydactyly, cleft palate, eye anomalies	Autosomal recessive
Rutledge (Rutledge et al., 1984)	Joint contractures, cerebellar hypoplasia, renal hypoplasia, ambiguous genitalia, urologic anomalies, tongue cysts, shortness of limbs, eye abnormalities, heart defects, gallbladder agenesis, ear malformations	Autosomal recessive
SCARF syndrome (Koppe et al., 1989)	*S*keletal abnormalities, *c*utis laxa, *c*raniosynostosis, *a*mbiguous genitalia, psychomotor *r*etardation, *f*acial abnormalities	Uncertain
Short rib-polydactyly, Majewski type (Cooper and Hall, 1982; Silengo et al., 1987)	Short stature; short limbs; cleft lip and palate; ear anomalies; limb anomalies, including pre-and postaxial polysyndactyly; narrow thorax; short horizontal ribs; high clavicles; ambiguous genitalia	Autosomal recessive
Smith-Lemli-Opitz (Bialer et al., 1987; Joseph et al., 1987; Tint et al., 1997; Nezanti et al., 2002)	Microcephaly, mental retardation, hypotonia, ambiguous genitalia, abnormal facies	Autosomal recessive (deficiency 7-OH cholesterol dehydrogenase)
Trimethadione teratogenicity (Feldman et al., 1977)	Mental deficiency, speech disorders, prenatal onset growth deficiency, brachycephaly, midfacial hypoplasia, broad and upturned nose, prominent forehead, eye anomalies, cleft lip and palate, cardiac defects, ambiguous genitalia	Teratogenicity
VATER association (Sofatzis et al., 1983; Källen et al., 2001)	*V*ertebral, *a*nal, *t*racheo*e*sophageal, and *r*enal; anomalies, subjects with ambiguous genitalia as part of the cloacal anomalies	Unknown (if valid entity); alleged progestational teratogeneicity unproved (see Simpson and Kaufman, 1998)

Updated from Simpson JL, Verp MS, Plouffe L: Female genital system. *In* Stevenson RE, Hall JG, Goodman RM (eds): Human Malformations and Related Anomalies, vol 2. London: Oxford Press, 1993.

(female phenotype). However, varied expressively exists, and these individuals may occasionally present as male pseudohermaphrodites (genital ambiguity).

Smith-Lemli-Opitz syndrome is a relatively common (1:10,000) autosomal recessive syndrome in which 46,XY individuals show genital abnormalities (from hypospadias to male pseudohermaphroditism). In Ontario, the incidence has been estimated at 1 per 22,700 among individuals of European ancestry (Nowaczyk et al., 2001). A wide phenotypical spectrum exists (Ryan et al., 1998). In Type I simple hypospadias is most common. In Type II external genitalia may be female (sex reversal) (Curry et al., 1987). Both Types I and II are caused by mutation of the gene whose enzyme is responsible for converting 7-hydroxycholesterol to cholesterol (Tint et al., 1994, 1997). The most common molecular explanation is a defect in exon-intronic splicing. Of interest is that in a consanguineous Syrian-Lebanese family three sibs with the same homozygous missense mutation (P467L) phenotype was variable (Nezarati et al., 2002). Considerable attention is being directed to the feasibility of postnatal as well as prenatal treatment with a high cholesterol diet. Given its low molecular weight, cholesterol should cross the placenta readily. During pregnancy, maternal serum estriol is low to nondetectable (Bradley et al., 1999), making feasible detection during maternal serum analyte screening. More specifically, presence of the novel compounds dehydro-estriol and dehydro-pregnanetriol in *maternal urine* indicate a Smith-Lemli-Opitz (SLO) fetus. In normal pregnancies these compounds are undetectable (Shackleton et al., 2001). Another multiple malformation syndrome associated with abnormal steroid metabolism is Antley-Bixler syndrome, of which several etiologically distinct subtypes exist among the some 40 affected subjects (Kelley et al., 2002). Some cases result from deficiency of lanosteral 14-alpha-demethylase (CYP51), an enzyme required in the synthesis of cholesterol.

In the genitopalatocardiac (Gardner-Silengo-Wachtel) syndrome, 46,XY individuals show phenotypical variability not only in external genitalia but also in gonads (Greenberg et al., 1987). Complete sex reversal can occur in 46,XY individuals, who may even have ovaries.

DEFICIENCIES IN TESTOSTERONE BIOSYNTHESIS

Male pseudohermaphroditism may result from deficiencies of the bifunctional enzyme 17α-hydroxylase/17,20 desmolase, from 3β-ol-dehydrogenase, from 17-ketosteroid reductase (17β-ol-dehydrogenase) or from any of the enzymes or requisite processes necessary to convert cholesterol to pregnenolone (congenital adrenal lipoid hyperplasia) (see Fig. 11–1). The common pathogenesis involves testosterone levels too low to virilize external genitalia. Deficiencies of 21- or 11β-hydroxylase, the most common causes of female pseudohermaphroditism, do not cause male pseudohermaphroditism; males (46,XY) show precocious masculinization.

Adrenal biosynthetic defects should be suspected if levels of testosterone or its metabolites are decreased. Diagnosis is not difficult in older children but may be hazardous during infancy because neonatal testosterone levels are physiologically low. Provocative tests (i.e., human chorionic gonadotropin [hCG] stimulation) may be necessary.

Congenital Adrenal Lipoid Hyperplasia

Male pseudohermaphrodites with congenital adrenal lipoid hyperplasia show ambiguous or female-like external genitalia, severe sodium wasting, and adrenals characterized by foamy-appearing cells filled with cholesterol (Chung et al., 1986; Frydman et al., 1986). Hyperpigmentation and respiratory distress are common (25%) in neonates. Accumulation of cholesterol has long indicated inability of cholesterol to be converted to pregnenolone (see Fig. 11–1). Levels of C18, C19, and C21 steroids are undetectable in plasma and urine. Thus, prenatal diagnosis is possible on the basis of low levels of certain hormones in amniotic fluid (Saenger et al., 1995). Inheritance has long been presumed to be autosomal recessive on the basis of observed parental consanguinity.

The cytochrome P-450 enzyme responsible for converting cholesterol to pregnenolone is P450scc (side chain cleavage); the gene is *CYP11A*. P-450scc converts cholesterol to pregnenolone via 20α-hydroxylase, 22α-hydroxylase, and 20,22-desmolase. Located on chromosome 15, *CYP11A* is 20 kb long and has 9 exons. Homozygous *CYP11A1* gene deletion in rabbits causes adrenal lipoid hyperplasia (Yang et al., 1993). Surprisingly, perturbations of *CYP11A1* have never been shown in human congenital adrenal lipoid hyperplasia (Lin et al., 1991).

Congenital adrenal lipoid hyperplasia in humans has instead proved to be the result of perturbation of the gene encoding *st*eroidogenic *a*cute *r*egulatory protein (*StAR*). The *StAR* protein delivers precursors for cholesterol side chain cleavage (see Fig. 11–1); thus, its perturbation would be predicted to have major consequences for hormone action in gonads and adrenals. The term "acute" reflects the necessity of responding rapidly ("acutely") to corticotropin stimulation, specifically by producing a 30 kd mitochondrial protein in adrenal cells. Mapped to 8p11.2, the gene coding for the *StAR* confers such a function. The gene spans 8kb and consists of seven exons (Bose et al., 1996) (Fig. 11–11). Among the nearly 100 reported cases, patients of Japanese and Korean descent predominate. In these ethnic groups the affected allele is usually (80%) Gln258X(Stop) (Bose et al., 1996). In Arabs the mutation is usually (75%) Arg182 Leu. However, molecular hetereogeneity exists, Bose and associates (1996) having found 15 different mutations in 14 cases. Different mutations have been found in other ethnic groups. Founder effects are presumably operative in different ethnic groups (Bose, 1996).

3β-Hydroxysteroid Dehydrogenase (3β-HSD) (3β-ol-Dehydrogenase Deficiency)

This enzyme deficiency is inherited in autosomal recessive fashion. Synthesis of both androgens and estrogens is decreased (see Fig. 11–1). The major androgen produced is dehydroepiandrosterone (DHEA), a relatively weaker androgen than testosterone. DHEA alone is not capable of adequately virilizing the male fetus; thus, genital ambiguity occurs. Diagnosis is usually established on the basis of increased serum DHEA levels before and after ACTH stimulation. In addition to genital abnormalities, 3β-ol-dehydrogenase deficiency is associated with severe sodium wasting, predictably given that both aldosterone and cortisol levels are decreased.

Incompletely developed external genitalia of males with 3β-ol-dehydrogenase (3β-HSD) deficiency are clinically similar to the external genitalia of most other male pseudohermaphrodites—small phallus, urethral opening proximal on the penis, and incomplete labioscrotal fusion. Testes and wolffian ducts differentiate normally. Affected females (46,XX) also show genital ambiguity; thus, 3β-HSD is the only enzyme that, when deficient, produces male pseudohermaphroditism in males and female pseudohermaphroditism in females.

Of the 5 3β-HSD genes, only Type II is expressed in the adrenal cortex and gonads. Gonadal expression is consistent with 3β-hydroxysteroid dehydrogenase (3β-HSD) being a microsomal enzyme, unlike the mitochondrial enzymes 21- or 11 β-hydroxylase. Predictably, male pseudohermaphroditism can result from Type II mutations. Mutations are scattered among the four exons (Simard et al., 1995a). Mutations have been observed in both salt-wasting and non–salt-wasting forms and were discussed above (Female Pseudohermaphroditism) (see Fig. 11–6).

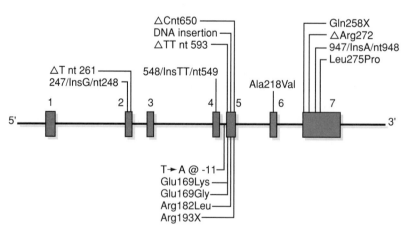

FIGURE 11–11 • Diagrammatic representation of the mutations identified in the *StAR* gene associated with congenital lipoid adrenal hyperplasia. 247/InsG/nt248 is an insertion causing a frameshift between nucleotides 247 and 248. ΔT nt261 is a deletion of a thymidine at nucleotide 261. 548/InsTT/nt549 is an insertion of two thymidines in exon 4 between nucleotides 548 and 549, causing a frameshift. ΔTT nt 593 is a deletion of two thymidines at nucleotide 593, causing a frameshift. ΔCnt650 is a deletion of a cytosine at nucleotide 650, causing a frameshift. T→A @ −11 is a thymidine-to-adenine transition minus 11 nucleotides from the intron 4/exon 5 junction. 947/InsA/nt948 is the insertion of an adenine between nucleotides 947, which results in a frameshift. (From Bose H, Sugawara T, Stauss JF, et al.: The pathophysiology and genetics of congenital lipoid adrenal hyperplasia. International Congenital Lipoid Adrenal Hyperplasia Consortium. N Engl J Med 335:1870, 1996.)

17α-Hydroxylase and 17,20-Desmolase (Lyase) Deficiency

17α-Hydroxylase/17,20 desmolase function is coded by a bidirectional cytochrome P-450 enzyme. Males deficient in 17α-hydroxylase/ 17,20 desmolase (lyase) usually show ambiguous external genitalia. Some even show female-like external genitalia (Heremans et al., 1976). Wolffian duct and testicular development are normal. Affected females (46,XX) show hypertension, but males deficient in 17α-hydroxylase usually display normal blood pressure. Both males and females are affected; thus, inheritance has long been accepted as autosomal recessive.

The P450c17 enzyme is coded by a gene (*CYP17*) on chromosome 10q24-25. *CYP17* consists of 8 exons and is structurally similar to *CYP21*. However, no pseudogene exists. Many different missense mutations have been observed (Kagimoto et al., 1989; Yanase et al., 1989, 1991; Rumsby et al., 1993; Yanase, 1995), usually abolishing P450c17. A four base duplication beginning in codon 480 explains cases in Mennonites (Imai et al., 1992).

When it became evident that a single enzyme fulfills both 17α-hydroxylase and 17,20-desmolase functions, considerable genetic and nosologic confusion was generated (Nebert et al., 1989). A single gene/enzyme responsible for both actions was a surprise because earlier studies had indicated two genetically distinct conditions, presumably encoded by two separate genes. In particular, Zachmann and coworkers (1972) reported a family in which two maternal cousins had genital ambiguity, bilateral testes, and no müllerian derivatives; a maternal "aunt" was said to have abnormal external genitalia and bilateral testes. The deficient enzyme was deduced to be 17,20-desmolase (lyase) on the basis of both cousins showing low plasma testosterone and DHEA levels despite normal urinary excretion of pregnanediol, pregnanetriol, and 17-hydroxycorticoids. In testicular tissue, testosterone could be synthesized from androstenedione or DHEA, excluding 17-ketosteroid reductase deficiency (see below) but suggesting isolated 17,20-desmolase deficiency. In other families only 17α-hydroxylase activity seemed deficient, and these families only involved affected sibs. Mutations have been observed in which only 17,20-lyase function is affected, which has partially clarified the confusion (Mendonca et al., 1995; Biason-Lauber et al., 1997; Geller et al., 1997), perhaps explaining the family studied by Zachmann and colleagues (1972). Indeed, in the rat, targeted mutagenesis and correction have pointed to regions responsible for these various functions (see Fig. 11–7). Zachmann (1995) reviewed the quandary of a single enzyme having disparate effects in different individuals.

Deficiency of 17β-Hydroxysteroid Dehydrogenase (17-Ketosteroid Reductase)

Inability to convert dehydroepiandrosterone to testosterone is the result of deficiency of the microsomal enzyme 17-ketosteroid reductase or 17-β hydroxysteroid dehydrogenase (17 β-ol dehydrogenase). The enzyme reaction is reversible; thus, designations connoting either oxidative or reductive functions could be appropriate (see Fig. 11–1).

Plasma testosterone is usually decreased, androstenedione and dehydroepiandrosterone are increased. Affected males show ambiguous or female-like external genitalia, wolffian derivatives, bilateral testes, and no müllerian derivatives. Breast development may or may not be present, apparently reflecting the estrogen-to-testosterone ratio (Imperato-McGinley et al., 1979). Pubertal virilization is greater than in many other enzyme deficiencies, and sometimes gynecomastia is not even evident (Caufriez, 1986). The sex of rearing of an affected individual has been changed from female to male after puberty (Imperato-McGinley et al., 1979; Mendonca, 2000).

It has been assumed that greater virilization at puberty than at birth reflects the placenta no longer being present to aromatize androstenedione to estrone; thus, unimpeded accumulation of androstenedione occurs.

Of the five isozymes of 17β-hydroxysteroid dehydrogenase, only type 3 is of interest here. The 17hydroxysteroid dehydrogenase-3 gene is located on chromosome 9 and consists of 11 exons (Fig. 11–12). The 17hydroxysteroid dehydrogenase-3 gene is, like 3β-HSD, microsomal and not mitochondrial, consistent with its action involving gonads rather than adrenals. Molecular perturbations typically involve single amino-acid substitutions (Geissler et al., 1994; Andersson et al., 1996) at a variety of positions; disruption of the splice junction involving intron 3 is also not uncommon. Exon or intron 3 is most commonly involved. Mutations may also involve exons 2, 8, 9, 10, 11, and 12.

The largest single aggregation of cases is found in Gaza Arabs (Rösler et al., 1983, 1992). In these cases, the phallus is typically bound down by chordee, reaching lengths of only 4 to 8 cm. Gynecomastia is not uncommon. In Gaza Arabs, the most frequent mutation is a missense mutation in exon 3 (Arg80Gln or R80Q), which reduces enzyme activity to 15 to 20% of normal

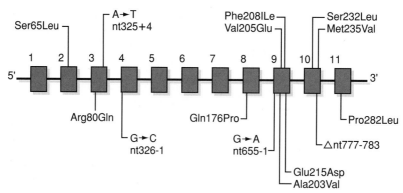

FIGURE 11–12 • Diagrammatic representation of the gene encoding 17β-hydroxysteroid dehydrogenase type 3 with the mutations reported to cause 17β-HSD deficiency. Nt325 + 4 is a splice junction mutation, a transition of adenine (A) to thymidine (T), located four nucleotides downstream 3′ of the boundary between exon 3 and intron 3; nucleotide 325 is the closest base pair in the exon to the mutation. Nt326 –1 is a splice junction mutation, a transition of guanine (G) to cytosine (C), located one nucleotide upstream 5′ of the splice junction between intron 8 and exon 9. Δnt777–783 indicates a deletion of nucleotides 777 to 783. (From Grumbach MM, Conte FA: Disorders of sex differentiation. *In* Wilson JD, Foster DW, Kronenberg HM, et al. (eds): Williams Textbook of Endocrinology, 9th ed. Philadelphia: WB Saunders, 1998.)

(Andersson et al., 1996). 46,XX Homozygous females having this mutation are completely asymptomatic, consistent with 17β-hydroxysteroid dehydrogenase-3 expression limited to testes.

Other aggregates have been studied in Brazil (Mendonca et al., 2000) and the Netherlands (Boehmer et al., 1999). In Brazil 10 subjects were studied; external genitalia usually showed a small phallus (perineoscrotal hypospodias), a bifid scrotum, and a separate vaginal pouch without müllerian derivatives. At puberty virilization occurred, with change in gender role (female and male) occurring in 30% of Brazilian cases (3/10). The R80Q mutation was observed as well as several other point mutations. In the Netherlands 18 cases were studied; the incidence was estimated at 1:147,000 with a heterozygote frequency of 1:135. Both point mutations and splice junction mutations were observed. Of interest, 12 of the 18 Dutch cases were originally diagnosed with partial androgen insensivity.

Overall, most affected individuals worldwide are homozygous, presumably reflecting parental consanguinity. Mutations have included frameshifts, splice junction alterations, and most often missense mutations. Some mutations exist worldwide (R80Q, N74T, 325 + 4; A→T, 655-1, G→A) whereas other are unique to certain populations (Boehmer et al., 1999). Nonsense mutation usually resulted in complete absence of 17β-hydroxysteroid dehydrogenase-3 activity and female external genitalia. They are spread throughout the 11 exons, with aggregation toward the 3′ end (exons 9 and 10, especially) (see Fig. 11–12). Several affected males have had sisters (46,XX) homozygous or compound heterozygous for the same mutation. These sisters have been phenotypically normal.

GLUCOCORTICOID RECEPTOR DEFECT

Mendonca et al. (2002) recently reported a new form of female pseudohermaphroditism due to homozygous mutation of the glucocorticoid gene (GR). This condition in this Brazilian mulatto girl (46,XX) was the product of a consanguineous mating. She presented with enlarged clitoris, posterior labial fusion and a vaginal opening common with the urethra (urogenital sinus). Blood pressure was elevated and serum potassium low. 17α-hydroxyprogesterone was elevated. Cortisol was elevated and did not suppress following dexamethasone administration. The specific mutation was missense, nt1844 T→C, yielding valine → alanine at codon 571 (V571A).

This case contrasts in many respects with all other individuals having mutations in the glucocorticoid receptor (GR) gene. The usual phenotype in 46,XX females includes hirsutism with male-pattern baldness, acne, oligomenorrhea; 46,XY males may be infertile and show precocious puberty. Mutations in these cases differed from those of Mendonca et al. (2002).

DEFICIENCY OF STEROIDOGENIC FACTOR-1 (SF-1)

Steroidogenic factor-1 (SF-1) plays a potentially pivotal role in hypothalamic-pituary gonadal axis. An orphan nuclear receptor related structurally to steroid receptors, SF-1 has no known ligand (hence the designation "orphan"). SF-1 gene product is encoded by the gene *FTZ1*, a zinc finger protein encoded on human 9q33. Prior to human cases being recognized, disruption of *FTZ1* in mice (gene knockouts) was known to cause not only perturbation of adrenal *and* gonadal development but also abnormalities of the hypothalamus and pituitary gonadotropes (Luo et al., 1994; Parker and Schimmer, 1997). The significance of the many interactions of SF-1 was not clear, but it was confidently predicted that human *FTZ1* mutations perturbing SF-1 receptors would cause abnormalities of sexual development.

The first ostensible human case of SF-1 deficiency attributable to mutant *FTZ-1* was reported by Achermann and coworkers (1999). This 46,XY individual showed primary adrenal failure, female external genitalia, streak gonads, and normal müllerian derivatives responsive to hormones. The diagnosis of congenital adrenal lipoid hyperplasia was originally entertained. The

proband was heterozygous for a 2bp substitution at codon 35. That the mutated glycine is the last amino acid of the first zinc finger of SF-1 suggests disturbance of a DNA binding site. In mice the same (G35E) mutation does not exert a dominant negative effect; thus, homozygous mutations in humans would be expected to be necessary. In the case described above, compound heterozygosity is presumed to exist, even though the second mutation could not be immediately detected; *SRY*, *StAR*, and *DAX1* were normal.

Of significance is the presence of a uterus in this 46,XY individual. This supports the hypothesis that SF-1 regulates repression of antimüllerian hormone (AMH).

COMPLETE ANDROGEN INSENSITIVITY (CAI) (COMPLETE TESTICULAR FEMINIZATION)

In complete androgen insensitivity (CAI) (complete testicular feminization), 46,XY individuals show bilateral testes, female external genitalia, a blindly ending vagina, and no müllerian derivatives (Fig. 11–13). Incidence is estimated to be 2 to 5 per 100,000 (Grumbach and Conte, 1998; Gottlieb et al., 1999). Phenotype is entirely predictable, given the underlying pathogenesis

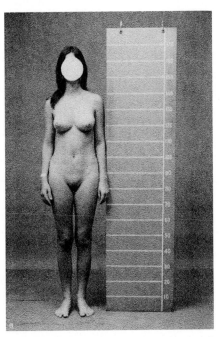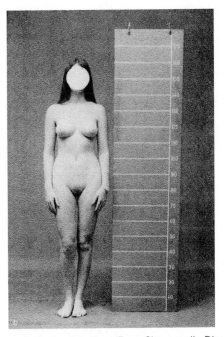

FIGURE 11–13 • Photograph of two sibs with complete testicular feminization. (From Simpson JL: Disorders of Sexual Differentiation: Etiology and Clinical Delineation. New York: Academic Press, 1976. Courtesy of Dr. Charles Hammond, Duke University.)

involving cellular inability to respond to testosterone. Antimüllerian hormone (AMH) is synthesized normally by Sertoli cells and the body responds normally to AMH; thus, no uterus is present. As predicted on the basis of the testes synthesizing estrogens in unimpeded fashion, affected individuals manifest breast development and pubertal feminization. Estrogen levels only approximate those of normal males, but feminization occurs because circulating androgen fails to antagonize estrogenic cellular action. LH is disproportionally increased, reflecting hypothalamic unresponsiveness to testosterone.

Despite pubertal feminization, some individuals with androgen insensitivity show clitoral enlargement and labioscrotal fusion; the term incomplete or partial androgen insensitivity (PAI) (incomplete testicular feminization) is applied to these patients. A still milder end of the spectrum consists of males manifesting only gynecomastia or oligospermia/azoospermia (mild androgen insensitivity or MAI). In mild androgen insensitivity (MAI) spermatogenesis may (Cundy et al., 1986) or may not occur (Grino et al., 1989; Pinsky et al., 1989; Tsukada et al., 1994); gynecomastia, impotence and poor virilization are more constant. Complete, partial and mild androgen insensitivity are all inherited in X-linked recessive fashion. All forms result from mutations of the androgen receptor gene located on the X long arm (Xq11).

This X-linked recessive condition is genetically lethal, for affected males cannot reproduce. Thus, one would predict that one third of all cases would be new (sporadic) mutations. This was indeed true in 8 of 30 (30%) cases studied by Hiort et al. (1998). In the remaining two thirds of cases the phenotypically normal mother must be heterozygous (see Chapter 2). Some obligate heterozygtes show decreased pubic hair and delayed puberty, but many are clinically normal.

Clinical. Adult individuals with complete androgen insensitivity have been described as quite attractive and showing excellent breast development. Despite this traditional textbook description, in reality most cases are similar in appearance to unaffected females in the general population. Breasts contain normal ductal and glandular tissue, but areolae are often pale and underdeveloped. Pubic and axillary hair (terminal) are usually sparse (e.g., only vellus hair is present). Scalp hair is normal. Pubic and axillary hair is not uncommonly observed and should not dissuade one from the diagnosis of CAI.

The vagina terminates blindly, usually foreshortened but still adequate in length. Uncommonly, the vagina may only be 1 to 2 cm long or represented merely by a dimple. Dilators to enlarge and elongate the vagina may be necessary. Surgery to create a neovagina is not usually necessary. Neither normal uterus nor fallopian tubes are ordinarily present, but occasionally there may be fibromuscular remnants, rudimentary fallopian tubes (Ulloa-Aguirre et al., 1990).

Testes are usually normal in size. Their location may be in the abdomen, inguinal canal, labia, or anywhere along the path of embryonic testicular descent. If arrested in descent in the inguinal canal, the testes may produce inguinal hernias. One half of all individuals with complete androgen insensitivity develop inguinal hernias. It is probably worthwhile to determine the cytogenetic status of prepubertal girls with inguinal hernias, although most will be 46,XX (German et al., 1973). Height is slightly increased compared with that of normal women but unremarkable compared with 46,XY males.

Frequency of gonadal neoplasia is increased but less than was once believed (Morris and Mahesh, 1963). Actual risk is probably no greater than 5% (Simpson and Photopulos, 1976; Verp and Simpson, 1987). Moreover, the risk of malignancy is low before 25 to 30 years of age. Benign tubular adenomas (Pick adenomas) are common in postpubertal patients, probably as a result of increased LH secretion. Orchiectomy is eventually necessary, but the testes may be left *in situ* until after spontaneous pubertal feminization. If herniorrhaphy proves necessary before puberty, it is logical to perform orchiectomy at the same time. There may also be some psychological benefit to prepubertal orchiectomies. Inguinal testes can often be removed by laparoscopy more efficiently than by open surgery (laparotomy).

Molecular Basis. The androgen receptor (*AR*) gene is localized to Xq11-12. This gene is about 90,000 base pairs (bp) long and consists of eight exons (Fig. 11–14). The gene encodes fewer than 2000 amino acids. Exon 1 appears to confer regulatory function. The DNA binding domain (DBD), amnio acids 552-616, is encoded by exons 2 and 3. The latter part of exon 3 and part

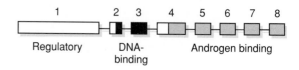

FIGURE 11–14 • Schematic diagram showing major structure/function domains of the androgen receptor gene. DNA-binding, black; androgen-binding, gray. Numbers above boxes refer to exons.

of exon 4 encodes a bipartite nuclear localization signal (amino acids 617-636). The C-terminal region of 250 amino acids extends over exons 4-8 and is the androgen binding domain (ABD) (Gottlieb et al., 1996). The *AR* gene contains two regions of homopolymeric amino acid "repeats" that vary in size: one polyglutamine (9–36 amino acids) and one polyglycine (10–31 amino acids) (Lambroso, 1997).

Many different mutations have been reported (Gottlieb et al., 1998, 1999) and are compiled in an international registry at McGill University, Canada (e-mail:mc33@musica.mcgill.ca). Mutations causing CAI and PAI are scattered throughout the gene. Deletions and insertions are rare (Quigley et al., 1992). Point mutations are far more common, and include deletion of three nucleotides with preservation of an open reading frame, single-nucleotide changes resulting in either substitution of an amino acid or changes generating a stop codon; this would result in premature message termination and production of a nonfunctional protein.

Table 11–6 summarizes types of mutations (Gottlieb et al., 1999). Exon 1 encompasses half of the *AR* gene but accounts for the fewest recognized mutations (10% of total). More common are mutations in exons 2 and 3 (the DNA binding domain), which can produce either CAI and PAI. The most common mutations site are exons 5–8, the androgen binding domain. Large deletions and mutations resulting in premature termination (stop codon) predictably cause complete androgen insensitivity (McPhaul et al., 1993; Gottlieb et al., 1998, 1999). However, the preponderance of mutations are missense (see Table 11–6), causing PAI, CAI, or MAI in seemingly near random fashion. Some point mutations may be compatible with production of some androgen receptors, but the receptor may be unstable or display poor binding (McPhaul et al., 1993). A given mutation may be associated with either PAI or MAI (Gottlieb et al., 1999).

Determining presence or absence of a specific molecular defect in the androgen receptor gene would be desirable. Unfortunately, this may become applicable only if the molecular defect is already known in another family member. Otherwise, molecular testing is available only on a research basis (Gottlieb et al., 1999). Multiplex PCR is potentially useful but again not readily available. Sequencing the entire gene is the eventual goal. Heterozygote detection would be useful for genetic counseling and prenatal genetic diagnosis. One could identify heterozygotes by finding that one of their two X's contains the same mutation as in affected cases in that family.

▼ **Table 11–6.** MUTATIONS CAUSING
• COMPLETE, PARTIAL, OR MILD ANDROGEN INSENSITIVITY SYNDROME (AIS)

Type	Phenotype	Mutation
Single Base Mutations		
Amino acid substitutions	Complete AIS	134
	Partial AIS	104
	Mild AIS	10
	Normal	4
Multiple amino acid substitutions	Complete AIS	2
Splice junction substitutions	Complete AIS	5
	Partial AIS	1
Splice junction insertion	Complete AIS	1
Intron substitution	Complete AIS	1
Premature termination codons	Complete AIS	22
	Partial AIS	1
Subtotal		285
Structural Defects		
Complete gene deletions	Complete AIS	3
Partial gene deletions (6-30 bp, 1-7 exons)	Complete AIS	8
	Mild AIS	1
1- to 4-bp deletions	Complete AIS	6
Intron deletion	Partial AIS	1
Splice junction deletion	Complete AIS	1
Insertions	Complete AIS	4
Duplications	Complete AIS	1
Total		25
Grand Total		310

*AIS, androgen insensitivity syndrome.
Modified from Gottlieb B, Pinsky L, Beitel LK, et al.: Androgen insensitivity. Am J Med Genet 89:210, 1999.

In families with only one affected male, it is difficult to distinguish between a new mutation or the first affected case in a family in which one or more females are heterozygous.

If a female is known to be heterozygous but the molecular basis is not known in that family, the probability that offspring will be affected (male) or heterozygous (female) can be estimated through linkage analysis. DNA from affected and unaffected male relatives is needed, and the family must further be informative for a linked marker.

PARTIAL ANDROGEN SENSITIVITY (PAI) (INCOMPLETE TESTICULAR FEMINIZATION AND REIFENSTEIN SYNDROME); MILD ANDROGEN INSENSITIVITY (MAI)

As alluded to above, some 46,XY individuals feminize at puberty (e.g., breast development), but their external genitalia are still characterized by phallic enlargement and partial labioscrotal fusion (Fig. 11–15). These individuals have incomplete or partial androgen insensitivity (PAI), also called incomplete testicular feminization. Partial (incom-

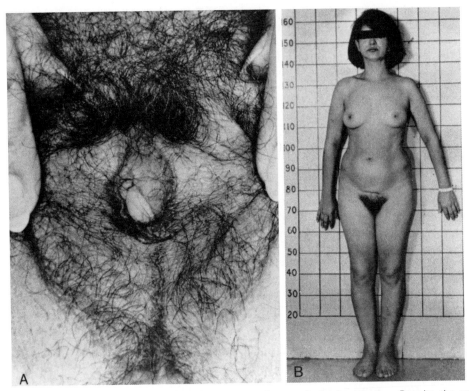

FIGURE 11–15 • Photographs of an individual with incomplete testicular feminization. Despite the enlarged phallus and labioscrotal fusion A, breast development occurred at puberty, B. (From Park IJ, Jones HW: Familial male hermaphroditism with ambiguous external genitalia. Am J Obstet Gynecol 108:1197, 1970.)

plete) and complete androgen insensitivity share many features: bilateral testes with Leydig cell hyperplasia, absence of müllerian derivatives, pubertal breast development, lack of pubertal virilization, normal (male) plasma testosterone, and failure to respond to androgen (Park and Jones, 1970). Cellular pathogenesis of partial androgen insensitivity may involve decreased numbers or qualitative defects of androgen receptors (Griffin et al., 1976; Pinsky and Kaufman, 1987; Pinsky et al., 1987). As noted above, there is poor correlation between phenotype (CAI vs PAI) and the exon or sequence of the *AR* gene involved.

To avoid nosologic confusion, it is worth recounting that incomplete (partial) androgen insensitivity encompasses several entities once considered genetically distinct—the erstwhile syndromes reported by Lubs and coworkers (1959), Gilbert-Dreyfus and colleagues (1957), and Reifenstein (1947). In 1974 Wilson and colleagues (1974) reported a single kindred in which both the Reinfenstein phenotype and the PAI phenotype as traditionally defined were segregating. In 1984 the same group confirmed PAI in two individuals with the Lubs syndrome phenotype (Wilson et al., 1984). Thus, the distinction once made between

the Reinfenstein syndrome, the Lubs syndrome, and PAI is not valid. All three disorders represent different spectrums of a single X-linked recessive disorder, now called partial androgen insensitivity (PAI). Variable expressivity should be expected in a kindred (Pinsky et al., 1996; Gottlieb et al., 1999). Affected individuals with opposite sex of rearing have even been reported (Rodien et al., 1996).

The clinical significance of PAI is that this disorder must be excluded in infants before a male sex of rearing can be assigned. Demonstrating a response to androgens excludes the condition; presence or absence of a specific molecular defect in the androgen receptor gene would be useful only if the molecular defect in an index case were already known or if the phenotype of that specific nucleotide change were known.

5α-REDUCTASE DEFICIENCY (PSEUDOVAGINAL PERINEOSCROTAL HYPOSPADIAS)

It has long been recognized that some genetic males show ambiguous external genitalia at birth

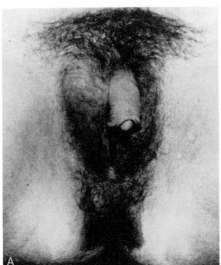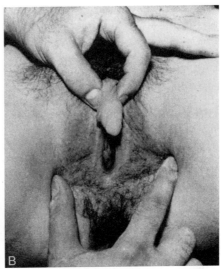

FIGURE 11–16 • Photographs of the external genitalia of an individual reported in 1972 to have pseudovaginal perineoscrotal hypospadias and now considered the result of 5α-reductase deficiency. At puberty, phallic enlargement occurred and breast development did not. (From Opitz JM, Simpson JL, Sarto GE, et al.: Pseudovaginal perineoscrotal hypospadias. Clin Genet 3:1, 1972.)

but at puberty undergo virilization like normal males. They experience phallic enlargement, increased facial hair, muscular hypertrophy, and voice deepening but no breast development. Their external genitalia consist of a phallus that resembles a clitoris more than a penis and a perineal urethral orifice. A separate, blindly ending, perineal orifice resembles a vagina (pseudovagina) (Fig. 11–16).

Initially called pseudovaginal perineoscrotal hypospadias (PPSH), this trait was shown in 1971 to be inherited in autosomal recessive fashion (Opitz et al., 1971; Simpson et al., 1971b). This disorder soon proved to be the result of deficiency of 5α-reductase (Imperato-McGinley et al., 1974; Walsh et al., 1974; Peterson et al., 1977), the enzyme that converts testosterone to dihydrotestosterone (DHT) (see Fig. 11–1). Intracellular 5α–reductase deficiency results in the PPSH phenotype, which is consistent with virilization of the external genitalia during embryogenesis requiring dihydrotestosterone; wolffian differentiation requires only testosterone. Pubertal virilization also can be accomplished by testosterone alone.

Affected males with 5α-reductase deficiency have a broader spectrum than most disorders discussed in this section. They may be more masculinized at birth, even having penile hypospadias or a penile urethra. Testes may be abdominal, inguinal, or scrotal. The prostate is very small, indicating the necessity of DHT for prostatic development. Plasma LH is elevated

despite elevated testosterone. Plasma FSH may be eliminated.

46,XX Females homozygous for 5α-reductase deficiencies are fertile and show normal ovarian function (Wilson et al., 1993). Breast development is normal (Katz et al., 1995). However, limb and pubic hair may be reduced and menarche delayed.

Diagnosis is best made on the basis of an elevated testosterone-to-DHT ratio following administration of hCG or testosterone propionate (Greene et al., 1987). The ratio of the respective urinary metabolites of testosterone and DHT (i.e., etiocholanolone and androsterone) is also elevated. In infants, baseline levels of testosterone and DHT are so low that distinguishing normal from affected individuals may be difficult. Elevated urinary tetrahydrocortisol-to-5α–tetrahydrocortisol ratio can also serve as the basis for diagnosis (Imperato-McGinley et al., 1986).

If fibroblasts are to be assayed for diagnosis, it is essential to study cells derived from external genitalia (e.g., foreskin). Considerable variability exists in 5α–reductase activity among control genital tissues, with overlap in values between controls and individuals known on clinical grounds to be deficient for 5α–reductase. Presence of 5α–reductase in cultured genital fibroblasts excludes 5α–reductase deficiency, whereas absence of 5α–reductase provides less confidence in confirming the diagnosis. Diagnosis may be difficult in infants, whose baseline levels of T and DHT are low.

Two 5α–reductase (*SRD5*) genes exist. The Type I gene is located on chromosome 5 (*SRD5A1*), Type II (*SRD5A2*) on chromosome 2p23. Only Type II is expressed in gonads; thus, only the Type II isoform is deficient in male pseudohermaphroditism. Consisting of 5 exons (Labrie et al., 1992), *SRD5A2* in affected individuals typically shows point mutations (Thigpen et al., 1992) (Fig. 11–17). Of 38 cases studied, there were 33 missense mutations, 3 nonsense mutations, and 2 splice-junction defects (Sultan et al., 2001). Different ethnic groups show different mutations, scattered among the 5 exons and presumably reflecting a

founder effect (see Fig. 11–16). There is little ostensible correlation between site of missense mutations and severity of phenotype. Cases in New Guinea show deletions (Mendonca et al., 1996). Within a given ethnic group the mutation is usually homozygous, presumably reflecting parental consanguinity with identity by descent (founder effect). Given specific mutations in different ethnic groups, a molecular strategy for prenatal diagnosis and genetic counseling could be devised once the index case has been characterized molecularly or the affected individual is known to be a member of an ethnic group characterized by a specific mutation.

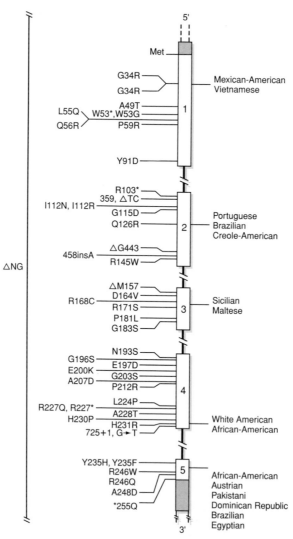

FIGURE 11–17 • Mutations in the steroid 5α-reductase 2 gene and protein. On the left are the locations of 45 different mutations, and the sites of several recurring mutations are shown on the right. (ΔNG represents the deletion of the gene in the New Guinea cohort. The initiating methionine is designated Met in exon 1, and the normal termination codon is designated with an asterisk in exon 5.) (From Griffin JE, McPaul J, Russel DW, et al.: The androgen resistance syndromes: Steroid 5 alpha-reductase 2 deficiency, testicular feminization, and related disorders. *In* Scriver CR, Beaudet AL, Sly WS, et al. (eds): The Metabolic and Molecular Bases of Inherited Disease, 8th ed, vol III. New York: McGraw-Hill, 2001.)

REFERENCES

Achermann JC, Ito M, Ito M, et al.: A mutation in the gene encoding steroidogenic factor-1 causes XY sex reversal and adrenal failure in humans. Nat Genet 22:125, 1999.

Andersson S, Geissler WM, Wu L, et al.: Molecular genetics and pathophysiology of 17 β–hydroxysteroid dehydrogenase 3 deficiency. J Clin Endocrinol Metab 81:130, 1996.

Angehrn V, Zachmann M, Prader A: Silver-Russell syndrome. Observations in 20 patients. Helv Paediatr Acta 34:297, 1979.

Antley R, Bixler D: Trapexoidocephaly, midfacial hypoplasia and cartilage abnormalities with multiple synostoses and skeletal fractures. Birth Defects Orig Artic Ser 11(2):397, 1975.

Araki S, Chikazawa K, Sekiguchi I, et al.: Arrest of follicular development in a patient with 17 alpha hydroxylase deficiency: Folliculogenesis in association with a lack of estrogen synthesis in the ovaries. Fertil Steril 47:169, 1987.

Aughton DJ, Cassidy SB: Physical features of Prader-Willi syndrome in neonates. Am J Dis Child 144:1251, 1990.

Ayme S, Julian C, Gambarelli D, et al.: Fryns syndrome: Report on 8 new cases. Clin Genet 35:191, 1989.

Beemer FA, von Ertbruggen I: Peculiar facial appearance, hydrocephalus, double-outlet right ventricle, genital anomalies and dense bones with lethal outcome. Am J Med Genet 19:391, 1984.

Bialer MG, Penchaszadeh VB, Kahn E, et al.: Female external genitalia and müllerian duct derivatives in a 46,XY infant with the Smith-Lemli-Opitz syndrome. Am J Med Genet 28:723, 1987.

Biason-Lauber A, Leiberman E, Zachmann M: A single amino acid substitution in the putative redox partner-binding site of P450c17 as cause of isolated 17,20-lyase deficiency. J Clin Endocrinol Metab 82:3807, 1997.

Bishop CE, Whitworth DJ, Qin Y, et al.: A transgenic insertion upstream of SOX9 is associated with dominant XX sex reversal in the mouse. Nat Genet 26:490, 2000.

Bobba A, Marra E, Giannattasio S, et al.: 21-Hydroxylase deficiency in Italy: A distinct distribution pattern of CYP21 mutations in a sample from southern Italy. J Med Genet 36:648, 1999.

Boehmer AL, Brinkmann AO, Sandkuijl LA, et al.: 17 Beta-hydroxysteroid dehydrogenase-3 deficiency: diagnosis, phenotypic variability, population genetics, and worldwide distribution of ancient and de novo mutations. J Clin Endocrinol Metab 84:4713, 1999.

Bongiovanni AM: Further studies of congenital adrenal hyperplasia due to 3β– hydroxysteroid dehydrogenase deficiency. In Vallet HL, Porter IH (eds): Genetic Mechanisms of Sexual Development. New York: Academic Press, 1979.

Bongiovanni AM, Di George AM, Grumbach MM: Masculinization of the female infant associated with estrogenic therapy alone during gestation: Four cases. J Clin Endocrinol Metab 19:1104, 1959.

Bose HS, Sugawara T, Strauss JF III, et al.: The pathophysiology and genetics of congenital lipoid adrenal hyperplasia. International Congenital Lipoid Adrenal Hyperplasia Consortium. N Engl J Med 335:1870, 1996.

Bosze P, Szamel I, Molnar F, et al.: Non-neoplastic gonadal testosterone secretion as a cause of vaginal cell maturation in streak gonad syndrome. Gynecol Obstet Invest 22:153, 1986.

Bowen P, Lee CNS, Zellweger H, et al.: A familial syndrome of multiple congenital defects. Bull Johns Hopkins Hosp 114:402, 1964.

Bradley LA, Palomaki GE, Knight GJ, et al.: Levels of unconjugated estriol and other maternal serum markers in pregnancies with Smith-Lemli-Opitz (RSH) syndrome fetuses. Am J Med Genet 82:355, 1999.

Brunskill PJ: The effects of fetal exposure to danazol. Br J Obstet Gynecol 99:212, 1992.

Carey JC: Exstrophy of the cloaca and the OEIS complex: One and the same. Am J Med Genet 1:270, 2001.

Carson SA, Simpson JL: Virilization of female fetuses following maternal ingestion of progestional and androgenic steroids. In Mahesh VB, Greenblatt RN (eds): Hirsutism and Virilization. Littleton MA: PSG Publishing, 1984, p 177

Caufriez A: Male pseudohermaphroditism due to 17-ketoreductase deficiency: Report of a case without gynecomastia and without vaginal pouch. Am J Obstet Gynecol 154:148, 1986.

Chang HJ, Clark RD, Bachman H: The phenotype of 45,X/46,XY mosaicism: An analysis of 92 prenatally diagnosed cases. Am J Hum Genet 46:156, 1990.

Chen H, Chang CH, Misra RP, et al.: Multiple pterygium syndrome. Am J Med Genet 7:91, 1980.

Chung BC, Matteson KJ, Voutilainen R, et al.: Human cholesterol side-chain cleavage enzyme P450scc:cDNA cloning assignment of the gene to chromosome 15 and expression in the placenta. Proc Natl Acad Sci USA 83:8962, 1986.

Cooper CP, Hall CM: Lethal short-rib polydactyly syndrome of the Majewski type: a report of three cases. Radiology 144:513, 1982.

Curry CJ, Carey JC, Holland JS, et al.: Smith-Lemli-Opitz syndrome-type II. Multiple congenital anomalies with male pseudohermaphroditism and frequent early lethality. Am J Med Genet 26:45, 1987.

Cundy TF, Rees M, Evans BA, et al.: Mild androgen insensitivity presenting with sexual dysfunction. Fertil Steril 46:721, 1986.

Day DJ, Speiser PW, Schulze E, et al.: Identification of non-amplifying CYP21 genes when using PCR-based diagnosis of 21-hydroxylase deficiency in congenital adrenal hyperplasia (CAH) affected pedigrees. Hum Mol Genet 5:2039, 1996.

Del Giudice SM, Nydorf ED: Cutis marmorata telangiectatica congenita with multiple congenital anomalies. Arch Dermatol 122:1060, 1986.

Diekmann L, Huther W, Pfeiffer RA: Unusual manifestations of neurofibromatosis (von Recklinghausen's disease) in childhood. Abnormal tumor with clitoris hypertrophy. Renal hypertension caused by renal artery stenosis. Monozygotic twins–plexiform neuroma in the head region and glaucoma. Z Kinderheilkd 101:191, 1967.

Donohue WL, Uchida IA: Leprechaunism: A euphemism for a rare familial disorder. J Pediatr 45:505, 1954.

Dougherty CM, Spencer R: Female Sex Anomalies. Hagerstown, MD: Harper & Row Publishers, 1972.

Duck SC, Katayama KP: Danazol may cause female pseudohermaphroditism. Fertil Steril 35:230, 1981.

Duncan NO III, Miller RH, Catlin FI: Choanal atresia and associated anomalies: The CHARGE association. Int J Pediatr Otorhinolaryngol 15:129, 1988.

el-Sahy N, Waters WR: The branchio-skeleto-genital syndrome. A new hereditary syndrome. Plast Reconstr Surg 48:542, 1971.

Elsas LJ, Endo F, Strumlauf E, et al.: Leprechaunism: An inherited defect in a high-affinity insulin receptor. Am J Hum Genet 37:73, 1985.

Falk HC, Hyman AB: Congenital absence of clitoris. A case report. Obstet Gynecol 38:269, 1971.

Feins NR, Cranley W: Bladder duplication with one exstrophy and one cloaca. J Pediatr Surg 21:570, 1986.

Feldman GL, Weaver DD, Lovrien EW: The fetal trimethadione syndrome: Report of an additional family and further delineation of this syndrome. Am J Dis Child 131:1389, 1977.

Frydman M, Kauschansky A, Zamir R, et al.: Familial lipoid adrenal hyperplasia: Genetic marker data and an approach to prenatal diagnosis. Am J Med Genet 25:319, 1986.

Fullana A, Garcia-Frias E, Martinez-Frias ML, et al.: Caudal deficiency and asplenia anomalies in sibs. Am J Med Genet Suppl 2:23, 1986.

Gattuso J, Patton MA, Baraitser M: The clinical spectrum of the Fraser syndrome: Report of three new cases and review. J Med Genet 24:549, 1987.

Geissler W, Davis DL, Wu L, et al.: Male pseudohermaphroditism caused by mutations of testicular 17β-hydroxysteroid dehydrogenase 3. Nat Genet 7:34, 1994.

Geley S, Kapelari K, Johrer K, et al.: CYP11B1 mutations causing congenital adrenal hyperplasia due to 11 beta-hydroxylase deficiency. J Clin Endocrinol Metab 81:2896, 1996.

Geller DH, Auchus RJ, Mendonca BB, et al.: The genetic and functional basis of isolated 17,20-lyase deficiency. Nat Genet 17:201, 1997.

German J, Simpson JL, Morillo-Cucci G, et al.: Testicular feminisation and inguinal hernia. Lancet 1:891, 1973.

Gilbert-Dreyfus S, Sébaoun AC, Belaisch J: Etude de'un cas familial d'androgynordisme avec hypospadias grave, gynecomastic et hyperoestrogénie. Ann Endocrinol 18:93, 1957.

Gottlieb B, Lehvaslaiho H, Beitel LK, et al.: The androgen receptor gene mutations database. Nucleic Acids Res 26:234, 1998.

Gottlieb B, Pinsky L, Beitel LK, et al.: Androgen insensitivity. Am J Med Genet 89:210, 1999.

Gottlieb B, Trifiro M, Lumbroso R, et al.: The androgen receptor gene mutations database. Nucleic Acids Res 24:151, 1996.

Greenberg F, Gresik WV, Carpenter RJ, et al.: The Gardner-Silengo-Wachtel or genito-palato-cardiac syndrome: Male pseudohermaphroditism with micrognathia, cleft palate, and conotruncal cardiac defects. Am J Med Genet 26:59, 1987.

Greenberg F, Keenan B, De Yanis V, et al.: Gonadal dysgenesis and gonadoblastoma in situ in a female with Fraser (cryptophthalmos) syndrome. J Pediatr 108:952, 1986.

Greene S, Zachmann M, Mannella B, et al.: Comparison of two tests to recognize or exclude 5α-reductase deficiency in prepubertal children. Acta Endocrinol (Copenh) 114:113, 1987.

Griffin JE, Punyashthiti K, Wilson JD: Dihydrotestestosterone binding by culture of human fibroblasts. Comparison of cells from control subjects and from patients with hereditary male pseudohermaphroditism due to androgen resistance. J Clin Invest 57:1342, 1976.

Grino PB, Isidro-Gutierrez RF, Griffin JE, et al.: Androgen resistance associated with a qualitative abnormality of the androgen receptor and responsive to high dose androgen therapy. J Clin Endocrinol Metab 68:578, 1989.

Grumbach MM, Conte FA: Disorders of sex differentiation. In Wilson JD, Foster DW, Kronenberg HM, et al. (eds): Williams Textbook of Endocrinology, 9th ed. Philadelphia: WB Saunders, 1998, p 1303.

Grumbach MM, Ducharme JR, Moloshak RE: On fetal masculinizing action of certain oral progestins. J Clin Endocrinol Metab 19:1369, 1959.

Habib R, Loirat C, Gubler MC, et al.: The nephropathy associated with male pseudohermaphroditism and Wilm's tumor (Drash syndrome): A distinctive glomerular lesion–report of 10 cases. Clin Nephrol 24:269, 1985.

Harada N, Ogawa H, Shozu M, et al.: Biochemical and molecular genetic analyses on placental aromatase (P-450AROM) deficiency. J Biol Chem 267:4781, 1992.

Heremans GF, Moolenaar AJ, van Gelderen HH: Female phenotype in a male child due to 17α-hydroxylase deficiency. Arch Dis Child 51:721, 1976.

Hiort O, Sinnecker GH, Holterhus PM, et al.: Inherited and de novo androgen receptor gene mutations: Investigation of single-case families. J Pediatr 132:939, 1998.

Hornblass A, Reifler DM: Ablepharon macrostomia syndrome. Am J Ophthalmol 15:552, 1985.

Hsu LYF: Prenatal diagnosis of chromosomal abnormalities through amniocentesis. In Milunsky A (ed): Genetic Disorders and the Fetus: Diagnosis, Prevention, and Treatment, 4th ed. Baltimore: The Johns Hopkins University Press, 1998, p 179.

Hsu LYF: Prenatal diagnosis of chromosome abnormalities through amniocentesis. In Milunsky A (ed): Genetic Disorders and the Fetus, 3rd ed. Baltimore: Johns Hopkins Press, 1986, p 155.

Huang B, Thangavelu M, Bhatt S, et al.: Prenatal diagnosis of 45,X and 45,X mosaicism: the need for thorough cytogenetic and clinical evaluations. Prenat Diagn 22:105, 2002.

Huang B, Wang S, Ning Y, et al.: Autosomal XX sex reversal caused by duplication of SOX9 Am J Med Genet 87:349, 1999.

Imai T, Yanase T, Waterman MR, et al.: Canadian Mennonites and individuals residing in the Friesland region of The Netherlands share the same molecular basis of 17 alpha-hydroxylase deficiency. Hum Genet 89:95, 1992.

Imperato-McGinley J, Gautier T, Pichardo M, et al.: The diagnosis of 5 alpha-reductase deficiency in infancy. J Clin Endocrinol Metab 63:1313, 1986.

Imperato-McGinley J, Guerrero L, Gauter T, et al.: Steroid 5α-reductase deficiency in man: An inherited form of male pseudohermaphroditism. Science 186:1213, 1974.

Imperato-McGinley J, Peterson RE, Stoller R, et al.: Male pseudohermaphroditism secondary to a 17 beta-hydroxysteroid dehydrogenase deficiency: Gender role with puberty. J Clin Endocrinol Metab 49:391, 1979.

Jiang M, Aittomaki K, Nilsson C, et al.: The frequency of an inactivating point mutation (^{566}C→T) of the human follicle-stimulating hormone receptor gene in four populations using allele-specific hybridization and time-resolved fluorometry. J Clin Endocrinol Metab 83:4338, 1998.

Jones HW: An anomaly of the external genitalia in female patients with exstrophy of the bladder. Am J Obstet Gynecol 117:748, 1973.

Jones HW, Park IJ: A classification of special problems in sex differentiation. Birth Defects Orig Ser 7(6):113,1971.

Joseph DB, Uehling DT, Gilbert E, et al.: Genitourinary abnormalities associated with the Smith-Lemli-Opitz syndrome. J Urol 137:719, 1987.

Kagimoto K, Waterman MR, Kagimoto M, et al.: Identification of a common molecular basis for combined 17 alpha-hydroxylase/17,20-lyase deficiency in two Mennonite families. Hum Genet 82:285, 1989.

Källén K, Mastroiacovo P, Castilla EE, et al.: VATER nonrandom association of congenital malformations: Study based on data from four malformation registers. Am J Med Genet 101:26, 2001.

Kaneko E, Kobayashi Y, Yasukochi Y, et al.: Genomic analysis of two siblings with 17α-hydroxylase deficiency and hypertension. Hypertens Res 17:143, 1994.

Kapoor R, Saha MM: Complete duplication of the bladder, urethra and external genitalia in a neonate—a case report. J Urol 137:1243, 1987.

Katz MD, Cai LQ, Zhu YS, et al.: The biochemical and phenotypic characterization of females homozygous for 5 alpha-reductase-2 deficiency. J Clin Endocrinol Metab 80:3160, 1995.

Kelley RI, Kratz LE, Glaser RL, et al.: Abnormal sterol metabolism in a patient with Antley-Bixler syndrome and ambiguous genitalia. Am J Med Genet 110:95, 2002.

Keppler-Noreuil KM: OEIS complex (omphalocele-exstrophy-imperforate anus-spinal defects): A review of 14 cases. Am J Med Genet 99:271, 2001.

Koppe R, Kaplan P, Hunter A, et al.: Ambiguous genitalia associated with skeletal abnormalities, cutis laxa, craniostenosis, psychomotor retardation, and facial abnormalities (SCARF syndrome). Am J Med Genet 34:305, 1989.

Labrie F, Sugimoto Y, Luu-The V, et al.: Structure of human type II 5 alpha-reductase gene. Endocrinology 131:1571, 1992.

Lambroso CT: Paroxysmal kinesigenic choreoathetosis. Neurology 49:642, 1997.

Lin D, Gitelman SE, Saenger P, et al.: Normal genes for the cholesterol side chain cleavage enzyme, P450scc, in congenital lipoid adrenal hyperplasia. J Clin Invest 88:1955, 1991.

Litwin A, Fisch B, Tadir Y, et al.: Limb-body wall complex with complete absence of external genitalia after in vitro-fertilization. Fertil Steril 55:634, 1991.

Lubinsky MS: Female pseudohermaphroditism and associated anomalies. Am J Med Genet 6:123, 1980.

Lubs HA Jr, Vilar O, Bergenstal DN: Familial male pseudo-hermaphroditism of labial testes and partial feminization: Endocrine studies and genetic aspects. J Clin Endocrinol Metab 19:1110, 1959.

Lukusa T, Fryns JP, van den Berghe H: Gonadoblastomoa and Y-chromosome fluorescence. Clin Gen 29:311, 1986.

Luo X, Ikeda Y, Parkee KL: A cell-specific nuclear receptor is essential for adrenal and gonadal development and sexual differentiation. Cell 77:481, 1994.

Martinez-Frias ML, Bermejo E, Rodriguez-Pinilla E, et al.: Exstrophy of the cloaca and exstrophy of the bladder: Two different expressions of a primary developmental field defect. Am J Med Genet 99:261, 2001.

Mazza V, Di Monte I, Ceccarelli PL, et al.: Prenatal diagnosis of female pseudohermaphroditism associated with bilateral luteoma of pregnancy. Hum Reprod 17:821, 2002.

McDonough PG, Tho PT: The spectrum of 45X/46,XY gonadal dysgenesis and its implications (a study of 19 patients). Pediatr Adolesc Gynecol 1:1, 1983.

McPhaul MJ, Marcelli M, Zoppi S, et al.: Genetic basis of endocrine disease. 4. The spectrum of mutations in the androgen receptor gene that causes androgen resistance. J Clin Endocrinol Metab 76:17, 1993.

Mendonca BB, Inacio M, Arnhold IJ, et al.: Male pseudoher-maphroditism due to 17 beta-hydroxysteroid dehydroge-nase 3 deficiency. Diagnosis, psychological evaluation, and management. Medicine 79:299, 2000.

Mendonca BB, Leite MV, de Castro M, et al.: Female pseudo-hermaphroditism caused by a novel homozygous missense mutation of the GR gene. J Clin Endocrinol Metab 87:1805, 2002.

Mendonca BB, Arnhold IJP, Pelegrinelli AC, et al.: Male pseudohermaphroditism due to isolated 17,20-lyase deficiency. Abstract P3-617. Proceedings of the 77th Annual Meeting of the Endocrine Society, Washington, DC, 1995.

Mendonca BB, Inacio M, Costa EM, et al.: Male pseudoher-maphroditism due to steroid 5α-reductase 2 deficiency. Diagnosis, psychological evaluation, and management. Medicine (Baltimore) 75:64, 1996.

Merrer ML, Briard ML, Girard S, et al.: Lethal acrodysgeni-tal dwarfism: A severe lethal condition resembling Smith-Lemli-Opitz syndrome. J Med Genet 25:88, 1988.

Miura K, Yasuda K, Yanase T, et al.: Mutation of cytochrome P-45017 α gene (CYP17) in a Japanese patient previously reported as having glucocorticoid-responsive hyperaldosteronism: With a review of Japanese patients with mutations of CYP17. J Clin Endocrinol Metab 81:3797, 1996.

Moisan AM, Ricketts ML, Tardy V, et al.: New insight into the molecular basis of 3beta-hydroxysteroid dehydroge-nase deficiency: Identification of eight mutations in the HSD3B2 gene eleven patients from seven new fami-lies and comparison of the functional properties of twenty-five mutant enzymes. J Clin Endocrinol Metab 84:4410, 1999.

Morel Y, Murena M, Nicolino M, et al.: Correlation between genetic lesions of the CYP21B gene and the clinical forms of congenital adrenal hyperplasia (CAH) due to 21-hydroxylase deficiency: Report of a large study of 355 CAH chromosomes. Horm Res 37:13, 1992.

Morishima A, Grumbach MM, Simpson ER, et al.: Aromatase deficiency in male and female siblings caused by a novel mutation and the physiological role of estro-gens. J Clin Endocrinol Metab 80:3689, 1995.

Mornet E, White PC: Analysis of genes encoding steroid 11-betahydroxylase. Cytogenetic Cell Genetic 15:1047, 1989.

Morris JM, Mahesh VB: Further observations on the syn-drome "testicular feminization." Am J Obstet Gynecol 87:731, 1963.

Mulaikal RM, Migeon CJ, Rock JA: Fertility rates in female patients with congenital adrenal hyperplasia due to 21-hydroxylase deficiency. N Engl J Med 316:178, 1987.

Mullis PE, Yoshimura N, Kuhlmann B, et al.: Aromatase deficiency in a female who is compound heterozygote for two new point mutations in the P450arom gene: Impact of estrogens on hypergonadotropic hypogonadism, multicys-tic ovaries, and bone densitometry in childhood. J Clin Endocrinol Metab 82:1739, 1997.

Naiki Y, Kawamoto T, Mitsuuchi Y, et al.: A nonsense muta-tion (TGG [Trp116]→TAG [Stop]) in CYP11B1 causes steroid 11 beta-hydroxylase deficiency. J Clin Endocrinol Metab 77:1677, 1993.

Nakagawa Y, Yamada M, Ogawa H, et al.: Missense muta-tion in CYP11B1 (CGA[Arg-384]→GGA[Gly]) causes steroid 11 beta-hydroxylase deficiency. Eur J Endocrinol 132:286, 1995.

Nebert DW, Nelson DR, Adesnik M, et al.: The P-450 superfamily: Updated listing of all genes and recommended nomenclature for the chromosomal loci. DNA 8:1, 1989.

New MI, White PC: Genetic disorders of steroid hormone syn-thesis and metabolism. Baillieres Clin Endocrinol Metab 9:525, 1995.

Nezarati M, Loeffler J, Yoon G, et al.: Novel mutation in the Δ-sterol reductase gene in three Lebanese sibs with Smith-Lemli-Opitz (RSH) syndrome. Am J Med Genet 110:103, 2002.

Nowaczyk MJ, McCaughey D, Whelan DT, et al.: Incidence of Smith-Lemli-Opitz syndrome in Ontario, Canada. Am J Med Genet 102:18, 2001.

Opitz JM, Howe JJ: The Meckel syndrome (dysencephalic splanchnocystica, the Gruber syndrome). Birth Defects 5:167, 1969.

Opitz JM, Simpson JL, Sarto GE, et al.: Pseudovaginal peri-neoscrotal hypospadias. Clin Genet 3:1, 1971.

Pang S, Clark A: Congenital adrenal hyperplasia due to 21-hydroxylase deficiency: Newborn screening and its rela-tionship to the diagnosis and treatment of the disorder. Screening 2:105, 1993.

Park IJ, Jones HW: Familial male hermaphroditism with ambiguous external genitalia. Am J Obstet Gynecol 108:1197, 1970.

Park IJ, Jones HW, Melhem RE: Nonadrenal familial female hermaphroditism. Am J Obstet Gynecol 112:930, 1972.

Parker KL, Schimmer BP: Steroidogenic factor 1: A key determinant of endocrine development and function. Endocrinol
Rev 18:361, 1997.

Passarge E, Lenz W: Syndrome of caudal regression in infants
of diabetic mothers: Observations of further cases.
Pediatrics 37:672, 1966.

Peixoto MA, Perpetuo FO, de Souza RP, et al.: LEOPARD
syndrome, a neural crest disorder: A case report. Arq
Neuropsiquiatr 39:214, 1981.

Perloff WH, Conger KB, Levy LM: Female pseudohermaphroditism: A description of 2 unusual cases. J Clin
Endocrinol Metab 13:783, 1953.

Peterson RE, Imperato-McGinley J, Gautier T, et al.: Male
pseudohermaphroditism due to steroid 5α-reductase
deficiency. Am J Med 62:170, 1977.

Phillips OP, Simpson JL: Contraception and congenital malformations. In Sciarra J (ed): Gynecology and Obstetrics,
vol VI. Philadelphia: Lippincott Williams and Wilkins,
2001.

Pinsky L, Beitel LK, Kazemi-Esfarjani P, et al.: Lessons from
androgen receptor gene mutations that cause androgen
resistance in humans. In Hughes IA (ed): Sex differentiation: Clinical and Biological Aspects. Cambridge, England:
Serono Symposia Series. [Frontiers in Endocrinology], vol
20, 1996, p 95.

Pinsky L, Erickson RP, Schimke RN: Genetic Disorders of
Human Sexual Development. New York: Oxford University
Press, 1999.

Pinsky L, Kaufman M: Genetics of steroid receptors and their
disorders. Adv Hum Genet 16:299, 1987.

Pinsky L, Kaufman M, Killinger DW: Impaired spermatogenesis is not an obligate expression of receeptor-defective
androgen resistance. Am J Med Genet 32:100, 1989.

Pinsky L, Kaufman M, Levitsky LL: Partial androgen resistance due to a distinctive qualitative defect of the androgen
receptor. Am J Med Genet 27:459, 1987.

Pisarska MD, Simpson JL, Zepeda DE, et al.: Laparoscopic
removal of streak gonads in 46,XY or 45,X/46,XY
gonadal dysgenesis. J Gynecol Tech 4:95, 1998.

Quigley CA, Friedman KJ, Johnson A, et al.: Complete deletion of the androgen receptor gene: Definition of the null
phenotype of the androgen insensitivity syndrome and
determination of carrier status. J Clin Endocrinol Metab
74:927, 1992.

Rabinovici J, Blankenstein J, Goldman B, et al.: In vitro fertilization and primary embryonic cleavage are possible in
17 alpha-hydroxylase deficiency despite extremely low
intrafollicular 17 beta-estradiol. J Clin Endocrinol Metab
68:693, 1989.

Rabinowitz R, Schillinger JF: Prune belly syndrome in the
female subject. J Urol 118:454, 1977.

Reinfenstein EC: Hereditary familial hypogonadism. Clin
Res 3:86, 1947.

Riccardi VM, Borges W: Aniridia, cataracts, and Wilms
tumor. Am J Ophthalmol 86:577, 1978a.

Riccardi VM, Sujansky E, Smith AC, et al.: Chromosomal
imbalance in the Aniridia-Wilms' tumor association: 11p
interstitial deletion. Pediatrics 61:604, 1978b.

Riddick DH, Hammond CB: Long-term steroid therapy in
patients with adrenogenital syndrome. Obstet Gynecol
45:15, 1975.

Rivkees SA, Crawford JD: Dexamethasone treatment of virilizing congenital adrenal hyperplasia: The ability to achieve
normal growth. Pediatrics 106:767, 2000.

Robinow M, Silverman FN, Smith HD: A newly recognized
dwarfing syndrome. Am J Dis Child 117:645, 1969.

Rodien P, Mebarki F, Mowszowicz I, et al.: Different phenotypes in a family with androgen insensitivity caused by the
same M780I point mutation in the androgen receptor
gene. J Clin Endocrinol Metab 81:2994, 1996.

Rodriguez JI, Palacios J, Omenaca F, et al.: Polyasplenia,
caudal deficiency, and agensis of the corpus callosum. Am
J Med Genet 38:99, 1991.

Rosenberg C, Frota-Pessoa O, Vianna-Morgante AM, et al.:
Phenotypic spectrum of 45,X/46,XY individuals. Am J
Med Genet 27:553, 1987.

Rösler A: Steroid 17β-hydroxysteroid dehydrogenase deficiency
in man: An inherited form of male pseudohermaphroditism.
J Steroid Biochem Mol Biol 43:989, 1992.

Rösler A, Kohn G: Male pseudohermaphroditism due to
17β-hydroxysteroid dehydrogenase deficiency: Studies on
the natural history of the defect and effect of androgens on
gender role. J Steroid Biochem 19:663, 1983.

Rumsby G, Skinner C, Lee HA, et al.: Combined 17
alpha-hydroxylase/17,20-lyase deficiency caused by heterozygous stop codons in the cytochrome P450 17 alpha-
hydroxylase gene. Clin Endocrinol (Oxf) 39:483, 1993.

Russu IG: Absence of clitoris. Endocrinol Ginecol Obstet
(Roumania) 5:23, 1938.

Rutledge JC, Friedman JM, Harrod MJ, et al.: A "new"
lethal multiple congenital anomaly syndrome: Joint con-
tractures, cerebellar hypoplasia, renal hypoplasia, urogenital anomalies, tongue cysts, shortness of limbs, eye
abnormalities, defects of the heart, gallbladder agenesis,
and ear malformations. Am J Med Genet 19:255, 1984.

Ryan AK, Bartlett K, Clayton P, et al.: Smith-Lemli-Opitz
syndrome: A variable clinical and biochemical phenotype.
J Med Genet 35:558, 1998.

Saenger P, Klonari Z, Black SM, et al.: Prenatal diagnosis of
congenital lipoid adrenal hyperplasia. J Clin Endocrinol
Metab 80:200, 1995.

Schapiro RL, Sandrock AR: Esophagogastric and vulvar
leiomyomatosis: A new radiologic syndrome. J Can Assoc
Radiol 24:184, 1973.

Schey WL, Kandel G, Charles AG: Female epispadias. Report
of a case and review of the literature. Clin Pediatr 19:212,
1980.

Seaver LH, Grimes J, Erickson RP: Female pseudohermaph-
roditism with multiple caudal anomalies: Absence of
Y-specific DNA sequences as pathogenetic factors. Am J
Med Genet 51:16, 1994.

Shackleton CH, Roitman E, Kratz L, et al.: Dehydro-oestriol
and dehydropregnanetriol are candidate analytes for prenatal diagnosis of Smith-Lemli-Opitz syndrome. Prenat
Diagn 21:207, 2001.

Shozu M, Akasofu K, Harada T, et al.: A new cause of female
pseudohermaphroditism: Placental aromatase deficiency. J
Clin Endocrinol Metab 72:560, 1991.

Silengo MC, Bell GL, Biagioli M, et al.: Oro-facial-digital
syndrome II. Transitional type between the Mohr and the
Majewski syndromes: Report of two new cases. Clin
Genet 31:331, 1987.

Simard J, Rheaume E, Mebarki F, et al.: Molecular basis of
human 3 beta-hydroxysteroid dehydrogenase deficiency. J
Steroid Biochem Mol Biol 53:127, 1995b.

Simard J, Sanchez R, Durocher F, et al.: Structure-function
relationships and molecular genetics of the 3 beta-hydroxysteroid dehydrogenase gene family. J Steroid Biochem
Mol Biol 55:489, 1995a.

Simpson ER, Michael MD, Agarwal VR, et al.: Cytochromes
P450 11: Expression of the CYP19 (aromatase) gene: An
unusual case of alternative promoter usage. FASEB J 11:29,
1997.

Simpson JL: Disorders of Sexual Differentiation: Etiology
and Clinical Delineation. New York: Academic Press,
1976.

Simpson JL, Kaufman R: Fetal effects of progestogens and
diethylstilbestrol. In Fraser IS, Jansen RPS, Lobo RA, et
al. (eds): Estrogens and Progestogens in Clinical Practice.
London: Churchill Livingstone, 1998.

Simpson JL, New M, Peterson RE, et al.: Pseudovaginal perineoscrotal hypospadias (PPSH) in sibs. Birth Defects Orig Artic Ser 7(6):140, 1971b.

Simpson JL, Photopulos G: The relationship of neoplasia to disorders of abnormal sexual differentiation. Birth Defects Orig Artic Ser 12(1):15, 1976.

Simpson JL, Verp MS, Plouffe L: Female genital system. *In* Stevenson RE, Hall JG, Goodman RM (eds): Human Malformations and Related Anomalies, vol. 2. London: Oxford Press, 1993, p 563.

Sirota L, Shabtai F, Landman I, et al.: New anomalies found in the 11q-syndrome. Clin Genet 26:569, 1984.

Skinner CA, Rumsby G: Steroid 11 beta-hydroxylase deficiency caused by a five base pair duplication in the *CYP11B1* gene. Hum Mol Genet 3:377, 1994.

Sofatzis JA, Alexacos L, Skouteli HN, et al.: Malformed female genitalia in newborns with VATER association. Acta Paediatr Scand 72:923, 1983.

Speiser PW, Dupont J, Zhu D, et al.: Disease expression and molecular genotype in congenital adrenal hyperplasia due to 21-hydroxylase deficiency. J Clin Invest 90:584, 1992.

Stevenson RE, Jones KL, Phelan MC, et al.: Vascular steal: The pathogenetic mechanism producing sirenomalia and associated defects of the viscera and soft tissues. Pediatrics 78:451, 1986.

Sultan C, Paris F, Terouanne B, et al.: Disorders linked to insufficient androgen action in male children. Hum Reprod Update 7:314, 2001.

Taijma T, Nishi Y, Takase A, et al.: No genetic mutation in the type II 3 beta-hydroxysteroid dehydrogenase gene in patients with biochemical evidence of enzyme deficiency. Horm Res 47:49, 1997.

Thigpen AE, Davis DL, Milatovich A, et al.: Molecular genetics of steroid 5α-reductase 2 deficiency. J Clin Invest 90:799, 1992.

Tint GS, Batta AK, Xu G, et al.: The Smith-Lemli-Opitz syndrome: A potentially fatal birth defect caused by a block in the last enzymatic step in cholesterol biosynthesis. Subcell Biochem 28:117, 1997.

Tint GS, Irons M, Elias ER, et al.: Defective cholesterol biosynthesis associated with the Smith-Lemli-Opitz syndrome. N Engl J Med 330:107, 1994.

Tsukada T, Inoue M, Tachibana S, et al.: An androgen receptor mutation causing androgen resistance in undervirilized male syndrome. J Clin Endocrinol Metab 79:1202, 1994.

Turleau C, Niaudet P, Sultan C, et al.: Partial androgen receptor deficiency and mixed gonadal dysgenesis in Drash syndrome. Hum Genet 75:81, 1987.

Tusie-Luna M-T, Traktman P, White PC: Determination of functional effects of mutations in the steroid 21-hydroxylase gene (*CYP21*) using recombinant vaccinia virus. J Biol Chem 265:20916, 1990.

Ulloa-Aguirre A, Carranza-Lira S, Mendez PJ, et al.: Incomplete regression of müllerian ducts in the androgen insensitivity syndrome. Fertil Steril 53:1024, 1990.

Van de Velde H, Sermon K, De Vos A, et al.: Fluorescent PCR and automated fragment analysis in preimplantation genetic diagnosis for 21-hydroxylase deficiency in congenital adrenal hyperplasia. Mol Hum Reprod 5:691, 1999.

Verhoeven AT, Mastboom JL, van Leusden HA, et al.: Virilization in pregnancy coexisting with an (ovarian) mucinous cystadenoma: A case report and review of virilizing ovarian tumors in pregnancy. Obstet Gynecol Surv 28:597, 1973.

Verp MS, Simpson JL: Abnormal sexual differentiation and neoplasia. Cancer Genet Cytogenet 25:191, 1987.

Wahlen T, Astedt B: Familial occurrence of coexisting leiomyoma of vulva and oesophagus. Acta Obstet Gynecol Scand 44:197, 1965.

Walsh C, Madden JD, Harrod MJ, et al.: Familial incomplete male pseudohermaphroditism, Type 2. Decreased dihydrotestosterone formation in pseudovaginal perineoscrotal hypospadias. N Engl J Med 291:944, 1974.

Wedell A: Molecular genetics of congenital adrenal hyperplasia (21-hydroxylase deficiency): implications for diagnosis, prognosis and treatment. Acta Paediatr 87:159, 1998.

White PC, Curnow KM, Pascoe L: Disorders of steroid 11 beta-hydroxylase isozymes. Endocr Rev 15:421, 1994.

White PC, Dupont J, New MI, et al.: A mutation in *CYP11B1* (Arg-448—His) associated with steroid 11 beta-hydroxylase deficiency in Jews of Moroccan origin. J Clin Invest 87:1664, 1991.

Wilson JD, Carlson BR, Weaver DD, et al.: Endocrine and genetic characterization of cousins with male pseudohermaphroditism: Evidence that the Lubs phenotype can result from a mutation that alters the structure of the androgen receptor. Clin Genet 26:363, 1984.

Wilson JD, Griffin JE, Russell DW: Steroid 5α-reductase 2 deficiency. Endocr Rev 14:577, 1993.

Wilson JD, Harrod MJ, Goldstein JL, et al.: Familial incomplete male pseudohermaphroditism, type 1. Evidence for androgen resistance and variable clinical manifestations in family with the Reifenstein syndrome. N Engl J Med 290:1097, 1974.

Yanase T: 17 Alpha-hydroxylase/17,20-lyase defects. J Steroid Biochem Mol Biol 53:153, 1995.

Yanase T, Kagimoto M, Suzuki S, et al.: Deletion of a phenylalanine in the N-terminal region of human cytochrome P-450(17 alpha) results in partial combined 17 alpha-hydroxylase/17,20-lyase deficiency. J Biol Chem 264:18076, 1989.

Yanase T, Simpson ER, Waterman MR: 17α-hydroxylase/17,20-lyase deficiency: From clinical investigation to molecular definition. Endocr Rev 12:91, 1991.

Yang X, Iwamoto K, Wang M, et al.: Inherited congenital adrenal hyperplasia in the rabbit is caused by a deletion in the gene encoding cytochrome P450 cholesterol side-chain cleavage enzyme. Endocrinology 132:1977, 1993.

Zachmann M: Defects in steroidogenic enzymes. Discrepancies between clinical steroid research and molecular biology results. J Steroid Biochem Mol Biol 53:159, 1995.

Zachmann M, Vollmin JA, Hamilton W, et al.: Steroid 17, 20-desmolase deficiency: A new cause of male pseudohermaphroditism. Clin Endocrinol 1:369, 1972.

Sex Chromosomal Polysomies (47,XXY; 47,XYY; 47,XXX), Sex Reversed (46,XX) Males, and Disorders of the Male Reproductive Ducts

In previous chapters we considered disorders of gonadal development (Chapter 10) and disorders of external genital development (Chapter 11). Disorders discussed in those chapters were usually caused by *absence* of part or all of a chromosome (usually X or Y) or a mutant gene (mendelian). Also important are disorders caused by the additional sex chromosomes.

Polysomy X or Y are not infrequent. 47,XXX, 47,XXY, and 47,XYY each have incidences in approximately 1:800–1000 females or males, respectively. Associated phenotypes invariably cause gonadal abnormalities in 47,XXY but only occasionally in 47,XXX and 47,XYY. Variants exist with additional X or Y chromosomes. The Klinefelter phenotype may occur in 46,XX males, which is also discussed in this chapter.

Finally, we discuss several disorders of the male reproductive tract that cause infertility and thus are of interest to the reproductive medicine specialist.

47,XXY Klinefelter Syndrome

In 1942, Klinefelter and colleagues (1942) delineated a syndrome in nine postpubertal males consisting of gynecomastia; normal external genitalia; lack of pubertal virilization; small, firm testes with tubular hyalinization but with a normal number of Leydig cells; azoospermia; elevated gonadotropin levels; and decreased 17-ketosteroid levels. Subsequently, several groups reported that patients with the Klinefelter phenotype were often X-chromatin–positive, and the presence of an extra X chromosome was hypothesized (Bradbury et al., 1956; Plunkett et al., 1956; Riis et al., 1956). Later, Jacobs and Strong (1959) showed that an X chromatin-positive male had the complement 47,XXY. Minimal diagnostic criteria for this syndrome are accepted to be the presence of at least one Y chromosome and two X chromosomes (Fig. 12–1). Variants with three or four X chromosomes are less common and are discussed separately.

The incidence of Klinefelter syndrome is 1:800 liveborn males. Incidence is only slightly higher (1%) in abortuses, indicating relatively little selection in utero. Klinefelter syndrome accounts for perhaps 5 to 15% of infertile males (Carothers et al., 1988) or needing intracytoplasmic sperm injection (ICSI), usually the group with oligospermia or azoospermia. Overt mental retardation is a feature in a portion of patients with Klinefelter syndrome, as indicated by the increased prevalence of 47,XXY males among residents of institutions for the mentally retarded compared with the general population (Patil et al., 1977).

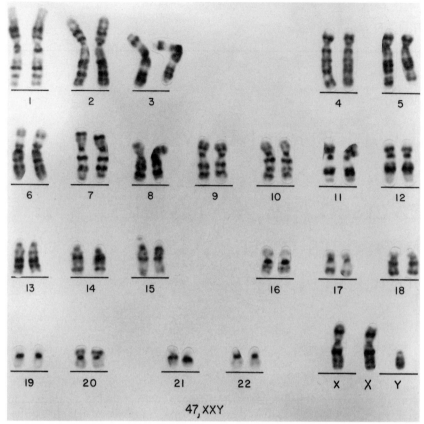

FIGURE 12–1 • Karyotype derived from a 47,XXY Klinefelter syndrome patient. (From Bischoff FZ, Elias S: Klinefelter Syndrome. *In* Sciarra JJ (ed): Gynecology and Obstetrics, Vol. 5. Philadelphia: Lippincott Williams & Wilkins, 1999.)

Klinefelter syndrome is also more prevalent among institutionalized patients with psychotic or neurotic disorders and/or a criminal history (Casey et al., 1966; Jacobs et al., 1968; MacLean et al., 1968; Nielsen, 1969).

CYTOLOGIC ORIGIN

Mean maternal age in 47,XXY has long been known to be increased (Hamerton, 1971). In 1964 Ferguson-Smith and coworkers (1964) reported mean maternal age in 45 cases to be 32.5 years compared with 28.7 years for controls and 36.1 years for mothers of children with Down syndrome. Patil and colleagues (1977) calculated that the highest risk of having 47,XXY offspring is for mothers over age 40; Carothers and Filippi (1988) reported that at age 40, the risk is two to three times that of a mother at age 30. By contrast, the consensus is that paternal age is not increased, even in those cases that are paternally derived (MacDonald et al., 1994; Thomas et al., 2000; Shi et al., 2002).

Using polymorphic DNA markers, the additional X chromosome has been shown to be paternal in origin in 50 to 60% of cases and maternal in origin in the remaining 40 to 50% of cases (Jacobs et al., 1988; Harvey et al., 1990; Lorda-Sanchez et al., 1992). Among maternal cases, nondisjunction occurs in meiosis I in 48% of cases and in meiosis II in 29% of cases; 16% show postzygotic origin, and in 7% origin is unknown (Harvey et al., 1990; Lorda-Sanchez et al., 1992; MacDonald et al., 1994; Thomas et al., 2000). In paternally derived 47,XXY cases, X-Y nondisjunction must occur in the first meiotic division. Increased maternal age is associated with errors in maternal meiosis I (Thomas et al., 2000), but not in meiosis II (Hassold et al., 1991).

Nondisjunction involving sex chromosomes reflects decreased crossing-over and, hence, increased nondisjunction analogous to autosomal trisomy. In 47,XXY, frequency of recombination in maternal cases ($47,X^mX^mY$) can be assessed by determining whether the number of exchanges (recombinants) between the two X's is that expected for the two homologous X's. In male origin cases ($47,X^mX^pY$) the frequency of exchange between X and Y in the pseudoautosomal region (PAR) can be assessed easily. In 65 maternal meiosis cases (54% of total cases studied by Hassold et al., 1991), there were 37 in which no recombination occurred (expected number 6). In 28 cases one recombinant was also observed versus the expected 60. In the 46% of cases arising from paternal meiosis I, recombination between paternal X and paternal Y was observed far less than expected, two thirds of $X^m\,X^p\,Y^p$ cases failing to show an exchange (Thomas et al., 2000). Consistent with the above, only a slight paternal age effect is observed in $X^m\,X^pY$, and no relationship between paternal age and X-Y recombination frequency (Shi et al., 2002). In conclusion, decreased recombination leads to sex chromosomal (XXY) aneuploidy, just as it leads to autosomal aneuploidy (trisomy).

GENITAL AND GONADAL PATHOLOGY

In Klinefelter syndrome, external genitalia are usually well differentiated (Fig. 12–2). The penis is normal in size in 80 to 90% of 47,XXY patients (Paulsen et al., 1968; Becker, 1972). However, development of the penis and scrotum may be abnormal. Presumably incomplete morphogenesis in the first 12 to 14 weeks' gestation produces anomalies such as hypospadias, chordee, and a small penis. 47,XXY Klinefelter syndrome is the most commonly known testicular disorder associated with a small penis, presumably the result of a moderate deficiency in testosterone production (Caldwell et al., 1972). The prostate is smaller than usual, also presumably owing to decreased testosterone levels (Carothers et al., 1988). Cryptorchidism occurs infrequently.

Prepubertal testes of 47,XXY patients are often described as approximately normal in size, but some report that even before puberty the testes are smaller than those of normal boys (Laron and Hochman, 1971). Irrespective of this, prepubertal 47,XXY patients display neither seminiferous tubule atrophy nor apparent Leydig cell (interstitial cell) hyperplasia; primary spermatogonia are reduced in number (Ferguson-Smith, 1959; Mikamo et al., 1968). To mitigate against this temporal sequence of germ cell failure, some physicians obtain sperm or testicular tissue from adolescent 47,XXY; the rationale is that cryopreserved sperm can permit pregnancies in the future, even if no

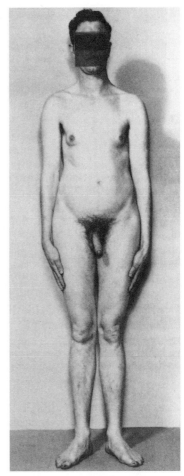

FIGURE 12–2 • Photograph of a 47,XXY male. Gynecomastia is present. (From Ferguson-Smith M: Testis and intersexuality. *In* Sorsby A (ed): Clinical Genetics, 2nd ed. London: Butterworth, 1973.)

sperm exists in situ at that time (Damani et al., 2002). At puberty germ cell attrition is dramatic, resulting in tubules containing only Sertoli cells. Inhibin A levels are normal, reflecting Sertoli cells. In a mouse model, Matzuk (2000) showed both X chromosomes to be active in Sertoli cells. Increased gene product attributable to two active X's, or parts thereof, is presumably pivotal to increased XXY germ cell attrition; however, the exact mechanism is unclear.

Testes of 47,XXY *adults* are rarely more than 2 cm in greatest diameter, compared with 3.5 cm in normal males. Usually 47,XXY testes are firmer than normal. Differences in consistency probably reflect differences in the extent of seminiferous tubule hyalinization. Adult 47,XXY testes show hyalinization and fibrosis of seminiferous tubules. There is a *relative* increase in the number of Leydig cells (interstitial cells), with

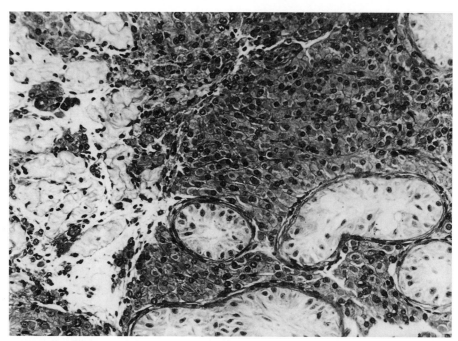

FIGURE 12–3 • Photomicrograph of a testicular biopsy of a 47,XXY patient. Seminiferous tubles contain Sertoli cells but no spermatogonia. Leydig cells are hyperplastic (x 200). (From Ferguson-Smith MA: Testis and intersexuality. *In* Hubble D (ed): Pediatric Endocrinology. Oxford: Blackwell Scientific, 1969.)

variable degrees of clumping (Fig. 12–3); the absolute number of Leydig cells is actually in the normal range or lower. Leydig cells are abnormal histologically, lacking crystalloids of Reinke. Interstitial regions of the testis contain increased fibroblasts and fat cells. Sertoli cells are present, and inhibin levels are normal.

Azoospermia or severe oligospermia is expected, but a few sperm can usually be recovered at testicular biopsy or, uncommonly, in the ejaculate. Prior to availability of ICSI, there were only a few instances of purported paternity (Warburg, 1963). These cases were often thought to have represented undetected 46,XY/47,XXY mosaicism.

With ICSI, pregnancy is now possible, although not easily (Palermo et al., 1998; Simpson et al., 2002). Offspring sired by 47,XXY men have low likelihood of being affected because sperm rarely shows hyperhaploidy (disomy XY). In XXY only 3.4% of gametes are 24,XY rather than the theoretical 50% (Guttenbach et al., 1997a; Okada et al., 1999). This figure is still higher than the 1% disomic XY sperm observed in XY infertile males or the 0.2% in fertile XY males (Bischoff et al., 1994; Moosani et al., 1995; Guttenbach et al., 1997b; Aran et al., 1999; Okada et al., 1999). It has been argued that XXY germ cells are not capable of proceeding through meiosis; thus, all spermatozoa would need to have been derived from a 46,XY spermatogonia (Egozcue et al., 2000).

SECONDARY SEXUAL DEVELOPMENT

Characteristic features of Klinefelter syndrome become more pronounced in adolescence, when delay of puberty is observed. This is clinically evident in perhaps half of 47,XXY men, whose penile size is reduced about 20% (Sorenson, 1988). Pubic hair may be feminine in distribution; facial and body hair are scanty, and few patients shave daily. Acne is rare during adolescence, and temporal hair recession usually does not occur. Obesity, gynecoid fat distribution, and poor muscular development are also frequent. Sexual activity is often reduced (Raboch, 1979), although libido and potency may be improved with testosterone therapy (Stewart et al., 1979).

Increased parenchymal breast tissue, as determined by palpation, is observed in 50 to 75% of 47,XXY patients (Warburg, 1963; Ferguson-Smith, 1969; Leonard et al., 1975; Wang et al., 1975; Raboch, 1979; Stewart et al., 1979; Sorenson, 1988); fewer, perhaps 20%, have overt gynecomastia (Becker, 1972). Breast enlargement in 47,XXY patients is characterized by increased collagenous material in interglandular spaces; the ductal epithelium is only slightly hyperplastic.

Longitudinal development in 47,XXY is intriguing. *Prepubertal* 47,XXY boys show no significant abnormalities in gonadotropin or testosterone serum levels (Stewart et al., 1979). Yet in adults, follicle-stimulating hormone (FSH) and luteinizing hormone (LH) levels are clearly elevated (Warburg, 1963; Leonard et al., 1975; Wang et al., 1975; Raboch, 1979; Stewart et al., 1979; Sorenson, 1988). Testosterone is usually below normal or in the lower part of the normal range (5–86 mg/100 ml). As in normal males, gonads are the principal source of testosterone in patients with Klinefelter syndrome; however, total plasma testosterone level is affected by peripheral metabolism, alterations in binding proteins, and diurnal changes. Thus, serum testosterone levels are not an inviolate indicator of testicular androgen *synthesis*, which explains why plasma testosterone levels vary in Klinefelter syndrome. Many experienced endocrinologists have the clinical impression that it is beneficial to administer testosterone even if blood levels are ostensibly normal (see Simpson et al., 2003).

Elevations in plasma LH and FSH levels reflect deficient testicular function and the consequent lack of feedback inhibition by sex steroids and inhibin on the pituitary and hypothalamus (Peterson et al., 1968; Means et al., 1976). The hypothalamic-gonadal axis itself is intact, as judged by normal response to gonadotropin-releasing hormone (GnRH) or exogenous testosterone.

HEIGHT AND BODY PROPORTIONS

The height of 47,XXY boys under age 3 falls within normal distributions, but after age 3 the distribution becomes skewed. Significantly fewer than expected 47,XXY boys have heights below the 25th percentile (Stewart et al., 1958). Adult 47,XXY patients are frequently taller than average and often have abnormal skeletal proportions, with relatively long legs and a decreased upper:lower segment ratio (Stewart et al., 1958; Milne et al., 1974). Shoulders are narrower than usual (2 cm decrease) and hips are wider (1 cm increase). Klinefelter syndrome patients differ from other eunuchoid patients in that their arm span is usually only 2 to 3 cm greater than their height, if at all; in most other types of eunuchoidism, arm span is usually at least 4 cm greater than the height. The cellular explanation for the abnormal proportions is not actually known. Perhaps epiphyses respond abnormally to androgens, consistent with their closing earlier in Klinefelter syndrome boys than in normal girls (Stewart, 1959). Bone age is usually normal.

SOMATIC ANOMALIES

No definite somatic phenotype exists, but a variety of findings are suggestive of Klinefelter syndrome. None are pathognomonic (Simpson et al., 2003). Facies shows midface underdevelopment and slightly decreased head circumference. Together with relative hypertelorism, facial appearance is sometimes said to be "handsome." Other skeletal anomalies include narrow wrists (25% decrease), scoliosis and kyphosis (S-curve) secondary to lax ligaments, cervical and other anomalous ribs, sacralization of the last lumbar vertebrae, pectus excavatum or carinatum, pes planus, 5th toe anomalies, and 5th finger clinodactyly. Overgrowth in the proximal radius and ulnar bones occurs, but not usually to an extent resulting in the radioulnar synostosis characteristic of 48,XXXY or 49,XXXXY.

Other structural anomalies exist, including cardiac anomalies in 10 to 15% (Gautier and Nouaille, 1964; Rosenthal, 1972). Robinson and colleagues (1979b) summarized findings in 63 47,XXY neonates prospectively ascertained through various chromosome surveys of unselected newborns. In 18%, one or more major congenital abnormalities were found. The most frequent were cleft palate and inguinal hernia. Minor anomalies (e.g., clinodactyly, strabismus, external rotation of legs, third fontanelle, upward slanted palpebral tissue antimongoloid obliquities) were found in 26% (Robinson et al., 1969). Of the probands' 224 siblings, only 2 (1%) had major anomalies and 15 (7.1%) had minor abnormalities.

ADULT-ONSET DISORDERS

Autoimmune diseases are not uncommon. These include systemic lupus erythematosus (Miller et al., 1983; Schlegelberger et al., 1986; Bizzarro et al., 1987), ankylosing spondylitis (Armstrong et al., 1985), Sjögren syndrome (keratoconjunctivitis, dry mouth, and arthritis) (Bizzarro et al., 1987), and rheumatologic disorders (Kobayashi et al., 1991). It has been hypothesized that testosterone protects normal males from autoimmune phenomena; therefore, hypogonadal males might be prone to defects in T-cell activity that lead to autoimmune disorders (Bizzarro et al., 1987).

Glucose tolerance tests (GTTs) may be abnormal, and both type 1 (juvenile) and type 2 (adult-onset) diabetes mellitus have long been recognized as more frequent among patients with Klinefelter syndrome and their parents than in the general population (Nielsen et al., 1969; Nielsen, 1972; Simpson et al., 2002). The autoimmune component is probably responsible for type 1 diabetes mellitus. Engelberth and colleagues (1965) reported elevated levels of autoantibodies against insulin and against pancreatic tissue in some patients with Klinefelter syndrome. Of 157 47,XXY cases reviewed by Nielsen (1972), 28 (29%) showed diabetic GTTs and 13 (18%) had overt diabetes mellitus compared with a 6% incidence of abnormal GTTs in a random population less than 50 years of age and 16% in a sample older than 50. However, far more common than type 1 diabetes mellitus is type 2, probably secondary to abdominal obesity and insulin resistance. Diabetes mellitus in patients with Klinefelter syndrome is usually mild (Nielsen, 1972).

Clinical hypothyroidism is rare, but decreased uptake and sluggish responsiveness to thyroid-stimulating hormone have been reported (Davis et al., 1963; Zuppinger et al., 1967). Thyroiditis is not rare (Tojo, 1998). Thyroid-binding globulin levels are usually normal, and antithyroid antibodies are not usually detectable (Carr et al., 1961).

Chronic leg ulcerations and varicose veins are associated with Klinefelter syndrome, with a prevalence as high as 13% (Verp et al., 1983; Downham and Mitek, 1986; Norris et al., 1987). Platelet hyperaggregability, rather than anatomic vascular changes, appears to be the major causative factor (Downham and Mitek, 1986). The etiology may involve plasminogen activator inhibition-1 (PAI-1), elevation of which leads to clotting secondary to platelet aggregation.

Klinefelter syndrome patients also have chronic pulmonary diseases (e.g., emphysema, bronchitis, asthma) (Rohde, 1964; Becker et al., 1966; Becker, 1972).

NEOPLASIA

Germ cell tumors of both gonadal (Carroll et al., 1988; Dexeus, 1988) and extragonadal origin (Lee and Stephens, 1987; Nichols et al., 1987) occur with increased frequency. Gonadal tumors include Leydig cell neoplasia (Sorio et al., 1999). Lee and Stephens (1987) suggested that dysgenetic germ cells might be arrested in their migration along the urogenital ridge, resulting in mediastinal and retroperitoneal germ cell rests from which tumors arise; there have also been rare reports of cerebral germ cell tumors (Nichols et al., 1987; Arens et al., 1988).

Gynecomastia predisposes to breast carcinoma, the frequency being 20 to 50 times more frequent than among normal males. Of males with breast cancer, 3 to 8% are 47,XXY patients (Stewart et al., 1979; Harnden et al., 1971; Cuenca and Becker, 1968); median age at diagnosis in 47,XXY is 72 years, similar to that in 46,XY subjects. The extent to which mammography is helpful or testosterone treatment decreases risk is unclear. For cosmetic purposes as well as to mitigate against neoplasia some investigators have advocated mastectomy (Becker, 1972).

Mediastinal tumors are 30-fold more common than in the general population (Lachman et al., 1986). Lymphoma (Becher, 1986) and leukemia (Ratcliffe and Paul, 1986; Horsman et al., 1987) have also been reported in 47,XXY patients, although no clear association between these malignancies and Klinefelter syndrome has been established.

INTELLIGENCE AND PSYCHOSOCIAL DEVELOPMENT

In 47,XXY Klinefelter syndrome IQ is definitely lowered, but not to the extent that occurs in 48,XXXY and 49,XXXXY. Overt mental retardation is uncommon. The consensus is that IQ is decreased about 15 points; with each additional X (e.g., 48,XXXY), an additional 15-point decrease occurs. That 47,XXY patients have an increased probability of being retarded was first deduced from observations that 1% of mentally retarded males are 47,XXY (Hambert, 1966; Hamerton, 1971). The prevalence of 47,XXY is higher among patients with an IQ between 50 and 85 than among those with a lower IQ (Robach and Sipova, 1961; Becker, 1972).

The largest standing cohort is the Denver Study of Sex Chromosomal Abnormalities. This cohort begun in 1964 with ascertainment through sex chromatin analysis of amniotic membranes and confirmation of full chromosomal complement through peripheral blood analysis. Many psychosocial investigations on this cohort have been reported (Robinson et al., 1979a; Bender et al., 1995). Many prior reports exist on intelligence, neuromuscular development, and psychosocial development (Bender et al., 1986; Robinson et al., 1991). Bender and coworkers (2001) recently updated information based on 11 47,XXY men, now 27.7 ± 2.76 years old. Verbal IQ was 90.1, performance IQ 94.9; mean years of education was 12.8 years. Although within the normal range, all the above were significantly different from sibling controls. All but one 47,XXY was employed, but none were professionals. By comparison, 3 of 16 sibs were; 4 of the 11 Klinefelter syndrome men were in skilled positions compared with 6 of 16 sibs.

Graham and coworkers (1988) and Samango-Sprouse (2001) reported that low IQ in Klinefelter syndrome is the result of expressive language deficits rather than global mental deficiency. Performance IQ scores did not significantly differ from those of controls in a study by Netley (1986). Samango-Sprouse and Suddaby (1997) and Samango-Sprouse (2001) estimate that two thirds of 47,XXY boys show expressive language difficulties. Those with normal overall IQ still show performance IQ > verbal IQ. Their problem is often dyspraxia or motor planning problems. They are unable to find the correct phase or response, even if thoughts are lucid ("tip of the tongue" phenomenon). Abnormalities of word finding, narrative formation, and syntactic production are common. Netley (1986) found a 10- to 20-point reduction in verbal skill during adolescence (Ratcliffe and Paul, 1986) and adult life (Sorenson, 1988). Inability to communicate effectively leads to fewer personal friends, difficulty relating to others, more withdrawn personalities, and paradoxically aggressive physical responses to frustration. Whether these difficulties could be ameliorated by early educational intervention, androgen therapy, or treatment is unknown. That the amygdala has been reported to be decreased in size in 47,XXY individuals bespeaks of an anatomic basis (Patwardhan et al., 2002).

Other behavioral characteristics include poor self-motivation, passivity, absence of anxiety, and bland facies (Hoaken et al., 1964; Federman, 1967; Money et al., 1974). Affected individuals adapt poorly to new situations, and as noted above, inappropriately aggressive behavior is common when they are confronted with stressful situations. All the above probably reflect difficulties in verbalizing. Among 47,XXY patients studied after being prospectively ascertained in newborn chromosome surveys, Robinson and colleagues (1979b) found that 32% had delayed emotional development, compared with 9% of their siblings ($P < 0.002$). Maladjustment to structured school situations was found in 20 of 45 cases (44%) of 47,XXY boys compared with 32 of 136 cases among siblings and controls (24%) ($P < 0.025$). Fortunately, only rarely does this behavior become overtly sociopathic.

MOLECULAR BASIS OF PHENOTYPE

In humans not all loci on X chromosomes in excess of one are inactivated. Thus, it is assumed that the abnormal phenotype in 47,XXY reflects inappropriate transcription of genes encoded on the X. Most (90%) of the genes that escape X inactivation are on the X short arm.

Several genetic mechanisms have been hypothesized to explain the variable phenotype among 47,XXY cases. Zang (1984) hypothesized that a nondisjunctional event in meiosis II or postzygotic division leading to two copies of the same X chromosome could induce a negative dosage effect as result of deleterious recessive genes on the X chromosome. Jacobs and colleagues (1988) postulated an imprinting effect depending upon parental origin of the extra chromosome. In a study of 80 females with Turner syndrome (45,X), Skuse and colleagues (1997) found that an imprinted locus on the long arm of the X chromosome appeared to play a role in cognitive and social development. However, no studies have yet demonstrated a difference in phenotype between 47,XXY paternally and maternally derived cases. Iitsuka and coworkers (2001) reported skewed X-inactivation in unusually high frequency in Klinefelter syndrome, possibly a clue as to why only a minority of Klinefelter syndrome cases manifest pronounced behavioral or learning problems.

TREATMENT

Treatment in Klinefelter syndrome is directed toward the androgen deficiency. Replacement can take the form of intramuscular testosterone injections (enanthate or cyclopentylpropionate esters), 25 mg every 3 weeks for 3 months, or topical application of testosterone. The earliest indication is treatment during infancy for a small penis, perhaps as early as 3 months after birth. At the time of anticipated puberty, androgen replacement therapy produces adequate sexual maturation with increased muscle mass, more masculine body contour, increased body hair, penile enlargement, hyperpigmentation of nipples, and bone age advancement. There is little amelioration in gynecomastia (Fromatin et al., 1974), a process that is difficult to reverse. Testicular size also remains unaffected (Myhre et al., 1970).

Testosterone treatment may mitigate against behavioral disturbances and learning disabilities, and some clinicians favor administration even in the 50% of XXY children whose plasma testosterone level is normal. After an average of 3.6 years of testosterone therapy, Nielsen and colleagues (1988) found most (77%) of their 30 patients showed improvement in mood, learning abilities, concentration, energy, and social interactions compared with their pretreatment status. This conclusion was derived from interviews with patients, parents, and physicians. Although the authors recommended that treatment begin at age 11 or 12 years, improvement was also noted in 20- to 30-year-old patients receiving testosterone.

Testosterone therapy may also ameliorate autoimmune disease. Bizzarro and colleagues (1987) described 47,XXY five patients, three 47,XXY cases with Sjögren's syndrome and two with systemic lupus erythematosus. While they were on oral testosterone therapy, serum antinuclear antibody levels, sedimentation rate, and rheumatoid factor all significantly decreased; the percentage of T-helper cells and T-suppressor-cytotoxic cells significantly increased compared with pretreatment values and to values while on placebo. Clinical features of their autoimmune disease decreased after initiation of testosterone therapy.

There is no *hormonal* treatment for the sterility caused by Klinefelter syndrome. Testes are unable to respond to either gonadotropin or androgen stimulation. However, fertility is possible even if the ejaculate is clinically azoospermic. Testicular biopsy may reveal a few sperm, and these sperm can be used in ICSI to achieve a pregnancy. Odds are low (Palermo et al., 1998), but successes have been recognized. The greatest experience comes from Brussels, where ICSI has been performed in 31 couples (41 cycles) with a XXY father. Data of Staessen were included by Simpson and coworkers (2003). Of 41 preimplantation genetic diagnosis (PGD) cycles, all involving ICSI, there were five fetuses (Staessen, 2001). Other reported ICSI pregnancies using sperm from 47,XXY men have been described (Ron-El et al., 2000), and in all offspring were normal. Nonetheless, preimplantation genetic diagnosis reveals over 50% of embryos to be cytogenetically abnormal. This number may or may not be higher than expected (see Chapters 5 and 16). In the Brussels 47,XXY experience, PGD revealed 50.4% abnormal embryos compared with 22.9% in cycles for mendelian disorders. Frequencies of gonosomal aneuploidy were 30.0% and 15.2%, respectively. Recall that ICSI per se is associated with 1% sex chromosomal abnormalities even when the father is presumptively 46,XY (see Chapter 16). Indeed, an 47,XXY embryo was detected at PGD (Ron-El et al., 2000). Thus, prenatal genetic diagnosis is recommended if PGD is not undertaken.

A key genetic question is whether 47,XXY cells actually complete meiosis. If they do, strong selection must exist against XY disomy or XX disomy gametes. Mroz and colleagues (1999) reported 1.7% disomic sperm in 41,XXY mice versus 0.2% in 40,XY mice. There was also an increase (0.51% versus 0.5%) in non-X, non-Y disomy. Bronson and coworkers (1995) studied two $X^m X^p Y$ mice, leading to the following predicted offspring: 11.1% XXY, 3% XYY, and 80% XY. Data from human XXY cases similarly reveals a dearth of disomic sperm, so much that some investigators have concluded that only XY spermatogenia (i.e., cryptic mosaicism) can lead to viable sperm in mice and humans.

46,XY/47,XXY

Approximately 15% of Klinefelter syndrome patients have two or more chromosomally distinct cell populations, two thirds being 46,XY/47,XXY (Ferguson-Smith, 1966). Frequency of cryptic mosaicism is probably much higher, as reflected by the above discussion concerning risk to offspring of ostensible 47,XXY fathers. Most patients with Klinefelter syndrome who have active spermatogenesis and fertility without ICSI are probably 46,XY/47,XXY mosaics (Warburg, 1963; Court-Brown et al., 1964). 46,XY/47,XXY Mosaicism probably arises by a nondisjunction or anaphase lag in the zygote or embryo. It is usually assumed that such an error involved a 47,XXY embryo (Sanger et al., 1971), consistent with advanced maternal age (Hamerton, 1971).

Clinical expression is variable as predicted for mosaicism, ranging from a nearly normal male phenotype to a moderate form of Klinefelter syndrome. 46,XY/47,XXY Patients are predictably less likely than 47,XXY patients to have gynecomastia, azoospermia, small testes, or decreased facial or pubic hair (Paulsen et al., 1968). Large-scale studies on the frequency of somatic abnormalities, intelligence, and psychological status in 46,XY/47,XXY have not been performed.

Other forms of sex chromosomal mosaicism have been reported, but data are insufficient to determine whether specific phenotypical features are associated.

48,XXXY

In 48,XXXY the Klinefelter syndrome phenotype (Court-Brown et al., 1964; Vormittag and Weninger, 1972; Ferrier et al., 1974; Simpson et al., 1974) is comparable to 47,XXY with respect to gonadal development but characterized by much more pronounced somatic anomalies and mental retardation. A generalization is that IQ decreases 15 points for each additional X chromosome. The expressive language deficiency observed in 47,XXY is accentuated in 48,XXXY. Additional X chromosomes are usually derived from a single parent, typically the mother (Hassold et al., 1990). Errors in successive meiotic divisions are assumed. There is no obvious parental age effect, in apparent contrast to 47,XXY.

Somatic anomalies occur more often in 48,XXXY (Fig. 12–4) than in 47,XXY. 47,XXY, 48,XXXY, and 49,XXXXY Patients show the same general spectrum of somatic anomalies, but frequencies are greater in 49,XXXXY than in 48,XXXY, and in turn both are greater than in 47,XXY (Table 12–1). About half of 48,XXXY patients have somatic developmental anomaly, the most frequent ones being hypertelorism, prognathism, simple ear, short neck, epicanthal folds, radioulnar synostosis, clinodactyly V, and cardiac anomalies. The skeletal anomalies in 47,XXY (e.g., scoliosis, hyphosis, pectus excavatum, clinodactyly V) are observed more frequently in 48,XXXY and 49,XXXXY.

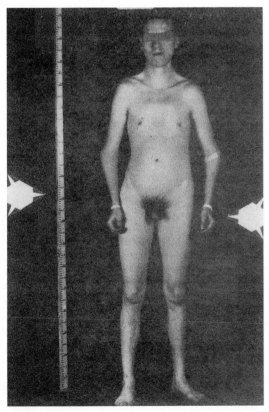

FIGURE 12–4 • Photograph of an 48,XXXY patient. Evident somatic anomalies are prominent zygoma, mandibular asymmetry, abnormal elbows, and pectus excavatum. (From Simpson JL, Morillo-Cucci G, Horwith M, et al.: Abnormalities of human sex chromosomes: VI. Monozygotic twins with the complement 48,XXXY. Humangenetik 21:301, 1974.)

49,XXXXY

XXXXY was first reported by Fraccaro and Lindsten (1960). The 49,XXXXY chromosomal complement may be explained by any of several mechanisms: (1) Successive nondisjunction at both the first and second meiotic division during spermatogenesis followed by syngamy of the resulting 25,XYY spermatozoon with a 23,X ovum. (2) Successive nondisjunction during maternal meiosis. (3) Nondisjunction during early cleavage with loss of nonmodal cell tines. (4) Nondisjunction at second meiotic division in both parents such that syngamy occurs between a 24,XX ovum and a 24,XY sperm. Usually all X's are derived from the same parent, pointing to successive meiotic errors followed by cleavage (mitotic) errors (Hassold et al., 1990). As in 48,XXXY, no obvious parental age effect exists.

Most cases have been ascertained in surveys of the mentally retarded; none were detected in prospective surveys of newborns. Nearly all reported patients are severely mentally retarded, IQ levels ranging from 20 to 60 (Terheggen et al., 1973). In contrast to the rarity of such features in 47,XXY, a small penis and cryptorchidism are often present in 49,XXXXY (Hamerton, 1971). 49,XXXXY Patients show seminiferous tubule dysgenesis, azoospermia, hypoplastic or absent Leydig cells, and androgen deficiency (Cunningham and Roigsdale, 1972). Somatic anomalies occur with increased frequency and severity compared with in 47,XXY patients (see Table 12–1).

48,XXYY and 49,XXXYY

48,XXYY was first reported by Muldal and Ockey (1960). Like 47,XXXY and 49,XXXXY, additional X chromosomes are derived from a single parent; no parental age effect exists. 48,XXYY subjects tend to be taller and more aggressive than those with 47,XXY Klinefelter syndrome (Borgaonkar et al., 1970; Barlow, 1973), but otherwise the phenotype is similar. Borgaonkar and colleagues (1970) found that 62% of 48,XXYY patients over 12 years old had gynecomastia, 18% a small penis, 12% cryptorchidism, and 74% elevated gonadotropin levels. Testicular histologic appearance was similar to that of 47,XXY.

Most 48,XXYY patients are mentally retarded, but the magnitude and frequency is uncertain. Because low intelligence is often the indication for cytogenetic evaluation, ascertainment bias surely exists. IQ is estimated to be 60

▼ **Table 12–1.** COMPARISON OF SOME CLINICAL FEATURES OF PATIENTS WITH 47,XXY, 48,XXXY,
• AND 49,XXXXY KLINEFELTER SYNDROME

Anomaly*	47,XXY†		48,XXXY‡		49,XXXXY§	
	Cases	N	Cases	N	Cases	N
Mental retardation	6	141•	29	29	28	28
Small testes	143	143	26	36	28	28
Hypoplastic penis	11	44¶	11	24	24	28
Gynecomastia	26	44¶	9	24	5	10#
Wide-set eyes	0	143	2	25	20	23
Epicanthal folds	1	143	6	25	16	19
Upturned nose	0	143	0	25	5	23
Low-set ears	0	143	1	25	2	21
Malformed ears	0	143	1	25	11	21
Strabismus	0	143	2	25	11	21
Prognathism	0	143	2	25	8	16
Webbed neck	0	143	2	25	4	19
Short neck	0	143	0	25	14	14
Kyphosis	1	143	3	25	9	13
Scoliosis	0	143	2	25	4	9**
Radioulnar synostosis	0	143	3	25	8	19
Abnormal ulnar or radius	0	143	0	25	4	19
Clinodactyly V	2	143	7	25	23	26
Coxa valga	0	143	1	25	12	14
Genu valgum	0	143	0	25	6	24
Pes planus	0	143	1	25	10	24
Malformed toes	0	143	0	25	5	24
Pes cavus	2	143	0	25	0	24
Wide gap, first and second toes	0	143	0	25	2	26
Talipes equinovarus	0	143	0	25	2	26

* An anomaly is listed if, in the data surveyed, it was found in any two persons with the same chromosomal complement. A number of minor radiographic anomalies detected in 49,XXXXY patients are not listed.
†Tabulated from patients of Court-Brown WM, et al. (1964) except as noted
‡Tabulated from the study by Simpson JL, et al. (1974)
§Tabulated from Zaleski WA, et al. (1966)
• Ascertained in surveys of the mentally retarded
¶Estimate of Froland A (1969)
#Estimate of Ferguson-Smith MA (1966)
**Estimate based on radiographic studies tabulated by Zaleski WA, et al. (1966)
N = total sample
From Simpson JL, Morillo-Cucci G, Horwith M, et al.: Abnormalities of human sex chromosomes: VI monozygotic twins with the complement 48,XXXY. Humangenetik 21:301, 1974.

to 80. Expressive language difficulties occur, but performance IQ is also low. Behavioral disturbances are more pronounced than in 47,XXY and perhaps have an anatomic basis. Electroencephalograms may be abnormal, and epilepsy is not uncommon (Borgaonkar et al., 1970; Hornstein et al., 1974). Few patients are socially well adjusted, and inappropriate aggression is common. Again, these findings may reflect ascertainment bias given the many cases ascertained in institutions for juvenile delinquents. As noted above, the incarceration could be the end point of frustration as a result of poor expressive skills.

Somatic anomalies reflect those with 47,XXY. Noteworthy are tall stature, long legs, and eunuchoid proportions. Peripheral vascular disease is frequent. The rare 49,XXXYY patients (Bray and Hosephine, 1963; Lecluse-van der Bilt et al., 1974) show mental retardation, delayed bone age, mandibular prognathism, and particularly small testes.

Polysomy X in Females

Females with 47,XXX females are relatively common, occurring 1 per 1000 (0.1%) liveborn females. The cytologic origin is usually maternal meiosis I. Paternal origin explains only about 5% of cases (MacDonald et al., 1994). Most 47,XXX individuals are normal in phenotype. However, as a group 47,XXY women are more likely to be mentally retarded or mentally ill than 46,XX women. The magnitude of the increased risk is difficult to estimate, for surprisingly few data exist. Limited prospective studies of 47,XXX patients ascertained at birth indicate an IQ 16 points below those of sibs (Robinson et al., 1979a). Perhaps one third show some mental or behavioral problems, but these are often minor. For counseling purposes, a minimum estimate might be that 5% of 47,XXX females are overtly retarded, having IQs between 45 and 70. Somatic anomalies are usually not present in 47,XXX patients. Occasionally, 47,XXX females have craniofacial anomalies reminiscent of those more consistently detected in 48,XXXX and 49,XXXXX patients (see below).

47,XXX Females have been reported to experience delayed menarche or premature ovarian failure. The basis for ovarian dysfunction is unknown, but if true it is probably related to the uneven number of X chromosomes (i.e., three) that interferes with meiotic segregation and only leads secondarily to cessation of oogenesis. (The same cytologic mechanism has been invoked to explain germ cell failure in 45,X and in 47,XXY.) A nonspecific deleterious effect of an uneven number of X's has also been invoked to explain germ cell failure in trisomy 13 and trisomy 18. Coincidental association of two common traits (47,XXX and ovarian failure) is the other possibility.

Most offspring of 47,XXX women have been chromosomally normal, despite theoretical expectations that 50% would be chromosomally abnormal. Analogous to comments made earlier in this chapter concerning whether meiosis can actually be completed in an XXY germ cell, whether an XXX oocyte can complete meiosis successfully is unclear. However, chromosomally abnormal offspring of 47,XXX or 45,X/47,XXX women have been reported (Dewhurst, 1978; Simpson, 1981). Thus, antenatal diagnosis should be offered the rare pregnant patient with a 47,XXX fetus who is ascertained antepartum.

48,XXXX

Almost all reported 48,XXXX females have been subnormal in intelligence. Some have shown esotropia, electroencephalographic abnormalities, or facies reminiscent of Down syndrome. Others have no somatic anomalies but manifest ovarian dysfunction. At least one affected female has had a normal child (Bialer et al., 1988).

49,XXXXX

The relatively few reported 49,XXXXX females invariably show mental retardation. Frequency of somatic anomalies is much higher than in 47,XXX and possibly also higher than in 48,XXXX. Anomalies most commonly present include hypertelorism, slanting palpebral fissures, a broad nasal bridge, exerted lips, esotropia, small hands and feet, abnormal teeth, clinodactyly of the fifth finger, and a short neck.

Polysomy Y in Males

Approximately 1 per 1000 (0.1%) liveborn males has a 47,XYY complement. The cytologic origin is paternal meiosis II. This complement has long been said to be associated with tall stature, mental retardation, and antisocial behavior. Early studies (Jacobs et al., 1965; Price et al., 1966) almost certainly overestimated the risk of aberrant behavior. Once this was recognized, it became fashionable in some circles to state that no increased risk exists. In reality, 47,XYY confers increased risk but not to the extent once believed.

Initial studies (Price et al., 1966; Price and Whatmore, 1967) involved inmates at a Scottish maximum security prison. The frequency of 47,XYY proved greater than expected in the general population. 47,XYY Inmates were first convicted at a younger age than 46,XY inmates, less often had a sib who had received a conviction, and more often committed crimes against property than crimes against persons. These observations suggested that 47,XYY inmates are incarcerated for reasons different from those of other inmates. The relatively few prospectively ascertained 47,XYY children have usually proved normal, although sometimes with behavioral difficulties. A useful estimate for counseling is that the likelihood of a 47,XYY male's becoming incarcerated is perhaps 1% compared with 0.1% for 46,XY males.

47,XYY Men usually have normal sized testes and normal external genitalia. Spermatogenic arrest is evident in approximately half the cases; histologically tubules may consist solely of Sertoli cells (Shakkebaek et al., 1973). Mean plasma testosterone levels are normal. Offspring of 47,XYY males are almost always chromosomally normal in contrast to theoretical predictions that half would be 47,XXY or 47,XYY. The likely explanation is that 24,XY hyperhaploid sperm are uncommon compared to 23,X or 23,Y. The principle of far fewer than expected aneuploid offspring in 47,XYY patients is consistent with observations in 47,XXY and 47,XXX. Nonetheless, it is prudent to offer antenatal diagnosis if a father is 47,XYY.

All reported 48,XYYY males have shown multiple somatic anomalies, as have the even rarer 49,XXYYY males. These complements presumably arise by nondisjunction in paternal meiosis, with nondisjunction in the zygote or embryo also occurring in certain cases.

46,XX and 47,XXX Sex-reversed Males

46,XX (Sex-reversed) males are phenotypical males with bilateral testes (de la Chapelle, 1972, 1981). This phenotype was alluded to in Chapter 10, where the cytologic basis was noted to usually (80%) involve Xp-Yp interchange during paternal meiosis, placing the *SRY* locus on the paternal X. This "experiment of nature" helped identify *SRY* as the Y-testis-determining factor (see Table 10–1). As also discussed in Chapter 10, several different X-Y interchanges exist, reflecting the several distinct regions of X-Y homology. The largest area of homology is the well-known pseudoautosomal region (PAR) shared between distal Xp and Yp. There also exists a smaller Xq/Yp homologous region and a similarly small Xp/Yq homology. Most XX males with normal external genitalia result from Xp/Yp interchange (McElreavey and Cortes, 2001). However, at least one XX true hermaphrodite (ambiguous external genitalia) has resulted from Yp/Xq interchange, the less severe phenotype possibly reflecting juxtaposition of *SRY* near the X-inactivation center (Margarit et al., 2000). Xp/Yq interchange may lead to duplication of Xp and, hence, dosage-dependent sex reversal in XY females (McElreavey and Cortes, 2001) (see Chapter 10).

Four 47,XXX males have been reported. The etiology is presumed to be X-Y interchange followed by maternal meiotic nondisjunction (Bigozzi et al., 1980; Annerén et al., 1987; Scherer et al., 1989; Ogata et al., 2001).

PHENOTYPE

Small testes and androgen deficiency are common in XX males, resembling those with 47,XXY Klinefelter syndrome. Facial and body hair are decreased and pubic hair may be distributed in the pattern characteristic of females. About one third have gynecomastia. Penis and scrotum may be small but traditionally are considered to be well differentiated (de la Chapelle, 1972, 1981). Wolffian derivatives are normal. Seminiferous tubules are decreased in number and size. Peritubular and interstitial fibrosis is present, Leydig cells are hyperplastic, and spermatogonia is usually detectable.

Virilization varies markedly among 46,XX males, more so than in 47,XXY. Some are well virilized and essentially indistinguishable from normal males except for their sterility. In other 46,XX males, genital ambiguity exists. The latter individuals probably reflect a different etiologic basis than XX males without genital ambiguity.

Multiple families are reported in which 46,XX males with genital ambiguity and 46,XX true hermaphroditism have been observed (see Chapter 10). XX Males with genital ambiguity are relatively more common among North Africans (from Morocco, Tunisia, Algeria).

ETIOLOGY

In the approximately 80% of XX males in whom *SRY* is detectable, the etiology is presumed to involve unequal crossing-over during paternal meiosis between homologous regions Xp and Yp. If this interchange occurs distal to *SRY*, *SRY* would become translocated from the potential Y to the paternal X. The varying length of aberrant X-Y interchanges in 46,XX males allowed a nested hierarchal approach to localize the testes determining region on the Y chromosome to a small region of the short curve (Yp) (Vergnaud et al., 1986; Page et al., 1987). Table 10–1 shows the strategy employed.

In the remaining 20% of 46,XX cases, other mechanisms must be postulated. These include mosaicism (46,XX/46,XY) or a mutant autosomal gene (de la Chapelle, 1988). Support for the latter includes familial aggregates of 46,XX males (de la Chapelle et al., 1975) (see Chapter 10) and familial aggregates in which both 46,XX males and 46,XX true hermaphrodites have been reported in single kindreds (Berger et al., 1970; Kasdan et al., 1973; Skordis et al., 1987). The relationship between gene(s) responsible for the above and other autosomal genes believed to perturb testicular development is unclear (see Chapter 10). The most attractive autosomal candidate region to date is that on chromosome 17 near *SOX9*. Duplication (gain of function mutation) in this region has produced an XX true hermaphrodite (Huang et al., 1999), complementary to the observation that deletions in XY individuals produce sex reversal. In the mouse, in Chapter 10 we noted the consequence of deletion of a 150 kb region near *SOX9* affected. XX Mice developed testes despite lacking *SRY* (Bishop et al., 2000). An XX transgenic mouse ectopically expressing *SOX9* also developed testes (Vidal et al., 2001).

PERSISTENT MÜLLERIAN DERIVATIVES (PMDS) IN MALES

The uterus and fallopian tubes (müllerian derivatives) may persist in ostensibly normal (46,XY) males. External genitalia, wolffian (mesonephric) derivatives, and testes develop as expected; pubertal virilization occurs. Infertility is common, and in about 5% of cases seminomas or other germ cell tumors arise. The disorder is sometimes ascertained because the uterus and fallopian tubes are found in inguinal hernias; thus, the appellation hernia uteri inguinale has been applied.

Testes initially differentiate normally, but this may not continue. One problem is that one or more testes may remain intra-abdominal or inguinal (Guerrier et al., 1989). The two sides may differ with respect to whether a testes is or is not present in the scrotum. Testes are abnormally mobile as result of not being anchored to the processus vaginalis (Hutson et al., 1994). This role is usually played by the male gubernaculum, but in PMDs it must be served by elongated thin ligaments. Increased mobility could predispose to testicular torsion and secondarily lead to testicular degeneration, which is frequent in PMDs (Imbeaud et al., 1995). Testicular tumors occur (Snow et al., 1985; Nishioka et al., 1992), presumably reflecting intra-abdominal location. Testes may also not be properly connected to male excretory ducts, as a result of aplasia of the epididymis and upper vas deferens (Imbeaud et al., 1996). This occurs in perhaps 10% of cases (Farag, 1993) and is reflected by the short free segment of spermatic cord. This problem further contributes to infertility.

Two genes are integral to pathogenesis of PMDs. One codes for antimüllerian hormone (AMH) (also called müllerian inhibitory substance or MIS). The other codes for the AMH receptor (AMHR).

ANTIMÜLLERIAN HORMONE (AMH) MUTATIONS

The AMH gene is located on 19p. Consisting of five exons, AMH is 3079 bp long (Fig. 12–5). AMH can be measured by enzyme-linked immunosorbent assay, but the assay is informative only before sexual maturation because thereafter AMH production is suppressed. When AMH is not detectable, a mutation in the structural gene can usually be demonstrated. Belville and coworkers (1999) recommend single-stranded conformational polymorphism (SSCP) screening to detect AMH mutations, given the small size of the gene and its high guanine-cytosine (GC) rich content; sequencing can be performed if SSCP reveals an abnormality. Direct sequencing is recommended only for exon 1.

Initially, Imbeaud and colleagues (1994) failed to find the same AMH mutation in more than one of their 19 PMDs families (molecular heterogeneity). However, this group's later compilation reported a few recurrent mutations. Twenty-eight different mutations were found in 31 families (Belville et al., 1999). In 52%, the mutation was homozygous. PMDs caused by an AMH mutation are relatively more likely (44%) to be found in cases of North African (Arab) or Mediterranean

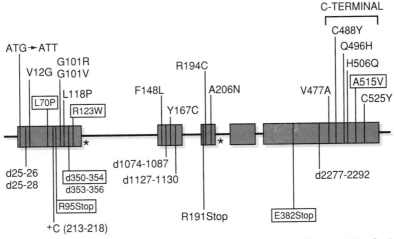

FIGURE 12–5 • AMH gene with location of known mutations causing PMDs. (From Belville C, Josso N, Picard JY: Persistence of müllerian derivatives in males. Am J Med Genet 89:218, 1999.)

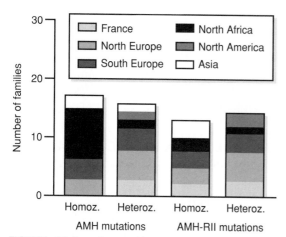

FIGURE 12–6 • Geographic origin of reported *AMH* and *AMHR II* mutations causing PMDs, stratified by homozygous (homoz.) or heterozygous (heteroz.) status. (From Belville C, Josso N, Picard JY: Persistence of müllerian derivatives in males. Am J Med Genet 89:218, 1999.)

origin (Fig. 12–6). This has especially proved true when the mutation was homozygous, presumably reflecting parental consanguinity.

AMH RECEPTOR MUTATIONS

The *AMH* receptor (*AMHR II*) gene is located on 12q13 and consists of 11 exons (Fig. 12–7). Most mutations are missense and occur throughout the gene except for exon 4. Mutations in exon 1 or in the 3' portion of exon 5 are most common. Imbeaud and colleagues (1996) were the first to report a mutation in the *AMHR*, initially finding only one case among 21 AMH-positive cases. Their latest update recorded 23 different *AMHR II* mutations in 27 families. Most were missense and half were compound heterozygotes (Fig. 12–7). Compared to *AMH*-negative cases, *AMH*-positive cases were relatively less likely to be derived from North

African Arab than from European populations (see Fig. 12–6).

First described by Imbeaud and coworkers (1996), the most frequent perturbation is deletion of 27 base pairs in exon 10. When present, the deletion exists in homozygous form in 42% of cases and is coupled with a missense mutation in the remaining 58% (Belville et al., 1999). If *AMH* is elevated, an *AMHR* mutation should be suspected. Belville and coworkers (1999) recommend polymerase chain reaction to detect the 27 bp mutation, followed by sequencing the entire *AMHR* gene if the deletion is not present in homozygous form.

That females with *AMHR* mutations undergo puberty normally (Belville et al., 1999) is a mild surprise because transgenic XX mice that express *AMH* show gonadal abnormalities (Behringer et al., 1990). Granulosa cells also normally produce *AMH* (Lee et al., 1996; Rey et al., 1996). For this reason a role for *AMH* in gonadal development probably exists.

An informative animal model exists. *AMH* receptor mutation occurs in miniature Schnauzer dogs (Meyers-Wallen et al., 1993).

OTHER PMDS CASES

In 20% of PMDs cases, mutations of neither *AMH* nor *AMHR II* are found (Belville et al., 1999). Etiology could involve the promoter region, translational process, or other molecular mechanisms.

One puzzling family exists in which maternal half-siblings were affected (Sloan and Walsh, 1976). Ordinarily this would suggest X-linked inheritance, but genes for both *AMH* and *AMHR* are encoded by autosomes. Further genetic hetereogeneity could exist, or the multiple individuals in the family could have been affected only coincidentally.

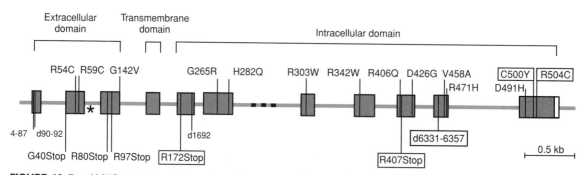

FIGURE 12–7 • *AMHR 11* gene, with location of known mutations causing PMDs: (From Belville C, Josso N, Picard JY: Persistence of müllerian derivatives in males. Am J Med Genet 89:218, 1999.)

URIOSTE SYNDROME AND PMD

Persistence of müllerian derivatives exists as part of a rare multiple malformation syndrome. Urioste et al. (1993) reported three unrelated males, and Bellini et al. (2001) reported two affected sibs. In addition to presence of uterus and fallopian tubes, somatic anomalies were present: dilated colon, intestinal and pulmonary lymphangiectasia, dysmorphic facial features (broad nasal bridge, bulbous nasal tip, long upper lip with smooth philtrum, high arched palate). Affected cases have manifested remarkable similar neonatal courses leading to early death within the first few months of life.

Wolffian Aplasia and Congenital Absence of the Vas Deferens (CAVD)

Wolffian ducts differentiate into vasa deferentia, epididymides, and seminal vesicles. Absence of wolffian derivates (wolffian aplasia) may be an isolated defect or may be associated with absence of the upper urinary tract. Absence of both wolffian duct derivatives and the upper urinary tract implies total failure of mesonephric development. By contrast, absence of wolffian derivatives without upper urinary tract anomalies implies resorption of wolffian elements after the wolffian duct reached the cloaca. Irrespective of whether absence of wolffian derivates is or is not accompanied by abnormalities of the upper urinary tract, gonads are only rarely involved. The upper urinary tract is usually normal in individuals who lack an epididymis, vas deferens, or seminal vesicle. If wolffian aplasia is bilateral, affected individuals are, of course, infertile. If the defect is unilateral, patients are usually asymptomatic.

Cystic fibrosis results from a mutation in the cystic fibrosis transmembrane regulation (CFTR), a gene on chromosome 7 that functions as a chloride channel. See Chapter 4 for a detailed discussion. Almost all cystic fibrosis homozygotes are infertile, usually because of congenital absence of the vas deferens (CAVD). Conversely, a relationship exists between CFTR mutations and CAVD in men with no pulmonary or pancreatic symptoms. Up to 70% of males with CAVD have cystic fibrosis, usually in the form of compound heterozygosity. In fact, two mutant CFTR alleles should be assumed in CAVD, even if only one can be detected molecularly. The most common mutations are ΔF508 and R117H.

A potentially deleterious polymorphism also exists involving five thymidines (5T) in intron 8 (Chillon et al., 1995). Presence of the five thymidines (5T) results in low (10%) transcription of CFTR protein as a result of improper exon-intron splicing and loss of exon 9. This truncated CFTR protein is poorly equipped to fulfill its function as a chloride channel, possessing only about 10% activity from the chromosome cis to the mutation (polymorphism). This is still more than the near zero for ΔF508, explaining why even homozygous 5T/5T men do not manifest lung or pancreatic abnormalities. The presence of seven thymidines has less deleterious effect, and the presence of nine thymidines has almost no effect. Many CBAVD individuals show ΔF508/5T, or homozygous 5T/5T. This assumes that there are no other cis CFTR perturbations. If so, a mild CFTR mutation like R117H can lose its low residual activity and result in the phenotype associated with ΔF508 (no CFTR activity).

Older reports describing affected sibs having CAVD suggested polygenic/multifactorial etiology (Schellen and Straaten, 1980; Budde et al., 1984; Czeizel, 1985). It seems more likely that mutations in the CFTR locus explain familial aggregates of CAVD. However, if upper tract anomalies coexist, this statement would not apply because unilateral renal agenesis with CAVD appears to be distinct from cystic fibrosis with CAVD (McCallum et al., 2001). This form constitutes about 10% of CBAVD cases. The etiology of renal aplasia/CAVD seems to be polygenic/multifactorial because recurrence risk for first-degree relatives is about 5%. Of 17 patients requiring ICSI, McCallum and associates (2001) achieved 10 conceptions in 26 cycles. In one pregnancy a male fetus had bilateral renal agenesis.

Failure of Fusion of Epididymis and Testes

Another relatively common urologic defect is failure of the testicular rete cords of the testis to fuse with the mesonephric tubules destined to form the ductule efferentia. As result, spermatozoa cannot egress. If the defect is bilateral, infertility results. One or both testes may also fail to descend.

Fusion defects of this type occur in about 1% of cryptorchid and in about 1% of azoospermic men. Familial aggregates have been reported. Fertility is now achievable by aspirating sperm from the testes of the epididymis and using assisted reproductive technologies such as ICSI.

REFERENCES

Annerén G, Andersson M, Page DC, et al.: An XXX male resulting from paternal X-Y interchange and maternal X-X nondisjunction. Am J Hum Genet 41:594, 1987.

Aran B, Blanco J, Vidal F, et al.: Screening for abnormalities of chromosomes X,Y, and 18 and for diploidy in spermatozoa from infertile men participating in an in vitro fertilization-intracytoplasmic sperm injection program. Fertil Steril 72:696, 1999.

Arens R, Marcus D, Engelberg S, et al.: Cerebral germinomas and Klinefelter syndrome. Cancer 61:1228, 1988.

Armstrong RD, Macfarlane DG, Panavi GS: Ankylosing spondylitis and Klinefelter's syndrome: Does the X-chromosome modify disease expression? Br J Rheumatol 24:277, 1985.

Barlow PW: X-chromosome and human development. Dev Med Child Neurol 15:205, 1973.

Becher R: Klinefelter syndrome and malignant lymphoma. Cancer Genet Cytogenet 1:271, 1986.

Becker KL, Hoffman DL, Underdahl LO, et al.: Klinefelter's syndrome: Clinical and laboratory findings in 50 patients. Arch Intern Med 118:314, 1966.

Becker KL: Clinical and therapeutic experiences with Klinefelter's syndrome. Fertil Steril 23:568, 1972.

Behringer RR, Cate RL, Froelick GJ, et al.: Abnormal sexual development in transgenetic mice chronically expressing müllerian inhibiting substance. Nature 345:167, 1990.

Bellini C, Bonioli E, Josso N, et al.: Persistence of Mullerian derivatives and intestinal lymphangiectasis in two newborn brothers. Am J Med Genet 104:74, 2001.

Belville C, Josso N, Picard JY: Persistence of müllerian derivatives in males. Am J Med Genet 89:218, 1999.

Bender BG, Harmon RJ, Linden MG: Psychosocial adaptation of 39 adolescents with sex chromosome abnormalities. Pediatrics 96:302, 1995.

Bender BG, Linden MG, Harmon RJ, et al.: Life adaptation in 35 adults with sex chromosome abnormalities. Genet Med 3:187, 2001.

Bender BG, Puck MH, Salbenblatt JA, et al.: Dyslexia in 47,XXY boys identified at birth. Behav Genet 16:343, 1986.

Berger R, Abonyi D, Nodot A: True hermaphroditism and "XX boy" in a sibship. Rev Eur Etud Clin Biol 15:330, 1970.

Bialer MG, Hogge WA, Atkin JF: A fertile woman with tetrasomy X and chromosomally normal offspring. Am J Hum Genet 43:A39, 1988.

Bigozzi U, Simoni G, Montali E, et al.: 47,XXX Chromosome constitution in a male. J Med Genet 17:62, 1980.

Bischoff FZ, Nguyen DD, Burt KJ, et al.: Estimates of aneuploidy using multicolor fluorescence in situ hybridization on human sperm. Cytogenet Cell Genet 66:237, 1994.

Bishop CE, Whitworth DJ, Qin Y, et al.: A transgenic insertion upstream of SOX9 is associated with dominant XX sex reversal in the mouse. Nat Genet 26:490, 2000.

Bizzarro A, Valentini G, Di Martino G, et al.: Influence of testosterone therapy on clinical immunological features of autoimmune diseases associated with Klinefelter's syndrome. J Clin Endocrinol Metab 64:32, 1987.

Borgaonkar DS, Mules E, Char F: Does the 48,XXYY male have a characteristic phenotype? Clin Genet 1:272, 1970.

Bradbury JT, Bunge RG, Boccabella RA: Chromatin test in Klinefelter's syndrome. J Clin Endocrinol Metab 16:689, 1956.

Bray P, Hosephine A: An XXXYY-sex chromosome anomaly. JAMA 184:179, 1963.

Bronson SK, Smithies O, Mascarello JT: High incidence of XXY and XYY males among the offspring of female chimeras from embryonic stem cells. Proc Natl Acad Sci USA 92:3120, 1995.

Budde WJ, Verjaal M, Hamerlynck JV, et al.: Familial occurrence of azoospermia and extreme oligozoospermia. Clin Genet 26:555, 1984.

Caldwell P, Smith DW: The XXY (Klinefelter's) syndrome in childhood: Detection and treatment. J Pediatr 80:250, 1972.

Carothers AD, Filippi G: Klinefelter's syndrome in Sardinia and Scotland. Comparative studies of parental age and other aetiological factors in 47,XXY. Hum Genet 81:71, 1988.

Carr DH, Barr ML, Plunkett ER, et al.: An XXXY sex chromosome complex in Klinefelter subjects with duplicated sex chromatin. J Clin Endocrinol 21:491, 1961.

Carroll PR, Morse MJ, Koduru PP, et al.: Testicular germ cell tumor in patient with Klinefelter syndrome. Urology 31:72, 1988.

Casey MD, Segall LJ, Street DR, et al.: Sex chromosome abnormalities in two state hospitals for patients requiring special security. Nature 209:641, 1966.

Chillon M, Casals T, Mercier B, et al.: Mutations in the cystic fibrosis gene in patients with congenital absence of the vas deferens. N Engl J Med 332:1475, 1995.

Court-Brown WM, Harnden DG, Jacobs PA, et al.: Abnormalities of the Sex Chromosome Complement in Man. Med Res Counc No. 305. London, Her Majesty's Stationery Office, 1964.

Cuenca CR, Becker KL: Klinefelter's syndrome and cancer of the breast. Arch Intern Med 121:159, 1968.

Cunningham MD, Ragsdale JL: Genital anomalies of an XXXXY male subject. J Urol 107:872, 1972.

Czeizel A: Congenital aplasia of the vasa deferentia of autosomal recessive inheritance in two unrelated sib-pairs. Hum Genet 70:288, 1985.

Damani MN, Mittal R, Oates RD: Testicular tissue extraction in a young male with 47,XXY Klinefelter's syndrome: potential strategy for preservation of fertility. Fertil Steril 76:1054, 2001.

Davis TE, Canfield CJ, Herman RH, et al.: Thyroid function in patients with aspermiogenesis and testicular tubal sclerosis. N Engl J Med 268:178, 1963.

de la Chapelle A, Koo GC, Wachtel SS: Recessive sex-determining genes in human XX male syndrome. Cell 15:837, 1975.

de la Chapelle A: Analytical review: Nature and origin of males with XX sex chromosomes. Am J Hum Genet 24:71, 1972.

de la Chapelle A: The complicated issue of human sex differentiation. Am J Hum Genet 43:1, 1988.

de la Chapelle A: The etiology of maleness in XX men. Hum Genet 58:105, 1981.

Dewhurst J: Fertility in 47,XXX and 45,X patients. J Med Genet 15:132, 1978.

Dexeus FH, Logothetis CJ, Chong C, et al.: Genetic abnormalities in men with germ cell tumors. J Urol 140:80, 1988.

Downham TF, Mitek FV: Chronic leg ulcers and Klinefelter's syndrome. Cutis 38:110, 1986.

Egozcue S, Blanco J, Vendrell JM, et al.: Human male infertility: Chromosome anomalies, meiotic disorders, abnormal spermatozoa and recurrent abortion. Hum Reprod Update 6:93, 2000.

Engelberth D, Charuat J, Jeykova H: Autoantibodies in chromatin-positive men. Lancet 2:1194, 1965.

Farag TI: Familial persistent müllerian duct syndrome in Kuwait and neighboring populations. Am J Med Genet 47:432, 1993.

Federman DD: Abnormal Sexual Development. Philadelphia: WB Saunders, 1967.

Ferguson-Smith MA: The prepubertal testicular lesion in chromatin-positive Klinefelter's syndrome (primary microorchidism) as seen in mentally handicapped children. Lancet 1:219, 1959.

Ferguson-Smith MA: Klinefelter's syndrome and mental deficiency. *In* More KL (ed): Sex Chromatin. Philadelphia: WB Saunders, 1966.

Ferguson-Smith MA: Testis and intersexuality. *In* Hubble D (ed): Pediatric Endocrinology. Oxford: Blackwell Scientific, 1969.

Ferguson-Smith MMA, Mack WS, Ellis PM, et al.: Parental age and the source of the X chromosomes in XXY Klinefelter syndrome. Lancet 1:46, 1964.

Ferrier PE, Ferrier SA, Pescia G: The XXXY Klinefelter syndrome in childhood. Am J Dis Child 127:104, 1974.

Fraccaro M, Lindsten J: A child with 49 chromosomes. Lancet 2:1303, 1960.

Froland A: Klinefelter's syndrome: Clinical, endocrinological, and cytogenetical studies. Dan Med Bull 16(suppl 6):1, 1969.

Fromatin M, Grutier D, Cuisinier JC, et al.: Resultats de l'androgene-therapie dans le syndrome de Klinefelter de l'adolescent. Ann Endocrinol (Paris) 35:305, 1974.

Gautier M, Nouaille J: Deux cas de syndrome de Klinefelter associe a une tetralogie de Fallot (etude systematique du corpuscule de Barr chez 210 mourrissons attiens de cardiopathies congenitales). Arch Fr Pediatr 21:761, 1964.

Graham JM, Bashir AS, Stark RE, et al.: Oral and written language abilities of XXY boys: Implications for anticipatory guidance. Pediatrics 81:795, 1988.

Guerrier D, Tran D, Vanderwinden JM, et al.: The persistent müllerian duct syndrome: A molecular approach. J Clin Endocrinol Metab 68:46, 1989.

Guttenbach M, Martinez-Expósito MJ, Michelmann HW, et al.: Incidence of diploid and disomic sperm nuclei in 45 infertile men. Hum Reprod 12:468, 1997b.

Guttenbach M, Michelmann HW, Hinney B, et al.: Segregation of sex chromosomes into sperm nuclei in a man with 47,XXY Klinefelter's karyotype: A FISH analysis. Hum Genet 99:474, 1997a.

Hambert G: Males with Positive Sex Chromatin. Gotenborg, Sweden: Akademiforlaget, 1966.

Hamerton JL: Human Cytogenetics, vol. 2 New York: Academic Press, 1971.

Harnden DG, MacLean N, Langlands AO: Carcinoma of the breast and Klinefelter's syndrome. J Med Genet 8:460, 1971.

Harvey J, Jacobs PA, Hassold T, et al.: The parental origin of 47,XXX males. Birth Defects Orig Artic Ser 26(4):289, 1990.

Hassold T, Arnovitz K, Jacobs PA, et al.: The parental origin of the missing or additional chromosome in 45,X and 47,XXX females. Birth Defects Orig Artic Ser 26(4):297, 1990.

Hassold TJ, Sherman SL, Pettay D, et al.: XY chromosome nondisjunction in man is associated with diminished recombination in the pseudoautosomal region. Am J Hum Genet 49:253, 1991.

Hoaken PCS, Clarke M, Breslin M: Psychopathology in Klinefelter's syndrome. Psychosom Med 26:207, 1964.

Hornstein OP, Rott HD, Schwanitz G, et al.: The variant of Klinefelter's syndrome. Dtsch Med Wochenschr 99:248, 1974.

Horsman DE, Pantzar JT, Dill FJ, et al.: Klinefelter's syndrome and acute leukemia. Cancer Genet Cytogenet 26:375, 1987.

Huang WJ, Lamb DJ, Kim ED, et al.: Germ-cell nondisjunction in testes biopsies of men with idiopathic infertility. Am J Hum Genet 64:1638, 1999.

Hutson JM, Davidson PM, Reece L, et al.: Failure of gubernacular development in the persistent müllerian duct syndrome allows herniation of the testes. Pediatr Surg Int 9:544, 1994.

Iitsuka Y, Bock A, Nguyen DD, et al.: Evidence of skewed X-chromosome inactivation in 47,XXY and 48,XXYY Klinefelter patients. Am J Med Genet 98:25, 2001.

Imbeaud S, Belville C, Messika-Zeitoun L, et al.: A 27 base-pair deletion of the anti-müllerian type II receptor gene is the most common cause of the persistent müllerian duct syndrome. Hum Mol Genet 5:1269, 1996.

Imbeaud S, Carre-Eusebe D, Rey R, et al.: Molecular genetics of the persistent müllerian duct syndrome: A study of 19 families. Hum Mol Genet 3:125, 1994.

Imbeaud S, Rey R, Berta P, et al.: Testicular degeneration in three patients with the persistent müllerian duct syndrome. Eur J Pediatr 154:187, 1995.

Jacobs PA, Brunton M, Melville MM, et al.: Aggressive behavior, mental subnormality and XYY male. Nature 208:1351, 1965.

Jacobs PA, Hassold TJ, Whittington E, et al.: Klinefelter's syndrome: An analysis of the origin of the additional sex chromosome using molecular probes. Ann Hum Genet 52:93, 1988.

Jacobs PA, Price WHH, Court-Brown WM, et al.: Chromosome studies on men in a maximum security hospital. Ann Hum Genet 31:339, 1968.

Jacobs PA, Strong JA: A case of human intersexuality having a possible XYY sex-determining mechanism. Nature 183:302, 1959.

Kasdan R, Nankin HR, Troen P, et al.: Paternal transmission of maleness in XX human beings. N Engl J Med 288:539, 1973.

Klinefelter HF Jr, Reifenstein EC Jr, Albright F: Syndrome characterized by gynecomastia, aspermatogenesis without a leydigism and increased excretion of follicle-stimulating hormone. J Clin Endocrinol 2:615, 1942.

Kobayashi S, Shimamoto T, Taniguchi O, et al.: Klinefelter's syndrome associated with progressive systemic sclerosis: Report of a case and review of the literature. Clin Rheumatol 10:84, 1991.

Lachman MF, Kim K, Koo BC: Mediastinal teratoma associated with Klinefelter's syndrome. Arch Pathol Lab Med 110:1067, 1986.

Laron Z, Hochman IH: Small testes in prepubetal boys with Klinefelter's syndrome. J Clin Endocrinol Metab 32:671, 1971.

Lecluse-van der Bilt FA, Hagemeijer A, Smit EM, et al.: An infant with an XXXYY karyotype. Clin Genet 5:263, 1974.

Lee MM, Donahoe PK, Hasegawa T, et al.: Müllerian inhibiting substance in humans: Normal levels from infancy to adulthood. J Clin Endocrinol Metab 81:571, 1996.

Lee MW, Stephens RL: Klinefelter's syndrome and extragonadal germ cell tumors. Cancer 60:1053, 1987.

Leonard JM, Bremner WJ, Capell PT, et al.: Male hypogonadism: Klinefelter and Reifenstein syndromes. Birth Defects Orig Artic Ser 11(4):17, 1975.

Lorda-Sanchez I, Binkert F, Maechler M, et al.: Reduced recombination and paternal age effect in Klinefelter syndrome. Hum Genet 89:524, 1992.

MacDonald M, Hassold T, Harvey J, et al.: The origin of 47,XXY and 47,XXX aneuploidy: Heterogeneous mechanisms and role of aberrant recombination. Hum Mol Genet 3:1365, 1994.

MacLean N, Brown WM, Jacobs PA, et al.: A survey of sex chromatin abnormalities in mental hospitals. J Med Genet 5:165, 1968.

Margarit E, Coll MD, Oliva R, et al.: *SRY* gene transferred to the long arm of the X chromosome in a Y-positive XX true hermaphrodite. Am J Med Genet 90:25, 2000.

Matzuk MM: In search of binding—identification of inhibin receptors. Endocrinology 141:2281, 2000.

McCallum T, Milunsky J, Munarriz R, et al.: Unilateral renal agenesis associated with congenital bilateral absence of the vas deferens: Phenotypic findings and genetic considerations. Hum Reprod 16:282, 2001.

McElreavey K, Cortes LS: Translocations and sex differentiation. Semin Reprod Med 19:133, 2001.

Means AR, Fakunding JL, Huckins C, et al.: Follicle-stimulating hormone, the Sertoli cell, and spermatogenesis. Recent Prog Horm Res 32:477, 1976.

Meyers-Wallen VN, Lee MM, Manganaro TF, et al.: Müllerian inhibiting substance is present in embryonic testes of dogs with persistent müllerian duct syndrome. Biol Reprod 48:1410, 1993.

Mikamo K, Aguercif M, Hazeghi P, et al.: Chromatin-positive Klinefelter's syndrome. A quantitative analysis of spermatogonial deficiency at 3, 4, and 12 months of age. Fertil Steril 19:731, 1968.

Miller MH, Urowitz MB, Gladman DD, et al.: Systemic lupus erythematosus in males. Medicine 62:327, 1983.

Milne JS, Lauder IJ, Price WH: Anthropometry in sex chromosome abnormality. Clin Genet 5:96, 1974.

Money J, Annecillo C, Van Orman B, et al.: Cytogenetics, hormones and behavior disability: Comparison of XYY and XXY syndromes. Clin Genet 6:370, 1974.

Moosani N, Pattinson HA, Carter MD, et al.: Chromosomal analysis of sperm from men with idiopathic infertility using sperm karyotyping and fluorescence in situ hybridization. Fertil Steril 64:811, 1995.

Mroz K, Hassold TJ, Hunt PA: Meiotic aneuploidy in the XXY mouse: Evidence that a compromised testicular environment increases the incidence of meiotic errors. Hum Reprod 14:1151, 1999.

Muldal S, Ockey CH: The "double male." A new chromosome situation in Klinefelter's syndrome. Lancet 2:492, 1960.

Myhre SA, Ruvalcaba RH, Johnson HR, et al.: The effects of testosterone treatment in Klinefelter's syndrome. J Pediatr 76:267, 1970.

Netley CT: Summary overview of behavioral development in individuals with neonatally identified X and Y aneuploidy. Birth Defects Orig Artic Ser 22(3):293, 1986.

Nichols CR, Heerema NA, Palmer C, et al.: Klinefelter's syndrome associated with mediastinal germ cell neoplasma. J Clin Oncol 5:1290, 1987.

Nielsen J: Diabetes mellitus in patients with aneuploid chromosome aberrations and in their parents. Humangenetik 16:165, 1972.

Nielsen J, Johansen K, Yde H: Frequency of diabetes mellitus in patients with Klinefelter's syndrome of different chromosome constitutions and the XYY syndrome: Plasma insulin and growth hormone levels after a glucose load. J Clin Endocrinol 29:1062, 1969.

Nielsen J, Pelsen B, Sorensen K: Followup of 30 Klinefelter males treated with testosterone. Clin Genet 33:4, 1988.

Nielsen J: Klinefelter's syndrome and the XYY syndrome: A genetical, endocrinological and psychiatric-psychological study of thirty-three severely hypogonadal male patients and two patients with karyotype 47,XXY. Acta Psychiatr Scand 45(suppl):209, 1969.

Nishioka T, Kadowaki T, Miki T, et al.: Persistent müllerian duct syndrome. Hinyokika Kiyo 38:89, 1992.

Norris PG, Rivers JK, Machin S, et al.: Platelet hyperaggregability in a patient with Klinefelter's syndrome and leg ulcers. Br J Dermatol 117:107, 1987.

Ogata T, Matsuo M, Muroya K, et al.: 47,XXX male: A clinical and molecular study. Am J Med Genet 98:353, 2001.

Okada H, Fujioka H, Tatsumi N, et al.: Klinefelter's syndrome in the male infertility clinic. Hum Reprod 14:946, 1999.

Page DC, Mosher R, Simpson EM, et al.: The sex-determining region of the human Y chromosome encodes a finger protein. Cell 51:1091, 1987.

Palermo GD, Schlegel PN, Sills ES, et al.: Births after intracytoplasmic injection of sperm obtained by testicular extraction from men with nonmosaic Klinefelter's syndrome. N Engl J Med 338:588, 1998.

Patil SR, Lubs HA, Kimberling WJ, et al.: Chromosomal abnormalities ascertained in a collaborative survey of 4,342 seven and eight year old children: Frequency, phenotype and epidemiology. *In* Hook EB, Porter IH (eds): Population Cytogenetics. New York: Academic Press, 1977.

Patwardhan AJ, Brown WE, Bender BG, et al.: Reduced size of the amygdala in individuals with 47,XXY and 47,XXX karyotypes. Am J Med Genet 114:93, 2002.

Paulsen CA, Gordon DL, Carpenter RW, et al.: Klinefelter's syndrome and its variants: A hormonal and chromosomal study. Recent Prog Horm Res 24:321, 1968.

Peterson NT, Midgley AR Jr, Jaffe RB: Regulation of human gonadotropins: III. Luteinizing hormone and follicle stimulating hormone in sera from adult males. J Clin Endocrinol Metab 28:1473, 1968.

Plunkett ER, Barr ML: Testicular dysgenesis affecting the seminiferous tubules principally, with chromatin-positive nuclei. Lancet 2:853, 1956.

Price WH, Strong JA, Whatmore PB, et al.: Criminal patients with XYY sex-chromosome complement. Lancet 1:565, 1966.

Price WH, Whatmore PB: Behavior disorders and pattern of crime among XYY males identified at a maximum security hospital. Br Med J 1:533, 1967.

Raboch J, Mellan J, Starka L: Klinefelter syndrome: Sexual development and activity. Arch Sex Behav 8:333, 1979.

Ratcliffe SG, Paul N: Prospective studies on children with sex chromosome aneuploidy. Birth Defects Orig Artic Ser 22(3):1, 1986.

Rey R, Lhommé C, Marcillac I, et al.: Anti-müllerian hormone as a serum marker of granulosa-cell tumors of the ovary: Comparative study with serum alpha-inhibin and estradiol. Am J Obstet Gynecol 174:958, 1996.

Riis P, Johnsen SG, Mosbeck J: Nuclear sex in Klinefelter syndrome. Lancet 1:962, 1956.

Robach J, Sipova I: The mental level in 47 cases of true Klinefelter's syndrome. Acta Endocrinol (Cophen) 36:404, 1961.

Robinson A, Bender B, Linden MG: Summary of clinical findings in children and young adults with sex chromosome anomalies. *In* Evans JA, Hamerton JL (eds): Children and Young Adults with Sex Chromosome Aneuploidy. New York: Wiley-Liss, for the March of Dimes Birth Defect Foundation. Birth Defects Orig Artic Ser 26(4):225, 1991.

Robinson A, Goad WB, Puck TT, et al.: Studies on chromosomal nondisjunction in man: III. Am J Hum Genet 21:466, 1969.

Robinson A, Lubs HA, Bergsma D: Sex chromosome aneuploidy: Prospective studies in children. Birth Defects Orig Artic Ser 15(1):1, 1979a.

Robinson A, Lubs HA, Nielsen J, et al.: Summary of clinical findings: Profiles of children with 47,XXY, 47,XXX and 47,XYY karyotypes. Birth Defects Orig Artic Ser 15(1):261, 1979b.

Rohde RA: Klinefelter's syndrome with pulmonary disease and other disorders. Lancet 2:149, 1964.

Ron-El R, Strassburger D, Gelman-Kohan S, et al.: A 47,XXY fetus conceived after ICSI of spermatozoa from a patient with non-mosaic Klinefelter's syndrome: case report. Hum Reprod 15:1804, 2000.

Rosenthal A: Cardiovascular malformations in Klinefelter's syndrome: Report of three cases. J Pediatr 80:471, 1972.

Samango-Sprouse C, Suddaby EC: Developmental concerns in children with congenital heart disease. Curr Opin Cardiol 12:91, 1997.

Samango-Sprouse C: Mental development in polysomy X Klinefelter syndrome (47,XXY; 48,XXXY): effects of incomplete X inactivation. Semin Reproad Med 19:193, 2001.

Sanger R, Tippett P, Gavin J: Xg groups and sex abnormalities in people of Northern European ancestry. J Med Genet 8:417, 1971.

Schellen TM, van Straaten A: Autosomal recessive hereditary congenital aplasia of the vasa deferentia in four siblings. Fertil Steril 34:401, 1980.

Scherer G, Schempp W, Fraccaro M, et al.: Analysis of two 47,XXX males reveals X-Y interchange and maternal or paternal nondisjunction. Hum Genet 81:247, 1989.

Schlegelberger T, Kekow J, Gross WL: Impaired T-cell independent B-cell maturation in systemic lupus erythematosus coculture experiments in monozygotic twins concordant for Klinefelter's syndrome but discordant for systemic lupus erythematosus. Clin Immunol Immunopathol 40:365, 1986.

Shakkebaek NE, Zeuthen E, Nielsen J, et al.: Abnormal spermatogenesis in XYY males: A report on 4 cases ascertained through a population study. Fertil Steril 24:390, 1973.

Shi Q, Spriggs E, Field LL, et al.: Absence of age effect on meiotic recombination between human X and Y chromosomes. Am J Hum Genet 71:254, 2002.

Simpson JL, de la Cruz F, Swerdloff R, et al.: Klinefelter Syndrome: Expanding the phenotype and identifying new research directions. (in preparation), 2002.

Simpson JL, Lamb D: Genetic effects of ICSI. Semin Reprod Med 19:239, 2001.

Simpson JL, Morillo-Cucci G, Horwith M, et al.: Abnormalities of human sex chromosomes: VI. Monozygotic twins with the complement 48,XXXY. Humangenetik 21:301, 1974.

Simpson JL: Pregnancies in women with chromosomal abnormalities. In Schulman JD, Simpson JL (eds): Genetic Diseases in Pregnancy. New York: Academic Press, 1981.

Skordis NA, Stetka DG, MacGillivray MH, et al.: Familial 46,XX males coexisting with familial 46,XX true hermaphrodites in same pedigree. J Pediatr 110:244, 1987.

Skuse DH, James RS, Bishop DV, et al.: Evidence from Turner's syndrome of an imprinted X-linked locus affecting cognitive function. Nature 387:705, 1997.

Sloan WR, Walsh PC: Familial persistent müllerian ducts syndrome. J Urol 115:459, 1976.

Snow BW, Rowland RG, Seal GM, et al.: Testicular tumor in patient with persistent müllerian duct syndrome. Urology 26:495, 1985.

Sorenson K: Klinefelter's Syndrome in Childhood, Adolescence and Youth. Carnforth: Parthenon, 1988.

Sorio C, Baron A, Orlandini S, et al.: The FHIT gene is expressed in pancreatic ductular cells and is altered in pancreatic cancers. Cancer Res 59:1308, 1999.

Staessen C: Fertility and assisted reproduction in XXY—ICSI and ART. In Simpson JL, et al.: Klinefelter Syndrome Conference Expanding the Phenotype and Identifying New Research Directions (in preparation, 2002).

Stewart DA, Netley CT, Bailey JD, et al.: Growth and development of children with X and Y chromosome aneuploidy: A prospective study. Birth Defects Orig Artic Ser 15(1):75, 1979.

Stewart JSS, Ferguson-Smith MA, Lenoz B, et al.: Klinefelter's syndrome: Genetic studies. Lancet 2:117, 1958.

Stewart JSS: Medullary gonadal dysgenesis (chromatin-positive Klinefelter's syndrome). Lancet 1:1176, 1959.

Terheggen HG, Pfeiffer RA, Haug H, et al.: The XXXXY syndrome. Report of 7 new cases and review of the literature. Z Kinderheilkd 115:209, 1973.

Thomas NS, Collins AR, Hassold TJ, et al.: A reinvestigation of non-disjunction resulting in 47,XXY males of paternal origin. Eur J Hum Genet 8:805, 2000.

Tojo K, Kaguchi Y, Tokudome G, et al.: 47 XXY/46 XY Mosaic Klinefelter's syndrome presenting with multiple endocrine abnormalities. Intern Med 35:396, 1998.

Urioste M, Rodriguez JI, Barcia JM, et al.: Persistence of Mullerian derivatives, lymphangiectasis, hepatic failure, postaxial polydactyly, renal and craniofacial anomalies. Am J Med Genet 47:494, 1993.

Vergnaud G, Page DC, Simmler MC, et al.: A deletion map of the human Y chromosome based on DNA hybridization. Am J Hum Genet 38:109, 1986.

Verp MS, Simpson JL, Martin AO: Hypostatic ulcers in 47,XXY Klinefelter's syndrome. J Med Genet 20:100, 1983.

Vidal VP, Chaboissier MC, de Rooij DG, et al.: *Sox9* induces testis development in XX transgenic mice. Nat Genet 28:216, 2001.

Vormittag V, Weninger W: XXXY Klinefelter's syndrome. Humangentik 15:327, 1972.

Wang C, Baker HW, Burger HG, et al.: Hormonal studies in Klinefelter's syndrome. Clin Endocrinol (Oxf) 4:399, 1975.

Warburg E: A fertile patient with Klinefelter's syndrome. Acta Endocrinol (Copenh) 43:12, 1963.

Zaleski WA, Houston CS, Pozsonyi J, et al.: The XXXXY chromosome anomaly: Report of three new cases and review of 30 cases from the literature. Can Med Assoc J 94:1143, 1966.

Zang KD: Genetics and cytogenetics of Klinefelter syndrome. In Bandmann HJ, Breit R (eds): Klinefelter syndrome. Berlin: Springer, 1984.

Zuppinger K, Engel E, Forbes AP, et al.: Klinefelter's syndrome: A clinical and cytogenetic study in twenty-four cases. Acta Endocrinol (Copenh) 54:5, 1967.

Prenatal Genetic Diagnosis

CHAPTER 13

Techniques For Prenatal Diagnosis

Prenatal diagnosis of genetic disorders usually requires analysis of fetal tissues. For over a quarter of a century and still today, the most commonly used invasive technique for prenatal diagnosis is amniocentesis performed at ≥ 15 weeks' gestation. However, in recent years additional invasive techniques have been introduced, including chorionic villus sampling (CVS), so-called early amniocentesis (<15 weeks' gestation), fetal blood sampling, fetal liver sampling, fetal muscle biopsy, and coelocentesis. Noninvasive techniques have proved invaluable, either alone, (for example high-resolution ultrasonography) or as an adjunct to invasive methods of screening. In this chapter we consider the techniques, applicability, and safety of these modalities. Common indications for prenatal genetic diagnosis are considered in Chapters 14 and 15.

Amniocentesis

TECHNICAL AMNIOCENTESIS (≥ 15 WEEKS' GESTATION)

Technique

Traditionally, amniocentesis has been performed at 15 to 17 weeks' gestation based on the onset of the last menses (Nadler and Gerbie, 1970). At this age of gestation, the volume of amniocentic fluid is approximately 200 mL and the ratio of viable to nonviable cells in the amniotic fluid is relatively high (Fuchs and Riis, 1956).

Immediately prior to amniocentesis, ultrasound examination is standard to evaluate fetal number and viability, to confirm gestational age by fetal biometric measurements, to establish placental location, and to estimate amniotic fluid volume. In our units a fetal anatomic survey also is routinely performed to screen for major anomalies.

Following the ultrasound examination, a needle insertion site is selected. Overall, we prefer to insert the needle in the midline; however, this is not always the site where the optimal pocket of amniotic fluid is located. Not infrequently, a lower uterine segment or lateral approach may be necessary. The placenta should be avoided when possible. If tapping the optimal pocket of fluid requires traversing the placenta, we select the thinnest portion of the placenta possible in which the needle can be directed. Transplacental amniocentesis has not been shown to increase the risk of the procedure (Tharmaratnam et al., 1998). The umbilical cord insertion site should be identified and avoided. Maternal bowel and bladder should be avoided.

Local anesthetic (e.g., 2–3 mL of 1% lidocaine) may or may not be used; however, local anesthesia does not appear to affect the level of pain of the procedure (Van Schoubroeck and Verhaeghe, 2000). The maternal skin is always cleaned with an iodine-based solution, and sterile drapes are placed around the needle-insertion site. We use a 22-gauge spinal needle. During the procedure ultrasonogrphic monitoring with continuous visualization of the needle should be performed. A real-time transducer is held in position adjacent to the insertion site by the operator or an assistant such that the ultrasound beam is directed parallel or at a slight angle to the planned needle track. Needle insertion should be performed with one smooth continuous motion until the needle tip is within the amniotic cavity (Fig. 13–1). Amniotic membrane "tenting" is rarely a problem in second-trimester amniocentesis and any difficulty can usually be resolved by rotating or advancing the needle. In theory, the first few milliliters of amniotic fluid are most likely to contain maternal cells from blood vessels, the abdominal wall, or the myometrium;

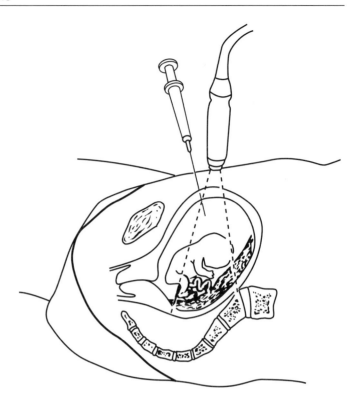

FIGURE 13–1 • Amniocentesis performed concurrently with ultrasound (From Simpson JL, Elias S: Techniques for prenatal diagnosis of genetic disorders. Reprod Genet 4:197, 1994, with permission.)

therefore, this initial sample should be discarded or set aside for alpha-fetoprotein (AFP) assay. For second-trimester amniocentesis performed between 17 and 20 weeks, 20 to 30 mL of amniotic fluid is usually aspirated. The specimen must be clearly labeled and transported at room temperature to the laboratory.

Occasionally, bloody amniotic fluid is aspirated. The blood, which is almost always maternal in origin, does not adversely affect amniotic cell growth. Brown or dark red or wine-colored amniotic fluid is associated with an increased likelihood of poor pregnancy outcome. Such a color indicates prior intra-amniotic bleeding. Hemoglobin breakdown products account for the pigment. Pregnancy loss eventually occurs in about one third of such cases (Milunsky, 1986). If the abnormally colored fluid is also associated with an elevated amniotic fluid AFP level, the outcome is almost always unfavorable (fetal death, anencephaly, spontaneous abortion, or fetal abnormality). Green-colored amniotic fluid is presumably due to meconium staining and apparently is not associated with poor pregnancy outcome (Karp and Schiller, 1977; Hess et al., 1986; Isada et al., 1990). Brown amniotic fluid was reported to be associated with increased risk of fetal aneuploidy (Isada et al., 1990).

Amniotic fluid and urine may be indistinguishable in appearance. Inadvertent aspiration of maternal urine is a risk when a suprapubic needle insertion site is chosen. Analysis of cells derived from maternal urine could obviously lead to diagnostic errors. If the origin of aspirated fluid is in doubt, a crystalline arborization test can be performed. If the fluid is allowed to dry on an acid-cleaned slide and examined under low power (x 11 magnification) microscopy, "ferning" characteristics of amniotic fluid can be sought (Elias et al., 1979). However, only rarely is any such test necessary.

Fetomaternal transfusion by disruption of the fetoplacental circulation logically might have an immunizing effect; however, the magnitude of the risk has not been determined. Administering Rh immunoglobulin (RhIG) to prevent Rh immunization in unsensitized women with Rh-positive fetuses is universally done but not completely proved to be efficacious. The dose to be administered is also controversial. In the United Kingdom, the recommended dose of RhIG is 50 µg before 20 weeks' gestation and 100 µg thereafter (Turnbull and MacKenzie, 1983). The American College of Obstetricians and Gynecologists (ACOG, 1999) recommends 300 µg of RhIG for every 1 mL of fetal blood in the maternal circulation. We routinely administer 300 µg of RhIG following genetic amniocentesis, irrespective of whether the needle has traversed the placenta.

Following amniocentesis fetal heart activity should be documented by ultrasonographic visualization. The patient is then observed briefly and instructed to report any vaginal fluid loss or bleeding, uterine cramping, or fever. We recommend that strenuous exercise (e.g., jogging or aerobic exercises) and coitus be avoided for a day or two; however, normal ambulatory activities may be resumed following the procedure.

Multiple Gestations

Amniocentesis can usually be performed readily in multiple gestations provided amniotic fluid volume is adequate (Elias et al., 1980a). Following aspiration of amniotic fluid from the first sac, 2 to 3 mL of indigo carmine, diluted 1:10 in bacteriostatic water, is injected prior to needle withdrawal. A second amniocentesis is performed. The second needle is then inserted into the sac of the second fetus, preferably determined after visualizing the membranes separating the two sacs. Aspiration of clear fluid confirms that the second sac has truly been entered (Fig. 13–2). Methylene blue should be avoided because it has been associated with jejunoileal atresia following intra-amniotic injection (Gluer, 1995). Although it is not well proved, the consensus is that amniocentesis in twins carries no increased risks over that in singleton pregnancies (Elias et al., 1980a; Anderson et al., 1991). Anderson and colleagues (1991) reported a postprocedure twin-loss rate of 3.57% up to 28 weeks, a rate interpreted as not increased over the sum of background twin-loss rate plus the loss rate associated with singleton amniocentesis. However, others (Yukobowich et al., 2001) interpreted the same study as showing an increased fetal loss rate, presumably based on the high absolute loss rate. Pruggmayer and coworkers (1991) also reported a high absolute loss rate. Ghidini and colleagues (1993a) concluded similar loss rates in a small sample of 101 twin gestations and 108 singleton controls. Yukobowich and coworkers (2001) retrospectively compared 476 twin gestations undergoing 17- to 18-week amniocentesis, 489 singleton gestations undergoing 17- to 18-week amniocentesis, and 477 twin gestations not undergoing 17- to 18-week amniocentesis. Loss rates up to 4 weeks postprocedure were 2.7%, 0.6%, and 0.6%, respectively. A problem with this and other studies is that maternal age was not taken into account by logistic regression, nor were indications and other variables.

Single-needle insertion under ultrasound guidance alone without instillation of dye to distin-

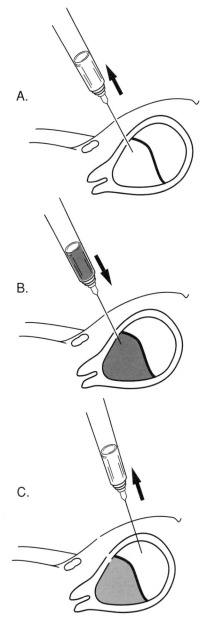

FIGURE 13–2 • Technique for amniocentesis in twin gestations. (*A*) Fluid is aspirated from the first amniotic sac. (*B*) Blue indigo carmine dye is injected into the first amniotic sac. (*C*) A second tap is made in the ultrasonographically determined location of the second fetus. Clear fluid confirms that the second amniotic sac was successfully aspirated. (From Elias TS, Gerbie AB, Simpson JL, et al.: Genetic amniocentesis in twin gestations. Am J Obstet Gynecol 138:169, 1980, with permission.)

guish both sacs in twins is advocated by some (Buscaglia et al., 1995; van Vugt et al., 1995), but we still prefer the dye technique described above. Yukobowich and associates (2001) used ultrasound only method in the study cited above.

Triplets and other multiple gestations can be managed similarly by sequentially injecting dye into successive sacs. As long as clear fluid is aspirated, a new amniotic sac has been entered.

Safety

Amniocentesis carries potential danger to both mother and fetus. Maternal risks are quite low, with symptomatic amnionitis occurring only rarely. Minor maternal complications such as transient vaginal spotting and minimal amniotic fluid leakage occur in 1% or fewer of cases, but almost always these are self-limited in nature.

Several large collaborative studies have addressed the safety of traditional amniocentesis. Unfortunately, the studies on which counseling is based were conducted decades ago. The first major prospective study of genetic amniocentesis, which included 1040 subjects and 992 matched controls, was conducted by the U.S. National Institute of Child Health and Human Development (1976). Of the 1040 women undergoing amniocentesis, 950 (91.3%) had the procedure performed for cytogenetic analysis and 90 (8.7%) to evaluate for the possible presence of inborn errors of metabolism. Of all women who underwent amniocentesis, 3.5% experienced fetal loss between the time of the procedure and delivery compared with 3.2% of controls; the small difference was not statistically significant and disappeared completely when corrected for maternal age. In Canada, a collaborative group conducted a cohort study but did not include a concurrent control group (Simpson et al., 1976; Medical Research Council, 1977). The pregnancy loss rate was 3.2%, a frequency similar to that reported in the U.S. collaborative study. Analysis was based on 1223 amniocentesis procedures performed during 1020 pregnancies in 900 women.

A British collaborative study found that the rate of fetal loss following amniocentesis was significantly higher than in controls (2.6% versus 1%) (United Kingdom Medical Research Council, 1978). In this study, however, a common indication for amniocentesis was elevated maternal serum alpha-fetoprotein (MSAFP), now recognized on its own as a factor associated with increased fetal loss and adverse perinatal outcome. After excluding subjects undergoing amniocentesis for that indication, the loss rates between subject and control groups narrowed to less than 1%, although still a statistically significant difference (National Institute of Child Health and Human Development Consensus Conference on Antenatal Diagnosis, 1979).

The relevance of the collaborative studies cited above has been questioned because they were not conducted with high quality ultrasonography as defined by today's standards, nor was concurrent ultrasonography even universally applied. This criticism was partially addressed in the 1980s by a Danish randomized controlled study that involved 4606 women aged 25 to 34 years who were without known risk factors for fetal genetic abnormalities (Tabor et al., 1986). Women with three or more previous spontaneous abortions, diabetes mellitus, multiple gestations, uterine anomalies, or intrauterine contraceptive devices were excluded. Maternal age, social group, smoking history, number of previous induced and spontaneous abortions, stillbirths, livebirths, and low birth weight infants were comparable in the study and control groups, as was gestational age at time of entry into the study. Amniocentesis was performed under real-time ultrasound guidance with a 20-gauge needle by experienced operators. Follow-up was available for all but three women. The spontaneous abortion rate after 16 weeks was 1.7% in amniocentesis patients compared with 0.7% in controls ($P < 0.01$), with a 2.6-fold relative risk of spontaneously abortion if the placenta was traversed. Respiratory distress syndrome was diagnosed more often (relative risk, 2.1) in the study group, and more infants were treated for pneumonia (relative risk, 2.5). The frequency of postural malformations in the infants in the two groups did not differ.

In a study from British Columbia, Baird and coworkers (1994) considered the question of whether children delivered of women who had midtrimester amniocentesis could be identified by a population-based database of congenital anomalies and disabilities at a different rate from that of matched controls (i.e., offspring of women who did not undergo amniocentesis). The authors studied 1296 cases (651 males and 645 females) and 3704 matched controls (1867 males and 1937 females) among live births (1972–1983) from the Health Surveillance Registry with data collected to 1990 to allow a follow-up of 7 to 18 years. Cases were children of mothers who had midtrimester amniocentesis for advanced maternal age (≥35 years) and whose results were normal for chromosomal disorders and neural tube defects. Using provincial birth records, three controls per case were matched for age of mother, sex, date of birth, and health. One hundred twenty-eight (9.9%) of the cases and 308 (8.3%) of the controls were registered (relative risk 1.23); this relative risk was not significantly different from 1. The children's likelihood of having disabilities was examined for cases as compared with controls, and no difference was found except for an increased ABO isoimmunization associated with amniocentesis. Overall, the study provides reassuring data for patients considering midtrimester amniocentesis with respect to long-term outcome.

Tongsong and coworkers (1998) from Thailand reported a large-scalecohort study among singleton pregnant women between 15 and 24 weeks' gestation undergoing amniocentesis and controls matched prospectively on a one-to-one basis for maternal age, parity, and socioeconomic status. A total of 2256 pairs were recruited. After excluding those pairs lost to follow-up, those with fetal malformations, and those with major chromosomal abnormalities, 2045 matched pairs were compared for pregnancy outcomes. There were no significant differences in fetal loss rates, premature deliveries, or placental abruptions between the two groups ($P > 0.5$). However, this study did not have enough statistical power to identify differences less than 1%.

Another data set suggesting very low loss rates following amniocentesis involves follow-up of 28,613 procedures. The total loss rate (background plus procedure-related) within 30 days was 1:362 and was similar between perinatologists and other obstetricians (Armstrong et al., 2002).

Sorely needed are large-scale randomized trials by skilled operators using modern ultrasonographic equipment. The sample would need to be very large (n = 5000 or 10,000) in each arm in order to distinguish between an increased loss rate of 0.5% (as usually stated) and the 0.2% or so that many have the clinical impression more closely approximates reality. Certainly, 0.5% increased loss after traditional amniocentesis strikes many as high.

In summary, in experienced hands the risk of pregnancy loss secondary to amniocentesis is perhaps 0.2–0.3%. Serious maternal complications and fetal injuries can be stated as "remote."

EARLY AMNIOCENTESIS (≤14 WEEKS' GESTATION)

After CVS was introduced, a trend occurred toward offering amniocentesis before 15 weeks' gestation. In some cases early amniocentesis has been recommended as an alternative to CVS for patients who desire prenatal diagnosis before the time in pregnancy when traditional amniocentesis is performed (i.e., ≥15 weeks' gestation). Early amniocentesis was also used to obviate the inconvenience of patients having to be rescheduled if they came in for CVS, and were determined to be beyond 12 weeks' gestation but under 15 weeks' gestation.

Technique

Early amniocentesis is performed using basically the same technique as that used for traditional amniocentesis. The exception is that a smaller amount of amniotic fluid is removed, usually 1 mL for each completed week of gestation. Concurrent ultrasound needle guidance is absolutely essential, given the relatively small target area and the need to avoid the bladder and bowel, which may interfere with the selected needle path into the uterus. It is also necessary to watch for tenting of the membranes as the needle enters. This is the most common cause of failing to obtain amniotic fluid in early amniocentesis. Membrane tenting becomes increasingly problematic the earlier in gestation amniocentesis is attempted, given incomplete fusion of the chorion and amnion (Henry and Miller, 1992).

It has been suggested that filtration and recirculation of amniotic fluid at early amniocentesis might increase cell yield and reduce the culture time before karyotyping (Kennerknecht et al., 1993; Sundberg et al., 1993; Byrne et al., 1995). However, such manipulations are probably not necessary. In a series reported by Hanson and coworkers (1992) of 936 amniocenteses performed at ≤12.8 weeks, the mean culture time was 8.8 days (SD 1.5 days); only a single patient required a retap because of inadequate cell growth. Among 1375 early amniotic fluid samples (≤14 weeks), Lockwood and Neu (1993) reported that 1356 of 1375 cases (98.6%) were successfully cultured and yielded cytogenetic results.

Another concern is whether interpretation of amniotic fluid AFP and acetylcholinesterase carries the same sensitivity and specificity for detecting neural tube defects (NTDs) in the midtrimester as it does at 12 weeks' gestation or less (Crandall et al., 1989; Watson and Craft, 1989; Wathen et al., 1993). Crandall and Chua (1995) identified 42 open NTDs among 7440 amniocentesis procedures between 11 and 15 weeks' gestation. Detection rate was 100% for anencephaly, 100% for spina bifida, and 78% for encephalocele using an amniotic fluid AFP ≥2.0 MOM and positive acetyl cholinesterase (AchE). Excluding fetal demise and other serious abnormalities, 43 (0.6%) false-positive results occurred with AFP alone but only 0.1% with AchE. Among amniotic fluid samples obtained prior to 13 weeks' gestation, the false-positive

AchE rate was 6.3%. Nearly all showed two very faint bands that could be distinguished from the true positive AchE bands seen in open NTDs. However, there are still insufficient data to determine the sensitivity of these tests prior to 12 weeks' gestation.

Safety

Initially, several programs reported experiences suggesting early amniocenteses to be a promising technique. Hanson and colleagues (1992) reported 936 amniocentesis procedures at ≤12.8 weeks' gestation; loss rates were 0.7% (7/936) within 2 weeks of amniocentesis, with an additional 2.2% before 28 weeks and an additional 0.5% stillbirths or neonatal deaths. Total losses (32/936 or 3.4%) were considered comparable to the 2.1 to 3.2% in ultrasonographically normal pregnancies in which a procedure was not undergone; however, lack of correction for maternal and gestational age renders comparisons less than exact. Henry and Miller (1992) also reported favorable results in amniocentesis at 12, 13, and 14 weeks' gestation. Pregnancy losses prior to 28 weeks were 5/193 (2.6%), 5/426 (1.2%), and 11/1172 (1.5%), respectively. Other early series were reported as well (Benacerraf et al., 1987; Elejalde et al., 1990, Penso et al., 1990, Stripparo et al., 1990; Hackett et al., 1991; Assel et al., 1992; Djalali et al., 1992; Eiben et al., 1993; Kerber and Held, 1993; Yang et al., 1993; Crandall et al., 1994).

Nicolaides and colleagues (1994a) performed early amniocentesis at 10 to 13 weeks' in 731 patients (493 by choice and 238 by randomization), and compared results with CVS in 570 patients (320 by choice and 250 by randomization). Both procedures were performed by transabdominal ultrasound-guided insertion of a 20-gauge needle. Spontaneous loss (intrauterine or neonatal death) was significantly higher after early amniocentesis (total group mean = 2.3%, CI 1.2–3.9; randomized subgroup: mean = 1.2%, 0.3–3.5). Vandenbussche and colleagues (1994) used a similar approach to that of Nicholaides and coworkers (1994a). Among 192 women with at least a follow-up of 6 weeks postprocedure, 102 were randomized and 66 and 24, respectively, chose early amniocenteses and CVS. There were eight unintended fetal losses among 120 early amniocenteses, as opposed to none among 64 CVS procedures, a difference of 6.7% (95% CI 2.2–11.1%). These investigators believed that the risks of early amniocenteses were so high that continuation of their trial could not be ethically justified.

Brumfield and coworkers (1996) reported 314 women undergoing early amniocentesis (11 to 14 weeks' gestation) who were matched to 628 controls undergoing traditional amniocentesis (16 to 19 weeks' gestation). Women who had early amniocenteses were significantly more likely to have postprocedure amniotic fluid leakage (2.9 versus 0.2%), postprocedure vaginal bleeding (1.9 versus 0.2%), and a fetal loss within 30 days of the amniocentesis (2.2 versus 0.2%) than were women undergoing traditional amniocentesis.

Most conclusively, a multicenter randomized trial was reported by The Canadian Early and Mid-Trimester Amniocenteses Trial (CEMAT) Group (CEMAT Group, 1998, Johnson et al., 1999). A precursor study by a member of the Canadian group had initially seemed promising. Johnson and colleagues (1996) compared early amniocentesis (11 weeks to 12 weeks, 6 days) to midtrimester amniocentesis (15 weeks to 16 weeks, 6 days). Among 638 women randomized and followed to pregnancy, fetal losses (spontaneous abortions) in the two groups were 27/344 (7.8%) and 25/399 (7.4%), respectively. They concluded that early amniocentesis appears to be as safe and accurate as midtrimester amniocentesis. However, results of the full Canadian study were different. Early amniocenteses (n = 2183) were performed between 11 weeks, 0 days, and 12 weeks, 6 days; midtrimester amniocenteses were performed between 15 weeks, 0 days, and 16 weeks, 6 days. In the early amniocentesis (n = 2185) cohort, 1916 women (87.8%) underwent amniocentesis before 13 weeks' gestation. First, there was a significant difference in total fetal losses for early amniocenteses compared with midtrimester amniocenteses (7.6% versus 5.9%); difference 1.7%, (one-sided CI 2.98%, P = 0.012). A significant increase in talipes equinovarus was found in the early amniocenteses group compared with the midtrimester amniocenteses group (1.3% versus 0.1%, P = 0.0001). Even more disturbingly, there was a significant difference in postprocedural amniotic fluid leakage (early amniocenteses 3.5% versus midtrimester amniocenteses 1.7%, P = 0.0007). Failed procedures, multiple needle insertions, and culture failures also occurred more frequently in the early amniocentesis group. More recently, Nikkilä et al. (2002) reported a series of 3469 genetic amniocenteses performed before 15 weeks gestation. They found a clear tendency of decreasing number of foot deformaties with increasing gestational age.

Our own clinical experience is in agreement with the Canadian experience. Our group (Shulman et al., 1994) had a less than sanguine early experience. When we compared our initial experience with 250 early amnioceteses (≤ 14 weeks) to that of our first 250 cases of transabdominal CVS (9.5 to 12.9 weeks), the loss rates for early amniocentesis and transabdominal CVS were 3.8% and 2.1%, respectively, despite the former's being performed later in gestation. Transplacental needle passage did not appear to increase the risk of pregnancy loss (Bravo et al., 1995).

In conclusion, we and ACOG (2001) have concluded CVS is safer than early amniocentesis, and the latter is not equal in safety to traditional amniocentesis. Early amniocentesis is not recommended.

Chorionic Villus Sampling

With traditional midsecond trimester amniocentesis (15 to 16 weeks' gestation), fetal diagnosis cannot usually be established prior to 17 to 18 weeks' gestation. Even early amniocentesis (12 to 14 weeks) does not provide a substantial advantage with respect to the gestational timing. A second-trimester termination would still be necessary after 2 to 3 weeks for culture and analysis. CVS is a technique that can be performed during the first trimester, thereby reducing the psychological stress of awaiting results until midpregnancy and allowing a safer method of pregnancy termination should an abnormality be detected.

Chorionic villi provide the same information as amniotic fluid cells, allowing cytogenetic, DNA, or biochemical analysis. Only assays requiring amniotic fluid, such as AFP, require amniocentesis and cannot be performed using CVS.

TECHNIQUES

1. *Transcervical* CVS is now usually performed at 10 to 12 gestational weeks, based on the onset of the last menstrual period. Absolute contraindications to transcervical CVS include active cervical or vaginal pathology (e.g., herpes, *Chlamydia*, or gonorrhea infection) or maternal blood group sensitization. Relative contraindications include leiomyomata obstructing the cervical canal, bleeding from the vagina within two weeks of scheduled CVS, and markedly retroverted, retroflexed uterus (Elias et al., 1985). Before CVS, fetal viability and normal fetal growth must be confirmed by ultrasound. The procedure is performed using catheters with a diameter of about 1.5 mm. CVS catheters consist of a plastic can-

nula enclosing a metal obturator that extends just beyond the catheter tip.

In transcervical CVS, the patient is positioned in the dorsal lithotomy position. The vagina is cleaned with an iodine preparation, the perineum draped with sterile towels, and a sterile vaginal speculum inserted. A tenaculum placed on the anterior lip of the cervix may be necessary to correct uterine anteflexion or retroflexion. The CVS catheter is introduced transcervically under simultaneous ultrasonographic visualization, with optimal catheter placement being parallel to the long axis of the placenta (Fig. 13–3). The obturator is then removed and the catheter attached by Luer-Lok to a 20- or 30-mL syringe. Chorionic villi are then aspirated by multiple, rapid aspirations of the syringe plunger to 20 to 30 mL negative pressure. The catheter is withdrawn under continuous maximum negative pressure. An adequate sample is at least 5 mg of villi, but 10 to 25 mg is preferred. We are successful in obtaining an adequate sample on the first attempt in about 95% of cases. Usually no more than two attempts are performed on a given day.

After the procedure, fetal heart activity is documented by ultrasonography. Patients are monitored for any untoward effects for approximately 30 minutes. Unsensitized Rh-negative patients are given 300 mg of Rh-immune globulin. Patients are asked to

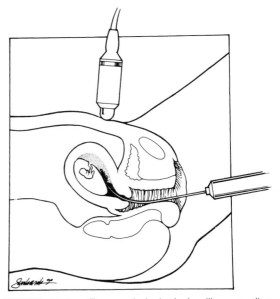

FIGURE 13–3 • Transcervical chorionic villus sampling. (From Simpson JL: Genetic counseling and prenatal diagnosis. *In* Gabbe SA, Niebyl JF, Simpson JL (eds): Obstetrics: Normal and Problem Pregnancies, 2nd ed. New York: Churchill Livingstone, 1991.)

refrain from sexual intercourse for several days. Otherwise, they can carry on with normal activities. Maternal serum AFP screening for fetal neural tube defects is performed at 16 to 18 weeks' gestation.

2. *Transabdominal CVS* is also applicable to 10 to 12 weeks of completed gestation; however, this procedure also can be performed later in pregnancy through to term (Holzgreve et al., 1987; Carroll et al., 1999). The transabdominal approach is particularly advantageous when the placenta is located in the fundus or located anteriorly in an anteflexed uterus. Transabdominal CVS is also an option when transcervical sampling is contraindicated (e.g., in active herpes or cervical lesions).

A needle insertion site is selected based on ultrasound findings. The overlying skin is infiltrated with a local anesthetic, cleaned with an iodine preparation, and draped with sterile towels. A 19- or 20-gauge spinal needle is inserted percutaneously through the maternal abdominal wall and myometrium under continuous ultrasound guidance. The tip is then guided into the long access of the placenta beneath the chorionic plate (Fig. 13–4). The needle stylet is removed, and the needle is attached to a syringe housed in an aspiration device (Cameco Syringe Pistol, Precision Dynamics, Inc., San Fernando, CA).

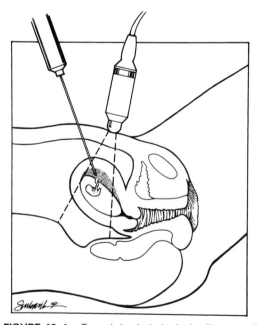

FIGURE 13–4 • Transabdominal chorionic villus sampling. (From Simpson JL: Genetic counseling and prenatal diagnosis. *In* Gabbe SA, Niebyl JF, Simpson JL (eds): Obstetrics: Normal and Problem Pregnancies, 2nd ed. New York: Churchill Livingstone, 1991.)

Chorionic villi are obtained by repetitive rapid aspirations of the syringe plunger to 20 mL of negative pressure. The needle is then withdrawn under continuous negative pressure. As with transcervical CVS, we are almost always successful in obtaining an adequate sample on the first attempt. No more than two attempts are performed on a given day. The same postoperative protocol is used as for transcervical CVS.

Some operators use a "guide-needle" or double-needle system device, which punctures the uterine wall once but permits multiple attempts at villus aspiration (Smidt-Jensen and Hahnemann, 1984). However, most physicians performing transabdominal CVS employ the aforementioned "free hand" technique.

3. In some women the only approach may be *transvaginal CVS*. This may be necessary in women having a retroverted, retroflexed uterus with a posterior placenta. Patients are positioned and prepared in a fashion similar to that for transcervical CVS. The wall of the vagina posterior to the cervix is infiltrated with a local anesthetic. We use a 35-cm 18-gauge spinal needle to aspirate chorionic villi. Transabdominal ultrasound is required for needle guidance through the vaginal mucosa and myometrium into the placenta. Once within the placenta, the needle stylet is removed, and villi are aspirated in a similar fashion to that for transabdominal CVS (Shulman et al., 1993).

Clinical judgment and patient individualization in choosing the optimal approach increase safety. For example, the transcervical approach would be favored over the transabdominal approach in a retroverted uterus with a posterior placenta. Sometimes CVS should be eschewed in favor of amniocentesis later in gestation. With conservation approach pregnancies, loss rates can be quite low.

SAFETY OF CHORIONIC VILLUS SAMPLING

Pregnancy Losses Following CVS

Pregnancy loss rate in transcervical CVS was not significantly higher than that for traditional amniocentesis in the United States Cooperative Clinical Comparison of Chorionic Villus Sampling and Amniocentesis Study and the Canadian Collaborative CVS-Amniocentesis Trial Group, respectively (Rhoads et al., 1989; Canadian Collaborative CVS-Amniocentesis Trial Group, 1991). In the U.S. study 2278 women self-selected transcervical CVS; 671 women similarly recruited in the first trimester selected amniocentesis. Randomization did not prove possible. Loss rates in the CVS group were 0.8% higher but not statistically significant. (Also see below for results of a follow-up study.) The Canadian study was randomized; 1391 subjects were assigned to transcervical CVS and 1396 to amniocentesis. Fetal loss rate was 0.6% higher in the CVS group. Factors found to adversely influence fetal loss rates included fundal placenta, number of catheter insertions, small sample size, and prior bleeding during the current pregnancy (Rhoads et al., 1989; Golbus et al., 1992). Almost all the above invariably reflect technical difficulty. Other obstetric complications (e.g., intrauterine growth restriction, placental abruption, premature delivery) did not exceed those in women not undergoing CVS.

In a later U.S. NICHD collaborative study, 1944 patients were randomized to transcervical CVS and 1929 patients randomized to transabdominal CVS. Loss rates of cytogenetically normal pregnancies through 28 weeks' gestation were 2.5% and 2.3%, respectively (Jackson et al., 1992). Thus, transcervical CVS and transabdominal CVS appear to be equally safe procedures for first-trimester diagnosis. Moreover, the overall loss rate (i.e., background plus procedure-related) following CVS decreased by about 0.8% during this 1988–1990 randomization trial in comparison with rates observed during the transcervical versus amniocentesis self-selection study (1985–1987). This decrease in procedure-related loss rate probably reflects increasing operator experience as well as availability of both transcervical and transabdominal approaches. In an Italian randomized trial, Brambati and coworkers (1990) also found no difference between transabdominal and transcervical CVS. By contrast, in a randomized comparison between amniocentesis, transabdominal CVS, and transcervical CVS in Denmark, Smidt-Jensen and colleagues (1992) found similar fetal loss rates after transabdominal CVS and amniocentesis but a significantly increased loss rate associated with transcervical CVS. However, Danish experience with transabdominal CVS was far greater prior to randomization than experience with transcervical CVS.

One major study has substantively differed from the above, the Medical Research Council Study (MRC Working Party on the Evaluation of Chorionic Villus Sampling, 1991). In this multi-center randomized study, first-trimester CVS was performed in whatever fashion deemed suitable by the obstetrician and compared with second-trimester amniocentesis. The outcome variable measured was completed pregnancies, including both unintended and intended pregnancy terminations. The latter group accounted for the 4.4% fewer completed pregnancies in the CVS cohort. Experience with CVS prior to randomization by MRC study operators was also considerably less than for operators in the U.S. studies. For example, the only requirement for participating in the MRC study was 30 "practice" CVS procedures. Some centers contributed very few cases.

No formal attempts to assess the safety of transvaginal CVS have been attempted. In the experience of Shulman and coworkers (1993) and Sidransky and coworkers (1990), neither major complications nor obvious excessive fetal loss rates were observed.

CVS in Multiple Gestations

Data now verify the safety of CVS in multiple gestations, an increasingly common indication because of assisted reproductive technologies. The technique involves transabdominal CVS, transcervical CVS, or a combination of the two approaches. In the major U.S. study involving four centers, the total loss rate of chromosomally normal fetuses (spontaneous abortions, stillborns, neonatal deaths) was 5.0% (Pergament et al., 1992), slightly higher than the 4.0% observed for singleton pregnancies (Rhoads et al., 1989). In comparing 81 women with twin pregnancies undergoing amniocentesis and 161 women with twin pregnancies undergoing CVS, Wapner and colleagues (1993) found the fetal loss rate following amniocentesis to be 2.9% and following CVS to be 3.2%. There were three cases of twin-twin villus contamination, one of which resulted in incorrect sex assignment. Van den Berg and coworkers (1999) reported a retrospective series of woman with multiple gestations who underwent either amniocentesis or CVS. Uncertain results in one or both samples that required further investigation were more frequent among the CVS cases (8/163 paired samples, 5%) compared to amniocentesis cases (1/298 paired samples, 0.3%). Sampling one fetus twice (erroneously) occurred only once in 163 pregnancies with two CVS samples. We now use CVS in multiple gestations when each placenta can be reliability visualized by ultrasound. When placental localizations preclude the reasonable obtaining of separate and distinct sampling, midtrimester amniocentesis is preferred.

Limb Reduction Defects

Safety concerns about CVS has now shifted focus less to risk of fetal loss than to CVS as a possible cause of limb reduction defects. The first claims were in 1991, when Firth and colleagues (1991a, b) reported that 5 of 289 (1.7%) infants exposed to CVS between 56 and 66 days of gestation (i.e., 42 to 50 days after fertilization) had severe limb reduction deformities (LRDs). Four of the five infants had oromandibular-limb hypogenesis; all mothers had undergone transabdominal CVS. The fifth case had isolated terminal transverse limb reduction after transcervical CVS. Subsequently, a number of reports followed both supporting and refuting such an association (Hsieh et al., 1991; Jackson et al., 1991; Mahoney and USNICHD Collaborators, 1991; Mastroiacovo and Cavalcanti, 1991; Monni et al., 1991; Scott, 1991). In the United States, Burton and coworkers (1992) reported a second cluster among 394 infants whose mothers had undergone CVS. Thirteen (3.3%) had major congenital abnormalities, including four with transverse LRDs (10/1000 or 1%). All four LRDs were transverse distal defects involving hypoplasia or absence of the fingers and toes. Three of these cases followed transcervical sampling, employing a device that in the hands of the reporting physicians was associated with a 11% fetal loss rate.

Teratogenic mechanisms by which CVS might cause LRDs are plausible (Simpson and Elias, 1994). Explanations include (1) hypoperfusion due to fetomaternal hemorrhage or release of pressor substances through disturbance of villi or the chorion; (2) embolization of chorionic villus material or maternal clots into the fetal circulation; and (3) amniotic puncture and limb entrapment in exocoelic gel. Los and coworkers (1996) suggested that fetomaternal transfusion following some cases of CVS may provoke congenital malformations on an immunologic basis.

After initial reports of Firth and coworkers (1991b) and Burton and coworkers (1992), various registries explored the potential association of LRDs with CVS. Using the Italian Multi-Center Birth Defects Registry, Mastroiacovo and colleagues (1992) reported that eight cases of oromandibular-limb hypogenesis complex were entered from January, 1988 through December, 1991. Of those with isolated transverse limb defects, four were exposed to CVS compared with 36 cases among 8445 controls. A 1994 update using this registry found 11 CVS-exposed cases and continued to indicate an association with transverse limb defects (Mastroiacovo and Botto, 1994). The highest risk was associated with procedures performed at less than 70 days' gestation (OR 23.2; 95% CI 1.31–41.0); a lower but still increased risk was found with procedures at 70 to 76 days (OR 17.1; 95% CI 6.7–44.0); after 84 days there were no exposed cases and the risk was interpreted as considerably lower. In contrast with the Italian registry, analysis of other European registries involving over 600,000 births showed that only four of 336 cases (1.2%) with limb reduction abnormalities had been exposed to CVS compared with 78 of 11,883 (0.66%) cases with other malformations (OR 1.8; 95% CI 0.7-5.0) (Dolk et al., 1992).

In combining their own cases with those reported in the literature, Firth and colleagues (1994) summarized LRDs in 75 infants exposed to CVS. The median gestational age at CVS ranged from 56 (range 49 to 65) postmenstrual days for the most severe defects to 72 (range 51 to 98) for the least severe. A correlation was believed to exist between the severity of the defects and the duration of gestation with CVS.

In an effort to quantify the risk for LRDs associated with CVS, Olney and coworkers (1995) reported results from a U.S. multistate case-controlled study. Case subjects consisted of 131 infants with nonsyndromic limb deficiency from seven population-based birth defects surveillance programs born to women 34 years or older from 1988 through 1992. Controls consisted of 131 infants with other birth defects, matched to case subjects by the infant's year of birth, mother's age, race, and state of residence. Odds ratio for limb deficiency after CVS from 8 to 12 weeks' gestation were not significant at 1.7 (85% CI 0.4-6.3). When LRDs were analyzed for specific anatomic subtypes, an association was found for transverse digital deficiency (OR 6.4; 95% CI 1.1–38.6). It was concluded that the absolute risk for such defects was approximately 1 in 3000.

The World Health Organization Committee on Chronic Villus Sampling has continued to analyze data collected through an international voluntary registry (Froster and Jackson, 1996; Kuliev et al., 1996). A total of 77 cases with LRDs found among 138,996 infants born after CVS were reported from 63 registering centers. Pattern analysis of the types of limb defects and overall frequencies of specific LRDs were compared with a background population study from British Columbia (Froster-Iskenius and Baird, 1989). The pattern of defects showed the upper limb to be affected in 65%, the lower limb in 13%, and both upper and lower limbs in 23% compared with general population frequencies of 68%, 23%, and 9%, respectively. Transverse limb defects occurred in 41% of infants in the cohort exposed to CVS compared to 43% in the general population, and longitudal limb deficiencies were found in 59% of cases, compared to 57% in the general population. Pattern analysis of the types of limb defects and calculation of overall incidences failed to find a difference between the CVS and background populations. The latest WHO report continued to show these same results (WHO/PAHO, 1999).

In 1995, the Committee on Genetics of the American College of Obstetricians and Gynecologists concluded the following:

1. Transcervical CVS and transabdominal CVS, when performed at 10 to 12 weeks of gestation, are relatively safe and accurate procedures and may be considered acceptable alternatives to midtrimester genetic amniocentesis.
2. CVS should not be performed before 10 weeks of gestation.
3. CVS requires appropriate genetic counseling before the procedure, an operator experienced in performing the technique, and a laboratory experienced in processing the villus specimen and interpreting the results. Counseling should include comparing and contrasting the risks and benefits of amniocentesis versus those of CVS.
4. Although further studies are needed to determine whether there is an increased risk of transverse digital deficiency following CVS performed at 10 to 12 weeks of gestation, it is prudent to counsel patients that such an outcome is possible and that the estimated risk may be on the order of 1 in 3000 births.

We counsel that in experienced hands fetal loss rates are comparable for traditional amniocentesis and CVS. We state that the rate of limb reduction defect *could* be as high as 1 in 3000 over the background of 6 per 10,000. However, like ACOG (2001) we believe after 9 menstrual weeks that "the risk is low and probably not higher than the general population risk."

Fetal Blood Sampling

Fetal blood sampling was first accomplished by fetoscopy, a technique of directly visualizing the fetus, umbilical cord, and chorionic surface of the placenta using endoscopic instruments (Hobbins and Mahoney, 1974; Elias, 1980). Fetoscopy for this purpose has now been replaced by ultrasound-directed percutaneous umbilical blood sampling (PUBS), also termed cordocenteis or funipuncture, or intrahepatic vein (IHV) fetal blood sampling.

Fetal blood chromosome analysis has help clarify purported chromosome mosaicism detected in cultured amniotic fluid cells (Gosden et al., 1988) or chorionic villi. Rapid assessment of the full fetal chromosome complement can also be performed by "direct" cytogenetic analysis of uncultured nucleated blood cells (Tipton et al., 1990). Short-term fetal lymphocyte cultures provide a cytogenetic result within 72 hours; direct analysis of spontaneously dividing fetal cells (probably nucleated red blood cells) can provide a karyotypic result within 24 hours. This is particularly useful for patients present late in the second trimester, when results from amniocentesis would be available too late for pregnancy termination to remain an option. In fetal structural abnormalities or intrauterine growth retardation first made known in the third trimester, rapid results may prove useful for decision-making concerning pregnancy management and the mode of delivery (Liou et al., 1993; Porreco et al., 1993; Claussen et al., 1995; Donner et al., 1995). Fluorescent *in situ* hybridization with chromosome-specific DNA probes has more recently replaced the above methods of rapid prenatal diagnosis of aneuploidy in umbilical cord blood, using of amniocentic fluid cells (Lapidot-Lifson et al., 1996; Pierluigi et al., 1996). However, metaphase analysis may be necessary for analysis of structural abnormalities (Thein et al., 2000).

Prenatal diagnosis for sickle cell disease, α- or β-thalassemia, or other hemoglobinopathies, once possible only by fetal blood sampling (Hobbins and Mahoney, 1974), can now be diagnosed by DNA analysis of chorionic villi or amniotic fluid cells. Fetal blood sampling may still be necessary to assess both platelet quantity and function (Donnenfeld et al., 1990) and hematologic indices (Nicolaides et al., 1987; Ryan and Rodeck, 1993). In PLA2 (platelet antigen) alloimmunization, PUBS is not only useful for diagnosis but allows access to the fetal circulation for *in utero* platelet transfusion or maternal immunotherapy with gamma globulin or steroids (Bussel et al., 1988; Kornfeld et al., 1996).

The prenatal diagnosis of blood factor abnormalities like hemophilia A, hemophilia B, or von Willebrand disease also began with fetal blood sampling (Forestier et al., 1988; Weiner et al., 1989). In the premolecular era, fetal blood samples were used to diagnose such autosomal recessive or X-linked immunologic deficiencies as severe combined immunodeficiency, Chédiak-Higashi syndrome, Wiskott-Aldrich syndrome, and chronic granulomatous disease (Durandy et al., 1982; Holmberg et al., 1983; Diukman et al., 1992). Thrombocytopenia-absent radius (TAR) syndrome was diagnosed demonstrating a low platelet count in fetal blood (Boute et al., 1996). In Blackfan-Diamond syndrome, an autosomal dominant or autosomal recessive disorder characterized by macrocytic anemia due to defective erythroid stem cells and variable presence of limb deformities (e.g., radial hypoplasia, thumb anomalies), short stature, and cardiac anomalies, PUBS was used to confirm fetal anemia in this condition as well as *in utero* transfusion therapy (McLennan et al., 1996). PUBS has also been utilized in the management of fetal goiter in maternal hypothyroidism (Bellini et al., 2000).

Fetal blood is still useful for assessment of viral, bacterial, or parasitic infections of the fetus. Detection of fetal viral or parasitic infection is usually made on the basis of maternal antibody titers or ultrasound-detected fetal structural abnormalities. Serum studies of fetal blood permit quantification of antibody titers (Daffos et al., 1988; Rodeck and Nicolini, 1988; Lecuru et al., 1995; Paidas et al., 1995; Newton, 1999). In addition to antibody studies, PUBS can be used for direct analysis of viral, bacterial, and parasitic infections by culture of fetal blood (Daffos, 1989; Hsieh et al., 1989; Peters and Nicolaides, 1990).

The real future for fetal blood sampling is likely to involve *in utero* vascular transfusion of blood products. Drug delivery is also possible. For example, fetal arrhythmias have been treated with direct administration of antiarrhythmic medications, and fetal paralysis may be induced to facilitate invasive procedures such as fetal transfusions or for magnetic resonance imaging (Moise et al., 1989; Elliott et al., 1994).

TECHNIQUES

PUBS or IHV fetal blood sampling can be safety undertaken from 18 weeks' gestation onward, although successful procedures have been reported as early as 12 weeks (Orlandi et al., 1987, 1990; Chinnaiya et al., 1998). Preliminary ultrasonographic examination of the fetus is performed to assess fetal viability, placental and umbilical cord location, fetal or placental anomalies, and fetal position. Maternal sedation is not usually required, but oral benzodiazepine shortly before the procedure may be of benefit to the anxious patient. A suitable site for needle insertion is selected, and skin over the site is anesthetized with 5 mL of 1% lidocaine. A sterile field is established; skin is cleansed with an iodine-based solution and sterile drapes are applied. The ultrasound transducer is placed on the abdomen away from the sterile insertion site, but at a location that permits visualization of the complete path of the needle from the skin to the fetal blood vessel.

There are various potential sampling sites. Given its fixed position, the placental cord root is usually the site of choice whenever it is clearly visible. Alternatively, free loops of cord or the intrahepatic vein are possibilities (Nicolini et al., 1990; Ryan and Rodeck, 1993; Chinnaiya et al., 1998). The spinal needle is percutaneously

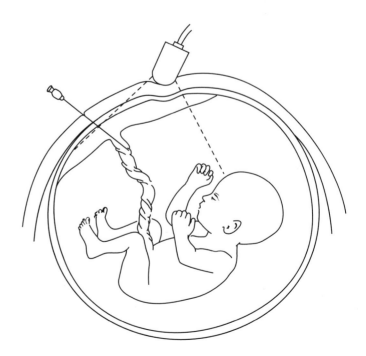

FIGURE 13–5 • Percutaneous umbilical blood sampling. (From Ryan R, Rodeck CH: Fetal blood sampling. *In* Simpson JL, Elias S (eds): Essentials of Prenatal Diagnosis. New York: Churchill Livingstone, 1993, with permission.)

inserted into the fetal blood vessel under direct ultrasound guidance, and a small sample of blood is aspirated (Fig. 13–5). Presence of fetal blood in this initial sample is confirmed using a Coulter counter and channelizer, which can differentiate fetal from maternal blood on the basis of erythrocyte volume. The amount of blood aspirated for diagnosis depends on the indication IHV for PUBS or fetal blood sampling; rarely is more than 5 mL required.

Upon completion of the fetal blood sampling, the spinal needle is withdrawn and an ultrasound examination is performed to evaluate fetal status. Women at risk for Rh-immunization receive 300 µg of Rh immune globin following the procedure. The woman and her fetus are monitored for about 1 hour following the procedure.

SAFETY

Maternal complications of PUBS and IHV are rare but include amnionitis and transplacental hemorrhage (Nicolini et al., 1988; Weiner et al., 1989). Data from large perinatal centers show the risk of *in utero* death or spontaneous abortion to be 3% or less following PUBS (Rodeck and Nicolini, 1988; Daffos, 1989; Hsieh et al., 1989; Weiner et al., 1989; Ghidini et al., 1993b; Wilson et al., 1994; Buscaglia et al., 1996; Weiner and Okamura, 1996). Collaborative data from 14 North American centers, sampling 1600 patients at varying gestational ages and for a variety of indications, revealed an uncorrected fetal loss rate of 1.6% (Nicolaides et al., 1990). Weiner and Okamura (1996) reported much lower loss rates. In two fetal diagnoses and treatment units in the United States (10 operators) and Japan (15 operators), the procedure-related fetal loss rate in 1260 cases was 0.9%; for all diagnoses other than chromosomal abnormalities and severe growth restriction, the procedure-related fetal loss rate was 2/1021 (0.2%). Chinnaiya and coworkers (1998) performed fetal blood sampling on 382 women over a seven-year period from 13 weeks' gestation onward. In 292 of 382 (76.4%) cases, the intrahepatic part of the umbilical vein was targeted; in 70 or 382 (18.3%) of cases, PUBS was performed; in 20 of 382 (5.2%) of cases, cardiocentesis was performed. Multivariate analysis showed increased odds of fetal loss for PUBS and cardiocentesis compared with the IVH fetal blood sampling group. It was statistically significant ($P < 0.01$) only in the cardiocentesis group, for fetal loss within 2 weeks of performing the procedure.

Four studies directly comparing loss rates in control and treated groups have been published. None were randomized studies. The only cohort comparison study is by Tongsong and coworkers (2001), who followed 1281 Thai women undergoing freehand cordocentesis between 16 and 24 weeks. Women with no overt fetal abnormalities served as controls. Indications were mostly risk of thalassemia (61%), rapid karyotyping (21%), or both karyotyping and thalassemia (8.7%). Exclusion of some matched pairs left 1029 pairs for comparisons. Loss rates were 3.2% versus 1.8%, with no differences in obstetric complications. An overall confounding factor is that baseline loss rates for patients undergoing PUBS or IVH fetal blood sampling vary greatly according to the indication of the procedure (Antsaklis et al., 1998). Loss rates are far greater for fetuses with ultrasound-detected anomalies than for fetuses evaluated for hemolytic diseases secondary to maternal blood group sensitization for late booking or for clarification of mosaicism at amniocentesis. Thus, additional data regarding loss rates in matched control and treated groups are necessary to determine the true safety of PUBS and IVH fetal blood sampling. Overall, procedure-related loss rates of at least 1% if not 1.5% should be assumed.

Potential fetal complications that may lead to fetal death or iatrogenic premature delivery include infection, premature rupture of the membranes, hemorrhage, severe bradycardia, cord tamponade or thrombosis, and abruptio placentae (Ryan and Rodeck, 1993). Estimation of risks associated with PUBS or IVH fetal blood sampling should include not only fetal and neonatal death but also risk of cesarean section for fetal distress, low Apgar scores, fetal anemia, and other indications of fetal and neonatal morbidity.

Fetal Skin Sampling

Prenatal diagnosis of serious genodermatoses (hereditary skin diseases) may occasionally require obtaining fetal skin samples (Elias et al., 1994; Bahado-Singh et al., 1995). Initially, this was the only method to detect anhidrotic ectodermal dysplasia (Arnold et al., 1984), bullous congenital ichthyosiform dystrophia (epidermolytic hyperkeratosis) (Golbus et al., 1980, Anton-Lamprecht, 1983; Jurkovic and Kurjak, 1989), epidermolysis bullosa dystrophia (Hallopean-Siemens) (Anton-Lamprecht et al., 1981), harlequin ichthyosis (Elias et al., 1980b; Blanchet-Bardon et al., 1983), hypohidrotic ectodermal dysplasia (Gilgenkrantz et al., 1989), epidermolysis bullosa lethalis

(Rodeck et al., 1980; Elias et al., 1994), nonbullous ichthyosiform erythroderma (Perry et al., 1987), and Sjögren-Larsson syndrome (Kousseff et al., 1982). In most families these disorders can now be detected by DNA analysis of chorionic villi, amniotic fluid cells, or even blastomeres or polar bodies (see Chapter 16).

TECHNIQUE

Fetal skin sampling was first performed by fetoscopy under direction visualization (Elias and Esterly, 1981; Golbus, 1984). The procedure-related loss rate was perhaps 2%. Later, ultrasound-directed biopsy forceps for fetal skin sampling was used, allowing a smaller caliber instrument to be introduced into the uterus. Presumably this latter technique is associated with lower risks to the woman and her fetus (Elias et al., 1994) than the fetoscopy approach, but available data are limited.

Fetal skin sampling is best performed between 17 and 20 weeks' gestation. An ultrasonographic examination must confirm fetal viability, diagnose multiple gestation, perform biometric measurements for gestational dating, localize the placenta and umbilical cord insertion site, and survey for fetal anomalies. A site of entry is then selected. The abdomen is prepared with an iodine-based antiseptic solution and appropriately draped. The patient is sedated with 10 mg of intravenous diazepam, which as a low molecular weight agent crosses the placenta and reduces fetal movement. Maternal skin is infiltrated with 1% lidocaine hydrochloride for local anesthesia, and a 5-mm stab incision is made with a No. 11 scalpel blade. A 14-gauge Angiocath with stylet (e.g., Deseret Medical Inc, Sandy, UT) is directed through the stab incision into the amniotic cavity, all under direct ultrasound visualization. The stylet is removed, and a 20-mL syringe is attached to the catheter; amniotic fluid is aspirated for chromosomal and AFP studies. After removal of the syringe, a biopsy forceps (e.g., Storz 270712; Karl Storz Endoscopy American Inc., Culver City, CA) is inserted through the catheter into the amniotic cavity. The biopsy forceps is placed against the fetus, preferably over the thorax, back, or buttocks, and a skin biopsy is taken (Fig. 13–6); each biopsy specimen is approximately 1 × 1 mm

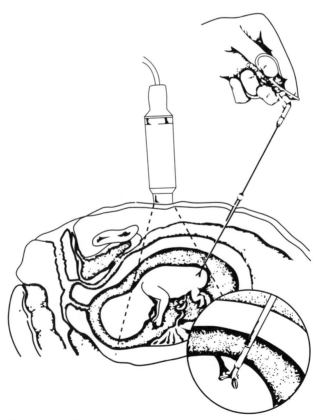

FIGURE 13–6 • Fetal skin sampling. (From Elias S, Emerson DS, Simpson JL, et al.: Ultrasound-guided fetal skin sampling for prenatal diagnosis of genodermatoses. Obstet Gynecol 83:337, 1994, with permission.)

in size. The umbilical cord insertion site, external genitalia, and head and neck region are avoided. Multiple biopsies (two to five) are taken to increase the probability of sampling an affected area of fetal skin.

When the procedure is completed, the cannula is removed and direct pressure is applied over the uterine insertion site for several minutes to help secure hemostasis. Women at risk for Rh immunization receive 300 µg of Rh-immune globulin. Maternal vital signs and fetal heart rate are monitored for about 1 hour postoperatively. Patients are instructed not to engage in strenuous activity (e.g., jogging) for several days after the procedure.

SAFETY

Far too few fetal skin sampling procedures are performed in the fashion described above to draw any firm conclusions with respect to their safety compared with that of the fetoscopy method. We reported 17 ultrasound-guided fetal skin sampling procedures (Elias et al., 1994). In five cases, a fetal skin disorder was diagnosed, and the pregnancies were terminated. In the remaining 12 cases all infants were delivered without complications at 37 weeks' gestation or later. Superficial scarring of the infant's skin has occasionally been noted after the use of biopsy forceps.

Fetal Liver Biopsy

Like skin biopsies, fetal liver biopsy for prenatal genetic diagnosis has now been supplanted by DNA-based analysis. However, fetal liver biopsy may rarely still be necessary to diagnose inborn errors of metabolism limited to liver parenchymal enzyme abnormalities not currently amenable to DNA analysis. Ornithine transcarbamylase deficiency, the most common enzyme defect in the urea cycle and an X-linked recessive disorder (Holzgreve and Golbus, 1984), was initially the disorder most frequently diagnosed by fetal liver biopsy. DNA mutations in the ornithine transcarbamylase gene (Rozen et al., 1985; Nussbaum et al., 1986) should now permit prenatal diagnosis to be performed by DNA analysis of any fetal nucleated cell (amniotic fluid cells, chorionic villi). Fetal liver biopsy may still be needed in families uninformative for a mutation. In addition to ornithine transcarbamylase deficiency, fetal live biopsy has been utilized in the diagnosis of glucose-6-phosphatase deficiency, glycogen storage disease type IA, nonketotic hyperglycemia, car-

bamoyl-phosphate synthetase deficiency, and primary hyperoxaluria type 1 (Golbus et al., 1988a, b; Piceni-Sereni et al., 1988; Illum et al., 1992; Murotsuki et al., 1994). DNA diagnoses of these disorders using chorionic villi or amniotic fluid cells are now usually possible (Qu et al., 1996; Wong, 1996).

TECHNIQUES

Fetal liver biopsy is best performed between 17 and 20 weeks' gestation. The preliminary ultrasound evaluation and maternal preparation are the same as for fetal skin sampling (see above). A disposable, thin-walled, 16.5-gauge biopsy needle (e.g., Becton-Dickinson, Rutherford, NJ) is then introduced into the amniotic cavity under continuous ultrasound guidance. The biopsy needle is ultrasonographically directed under the right costal margin of the fetus. Once the needle is within the liver parenchyma, a syringe (10 or 20 mL) is attached to exert continuous negative pressure; a fetal liver specimen is recovered from the needle and syringe by flushing with saline. An ultrasound examination is performed immediately following the procedure to assess fetal viability; maternal vital signs should be monitored. In Rh-negative unsensitized women, 300 µg Rh-immune globulin is given postoperatively. Postoperatively the patient should avoid strenuous activity for several days.

SAFETY

Only about two dozen fetal liver biopsies have been performed. There were no fetal losses, but the investigational nature of this procedure should be emphasized. Potential complications include (1) spontaneous abortion; (2) fetal or maternal hemorrhage; (3) fetal injury; (4) maternal infection; (5) leakage of fluid; (6) premature delivery; and (7) inability to obtain accurate prenatal diagnostic results either by failure to recover fetal liver or by inaccuracies in enzyme assays.

Fetal Muscle Sampling

Prenatal diagnosis of Becker-Duchenne muscular dystrophy is usually possible by DNA analysis using chorionic villi or amniotic fluid cells. However, in a few families homozgosity for all readily available polymorphic DNA variants precludes a DNA-based diagnosis. In these cases fetal muscle biopsies may be necessary, employing immunohistochemical analysis with a fluorescent antidystrophin antibody (Nevo et al., 1999). Males with Becker-Duchenne muscular dystrophy lack dystrophin staining, whereas muscle biopsies from unaffected male fetuses show abundant dystrophin.

TECHNIQUE

Fetal muscle sampling is usually performed at around 18 weeks' gestation using a technique analogous to that for fetal sampling or fetal liver sampling. Under direct ultrasound guidance, a Klear Kut (Baxter, Los Angeles, CA) kidney forceps gun can be inserted percutaneously into the uterine cavity. The instrument is directed toward the fetal buttock, and muscle biopsies are taken from the gluteal region.

SAFETY

Very few fetal muscle sampling procedures have been reported (Gustavii et al., 1983; Evans et al., 1991, 1994, 1995; Nevo et al., 1999); thus, definitive statements cannot be made concerning the safety of this procedure. Evans and colleagues (1994) reported the combined experience from the two centers and one reference laboratory in ten cases at risk for Duchenne muscular dystrophy, one for Becker muscular dystrophy and one for mitochondrial myopathy. Samples were obtained in 11 of 12 (92%) cases; spontaneous abortion occurred after the procedure in 2 of the 12 (17%) cases.

Embryoscopy

Embryoscopy is a relatively new and investigational technique that allows direct visualization of the fetus as early as the first trimester (Reece, 1992; Reece et al., 1997). Initially, a rigid fiberoptic endoscope was passed transcervically into the extracoelomic cavity, permitting inspection of fetal anatomic structures; fetal blood sampling was also feasible by this method (Reece, 1997). However, improvements and advancements in fiberoptic technology have led to the performance of thin-gauge transabdominal and transcervical embryoscopy (Quintero et al., 1993; Ville et al., 1997), allowing visualization as early as 4 weeks after conception (Reece, 1999).

This technique allows inspection of fetal anatomic structures. For example, Dommergues and coworkers (1995) used embryoscopy to diagnose fetal van der Woude syndrome (lip-pit syndrome) at 11 weeks' gestation. Fetal blood sampling and fetal cystoscopy and endoscopic fulguration of posterior urethral valves have also been reported (Quintero et al., 1995; Reece et al., 1995).

The initial procedures of embryoscopy were performed only on women who had elected pregnancy termination; however, embryoscopy has since been performed on those with continuing pregnancies (Reece et al., 1997; Ville et al., 1997). Ville and colleagues reported a procedure-related loss rate of 12% when the procedure was performed in the first trimester. Embryoscopy has also been used to detect neural tube defects in missed abortions, which may be helpful in genetic counseling for future pregnancies (Philipp and Kalousek, 2002).

Further studies of the safety, accuracy, and applications of this new modality are needed before embryoscopy is used as a routine prenatal diagnostic tool. However, the ability to access the embryonic circulation may have important applications for therapeutic interventions such as drugs and gene and cell therapy.

Other Fetal Tissue Sampling Techniques

COELOCENTESIS

Jurkovic and coworkers (1993) reported a technique called coelocentesis, performed between 6 and 12 weeks' gestation. A 20-gauge needle is introduced transvaginally into the coelomic cavity under continuous ultrasound monitoring, and fluid is aspirated. Among 100 women undergoing termination of pregnancy, coelomic fluid was successfully aspirated in 96%. Metaphase analysis is not possible with coelomic fluid, but fluorescence in situ hybridization (FISH) and polymerase chain reaction (PCR) can be performed. Later, this same group showed that these techniques could also be used for prenatal detection of sickle cell disease (Jurkovic et al., 1995). No continuing pregnancies in humans have been reported following coelocentesis.

Of interest is the work of Santolya-Forgas and colleagues. This group has investigated coelocentesis in baboons to determine its potential applicability for fetal therapy. In one series, coelocentesis was performed in 9 baboons; fluid aspiration (1 to 5 mL) was successful in eight cases and seven of the eight pregnancies were continuing 140 days after the procedure (Santolya-Forgas et al., 1998a). Coelocentesis was subsequently performed in six other baboons; assessment of the extracoelomic fluid osmometry and electrolyte composition in these six samples revealed that the chorion behaves as a semipermeable membrane at 40 days' gestation (Santolaya-Forgas et al., 1998b), suggesting that it may be useful for maternal-fetal transfer of some substances that could be used for fetal therapy.

Endocervical Sampling

Kingdom and associates (1995) described two methods for collecting trophoblasts from the endocervical canal: lavage with sterile physiologic saline and endocervical passage of a cytobrush. In 22 cases prior to pregnancy termination these techniques were shown to be efficacious in obtaining cells from fetal sex determination by FISH and PCR. The authors concluded that both methods are potentially suitable for molecular prenatal diagnosis. Cirigliano and coworkers (1999a) used endocervical fetal cell aspiration in ten women prior to CVS. In each case both parents were carriers for hemoglobinopathies (thalassemia or HbS). Fluorescent PCR analysis of trophoblast clumps allowed detection of the possibility that sperm contaminating the specimen could be a major limiting factor in the application of such techniques in clinical practice.

Ultrasonography

Ultrasonography is obviously pivotal for prenatal genetic diagnosis and detection of fetal malformations. Volumes on indications and techniques are available and need not be reported here. Of relevance is evidence that ultrasound is safe. At intensities usually produced by diagnostic equipment, ultrasound has not been found to cause any harmful effects on operators, pregnant women, fetuses, or other patients (Stark et al., 1984; Lyons et al., 1988; American Institute of Ultrasound in Medicine, 1993).

How accurate is ultrasound for anomaly assessment? Many major and even some minor fetal structural anomalies can be detected. It is unrealistic, however, to expect 100% accuracy in detecting fetal anomalies, even with the most expert and thorough scanning. Some anomalies are more readily diagnosed than others. Anencephaly and marked hydrocephaly are rarely misdiagnosed, whereas others are more difficult—cardiac defects, facial clefts, diaphragmatic hernias, skeletal abnormalities, and small neural tube defects (ACOG Technical Bulletin No. 187, 1993).

Accuracy of diagnosis of fetal anomalies reflects the experience of the sonographer, equipment, available gestational age at time of scanning, and the *a priori* risk of the abnormality in question (Sabbagha, 1993). Limitations of diagnostic ultrasonography must be recognized and discussed. For example, Platt and colleagues (1992) reviewed the ultrasound findings in 161 fetuses with spina bifida identified in the California maternal serum AFP scanning program, a program in which only regional referral centers performed the ultrasound. Before information regarding elevated maternal serum AFP levels was made available to the examiner, spina bifida was not initially visualized in 13 of the 161 cases. Subsequently, the defect was found in 10 of the 13 fetuses; in the remaining 3 cases, amniocentesis was declined, and the spina bifida was only diagnosed at birth. Not only is accuracy with ultrasound not 100%, or close, but it is inappropriate for a given unit to make claims about diagnostic accuracy unless they have analyzed their own experience. Data concerning the sensitivity, specificity, and predictive values of diagnostic ultrasound are usually not available (Philip, 1993).

Should ultrasound screening of all obstetric patients for prenatal diagnosis of structural birth defects be routine? The rationale for such a policy would be to allow couples the option of pregnancy termination for lethal or severely handicapping disorders and possibly to improve the chances of survival for infants with life-threatening but treatable conditions by delivery in a tertiary center. These issues were addressed in the well-cited RADIUS study, *Routine Antenatal Diagnostic Imaging with Ultrasound Study* (Crane et al., 1994). Utilizing several referral sites, low-risk pregnant women with no indication for ultrasonography were randomly assigned to have either two ultrasound scans (15 to 22 weeks' gestation plus 31 to 35 weeks) or the conventional obstetric care with ultrasonography performed only as determined by the clinical judgment of the patient's physician. Major congenital anomalies occurred in 2.3% of the 15,281 all fetuses and infants in the study. Antenatal ultrasonography detected 35% of the anomalous fetuses in the screened group versus only 11% of the control population (relative detection rate 3.1%, CI 2.0 to 5.1). Surprisingly, however, ultrasonography did not significantly influence the management or outcome of pregnancies complicated by fetuses with congenital malformations. Moreover, ultrasonography screening had no significant impact on survival rates among infants with potentially treatable, life-threatening anomalies despite the opportunity to take precautionary measures such as delivery in a tertiary center. It was estimated that a public health policy of routine ultrasonographic screening would increase U.S. health care costs by at least $500 million. This study concluded that "given this extraordinary cost and the lack of measurable benefit, ultrasonographic screening for fetal anomaly detection cannot be justified." The RADIUS study also provided some insight into the content and limitations of obstetric ultrasound examinations. For example, a four-chamber view of the heart allowed detection of only 43% of fetuses with complex heart disease, and only 30% of fetuses with cleft lip and palate were detected.

Many groups and centers have re-evaluated the RADIUS finding as well as their own experience and have come to the opposite conclusion. DeVore (1994) concluded that the RADIUS study actually demonstrated that second-trimester ultrasonography could be provided in a cost-effective fashion to low-risk pregnant women. Skupski and colleagues (1996) reported on their experience with ultrasound in a low-risk population and found that the detection of major and minor malformations had a profoundly positive impact. The Eurofetus Study (Grandjean et al., 1999) combined the ultrasound and clinical outcomes of 61 European centers over a three-year period and found that systematic ultrasound pregnancy detected a large proportion of fetal malformations. Providing ultrasonographic services to all women regardless of risk will continue to be a controversial issue.

The other new application of ultrasound that may have a considerable effect on prenatal diagnosis is three-dimensional and four-dimensional ultrasonography. The investigational technology has been introduced for use in selected centers for only the past 2 to 3 years. Reports from individual centers have demonstrated the potential positive impact of three- and four-dimensional ultrasonography on the ability to detect major and minor malformations in all three trimesters of pregnancy (Hata et al., 1998a; Platt et al., 1998; Chung et al., 2000; Lai et al., 2000), especially with regard to the fetal face (Hata et al., 1998b), heart (Sklansky et al., 1999), and skeleton (Yanagihara and Hata, 2000). Although three- and four-dimensional ultrasonography shows promise in improving our ability to diagnose fetal abnormalities prenatally, further and considerable study is needed not only to assess the sensitivity and specificity of this technology but also to evaluate the feasibility and cost-effectiveness of using this diagnostic tool in high and low-risk populations.

Detection of Down Syndrome by Ultrasound

SECOND TRIMESTER

In 1987, Benacerraf and colleagues (1987) reported that fetuses with Down syndrome are more likely than normal fetuses to have a thickened nuchal skin fold (≥ 6 mm) and relatively short femurs (ratio to actual expected femur length of 0.91) on ultrasound examination in the second trimester. Among more than 5500 fetuses evaluated, 28 were later shown to have Down syndrome; the sensitivity (detection rate) was 75% with a specificity of 98%. When other anomalies were added to these two criteria (e.g., atrioventricular canal, meconium peritonitis), sensitivity rose to 82%. Although these ultrasound "markers" for fetal Down syndrome have been confirmed by others, such correlations have not been universally observed (LaFollette et al., 1989; Biagiotti et al., 1994; Campbell et al., 1994; Donnenfeld et al., 1994; Watson et al., 1994; Grandjean et al., 1995; Johnson et al., 1995). In a meta-analysis of 10 studies, Vintzileos and Egan (1995) suggested that ultrasound markers for trisomy 21 can be used by experienced ultrasonographers to modify Down syndrome risk in both high- and low-risk pregnancies. However, Palomaki and Haddow (1995) suggested that this recommendation may be premature because (1) statistical methods for combining studies were inappropriate, (2) analysis was inappropriate because of unexplained heterogeneity, and (3) most studies dealt with high-risk pregnancies but conclusions were applied to low-risk populations. Thus, second-trimester ultrasound should not supplement maternal serum analyte screening (see Chapter 14) or invasive diagnostic procedure. Smith-Bindman and coworkers (2001) performed a meta-analysis of 56 articles using second-trimester ultrasound to detect Down syndrome. Markers evaluated included echogenic bowel, femur or humeral shortening, nuchal thickening, renal pyelectasis, echogenic bowel, and echogenic cardiac focus. Except for nuchal thickening, sensitivity for these markers was low (1 to 16%) in the absence of overt anomalies. Nuchal fold thickening showed by far the greatest sensitivity of second-trimester markers, but only a minority of fetuses showed this. Meta-analysis may or may not be appropriate in assessing ultrasound sensitivities, given differences in equipment and sonographers. However, conclusions were consistent with those of most individual reports. Particular caution needs to be raised about applying ultrasonographically based risk modification to pregnancies with high *a priori* risk for Down syndromes; if correction means avoiding an invasive test, women reclassified as low risk would help reduce the false-positive rate, but the detection rate would also fall by an undefined amount. The latter is probably of most importance to patients.

FIRST TRIMESTER

First-trimester ultrasonography seems more promising. In 1994, Nicolaides and colleagues (1994b) proposed a new method of screening for fetal trisomies based on the combination of maternal age and nuchal translucency (NT) thickness at 10 to 13 weeks' gestation (Fig. 13–7). The first study consisted of 1273 women with singleton pregnancies undergoing first-trimester cytogenetic studies because of advanced maternal age, parental anxiety, or family history of numerical chromosomal abnormalities. Estimates of maternal age-related risks for trisomy 21, 18, and 13 at this gestation were used to derive expected incidence of these trisomies with NT of ≥3 mm; the ratio of observed to expected number of cases was calculated. NT was ≥3 mm in 86% of all three trisomies (n = 36), in 85% of trisomy 21 fetuses (n = 25), and in 4.5% of the chromosomally normal fetuses. It could be predicted that a policy of offering fetal karyotyping to women younger than 40 years old could potentially identify more than 85% of trisomy fetuses with a false-positive rate of approximately 5%.

In order to standardize this method, the Fetal Medicine Foundation in London, a registered charity, set up a comprehensive training, support, and audit program for the proper implementation of the 10 to 14 week scan (Snijders et al., 1996). By January 1996, 66,600 singleton pregnancies with live fetuses had been examined in 20 approved centers in Britain. The first 42,619 completed pregnancies included 147 with trisomy 21; using a cut-off risk of 1/300 estimated from the maternal age and NT thickness, the sensitivity for trisomy 21 was 84%. Data continue to be salutary, and many U.S. centers are now offering NT scanning.

In Chapter 14 we learn that the first-trimester screening for Down syndrome can also be accomplished by maternal serum markers, namely, pregnancy-associated placental protein A (PAPP-A), and the free β subunit of human chorionic gonadotropin (hCG). Serum screening can be combined with ultrasound measurement of NT into a single measure of risk and so achieve the best possible screening performance (Wald et al., 1998; Spencer et al., 1999; Bahado-Singh et al., 2000). If NT, PAPP-A, and β-hCG are independent markers of Down syndrome, using both serum screening and NT will increase the detection rate to 91%. The real benefit of combining the two modalities would be in reducing the false-positive rate (Schuster et al., 2002). If the detection rate is expected to be 80%, the false-positive rate would be predicted to decline from 3 to 1.2%, a 50% reduction in the number of false-positives for Down syndrome (Wald et al., 1998).

Currently, two major trials are under way. These should help clarify the role of first-trimester screening in clinical practice. The SURUSS (Serum Urine and Ultrasound Screening Study) trial in the United Kingdom is funded by the Medical

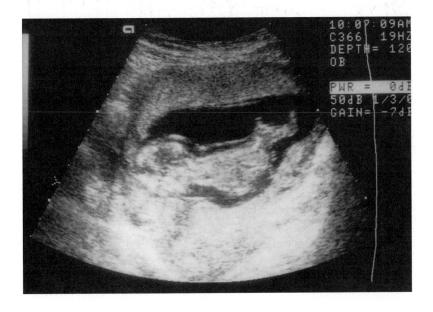

FIGURE 13–7 • Ultrasound at 12 weeks' gestation showing nuchal translucency thickness of 5.0 mm in the fetus with trisomy 21. (Courtesy of Isabelle Wilkins, MD.)

Research Council. A North American Study trial—FASTER (First and Second Trimester Evaluation for Risk of Aneuploidy)—is funded by the National Institute of Child Health and Human Development. Until the results of these major multicenter trials are available, Malone and coworkers (2000) believe that first-trimester methods of screening for aneuploidy should be considered investigational and should not be accepted as an alternative to second-trimester serum screening as the current standard of care. However, the promising results of Krantz and colleagues (2000) (see Chapter 16), indicate that centers with the requisite ability to perform ultrasound and assays can offer first-trimester screening confident of 80–85% sensitivity.

REFERENCES

ACOG Committee Opinion No. 160, October 1995 Chorionic Villus Sampling. Washington DC 20024–2188: The American College of Obstetricians and Gynecologists.

ACOG Technical Bulletin, No. 187, December 1993 Ultrasonography in Pregnancy. Washington DC 20024–2188: The American College of Obstetricians and Gynecologists.

ACOG Practice Bulletin, No. 4, 1999 Prevention of RhD Isoimmunization. Washington DC 20024–2188: American College of Obstetricians and Gynecologists.

ACOG Pratice Bulletin, No. 27, May 2001 Prenatal diagnosis of fetal chromosomal abnormalities. Washington DC 20024–2188: American College of Obstetricians and Gynecologists.

American Institute of Ultrasound in Medicine. Bioeffects and safety of diagnostic ultrasound. Rockville, MD: AIUM, 1993.

Anderson RL, Goldberg JD, Golbus MS: Prenatal diagnosis in multiple gestations: 20 years's experience with amniocentesis. Prenat Diagn 11:263, 1991.

Anton-Lamprecht I: Genetically induced abnormalities of epidermal differentiation and ultra-structure in ichthyoses and epidermolyses: Pathogenesis, heterogeneity, fetal manifestation and prenatal diagnosis. J Invest Dermatol 81: 149A, 1983.

Anton-Lamprecht I, Rauskolb R, Jovanovic V, et al.: Prenatal diagnosis of epidermolysis bullosa dystrophica Hallopeau-Siemens with electron microscopy of fetal skin. Lancet 2:1077, 1981.

Antsaklis A, Daskalakis G, Papantoniou N, et al.: Fetal blood sampling-indication-related losses. Prenat Diagn 18:934, 1998.

Arnold ML, Rauskolb R, Anton-Lamprecht I, et al.: Prenatal diagnosis of anhidrotic ectodermal dysplasia. Prenat Diagn 4:85, 1984.

Assel BG, Lewis SM, Dickerman LH, et al.: Single-operator comparison of early and midsecond trimester amniocentesis. Obstet Gynecol 79:940, 1992.

Bahado-Singh RO, Morotti R, Pirhonen J, et al.: Invasive techniques for prenatal diagnosis: Current concepts. J Assoc Acad Minor Phys 6:28, 1995.

Bahado-Singh RO, Oz AU, Gomez K, et al.: Combined ultrasound biometry, serum markers and age for Down syndrome risk estimation. Ultrasound Obstet Gynecol 15:199, 2000.

Baird PA, Yee IM, Sadovnick AD: Population-based study on long-term outcomes after amniocentesis. Lancet 344:1134, 1994.

Bellini P, Marinetti E, Arreghini A, et al.: Treatment of maternal hyperthyroidism and fetal goiter. Minerva Ginecol 52:25, 2000.

Benacerraf BR, Gelman R, Frigoletto FD Jr: Sonographic identification of second-trimester fetuses with Down's syndrome. N Engl J Med 317:1371, 1987.

Biagiotti R, Periti E, Cariati E: Humerus and femur length in fetuses with Down syndrome. Prenat Diagn 14:429, 1994.

Blanchet-Bardon C, Dumez Y, Labbe F, et al.: Prenatal diagnosis of harlequin fetus (letter). Lancet 1:132, 1983.

Boute O, Depret-Mosser S, Vinatier D, et al.: Prenatal diagnosis of thrombocytopenia-absent radius syndrome. Fetal Diagn Ther 11:224, 1996.

Brambati B, Lanzani A, Tului L: Transabdominal and transcervial chorionic villus sampling: Efficiency and risk evaluation of 2,411 cases. Am J Med Genet 35:160, 1990.

Bravo RR, Shulman LP, Phillips OP, et al.: Transplacental needle passage in early amniocentesis and pregnancy loss. Obstet Gynecol 86:437, 1995.

Brumfield CG, Lin S, Conner W, et al.: Pregnancy outcome following genetic amniocentesis at 11–14 versus 16–19 weeks' gestation. Obstet Gynecol 88:114, 1996.

Burton BK, Schulz CJ, Burd LI: Limb anomalies associated with chorionic villus sampling. Obstet Gynecol 79:726, 1992.

Buscaglia M, Ghisoni L, Bellotti M, et al.: Genetic amniocentesis in biamniotic twin pregnancies by a single transabdominal insertion of the needle. Prenat Diagn 15:17, 1995.

Buscaglia M, Ghisoni L, Levi-Setti PE: Alpha-fetoprotein elevation in maternal serum after percutaneous umbilical blood sampling (PUBS). Prenat Diagn 16:375, 1996.

Bussel JB, Berkowitz RL, McFarland JG, et al.: Antenatal treatment of neonatal alloimmune thrombocytopenia. N Engl J Med 319:1374, 1988.

Byrne DL, Penna L, Marks K, et al.: First trimester amnifiltration: Technical, cytogenetic and pregnancy outcome of 104 consecutive procedures. Br J Obstet Gynaecol 102:220, 1995.

Campbell WA, Vintzileos AM, Rodis JF, et al.: Efficacy of the biparietal diameter/femur length ratio to detect Down syndrome in patients with an abnormal biochemical screen. Fetal Diagn Therapy 9:175, 1994.

Carroll SG, Davies T, Kyle PM, et al.: Fetal karyotyping by chorionic villus sampling after the first trimester. Br J Obstet Gynaecol 106:1035, 1999.

Canadian Collaborative CVS-Amniocentesis Clinical Trial Group: Multicentre randomized clinical trial of chorion villus sampling. Lancet 337:1491, 1991.

CEMAT Group: Randomized trial to assess safety and fetal outcome of early and midtrimester amniocentesis. The Canadian Early and Mid-Trimester Amniocentesis Trial (CEMAT) Group. Lancet 351:242, 1998.

Chinnaiya A, Venkat A, Dawn C, et al.: Intrahepatic vein fetal blood sampling: Current role in prenatal diagnosis. J Obstet Gynaecol Res 24:239, 1998.

Cirigliano V, Sherlock J, Petrou M, et al.: Transcervical cells and the prenatal diagnosis of haemoglobin (Hb) mutations. Clin Genet 56:357, 1999.

Chung BL, Kim HJ, Lee KH: The application of three-dimensional ultrasound to nuchal translucency measurement in early pregnancy (10–14 weeks): A preliminary study. Ultrasound Obstet Gynecol 15:122, 2000.

Claussen U, Voigt HJ, Ulmer R, et al.: Rapid karyotyping in the 2nd and 3rd trimester; results and experiences. Geburtshilfe Frauenheilkd 55:41, 1995.

Crandall BF, Kulch P, Tabsh K: Risk assessment of amniocentesis between 11 and 15 weeks: Comparison to later amniocentesis controls. Prenat Diagn 14:913, 1994.

Crandall BF, Hanson FW, Tennant F: Acetylcholinesterase (AchE) electrophoresis and early amniocenteses. Am J Hum Genet 45:A257, 1989.

Crandall BF, Chua C: Detecting neural tube defects by amniocentesis between 11 and 15 weeks' gestation. Prenat Diagn 15:339, 1995.

Crane JP, LeFevre ML, Winborn RC, et al.: A randomized trial of prenatal ultrasonographic screening: Impact on the detection, management, and outcome of anomalous fetuses. Am J Obstet Gynecol 171:392, 1994.

Daffos F: Fetal blood sampling. Annu Rev Med 40:319, 1989.

Daffos F, Forestier F, Capella-Pavlovsky M, et al.: Prenatal management of 746 pregnancies at risk for congenital toxoplasmosis. N Engl J Med 318:271, 1988.

DeVore GR: The routine antenatal diagnostic imaging with ultrasound study: Another perspective. Obstet Gynecol 84:622, 1994.

Diukman R, Tanigawara S, Cowan MJ, et al.: Prenatal diagnosis of Chédiak-Higashi syndrome. Prenat Diagn 12:877, 1992.

Djalali M, Barbi G, Kennerknecht I, et al.: Introduction of early amniocentesis to routine prenatal diagnosis. Prenat Diagn 12:661, 1992.

Dolk H, Bertrand F, Lechat MF (Eurocat): Chorionic villus sampling and limb abnormalities. The EUROCAT Working Group. Lancet 339:876, 1992.

Dommergues M, Lemerrer M, Couly G, et al.: Prenatal diagnosis of cleft lip and 11 menstrual weeks using embryoscopy in the van der Woude syndrome. Prenat Diagn 15:378, 1995.

Donnenfeld AE, Carlson DE, Palomaki GE, et al.: Prospective multicenter study of second trimester nuchal skinfold thickness in unaffected and Down syndrome pregnancies. Obstet Gynecol 84:844, 1994.

Donnenfeld AE, Wiseman B, Lavi E, et al.: Prenatal diagnosis of thrombocytopenia absent radius syndrome by ultrasound and cordocentesis. Prenat Diagn 10:29, 1990.

Donner C, Rypens F, Paquet V, et al.: Cordocentesis for rapid karyotype: 421 consecutive cases. Fetal Diagn Ther 10:192, 1995.

Durandy A, Dumez Y, Guy-Grand D, et al.: Prenatal diagnosis of severe combined immunodeficiency. J Pediatr 101:995, 1982.

Eiben B, Goebel R, Rutt G, et al.: Early amniocentesis between 12th–14th week of pregnancy. Clinical experience with 1,100 cases. Geburtshilfe-Frauenheilkd 53:554, 1993.

Elejalde BR, de Elejalde MM, Acuna JM: Prospective study of amniocentesis performed between weeks 9 and 16 gestation: Its feasibility, risks, complications and use in early genetic prenatal diagnosis. Am J Med Genet 35:188, 1990.

Elias S, Emerson DS, Simpson JL, et al.: Ultrasound-guided fetal skin sampling for prenatal diagnosis of genodermatoses. Obstet Gynecol 83:337, 1994.

Elias S, Martin AO, Patel VA, et al.: Analysis for amniotic fluid crystallization in second-trimester amniocentesis. Am J Obstet Gynecol 133:401, 1979.

Elias S, Simpson JL, Martin AO, et al.: Chorionic villus sampling for first trimester prenatal diagnosis: Northwestern University Program. Am J Obstet Gynecol 152:204, 1985.

Elias S, Esterly NB: Prenatal diagnosis of hereditary skin disorders. Clin Obstet Gynecol 24:1069, 1981.

Elias S: The role of fetoscopy in antenatal diagnosis. Clin Obstet Gynaecol 7:73, 1980.

Elias S, Mazur M, Sabbagha R, et al.: Prenatal diagnosis of harlequin ichthyosis. Clin Genet 17:275, 1980b.

Elias S, Gerbie AB, Simpson JL, et al.: Genetic amniocentesis in twin gestations. Am J Obstet Gynecol 138:169, 1980a.

Elliott JP, Foley MR, Finberg HJ: In utero fetal cardiac resuscitation: A case report. Fetal Diagn Ther 9:226, 1994.

Evans MI, Greb A, Kunkel LM, et al.: In utero fetal muscle biopsy for the diagnosis of Duchenne muscular dystrophy. Am J Obstet Gynecol 165:728, 1991.

Evans MI, Krivchenia EL, Johnson MP, et al.: In utero fetal muscle biopsy alters diagnosis and carrier risks in Duchenne and Becker muscular dystrophy. Fetal Diagn Ther 10:71, 1995.

Evans MI, Hoffman EP, Cadrin C, et al.: Fetal muscle biopsy: Collaborative experience with varied indications. Obstet Gynecol 84:913, 1994.

Firth HV, Boyd PA, Chamberlain PF, et al.: Analysis of limb reduction defects in babies exposed to chorionic villus sampling. Lancet 343:1069, 1994.

Firth HV, Boyd PA, Chamberlain P, et al.: Severe limb abnormalities after chorion villus sampling at 55-66 days' gestation. Lancet 337:762, 1991a.

Firth HV, Boyd PA, Chamberlain P, et al.: Limb abnormalities and chorion villus sampling. Lancet 338:51, 1991b.

Forestier F, Cox WL, Daffos F, et al.: The assessment of fetal blood sample. Am J Obstet Gynecol 158:1184, 1988.

Froster-Iskenius UG, Baird PA: Limb reduction defects in over one million consecutive live births. Teratology 39:127, 1989.

Froster UG, Jackson L: Safety of chorionic villus sampling: Limb defects and chorionic villus sampling: Results from an international registry (1992 to 1994). Lancet 347:489, 1996.

Fuchs F, Riis P: Antenatal sex determination. Nature 117:330, 1956.

Ghidini A, Lynch L, Hicks C, et al.: The risk of second trimester amniocentesis in twin gestations: A case-control study. Am J Obstet Gynecol 169:1013, 1993a.

Ghidini A, Sepulveda W, Lockwood CJ, et al.: Complications of fetal blood sampling. Am J Obstet Gynecol 168:1339, 1993b.

Gilgenkrantz S, Blanchet-Bardon C, Nazzaro V, et al.: Hypohidrotic ectodermal dysplasia: Clinical study of a family of 30 over three generations. Hum Genet 81:120, 1989.

Gluer S: Intestinal atresia following intraamniotic use of dyes. Eur J Pediatr Surg 5:240, 1995.

Golbus MS: For the International Fetoscopy Group: Special report: The status of fetoscopy and fetal tissue sampling. Prenat Diagn 4:79, 1984.

Golbus MS, Simpson JL, Fowler SE, et al.: Risk factors associated with transcervical CVS losses. Prenat Diagn 12:373, 1992.

Golbus MS, McGonigle KF, Goldberg JD, et al.: Fetal tissue sampling. The San Francisco experience with 190 pregnancies. West J Med 150:423, 1988a.

Golbus MS, Simpson TJ, Koresawa M, et al.: The prenatal determination of glucose 6-phosphatase activity by fetal liver biopsy. Prenat Diagn 8:401, 1988b.

Golbus MS, Sagebiel RW, Filly RA, et al.: Prenatal diagnosis of congenital bullous ichthyosiform erythroderma (epidermolytic hyperkeratosis) by fetal skin biopsy. N Engl J Med 302:93, 1980.

Gosden C, Nicholaides KH, Rodeck CH: Fetal blood sampling in investigation of chromosome mosaicism in amniotic fluid cell culture. Lancet 11:613, 1988.

Grandjean H, Sarramon MF: Sonographic measurement of nuchal skinfold thickness for detection of Down syndrome in the second-trimester fetus: A multicenter prospective study. The AFDPHE Study Group. Association Francaise pour le Depistage et la Prevention des Handicaps de l'Enfant. Obstet Gynecol 85:103, 1995.

Grandjean H, Larroque D, Levi S: The performance of routine ultrasonographic screening of pregnancies in the Eurofetus Study. Am J Obstet Gynecol 181:446, 1999.

Gustavii B, Lofberg L, Henriksson KG: Fetal muscle biopsy. Acta Obstet Gynecol Scand 62:369, 1983.

Hackett GA, Smith JH, Rebello MT, et al.: Early amniocentesis at 11-14 weeks' gestation for the diagnosis of fetal chromosomal abnormality—a clinical evaluation. Prenat Diagn 11:311, 1991.

Hanson FW, Tennant F, Hune S, et al.: Early amniocentesis: Outcome, risks and technical problems at less than or equal to 12.8 weeks. Am J Obstet Gynecol 166:1707, 1992.

Hata T, Manabe A, Aoki S, et al.: Three-dimensional intrauterine sonography in the early first trimester of pregnancy: Preliminary study. Hum Reprod 13:740, 1998a.

Hata T, Yonehara T, Aoki S, et al.: Three-dimensional sonographic visualization of the fetal face. Am J Roentgenol 170:481, 1998b.

Henry GP, Miller WA: Early amniocentesis. J Reprod Med 37:396, 1992.

Hess LW, Anderson RL, Golbus MS: Significance of opaque discolored amniotic fluid at second-trimester amniocentesis. Obstet Gynecol 67:44, 1986.

Hobbins JC, Mahoney MJ: In utero diagnosis of hemoglobinopathies: Technic for obtaining fetal blood. N Engl J Med 290:1065, 1974.

Holmberg L, Gustavii B, Jonsson A: A prenatal study of fetal platelet count and size with application to fetus at risk for Wiskott-Aldrich syndrome. J Pediatr 102:773, 1983.

Holzgreve W, Miny P, Basarans S, et al.: Safety of placental biopsy in the second and third trimesters. N Engl J Med 317:1159, 1987.

Holzgreve W, Golbus MS: Prenatal diagnosis of ornithine transcarbamylase deficiency utilizing fetal liver biopsy. Am J Hum Genet 36:320, 1984.

Hsieh F-J, Chen D, Tseng L-H, et al.: Limb-reduction defects and chorion villus sampling. Lancet 337:1091, 1991.

Hsieh F-J, Ko TM, Chang FM, et al.: Percutaneous ultrasound-guided fetal blood sampling. Lancet 337:1091, 1989.

Illum N, Lavard L, Danpure CJ, et al.: Primary hyperoxaluria type 1: Clinical manifestations in infancy and prenatal diagnosis. Child Nephrol Urol 12:225, 1992.

Isada NB, Koppitch FC III, Johnson MP, et al.: Does the color of amniotic fluid still matter? Fetal Diagn Ther 5:165, 1990.

Jackson LG, Zachary JM, Fowler SE, et al.: A randomized comparison of transcervical and transabdominal chorionic villus sampling. N Engl J Med 327:594, 1992.

Jackson LG, Wapner RJ, Brambai B: Limb abnormalities and chorionic villus sampling. Lancet 337:1423, 1991.

Johnson J, Wilson RD, Winsor EJ, et al.: The Early Amniocentesis Study: A randomized clinical trial of early amniocentesis versus midtrimester amniocentesis. Fetal Diagn Ther 11:85, 1996.

Johnson JM, Wilson RD, Singer J, et al.: Technical factors in early amniocentesis predict adverse outcome. Results of the Canadian Early (EA) versus Midtrimester (MA) Amniocentesis Trial. Prenat Diagn 19:732, 1999.

Johnson MP, Michaelson JE, Barr M Jr, et al.: Combining humerus and femur length for improved ultrasonographic identification of pregnancies at increased risk for trisomy 21. Am J Obstet Gynecol 172:1229, 1995.

Jurkovic D, Kurjak A: Prenatal diagnosis of hereditary epidermolysis bullosa using ultrasonically guided biopsy of the fetal skin. Lijec Vjesn 111:60, 1989.

Jurkovic D, Jauniaux E, Campbell S, et al.: Coelocentesis: A new technique for early prenatal diagnosis. Lancet 341:1623, 1993.

Jurkovic D, Jauniaux E, Campbell S, et al.: Detection of sickle gene by coelocentesis in early pregnancy: A new approach to prenatal diagnosis of single gene disorders. Hum Reprod 10:1287, 1995.

Karp LE, Schiller HS: Meconium staining of amniotic fluid at mid-trimester amniocentesis. Obstet Gynecol 50:47s, 1977.

Kennerknecht I, Kramer S, Grab D, et al.: Evaluation of amniotic fluid cell filtration: An experimental approach to early amniocentesis. Prenat Diagn 13:247, 1993.

Kerber S, Held KR: Early genetic amniocentesis—4 years' experience. Prenat Diagn 13:21, 1993.

Kingdom J, Sherlock J, Rodeck C, et al.: Detection of trophoblast cells in transcervical samples collected by lavage or cytobrush. Obstet Gynecol 86:283, 1995.

Kornfeld I, Wilson RD, Ballem P, et al.: Antenatal invasive and noninvasive management of alloimmune thrombocytopenia. Fetal Diagn Ther 11:210, 1996.

Kousseff BG, Matsuoka LY, Stenn KS, et al.: Prenatal diagnosis of Sjogren-Larsson syndrome. J Pediatr 101:998, 1982.

Krantz DA, Hallahan TW, Orlandi F, et al.: First-trimester Down syndrome screening using dried blood biochemistry and nuchal translucency. Obstet Gynecol 96:207, 2000.

Kuliev A, Jackson L, Froster UG, et al.: Chorionic villus sampling safety. Report of World Health Organization/EURO meeting in association with the Seventh International Conference on Early Prenatal Diagnosis of Genetic Disease, Tel-Aviv, Israel, May 21, 1994. Am J Obstet Gynecol 174:807, 1996.

LaFollette L, Filly RA, Anderson R, et al.: Fetal femur length to detect trisomy 21. A reappraisal. J Ultrasound Med 8:657, 1989.

Lai TH, Chang CH, Yu CH, et al.: Prenatal diagnosis of alobar holoprosencephaly by two-dimensional and three-dimensional ultrasound. Prenat Diagn 20:400, 2000.

Lapidot-Lifson Y, Lebo RV, Flandermeyer RR, et al.: Rapid aneuploid diagnosis of high-risk fetuses by fluorescence in situ hybridization. Am J Obstet Gynecol 174:886, 1996.

Lecuru F, Bernard JP, Parrat S, et al.: Varicella in pregnancy. Presse Med 24:1352, 1995.

Lockwood DH, Neu RL: Cytogenetic analysis of 1375 amniotic fluid specimens from pregnancies with gestational age less than 14 weeks. Prenat Diagn 13:801, 1993.

Liou JD, Chen CP, Breg WR, et al.: Fetal blood sampling and cytogenetic abnormalities. Prenat Diagn 13:1, 1993.

Los FJ, Noomen P, Vermeij-Keers C, et al.: Chorionic villus sampling in materno-fetal transfusions: An immunological pathogenesis of vascular disruptive syndromes? Prenat Diagn 16:193, 1996.

Lyons EA, Dyke C, Toms M, et al.: In utero exposure to diagnostic ultrasound. A 6-year follow-up. Radiology 166:687, 1988.

MRC Working Party on the Evaluation of Chorionic Villus Sampling: Medical Research Council European Trial of Chorionic Villus Sampling. Lancet 337:1491, 1991.

Mahoney MJ, USNICHD collaborators: Limb abnormalities and chorionic villus sampling. Lancet 337:1422, 1991.

Malone FD, Berkowitz RL, Canick JA, et al.: First-trimester screening for aneuploidy: Research or standard of care? Am J Obstet Gynecol 182:490, 2000.

Mastroiacovo P, Botto LD: Chorionic villus sampling and limb deficiencies. Review of case control and cohort studies. In Zakut H (ed): Seventh International Conference on Early Prenatal Diagnosis of Genetic Disease. Jerusalem, Israel 22-27 May 1994, 1994, p 71.

Mastroiacovo P, Botto LD, Cavalcanti DP, et al.: Limb anomalies following chorionic villus sampling: A registry based case-control study. Am J Med Genet 44:856, 1992.

Mastroiacovo P, Cavalcanti DP: Limb reduction defects and chorion villus sampling. Lancet 337:1091, 1991.

McLennan AC, Chitty LS, Rissik J, et al.: Prenatal diagnosis of Blackfan-Diamond syndrome: Case report and review of the literature. Prenat Diagn 16:349, 1996.

Medical Research Council: Diagnosis of Genetic Disease by Amniocentesis During the Second Trimester of Pregnancy. Ottawa, Canada, 1977.

Milunsky A: The prenatal diagnosis of neural tube and other congenital defects. *In* Milunsky A (ed): Genetic Disorders and the Fetus. New York: Plenum Press, 1986, p 453.

Moise KJ, Deter RL, Kishorn B, et al.: Intravenous pancuronium bromide for fetal neuromuscular blockage during intrauterine transfusion for red cell alloimmunization. Obstet Gynecol 74:905, 1989.

Monni G, Ibba RM, Lai R, et al.: Limb-reduction effects and chorion villus sampling. Lancet 337:1091, 1991.

Murotsuki J, Uehara S, Okamura K, et al.: Fetal liver biopsy for prenatal diagnosis of carbamoyl phosphate synthetase deficiency. Am J Perinatol 11:160, 1994.

Nadler HL, Gerbie AB: Role of amniocentesis in the intrauterine detection of genetic disorders. N Engl J Med 282:596, 1970.

National Institute of Child Health and Human Development Consensus Conference on Antenatal Diagnosis December 1979, 1997 NIH Publication No. 80-1973, 1979.

National Institute of Child Health Development National Registry for Amniocentesis Study Group 1976. Midtrimester amniocentesis for prenatal diagnosis: safety and accuracy. JAMA 236:1471, 1976.

Nevo Y, Shomrat R, Yaron Y, et al.: Fetal muscle biopsy as a diagnostic tool in Duchenne muscular dystrophy. Prenat Diagn 19:921, 1999.

Newton ER: Diagnosis of perinatal TORCH infections. Clin Obstet Gynecol 42:59, 1999.

Nicolaides K, Brizot MD, Patel F, et al.: Comparison of chorionic villus sampling and amniocentesis for fetal karyotyping at 10-13 weeks gestation. Lancet 344:435, 1994a.

Nicolaides KH, Brizot MD, Snijders RJ: Fetal nuchal translucency: Ultrasound screening for fetal trisomy in the first trimester of pregnancy. Br J Obstet Gynaecol 101:782, 1994b.

Nicolaides KH, Thrope-Beeston JG, Noble P: Cordocentesis in assessment and care of the fetus. *In* Eden RD, Boehm FH (eds): Assessment and Care of the Fetus. Norwalk, CT: Appleton Lange, 1990, p 291.

Nicolaides KH, Clewell WH, Rodeck CH: Measurement of human fetoplacental blood volume in erythroblastosis fetalis. Am J Obstet Gynecol 157:50, 1987.

Nicolini U, Nicolaidis P, Fisk NM, et al.: Fetal blood sampling from the intrahepatic vein: Analysis of safety and clinical experience with 214 procedures. Obstet Gynecol 76:47, 1990.

Nicolini U, Kochenour NK, Greco P, et al.: Consequences of fetomaternal haemorrhage after intrauterine transfusion. BMJ 297:1379, 1988.

Nikkilä A, Valentin L, Thelan A: Early amniocentesis and congenital foot deformaties. Fetal Diagn Ther 17:129, 2002.

Nussbaum RL, Boggs BA, Beaudet AL, et al.: New mutation and prenatal diagnosis in ornithine transcarbamylase deficiency. Am J Hum Genet 38:149, 1986.

Olney RS, Khoury MJ, Alo CJ, et al.: Increased risk for transverse digital deficiency after chorionic villus sampling (CVS): Results of the United States Multistate Case-Control Study, 1988-1992. Teratology 51:20, 1995.

Orlandi F, Damiani G, Jakil C, et al.: The risks of early cordocentesis (12–21 weeks): Analysis of 500 procedures. Prenat Diagn 10:425, 1990.

Orlandi F, Damiani G, Jakil C, et al.: Clinical results and fetal biochemical data on 140 early second trimester diagnostic cordocentesis. Acta Eur Fertil 18:329, 1987.

Paidas MJ, Berkowitz RL, Lynch L, et al.: Alloimmune thrombocytopenia: Fetal and neonatal losses related to cordocentesis. Am J Obstet Gynecol 172:475, 1995.

Palomaki GE, Haddow JE: Can the risk for Down syndrome be reliably modified by second-trimester ultrasonography? Am J Obstet Gynecol 173:1639, 1995.

Penso CA, Sandstrom MM, Garber MF, et al.: Early amniocentesis: Report of 407 cases with neonatal follow-up. Obstet Gynecol 76:1032, 1990.

Pergament E, Schulman JD, Copeland K, et al.: The risk and efficacy of chorionic villus sampling in multiple gestations. Prenat Diagn 12:377, 1992.

Perry TB, Holbrook KA, Hoff MS, et al.: Prenatal diagnosis of congenital non-bullous ichthyosifrom erythroderma (lamellar ichthyosis). Prenat Diagn 7:145, 1987.

Peters MT, Nicolaides KH: Cordocentesis for the diagnosis and treatment of human fetal parvovirus infection. Obstet Gynecol 75:501, 1990.

Philip J: Sensitivity and specificity in ultrasonographic screening. *In* Simpson JL, Elias S (eds): Essentials of Prenatal Diagnosis. New York: Churchill Livingstone, 1993, p 1410.

Philipp T, Kalousek DK: Neural tube defects in missed abortions: embryoscopic and cytogenetic findings. Am J Med Genet 107:52, 2002.

Piceni-Sereni L, Bachman C, Pfister U, et al.: Prenatal diagnosis of carbamoyl-phosphate synthetase deficiency by fetal liver biopsy. Prenat Diagn 8:307, 1988.

Pierluigi M, Pefumo C, Cavani S, et al.: An improved method for the detection of Down's syndrome aneuploidy in uncultured amniocytes. Clin Genet 49:32, 1996.

Platt LD, Feuchtbaum L, Filly R, et al.: The California Maternal Serum Alpha-Fetoprotein Program: The role of ultrasonography in the detection of spina bifida. Am J Obstet Gynecol 166:1328, 1992.

Platt LD, Santulli T Jr, Carlson DE, et al.: Three dimensional ultrasonography in obstetrics and gynecoloogy: Preliminary experience. Am J Obstet Gynecol 178:1199, 1998.

Porreco RP, Harshbarger B, McGavran L: Rapid cytogenetic assessment of fetal blood samples. Obstet Gynecol 82:242, 1993.

Pruggmayer M, Baumann P, Schutte H, et al.: Incidence of abortion after genetic amniocentesis in twin pregnancies. Prenat Diagn 11:637, 1991.

Qu Y, Abdenur JE, Eng CM, et al.: Molecular prenatal diagnosis of glycogen storage disease type Ia. Prenat Diagn 16:333, 1996.

Quintero RA, Hume R, Smith C, et al.: Percutaneous fetal cystoscopy and endoscopic fulguration of posterior urethral valves. Am J Obstet Gynecol 172:206, 1995.

Quintero RA, Puder KS, Cotton DB: Embryoscopy and fetoscopy. Obstet Gynecol Clin North Am 20:563, 1993.

Reece EA: Embryoscopy: New developments in prenatal medicine. Curr Opin Obstet Gynecol 4:447, 1992.

Reece EA, Homko C, Goldstein I, et al.: Toward fetal therapy using needed embryofetoscopy. Ultrasound Obstet Gynecol 5:281, 1995.

Reece EA: First trimester prenatal diagnosis: Embryoscopy and fetoscopy. Semin Perinatol 23:424, 1999.

Reece EA, Homko CJ, Koch S, et al.: First-trimester needle embryofetoscopy and prenatal diagnosis. Fetal Diagn Ther 12:136, 1997.

Reece EA: Embryoscopy and early prenatal diagnosis. Obstet Gynecol Clin North Am 24:111, 1997.

Rhoads GG, Jackson LG, Schlesselman SE, et al.: The safety and efficacy of chorionic villus sampling for early prenatal diagnosis of cytogenetic abnormalities. N Engl J Med 320:609, 1989.

Rodeck CH, Nicolini U: Fetal blood sampling. Eur J Obstet Gynecol Reprod Biol 28:85, 1988.

Rodeck CH, Eady RAJ, Gosden CJ: Prenatal diagnosis of epidermolysis bullosa letalis. Lancet 1:949, 1980.

Rozen R, Fox J, Fenton WA, et al.: Gene deletion and restriction fragment length polymorphisms at the human ornithine transcarbamylase locus. Nature 313:815, 1985.

Ryan R, Rodeck CH: Fetal blood sampling. In Simpson JL, Elias S (eds): Essentials of Prenatal Diagnosis. New York: Churchill Livingstone, 1993, p 63.

Sabbagha RE: Ultrasound diagnosis of fetal structural anomalies. In Simpson JL, Elias S (eds): Essentials of Prenatal Diagnosis. New York: Churchill Livingstone, 1993, p 91.

Santolaya-Forgas J, Vengalil S, Kushwaha A, et al.: Assessment of the risk of fetal loss after coelocentesis procedure using a baboon model. Fetal Diagn Ther 13:257, 1998a.

Santolya-Forgas J, Duval J, Prespin C, et al.: Extracoelomic fluid osmometry and electrolyte composition during early gestation in the baboon. Am J Obstet Gynecol 179:1124, 1998b.

Schuster K, Hafner E, Stangl G: The first trimester 'combined test' for the detection of Down syndrome pregnancies in 4939 unselected pregnancies. Prenat Diagn 22:211, 2002.

Scott R: Limb abnormalities after chorionic villus sampling. Lancet 337:1038, 1991.

Shulman LP, Elias S, Phillips OP, et al.: Amniocentesis performed at 14 weeks' gestation or earlier: Comparison with first-trimester transabdominal chorionic villus sampling. Obstet Gynecol 83:543, 1994.

Shulman LP, Simpson JL, Elias S, et al.: Transvaginal chorionic villus sampling using transabdominal ultrasound guidance. A new technique for first-trimester prenatal diagnosis. Fetal Diagn Ther 8:144, 1993.

Sidransky E, Black SH, Soenksen DM, et al.: Transvaginal chorionic villus sampling. Prenat Diagn 10:583, 1990.

Simpson JL, Elias S: Techniques for prenatal diagnosis of genetic disorders. Reprod Genet 4:197, 1994.

Simpson NE, Dallaire L, Miller JR, et al.: Prenatal diagnosis of genetic disease in Canada: Report of a collaborative study. Can Med Assoc J 115:739, 1976.

Sklansky MS, Nelson T, Strachan M, et al.: Real-time three-dimensional fetal echocardiography: Initial feasibility study. J Ultrasound Med 18:745, 1999.

Skupski DW, Newman S, Edersheim T, et al.: The impact of routine obstetric ultrasonographic screening in a low-risk population. Am J Obstet Gynecol 175:1142, 1996.

Smidt-Jensen S, Permin M, Philip J, et al.: Randomized comparison of amniocentesis and transabdominal and transcervical chorionic villus sampling. Lancet 340:1237, 1992.

Smidt-Jensen S, Hahnemann N: Transabdominal fine needle biopsy from chorionic villi in the first trimester. Prenat Diagn 4:163, 1984.

Smith-Bindman R, Hosmer W, Feldstein VA, et al.: Second-trimester ultrasound to detect fetuses with Down syndrome: A meta-analysis. JAMA 285:1044, 2001.

Snijders RJ, Johnson S, Sebire NJ, et al.: First trimester ultrasound screening for chromosomal defects. Ultrasound Obstet Gynecol 7:216, 1996.

Spencer K, Souter V, Tul N, et al.: A screening program for trisomy 21 to 10–14 weeks using fetal nuchal translucency, maternal serum free beta-human chorionic gonadotropin and pregnancy-associated plasma protein A. Ultrasound Obstet Gynecol 13:231, 1999.

Stark CR, Orleans M, Haverkamp AD, et al.: Short-and long-term risks after exposure to diagnostic ultrasound in utero. Obstet Gynecol 63:194, 1984.

Stripparo L, Buscaglia M, Longatti L: Genetic amniocentesis: 505 cases performed before the sixteenth week of gestation. Prenat Diagn 10:359, 1990.

Sundberg K, Smidt-Jensen S, Lundsteen C, et al.: Filtration and recirculation of early amniotic fluid. Evaluation of cell cultures from 100 diagnostic cases. Prenat Diagn 13:1101, 1993.

Tabor A, Philip J, Madsen M, et al.: Randomized controlled trial of genetic amniocentesis in 4,606 low-risk women. Lancet 1:1287, 1986.

Tharmaratnam S, Sadek S, Sreele EK, et al.: Transplacental early amniocentesis and pregnancy outcome. Br J Obstet Gynecol 105:228, 1998.

Thein AT, Abdel-Fattah SA, Kyle PM, et al.: An assessment of the use of interphase FISH with chromosome specific probes as an alternative to cytogenetics in prenatal diagnosis. Prenat Diagn 20:275, 2000.

Tipton RE, Tharapel AT, Chang HH, et al.: Rapid chromosome analysis using spontaneously dividing cells derived from umbilical cord blood (fetal and neonatal). Am J Obstet Gynecol 161:1546, 1990.

Tongsong T, Wanapirak C, Sirivatanapa P, et al.: Amniocentesis-related fetal loss: A cohort study. Obstet Gynecol 92:64, 1998.

Tongsong T, Wanapirak C, Kunavikatikul C, et al.: Fetal loss rate associated with cordocentesis at midgestation. Am J Obstet Gynecol 184:719, 2001.

Turnbull AC, MacKenzie IZ: Second-trimester amniocentesis and termination of pregnancy. Br Med Bull 39:315, 1983.

United Kingdom Medical Research Council: Working Party on Amniocentesis. An assessment of the hazards of amniocentesis. Br J Obstet Gynecol 85(suppl 21):1, 1978.

Van den Berg C, Braat AP, Van Opstal D, et al.: Amniocentesis or chorionic villus sampling in multiple gestations? Experience with 500 cases. Prenat Diagn 19:234, 1999.

Vandenbussche FP, Kanhai HH, Keirse MJ: Safety of early amniocentesis. Lancet 344:1032, 1994.

Van Schoubroeck D, Verhaeghe J: Does local anesthesia at mid-trimester amniocentesis decrease pain experience? A randomized trial in 220 patients. Ultrasound Obstet Gynecol 16:536, 2000.

van Vugt JM, Nieuwint A, van Geijn HP: Single-needle insertion: An alternative technique for early second trimester genetic twin amniocentesis. Fetal Diagn Ther 10:178, 1995.

Ville Y, Khalil A, Homphray T, et al.: Diagnostic embryoscopy and fetoscopy in the first trimester of pregnancy. Prenat Diagn 17:1237, 1997.

Vintzileos AM, Egan JF: Adjusting the risk for trisomy 21 on the basis of second-trimester ultrasonography. Am J Obstet Gynecol 172:837, 1995.

Wald NJ, Kennard A, Hackshaw A, et al.: Antenatal screening for Down's syndrome. J Med Screen 5:181, 1998.

Wapner RJ, Johnson A, Davis G, et al.: Prenatal diagnosis in twin gestations: A comparison between second-trimester amniocentesis and first-trimester chorionic villus sampling. Obstet Gynecol 82:49, 1993.

Wathen NC, Campbell DJ, Kitau MJ, et al.: Alpha-fetoprotein levels in amniotic fluid from 8 to 18 weeks of pregnancy. Br J Obstet Gynecol 100:380, 1993.

Watson JD, Craft P: Acetylcholinesterase determination in early amniocentesis. Am J Hum Genet 45:A272, 1989.

Watson WJ, Miller RC, Menard MK, et al.: Ultrasonographic measurement of fetal nuchal skin to screen for chromosomal abnormalities. Am J Obstet Gynecol 170:583, 1994.

Weiner CP, Grant SS, Huson J, et al.: Effect of diagnostic and therapeutic cordocentesis upon maternal serum alpha fetoprotein concentration. Am J Obstet Gynecol 161:706, 1989.

Weiner CP, Okamura K: Diagnostic fetal blood sampling technique related losses. Fetal Diagn Ther 11:169, 1996.

WHO/PAHO consultation on CVS: Evaluation of chorionic villus sampling safety. Prenat Diagn 19:97, 1999.

Wilson RD, Farquharson DF, Wittmann BK, et al.: Cordocentesis: Overall pregnancy loss rate as important as procedure loss rate. Fetal Diagn Ther 9:142, 1994.

Wong LJ: Prenatal diagnosis of glycogen storage disease type 1a by direct mutation detection. Prenat Diagn 16:105, 1996.

Yanagihara T, Hata T: Three-dimensional sonographic visualization of fetal skeleton in the second trimester of pregnancy. Gynecol Obstet Invest 49:12, 2000.

Yang CH, Chu-Ho ES, Liu CC, et al.: Prenatal cytogenetic diagnosis by amniocentesis before 15 weeks' gestation. Zhonghua Yi Xue Za Zhi 52:81, 1993.

Yukobowich E, Anteby EY, Cohen SM, et al.: Risk of fetal loss in twin pregnancies undergoing second trimester amniocentesis (1). Obstet Gynecol 98:231, 2001.

Prenatal Cytogenetic Diagnosis and Maternal Serum Analyte Screening

The most common types of fetal tissue used for prenatal cytogenetic studies include amniotic fluid, chorionic villi, fetal blood, and fetal skin. Techniques used to obtain these tissues are described in Chapter 13. With these tissues, all chromosomal aneuploidies (trisomy, monosomy, triploidy, tetraploidy) and most structural chromosomal abnormalities (translocations, inversions, duplications, deletions) can be detected prenatally. In this chapter we consider the currently accepted indications and the accuracy of prenatal cytogenetic diagnosis. We also discuss the powerful new technology of fluorescence *in situ* hybridization (FISH), which combines cytogenetic and molecular techniques.

Common Indications for Prenatal Cytogenetic Diagnosis

ADVANCED MATERNAL AGE

By far the most common indication for prenatal cytogenetic studies is advanced maternal age. The overall incidence of Down syndrome is one per 800 liveborn births in the United States, but it is well known that the frequency increases with maternal age (Table 14–1). The occurrence of trisomy 21, trisomy 13, trisomy 18, 47,XXX, and 47,XXY increases with advanced maternal age, but 47,XYY, 45,X and translocation do not (Schreinemachers et al., 1982; Ferguson-Smith et al., 1984).

The prevalence of abnormalities at the stage of gestation when chorionic villus sampling (CVS) or amniocentesis is performed is higher than at term (see Table 14–1). For example, the risk of any fetal chromosome abnormality for a 35-year-old woman is 1 in 118 at the time of CVS (first trimester), 1 in 141 at the time of amniocentesis (second trimester), and 1 in 202 at birth. The frequency of chromosomal abnormalities is lower in liveborn infants than in first- or second-trimester fetuses, reflecting the disproportionate likelihood that fetuses lost spontaneously between the time of prenatal testing (9 to 16 weeks' gestation) and term (40 weeks' gestation) have chromosomal abnormalities (Hook, 1983; Hook et al., 1987). In fact, 5% of stillborn infants show chromosomal abnormalities. It follows that some abnormal fetuses would have died *in utero* had iatrogenic intervention (e.g., amniocentesis) not occurred in the second trimester.

The underlying mechanism of the age effect is not clear, as discussed in Chapter 1. Reduced chiasma formation as reflected by decreased recombination is associated with and probably causes nondisjunction (Warren et al., 1987; Sherman et al., 1991). (See Chapter 1 for further discussion.) DNA studies utilizing polymorphic markers have shown that 90 to 95% of trisomy 21 cases occur because of maternal meiotic nondisjunction; the vast majority of these errors occur at meiosis I (Antonarakis, 1991; Sherman et al., 1991; Lorber et al., 1992; Peterson et al., 1992).

The choice of a particular age threshold above which an invasive procedure is recommended is largely arbitrary because the risk of a chromosomally abnormal child increases steadily year by year. Simpson (1997) reviewed events that led to the choice of age 35 as the cutoff in the 1960s and early 1970s. In the United States, the definition of "advanced maternal age" is still accepted as 35 years and older at the estimated delivery date.

▼ **Table 14–1.** REGRESSION-DERIVED RATES OF CHROMOSOME ABNORMALITIES* AT BIRTH, AT
• AMNIOCENTESIS, AND AT CHORIONIC VILLUS SAMPLING†

Maternal Age	Risk of Down syndrome at Birth	Risk of any Chromosome Abnormality at Birth‡	Risk of any Chromosome Abnormality at Amniocentesis	Risk of any Chromosome Abnormality at Chorionic Villus Sampling
20	1:1667	1:526		
21	1:1667	1:526		
22	1:1429	1:500		
23	1:1429	1:500		
24	1:1250	1:476		
25	1:1250	1:476		
26	1:1176	1:476		
27	1:1111	1:455		
28	1:1053	1:435		
29	1:1000	1:417		
30	1:952	1:385		
31	1:909	1:385		
32	1:769	1:323		
33	1:602	1:312		
34	1:482	1:253		
35	1:375	1:202	1:141	1:118
36	1:289	1:163	1:112	1:93
37	1:224	1:129	1:88	1:72
38	1:173	1:103	1:70	1:56
39	1:136	1:82	1:56	1:44
40	1:106	1:65	1:45	1:34
41	1:82	1:51	1:35	1:27
42	1:63	1:40	1:28	1:21
43	1:49	1:32	1:22	1:16
44	1:38	1:25	1:18	1:13
45	1:30	1:20	1:14	1:10
46	1:23	1:16	1:11	1:8
47	1:18	1:12	1:9	1:6
48	1:14	1:10	1:7	
49	1:11	1:8		

*Mosaics, balanced rearrangements, and lethal abnormalities excluded.
†Because sample size for some intervals is relatively small, 95% confidence limits are sometimes relatively large.
Nonetheless, these figures are suitable for genetic counseling.
Data are from Hook EB, 1981; Hook EB, 1988; Hook EB, Cross PK, Jackson LG, et al., 1988; Hook EB, Cross PK, Schreinemachers DM, et al., 1983.
‡Estimated rates based on rate at amniocentesis and spontaneous loss rate of cytogenetically abnormal fetuses.
For ages 20 to 32 years, 47,XXX is excluded (data not given).

At age 35 (at delivery) the American College of Obstetricians and Gynecologists recommends that a woman be informed of the availability of prenatal cytogenetic diagnosis (Guidelines for Women's Health, 1996; ACOG, 2001). In twin gestations ACOG (2001) recommends offering amniocentesis at age 33, given that the cumulative likelihood of one of the two fetuses being affected is similar to that of a 35-year-old with a singleton pregnancy. Some woman under age 35 may be relatively less concerned about the risk of abortion than the risk of a chromosomally abnormal liveborn and may wish to have a diagnostic procedure despite the ostensibly unfavorable risk/benefit ratio.

In contrast to advanced maternal age, there appears to be no substantive increased risk for trisomy 21 with advancing *paternal* age (de Michelena et al., 1993). Some studies indicate the frequency of disomy in sperm may be increased up to twofold at older paternal age (~0.2 to 0.4%), but this has little practical significance. There is greater evidence that advancing paternal age predisposes to fresh mutations leading to autosomal dominant diseases, e.g., achondroplasia, neurofibromatosis, Marfan syndrome (Friedman, 1981). However, new autosomal dominant mutations are individually rare, and no specific prenatal testing is warranted. We counsel couples concerning increased risk when the father is ≥ 55 years old, recommending a comprehensive ultrasound evaluation around 18 weeks' gestation.

PREVIOUS OFFSPRING WITH ANEUPLOIDY

Following the birth of one child with an autosomal trisomy or a sex chromosome abnormality,

▼ **Table 14–2.** RECURRENCE RISK FOR A CHROMOSOME ABNORMALITY AFTER BIRTH
● OF A CHILD WITH A CHROMOSOME ABNORMALITY OTHER THAN TRISOMY 21*

Proband	Number of Cases	Number and Type of Abnormalities (at Amniocentesis or CVS)
Trisomy 13	175	1 t(Y;22)
Trisomy 18	294	4 (47,+18), [inv(18)], (47, +21), (47, +13)
Sex chromosome abnormality	180	3 (47, +13), (47,XYY), (45,X)
Total	649	8 (1.2%)
Deletion	70	2 (47,XXY), [mos t(B;G)]
De novo translocation	93	1 (47, +21)
Polyploidy	12	1 (47,XXY)
Other†	88	0
Total	263	4 (1.5%)

*Data from Mikkelson M, Stene J, 1979; Simoni G, Fraccaro M, Arslanian A, et al., 1982; Stene J, Stene E, Mikkelsen M, 1984.
†Other autosomal trisomies, double trisomies, partial trisomies, markers, mosaics, inversions, and rings.

the likelihood that subsequent progeny will have a chromosome abnormality is increased, even if parental chromosome complements are normal (Table 14–2).

Data on the chance of recurrence of trisomy 21 in children of parents who have had one live-born affected infant have been summarized by Hook (1992). If the mother in the at-risk pregnancy was less than 30 years old, recurrence risk was 1.4%. If she was 30 years or older, the risk was 0.5%, arguably not increased over expectations for that maternal age. Using cases ascertained by nuchal translucency screening (see Chapter 13), Snijders and colleagues (1999) calculated a 0.75% *increased* risk for another trisomy following an index case with trisomy 21. For counseling purposes, the likelihood of recurrence for Down syndrome can be rounded up to 1% greater than the maternal age-specific risk. This represents a significantly increased risk over age-specific risk in women under age 35 but a relatively less significant risk for women over 35 years.

Information concerning recurrence risk following the birth of a child with a chromosomal abnormality other than trisomy 21 is more limited, but data from four collaborative studies suggest a risk of 1 to 2% for either the same or a different chromosomal abnormality (Mikkelsen and Stene, 1979; Simoni et al., 1982; Stene et al., 1984) (see Table 14–2). Snijders and coworkers (1999) reported a 0.75% increase following trisomy 18 ascertained by nuchal translucency. Thus, prenatal diagnosis should also be offered to such couples.

Recurrence risk data discussed above are largely derived from rates at prenatal diagnosis following the birth of an affected liveborn child or more recently from cases detected *in utero* with increased nuchal translucency. Is the risk of recurrence after spontaneous abortion of autoso-

mal trisomy the same as the risk following an affected livebirth? Warburton and colleagues (1987) questioned whether the karyotype of a trisomic spontaneous abortion predicts the karyotype of a subsequent spontaneous abortion, believing that no such trend exists after information on maternal age has been taken into account. However, in Chapter 5 we voiced support for the concept of recurrent aneuploidy. Conservative advice best assumes the same recurrence risk after a trisomic abortus as after liveborn trisomy, i.e., 1% above the maternal age-specific and gestation-specific risk. No single biologic explanation for the recurrence is excepted. Cryptic parental gonadal mosaicism is one attractive hypothesis; genes predisposing to aneuploid gametes is another. See Chapter 1 for further discussion.

STRUCTURAL CHROMOSOMAL REARRANGEMENTS

Robertsonian Translocations

In robertsonian translocations, two acrocentric chromosomes (Nos. 13, 14, 15, 21, and 22) undergo centrometric fusion, i.e., the two chromosomes lose their short arms and their long arms fuse. In many cases, an exchange occurs between repeated elements within the short arms, and the result is a dicentric chromosome and a tiny acentric fragment (containing the ribosomal RNA genes but no other transcribed sequence). The acentric fragment is eliminated in subsequent cell divisions; thus, balanced carriers of robertsonian translocations typically have only 45 chromosomes, showing no phenotypical effects of loss of short arm. (Sufficient ribosomal RNA genes are presumed present in the other acrocentric chromosomes.)

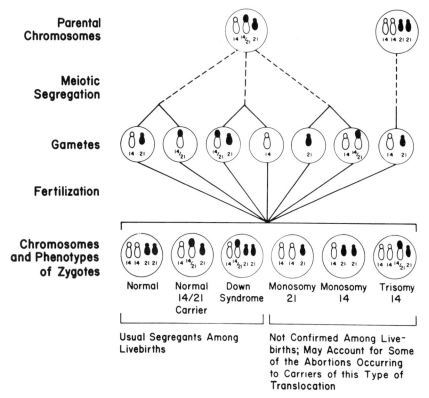

FIGURE 14–1 • Diagram of possible gametes and progeny of a phenotypically normal individual heterozygous for a robertsonian translocation between chromosomes 14 and 21. Three of the six possible gametes are incompatible with life. The likelihood that an individual with such a translocation would have a child with Down syndrome is theoretically 33%. However, the empirical risk is considerably less. (From Gerbie AB, Simpson JL: Antenatal detection of genetic disorders. Postgrad Med 59:129, 1976.)

The most common robertsonian translocation involves chromosomes 14 and 21, which leads to an increased risk of Down syndrome (Fig. 14–1). In theory, a balanced carrier has a one-third risk of having an affected offspring. However, empirical data show that for female carriers the risk of having an offspring with Down syndrome is 10 to 15%, whereas for male carriers the risk is 2 to 4% (Boué and Gallano, 1984; Daniel et al., 1989) (Table 14–3). Presumably this difference reflects perturbations in chromosome pairing and segregation between the two sexes.

Overall, only about 5% of Down syndrome cases involve unbalanced robertsonian translocations. Of these, 40% are inherited from a parent who is a balanced carrier. Among inherited cases, the mother is the carrier parent in more than 90% (Hook, 1981). All *de novo* robertsonian translocations involving chromosomes 14 and 21 that have been studied have had their origins in a maternal germ cell. The mean maternal age (29.2 years) in such cases is predictably only slightly raised above the population mean (27 years) (Petersen et al., 1991; Shaffer et al., 1992).

Risks are lower for robertsonian translocations not involving a chromosome 21 (e.g., t[13q;21q], t[15q;21q], t[21q;22q], Table 14–4). In the rare, unfortunate, event of a parent having a balanced t(21;21), virtually all offspring will be either monosomic or trisomic for chromosome 21. All monosomic and most trisomic conceptuses will spontaneously abort; all remaining conceptuses will have translocation Down syndrome. Robertsonian translocations that do not include chromosome 21 apparently carry much lower risks for liveborn unbalanced offspring. In fact, t(13q;14q), the most common robertsonian translocation found in normal individuals, apparently confers less than a 1% risk for liveborns or midtrimester fetuses (Boué and Gallano, 1984).

Reciprocal Translocations

Reciprocal translocations involve exchange of chromosome material between two and sometimes more nonhomologous chromosomes. They do not involve centrometric fusion and, hence,

▼ **Table 14–3.** FREQUENCIES OF UNBALANCED FETAL CHROMOSOMES IN PREGNANCIES OF
• CARRIERS WITH A ROBERTSONIAN TRANSLOCATION INVOLVING CHROMOSOME 21 BY
AMNIOCENTESIS

	Mother Carrier			Father Carrier	
	Total	Unbalanced	Percent	Total	Unbalanced
13q21q	20	2	10.0	11	0
14q21q	137	21	15.3	51	0
15q21q	9	1	11.1	5	0
21q22q	19	3	15.8	3	0

Data from Boué A, Gallano P, 1984.

▼ **Table 14–4.** SEGREGATION OF
• ROBERTSONIAN TRANSLOCATIONS
NOT INVOLVING CHROMOSOME 21*

Type of Translocation	Number of Diagnosis	Offspring		
		Normal	Balanced	Unbalanced
13q14q	230	96	134	–
13q15q	15	4	11	–
14q15q	6	4	2	–
13q22q	3	–	2	1†
14q22q	3	–	3	–
15q22q	5	2	3	–

*Data from amniocentesis only.
†Mother is the carrier.
Data from Boué A, Gallano P, 1984.

usually do not involve the acrocentric chromosomes. The risk of unbalanced offspring at amniocentesis is 10 to 15% if either father or mother has a balanced translocation (Table 14–5), but this depends on mode of ascertainment. Empirical data specific for most reciprocal translocations are not available. Generalizations must be based on pooled data derived from many different translocations. The risk of an abnormal liveborn versus a spontaneous abortion depends on the size of the chromosome segments involved and what genes are included in those segments. Translocations that result in short unbalanced segments are more likely to result in abnormal offspring than translocations leading to long unbalanced segments (Daniel et al., 1989) (see Chapter 1).

Mode of ascertainment is very important. If a balanced reciprocal translocation is ascertained through an unbalanced child or another liveborn relative, the likelihood of unbalanced liveborns is approximately 20%. If the balanced translocation is ascertained through a history of repeated miscarriage, the risk for an abnormal liveborns is much lower (1 to 5%) (Daniel et al., 1989). The lower empirical risk for anomalous liveborns

may reflect selective spontaneous abortion of unbalanced products or failure of fertilization of unbalanced gametes.

Inversions

An inversion is a chromosomal rearrangement in which a segment of a chromosome is reversed 180° (i.e., end-to-end). The reversed orientation of the chromosome segment changes the position and order of the genes on the chromosome. If the centromere is included in the inversion, the inversion is *pericentric*; if not, it is *paracentric*. Further details are provided in Chapter 1.

Although individuals with inversions are phenotypically normal, they may produce unbalanced gametes if during meiosis crossing-over (recombination) occurs within the inverted sequence. Crossing-over within a pericentric inversion gives rise to two duplication-deficiency products and two normal products. Crossing-over within a paracentric inversion loop leads to one dicentric, one acentric, and two normal products. Because acentric and dicentric products are generally lost, all aberrant products of paracentric inversion are usually lethal. Abnormal liveborns are correspondingly rare. However, individuals with a paracentric inversion may experience repeated spontaneous abortions and occasionally liveborn anomalous offspring.

Although empirical risk data for specific inversions are rarely available, pooled data indicate considerable risks to progeny. Females with an inversion are at a greater risk (8%) for abnormal unbalanced progeny than are males (4%) (Boué and Gallano, 1984). Risk is also influenced by sex (Table 14–6) and the length of chromosome involved in the inversion. Individuals with inversions involving relatively longer segments (30 to 60% of the total chromosomal length) are, paradoxically, more likely to produce anomalous offspring than are those with pericentric inversion involving shorter or longer segments. A relatively

▼ **Table 14–5.** OUTCOME OF PRENATAL DIAGNOSIS FOR PREGNANCIES IN RECIPROCAL TRANSLOCATION CARRIERS (N = 596), FREQUENCIES (%) OF NORMAL AND BALANCED VERSUS UNBALANCED FETAL CHROMOSOMES IN RELATION TO METHODS OF ASCERTAINMENT

Method of Ascertainment	Father Carrier (n = 243)		Mother Carrier (n = 353)		Total Number of Cases
	Balanced and Normal (%)	Unbalanced (%)	Balanced and Normal (%)	Unbalanced (%)	
By unbalanced progeny	71.4	28.6	81.9	18.1	235
By recurrent miscarriages	97.3	2.7	95.3	4.7	180
By other means	93.7	6.3	92.2	7.8	181
Overall	86.4	13.6	88.9	11.1	596

Prospective risk in reciprocal translocation in heterozygotes at amniocentesis as determined by potential chromosome imbalance sizes. Data of the European collaborative prenatal diagnosis centers.
From Daniel A, Boué A, Gallano P: A collaborative study of the segregation of inherited chromosome structure rearrangements in 1356 prenatal diagnosis. Prenat Diagn 6:315, 1986.

▼ **Table 14–6.** PRENATAL RESULTS FOR PERICENTRIC INVERSIONS*

Method of Ascertainment	Maternal Carrier				Paternal Carrier				Grand Total
	Balanced	Normal	Unbalanced	Total	Balanced	Normal	Unbalanced	Total	
Through term unbalanced progeny	6	1	1 (12.5%)	8	2	3	0	5	13
Through recurrent miscarriages	10	4	0	14	4	2	0	6	20
Other	63	4	2 (2.9%)	69	68	3	0	71	140
Total	79	9	3 (3.3%)	91	74	8	0	82	173

*n = 173.
Data from Kleijer WJ, Thompson EJ, Niermeijer MF, 1983.

short pericentric inversion segment is associated with decreased likelihood of recombination within the segment. Recombination within both relatively long or relatively short inversions yields such large imbalances that lethality usually results.

Of special note is pericentric inversion of chromosome 9, with break points p11 and q11. This aberration is very common in the general population and should be considered a normal variant. Whether such an inversion of chromosome 9 predisposes to nondisjunction is arguable. If an increased risk does occur, it appears to be very small (Mikkelson et al., 1979).

Noninvasive Screening for Chromosome Abnormalities

REVISING RISKS BASED ON MATERNAL SERUM ANALYTE VALUES

In 1984, Merkatz and coworkers first reported that pregnant women carrying fetuses with chromosome abnormalities, particularly Down syndrome, tended to have lower maternal serum alpha-fetoprotein (MSAFP) levels than those with unaffected pregnancies (Merkatz et al., 1984). Because only 25% of infants with Down syndrome are born to women aged 35 years and older, low MSAFP values were suggested as a way to identify younger women at sufficient increased risk for fetal chromosomal anomalies to make them candidates for amniocentesis.

Screening for Down syndrome is more complicated than screening for neural tube defects (Chapter 15) because the risk of Down syndrome is age-specific and because greater overlap exists between the distribution of values in mothers carrying normal fetuses compared with mothers carrying Down syndrome fetuses. The median MSAFP in the midtrimester for a woman carrying a Down syndrome fetus is approximately 0.8 multiples of the normal gestation-specific median (MoM) of the normal pregnancy median. MSAFP is therefore only about 20% lower on average in women carrying fetuses with Down syndrome.

This provides useful information, but applying a simple threshold cutoff above or below which an invasive procedure can be recommended does not suffice. Instead, one must adjust the patient's maternal age risk for Down syndrome on the basis of specific MoM, using a likelihood ratio (Cuckle et al., 1987) (Fig. 14–2). Likelihood risks for various markers can be multiplied to yield an overall risk, which could be greater or less than the *a priori* maternal age and gestational week specific risk. Women whose risk equals or is greater than the age-specific risk for Down syndrome at 16 weeks in a 35-year-old woman (1 in 270) are said to be "screen-positive" and are offered further evaluation (amniocentesis). Among women under 35 years of age, 25 to 35% of pregnancies with fetuses affected by Down syndrome may be detected by MSAFP screening alone (New England Regional Genetics Group, 1989; Wald et al., 1997).

If ultrasonographic examination offers no explanation (e.g., underestimated gestational age) for being screen-positive, the patient should undergo genetic counseling and be offered an amniocentesis procedure to exclude Down syndrome and other chromosomal abnormalities. If the amniocentesis is normal, an association between abnormal serum analytes and poor prenatal outcome (e.g., spontaneous abortion or stillbirths) still exists (Waller et al., 1994). However, predictive value is too low for this to be useful, even if third-trimester values are also taken into account (Simpson et al., 1991).

Using MSAFP as the only serum marker increases the ability to detect Down syndrome only modestly. Table 14–7 shows median values for seven useful analytes. Using more than one serum analyte can progressively increase detection rates (Table 14–8). The most informative analyte is human chorionic gonadotropin (hCG), which consists of an α-subunit that is the same for each of the four glycoproteins and a β-subunit that is unique to each hormone. The β-subunit provides the specificity of hormone action. Levels of hCG rise from implantation to 8 weeks' gestation, plateau between 8 and 12 weeks' gestation, decrease from 12 to 18 weeks, and then plateau until term. In the 1980s, studies found that serum hCG levels from women carrying Down syndrome fetuses were often ≥2.5 MoM (Bogart et al., 1987; Petrocik et al., 1989). Controversy exists as to whether the free β-subunit of hCG is preferable to total hCG in Down syndrome screening. Some believe free β-subunit increases the detection rate for fetal Down syndrome and lowers the false-positive rate (Wenstrom et al., 1997; Extermann et al., 1998). Others believe that similar performance exists with either hCG or free β-subunit measures, provided that samples are properly collected and transported (Valerio et al., 1996a; Knight et al., 1998).

Another widely used analyte is unconjugated estriol (uE_3). This hormone is synthesized from dehydroepiandrosterone sulfate (DHEAS) after being converted to 16αOH-DHEAS in the fetal liver and then to uE_3 in the placenta. Like MSAFP, levels of uE_3 in maternal serum were shown to be lower (about 25%) in pregnancies affected with Down syndrome compared with in unaffected pregnancies (Canick et al., 1988). That is, the distribution of values in Down syndrome pregnancies shifts to the left (lower

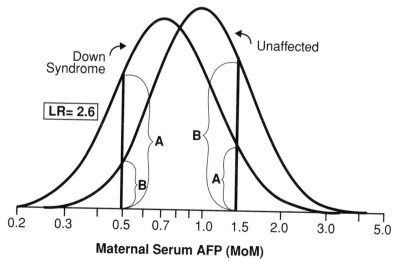

FIGURE 14–2 • Schematic diagram illustrating likelihood ratio, which for Down syndrome at MoM 0.5 is 2.6 (A/B = 2.6) and for MoM 1.5 is 0.4 (A/B = 0.4).

▼ **Table 14–7.** AVERAGE LEVEL IN DOWN SYNDROME FOR VARIOUS SERUM ANALYTES

Marker	Effective Screening Range (Weeks)	Down Syndrome	Average (MoM)	95% CI	Mahalanobus Distance*
NT	11–13	326	2.02	1.93–2.12	1.72
PAPP-A	6–8	31	0.35	0.25–0.49	1.52
	9–11	197	0.40	0.35–0.46	1.33
	12–14	113	0.62	0.52–0.74	0.69
Free β–hCG	<14	579	1.98	1.83–2.10	1.05
	14+	477	2.30	2.13–2.49	1.29
hCG	14+	850	2.02	1.91–2.13	1.15
Inhibin A	13+	585	1.84	1.73–1.95	1.12
AFP	<14	542	0.79	0.75–0.84	0.49
	14+	1140	0.73	0.71–0.75	0.86
uE₃	<14	226	0.74	0.67–0.82	0.56
	14+	613	0.73	0.70–0.76	0.86

AFP, alpha-fetoprotein; CI, confidence interval; hCG, human chorionic gonadotropin; MoM, multiples of the normal gestation-specific median; NT, nuchal translucency; uE₃, unconjugated estriol.
*Deviation of average from 1 MoM in standard deviations (mean of Down syndrome and unaffected value).
From Cuckle H: Integrating antenatal Down syndrome screening. Curr Opin Obstet Gynecol 13:175, 2001.

values). It has been suggested that the uE₃ measurements are dispensable with because the contribution to Down syndrome detection is less than that of MSAFP or hCG; others believe that the range of error in uE₃ measurement is greater than that of MSAFP and hCG (Spencer et al., 1994). In most U.S. programs, uE₃ continues to be included in triple marker screening in order to lower the false positive (procedure) rate.

The fourth useful second trimester analyte is inhibin A, which like hCG is elevated in Down syndrome pregnancies. Inhibin A can be added to the triple screening analytes described above to produce a quadruple test (Haddow et al., 1998a; Wenstrom et al., 1999). Inhibin A is a dimeric glycoprotein with an α-subunit and a βA-subunit linked by a disulfide bond. During pregnancy, inhibin is produced by the corpus luteum and then the placenta. Wald and coworkers (1996a) compared inhibin A levels in the maternal serum from 77 pregnancies affected with Down syndrome with 1355 control preg-

▼ **Table 14–8.** DETECTION RATES IN SINGLETON PREGNANCIES USING SECOND TRIMESTER MARKERS*

Marker(s)	Detection Rate (%) for a 5% False-Positive Rate
Maternal age alone:	
≥36 years	30
Maternal age with one marker:	
AFP	36
uE₃	41
hCG	49
Free α-hCG	38
Free β-hCG	49
Inhibin A	44
Maternal age with two markers:	
AFP, hCG	54
AFP, free β-hCG	53
AFP, inhibin A	
Maternal age with three markers:	
AFP, uE₃, hCG	59
AFP, uE₃, free β-hCG	60
AFP, uE₃, inhibin A	60
AFP, hCG, inhibin A	64
Maternal age with four markers:	
AFP, uE₃, hCG, inhibin A	67
AFP, uE₃, free β-hCG, inhibin A	67

*Gestational age estimated by dates.
From Wald NJ, Kennard A, Hackshaw S, et al.: Antenatal screening for Down's syndrome. J Med Screen 4:181, 1997.

nancies. Serum inhibin A levels from women carrying fetuses with Down syndrome had a median MoM of 1.79. At a 5% false-positive (amniocentesis) rate, the combination of serum AFP, hCG, uE_3, and inhibin A gave a 70% detection rate for Down syndrome. However, Lam and Tang (1999) believe that inhibin A levels are strongly correlated with hCG levels; thus, the value of adding inhibin A to existing hCG and AFP screening protocols would be limited.

DOWN SYNDROME SCREENING PROGRAMS (SECOND TRIMESTER)

In the early 1990s the first two prospective studies in the U.S. examined the efficacy of MSAFP, hCG, and μE_3 in serum screening for fetal Down syndrome. Haddow and colleagues (1992) prospectively screened women for fetal Down syndrome during the second trimester with MSAFP, hCG, and μE_3. Of the 25,207 women screened, 1661 (6.6%) were defined as being at increased risk ($\geq$ 1:190) for infants with Down syndrome and confirmed for gestational dates by ultrasound once reinterpreted for risk. Of these women, 760 ultimately underwent amniocentesis; 20 Down syndrome cases and 7 other chromosomal abnormalities were detected. The rate of detection for fetal Down syndrome was 58% (21/36), with a false-positive rate of 3.8%. Concurrently, our group (Phillips et al., 1992) examined serum MSAFP, hCG, and uE_3 from women under the age of 35 years who were not at increased risk for having a fetus with a chromosomal abnormality. Of 9530 women screened between 15 and 20 weeks' gestation, amniocentesis was offered to those whose newly calculated risk (based on multiplying likelihood rates for hCG, AFP, uE_3) equaled or exceeded that of a woman age 35. Fetal Down syndrome was detected in 57% (4/7) of cases. No case would have been detected by MSAFP alone. Using these three analytes (MSAFP, uE_3, and hCG) results in a slightly higher false-positive rate than using MSAFP alone but detects 2.3 times more Down syndrome cases (Haddow and Palomaki, 1993). Many other studies have confirmed enhanced Down syndrome detection using maternal age plus triple marker screening (Chao et al., 1999; Spencer, 1999; Jou et al., 2000).

In contrast to management after finding one elevated MSAFP level, a positive screen for Down syndrome should not be repeated (Hackshaw et al., 1995). An ultrasound examination performed to confirm gestational age should rely on biparietal diameter (BPD) and not femur length measurement because femurs are on average shorter in fetuses with Down syndrome.

Bahado-Singh and coworkers (2000) compared Down syndrome screening using a triple analyte approach to a four-component screen consisting of ultrasound biometry (humerus length and nuchal thickness), AFP, hCG, and maternal age. There were 46 cases of Down syndrome (1.9%) with 2391 normal pregnancies at this referral center. At a 10% false-positive rate, Down syndrome detection was 45.7% for the triple screen and 80.4% for the four-marker screen. In the United Kingdom, Howe and coworkers (2000) detected 68% of cases (adjusted to 61% after taking into account the likelihood of fetal demise).

On the other hand, an extensive meta-analysis by Smith-Bindman and coworkers (2001) covering 56 articles found that only nuchal thickening was possibly predictive, and here too low to be a practical screening test for Down syndrome. When present, nuchal thickening was useful (17-fold increase in Down syndrome), but few fetuses with Down syndrome showed this finding. Sensitivity was even lower for other ultrasound markers, alone or in combination. Bricker and coworkers (2000) concluded that only 16% of Down syndrome cases could be detected by ultrasound, and Jorgensen and colleagues (1999) detected only 2 of 32 cases. ACOG (2001) recommends offering amniocentesis if choroid plexus cyst is found in a woman age 32 years or older, but this could be arguable.

PROGRAMMATIC RECOMMENDATIONS (ACOG)

The American College of Obstetricians and Gynecologists has made the following recommendations with regard to screening methods for fetal Down syndrome (ACOG, 1994, 2002):

1. Women who are less than 35 years of age and who are between 15 and 18 weeks' gestation by menstrual dating should be offered serum screening to assess Down syndrome risk.
2. Screening should be voluntary and based on informed consent. Various options for screening are available and the detection rates expected should be discussed with the patient. Prior to screening, patients should be provided with information regarding the nature and purpose of the tests, the predictive value of the tests, and the limitations of screening tests in contrast to diagnostic tests.

3. No specific panel of analytes can be exclusively recommended. However, each laboratory should be able to confirm that the specific combination of tests and the particular assays that are performed will yield a Down syndrome detection rate comparable to that of the published expectations (i.e., 20 to 25% with MSAFP alone and at least 55 to 60% with MSAFP, hCG, and unconjugated estriol). The false-positive rate, after ultrasound correction of gestational age, should be 5% or less.

4. The laboratory should provide information regarding its actual rates of positive screening after ultrasound correction. For new programs, the detection rate of Down syndrome may need to be based initially on measurements of samples obtained retrospectively. Programs with a large prospective screening experience may provide actual rates of their Down syndrome detection.

5. The screening program should provide information needed to interpret the test result: date of the patient's last menstrual period, age, weight, race, and relevant obstetric and family history.

6. The obstetrician should be familiar with the reporting method of the laboratory. Reporting should include information about (1) the patient's age-related risk, (2) the patient's adjusted risk, and (3) an indication of whether the patient's adjusted risk exceeds a preset cutoff (e.g., greater or less than that of a 35-year-old woman). The cutoff selected for counseling the patient should be consistent with the Down syndrome risk at which the obstetrician routinely offers prenatal cytogenetic diagnosis based on maternal age alone.

7. All patients who have a Down syndrome risk higher than the selected cutoff should have ultrasonography performed to confirm gestational age and to revise the risk estimate when dating errors are detected prior to performing amniocentesis. Revision of gestational age should be based on BPD and not femur length measurement, given that femurs are shortened in some fetuses with Down syndrome.

8. Multiple marker testing in women over the age of 35 years is not yet recommended routinely in lieu of offering an invasive test for prenatal cytogenetic diagnosis (not all countries agree with the U.S. policy). Serum screening may be offered as an option for those women who either do not accept the risk of amniocentesis or who wish to have this additional information prior to making a decision about having amniocentesis. If serum screening for Down syndrome is requested by a patient over the age of 35 years, the patient should be informed of the higher rate of a positive screening test result in this age group. The patient should also be informed of the diminished ability of screening to detect Down syndrome and certain other chromosome abnormalities, such as 47,XXX and 47,XXY, when screening with this approach is compared with diagnostic testing with CVS or amniocentesis.

SCREENING FOR TRISOMY 18

Trisomy 18 can also be detected with the triple marker screening. Pregnancies with trisomy 18 fetuses show decreased hCG, decreased AFP, and decreased uE_3 levels. It is possible to offer invasive prenatal diagnosis simply by recommending amniocentesis when each of these three markers fall below certain thresholds: AFP ≤0.75 MoM; hCG ≤0.55 MoM; unconjugated estriol ≤0.60 MoM (Palomaki et al., 1992). Using these thresholds would detect 60% to 80% of trisomy 18 fetuses with a 0.4% false-positive (amniocentesis) rate (Haddow et al., 1993). Using a method providing an individual risk estimation derived from the exact value of the three analytes, Palomaki and associates (1995) reported that 60% of trisomy 18 pregnancies can be detected with a false-positive rate of 0.4%. One in nine pregnancies identified as at increased risk for trisomy 18 would be expected to be affected. Benn and colleagues (1999) reviewed second trimester screening results for 41,565 women, comparing results of using a fixed cutoff (MSAFP ≤0.75 MoM, hCG ≤0.55 MoM, and uE_3 ≤0.60 MoM) versus results with patient-specific risk protocol for trisomy 18 screening. The fixed cutoff method showed a 23% detection rate with a 0.19 false-positive rate; the patient-specific approach showed a 69% detection rate with a 0.45% false-positive rate. The risk-based method was obviously more effective.

Brumfield and colleagues (2000) found that ultrasound was more likely to be abnormal than multiple-marker screening in fetuses with trisomy 18 (70%) (95% confidence interval [CI] 54.86 versus 43% CI 25.61). Combining ultrasound and serum screening yielded the highest detection rate (80% [CI 60%, 94%]).

URINARY AND OTHER MATERNAL SERUM MARKERS FOR DOWN SYNDROME

Urinary metabolites may be used to detect fetal Down syndrome (Cuckle et al., 1994, 1995).

Canick and coworkers (1995) compared urinary gonadotropin peptide (UGP) levels from 14 women carrying fetuses affected with Down syndrome with urinary samples from 91 control pregnancies. The median UPG level in Down syndrome cases was 5.34 MoM. A smaller initial study (Cuckle et al., 1994; Cuckle, 1995) examined use of the β-core fragment of hCG (another name for UGP), total urinary estrogen (tE), and free α-subunit of hCG in urine samples as a method for detecting fetal Down syndrome. Levels were examined from 24 pregnancies with fetal Down syndrome and 294 control pregnancies. The median values in Down syndrome pregnancies were 6.02 MoM for β-core hCG; 0.74 MoM for tE; and 1.08 MoM for α-hCG. α-hCG levels were not significantly different between the two groups. Given a 5% false-positive rate, the calculated detection rate for fetal Down syndrome was 79.6% using β-core hCG and 82.3% using both β-core hCG and tE. In a prospective study involving 23 cases of fetal Down syndrome among 1016 singleton pregnancies, Bahado-Singh and associates (2000) used urinary hyperglycosylated hCG plus ultrasound biometry for second-trimester screening. Detection rate for Down syndrome was 91.3% at a 3.2% false-positive rate and 100% at a 10.7% false-positive rate.

Other second-trimester maternal serum analytes still being considered for fetal Down syndrome screening include various hCG glycoforms, superoxide dismutase, eosinophil major basic protein, prostate-specific antigen, activin A, and follistatin (Christiansen et al., 1999; Cuckle et al., 1999; Ognibene et al., 1999; Wald et al., 1999a; Abushoufa et al., 2000).

CONFOUNDING VARIABLES IN MATERNAL SERUM SCREENING

Increasing maternal weight decreases serum AFP, uE_3 and hCG because of the dilutional effect. Race-ethnicity-specific variations also exist in all these analytes, to greater or lesser extent. AFP levels are generally higher in Asian and black women than in Hispanic and white women; hCG and uE_3 are highest in Asian women (O'Brien et al., 1997a). hCG levels are increased in African-Americans (Simpson et al., 1990). Insulin-dependent diabetes is associated with slightly decreased uE_3 and hCG levels (Wald et al., 1994a). Maternal smoking increases MSAFP by 3% and decreases maternal serum uE_3 and hCG levels by 3% and 23%, respectively (Palomaki et al., 1993; Perona et al., 1998). Ribbert and coworkers (1996) found that mater-

nal serum hCG was significantly higher and MSAFP significantly lower in pregnancies conceived by *in vitro* fertilization compared with pregnancies conceived spontaneously. Maymon and colleagues (1999a) reviewed the topic and concluded that a lack of consensus exists. Later, Bar-Hava and coworkers (2001) found second-trimester maternal serum hCG levels to be higher than in spontaneously conceived pregnancies. Liao (2001) found first trimester free β-hCG to be increased and PAPP-A decreased; NT was unchanged. Failing to adjust for these changes would result in a 1% higher false-positive rate. In general adjustments are recommended for weight and ethnicity but not for smoking, prior in vitro fertilization (IVF) or maternal disease status (Heinonen et al., 1996; Frishman et al., 1997; Wald et al., 1999b).

SCREENING IN MULTIPLE GESTATIONS

Down syndrome is more frequent in twin pregnancies than in singleton pregnancies (Wald et al., 1994b). This reflects both twinning and Down syndrome being correlated with advanced maternal age. Because this increase is accounted for by dizygotic twinning, twins usually are discordant if trisomy 21 is present. This increases difficulty in detecting Down syndrome by maternal serum screening, for which reason noninvasive screening was restricted to singleton pregnancies for years. Indeed, Neveux and coworkers (1996) calculated on the basis of modeling that with singleton cutoffs 73% of monozygotic twin pregnancies but only 43% of dizygotic twin pregnancies with a Down syndrome fetus could be detected, given a 5% false-positive rate. Applying second-trimester distributions of free β-hCG and AFP levels in 420 twins compared with 6661 singleton pregnancies, Spencer and colleagues (1994) showed that after twin correction of the multiple of the medians, these two analytes produced a 51% detection rate at a 5% false-positive rate. O'Brien and associates (1997b) compared serum AFP, hCG, and uE_3 levels from 4443 twin pregnancies with those from 258,885 singleton pregnancies from 14 to 21 weeks' gestation. Median AFP levels for twins were approximately double those of singletons, but median increases for hCG and uE_3 were less than double (see Table 14–9). Thus, mere mathematical conversion from singleton Down syndrome risks cannot be applied with equal accuracy to twins. Couples should be counseled that detection rates are lower than those for singleton pregnancies.

▼ **Table 14–9.** MEDIAN SECOND TRIMESTER SERUM MARKER LEVELS IN UNAFFECTED TWIN
• PREGNANCIES RELATIVE TO SINGLETON PREGNANCIES

| Serum Marker | Number of Women | | Median Marker Level in Twins Relative to Singletons |
	Singleton Pregnancy	Twin Pregnancy	
AFP	58,572	1892	2.23
uE$_3$	38,360	739	1.65
hCG	42,730	1211	2.01
Free α-hCG	600	199	1.66
Free β-hCG	7261	619	2.08
Inhibin A	600	199	1.99

Data from Wald NJ, Kennard A, Hackshaw S, et al., 1997.

Nonetheless, most laboratories offer second-trimester Down syndrome screening risks in twin pregnancies using multiples analytes.

The alternative is to offer an invasive procedure directly. Given the independent likelihood of risk of each of the two dizygotic twins having trisomy 21, the additive risk for one to have Down syndrome is comparable for a 32-year-old with twins and a 35-year-old with a singleton pregnancy (Rodis et al., 1991). For this reason the ACOG (2001) recommends amniocentesis be offered to 33-year-old women with twin gestations. However, this calculation assumes the one-third of twins who are monozygotic cannot be distinguished from the dizygotic twins. If dichorionicity is verified, the risk is 1:315 at age 31, nearly that of a 35-year-old.

FIRST-TRIMESTER MATERNAL SERUM ANALYTES

Serum screening in the first trimester would be highly desirable because privacy is greater and first-trimester pregnancy termination is safest. Women at increased risk could be offered either CVS or amniocentesis at 14 or 15 weeks, avoiding late-pregnancy terminations if fetal abnormalities are detected. Screening in the first trimester would help ensure privacy for women with affected pregnancies. Early evidence appears quite strong that screening in the first trimester also allows detection of fetal Down syndrome. A caveat is that first-trimester screening does not allow detection of open neural tube defects because maternal serum AFP is not a useful discriminator prior to 15 weeks' gestation. Thus, if serum screening for Down syndrome were to be performed in the first trimester, it would become necessary to carry out a second-trimester screening to detect neural tube defects in the second trimester.

Numerous fetoplacental products have been investigated for *first trimester* Down syndrome screening; AFP, uE$_3$, hCG, free β-hCG, free α-hCG, pregnancy-associated plasma protein A (PAPP-A), CA-125, dimeric inhibin A, inhibin A, progesterone, and placental alkaline phosphatase. Eventually, the conclusion has been reached that PAPP-A and free β-hCG are most useful for detecting Down syndrome in the first trimester (Table 14–10). In the first trimester (8 to 14 weeks) Down syndrome is associated with decreased levels of maternal serum PAPP-A; 42% of the PAPP-A values from affected pregnancies are less than the fifth percentile of unaffected pregnancies. Maternal serum levels of free β-hCG are increased in Down syndrome; 18% of the free β-hCG values from affected pregnancies are greater than the 95th percentile of unaffected pregnancies (Wald et al., 1996b). Using PAPP-A and free β-hCG permits a mean detection rate of 60% (range 55 to 63%) at a 5% false-positive rate (Wald et al., 1995; Krantz et al., 1996; Berry et al., 1997; Biagiotti et al., 1998; Haddow et al., 1998b) (see Table 14–10). In twins Spencer (2002) calculated that hCG was almost twice as high in twins as singletons; PAPP-A was 1.86 higher modeling on the basis of a 5% false-positive rate. There was a 52% detection rate for Down syndrome in discordance and 55% in concordance.

FIRST-TRIMESTER ULTRASOUND SCREENING (NUCHAL TRANSLUCENCY)

In Chapter 13 we first discussed the association of nuchal translucency (NT) as a first-trimester marker in fetal Down syndrome screening. In eight studies, NT screening in general populations was found by Malone and coworkers (2000) to show Down syndrome detection rates ranging from 29 to 91%. This variable range is

▼ **Table 14–10.** FIRST TRIMESTER SERUM SCREENING: PREDICTED EFFICIENCY

| | | Cutoff Risk (at Term) | | | | | |
| | DR for 5% | 1 in 200 | | 1 in 250 | | 1 in 300 | |
Combination	FPR	DR	FPR	DR	FPR	DR	FPR
PAPP-A and free β-hCG	71.5	68.9	4.2	72.1	5.2	74.6	6.2
PAPP-A, free β-hCG, and AFP	73.7	70.9	4.1	73.9	5.1	76.3	5.1
PAPP-A, free β-hCG, and uE₃	75.6	71.7	3.6	74.1	4.5	76.4	5.4

AFP, alpha-fetoprotein; DR, detection rate; FPR, false-positive rate; hCG, human gonadotropin; PAPP-A, pregnancy-associated plasma protein A; uE_3, unconjugated estriol.
Modified from Cuckle H: Integrating antenatal Down syndrome. Curr Opin Obstet Gynecol 13:175, 2001.

best explained by the methods used for defining abnormal NT. For example, use of an absolute cutoff (e.g., 2.5 mm) yields different results compared with applying a 95th percentile NT value according to fetal crown-rump length (Snijders et al., 1998). Differences in ultrasonographic measurements can readily explain some discrepancies.

The best data are those of Snijders and coworkers (1998) from the Fetal Medicine Foundation. In that study, 96,127 pregnant women at both high and low risk for fetal aneuploidy had NT screening performed at one of 22 certified centers in the United Kingdom. With an NT measurement cutoff of >95th percentile according to fetal crown-rump length, Down syndrome detection was 75%. After addition of maternal age to the risk assessment calculation, 82% of cases of Down syndrome would have been detected with a 1 in 30 risk cutoff, resulting in an 8% false-positive rate. The Down syndrome detection rate would have been 77% if the false-positive rate were kept at 5%. Nuchal translucency (NT) can be as reliably measured in twins as in singleton pregnancies (Sebire et al., 1996; Maymon et al., 1999b).

COMBINING FIRST-TRIMESTER MATERNAL SERUM ANALYTES AND NUCHAL TRANSLUCENCY MEASUREMENTS

First-trimester maternal serum free β-hCG and PAPP-A analyte may be combined with NT screening to yield improved detection rates (Table 14–11) for Down syndrome screening. Spencer and coworkers (1999) used free β-hCG and PAPP-A values in 210 singleton pregnancies with trisomy 21 and 946 chromosomally normal controls, matched for maternal age, gestation, and sample storage time. In all cases the fetal crown-rump length and NT had been measured by ultrasonography at 10 to 14 weeks' gestation;

maternal blood had been obtained at the time of the scan. Combining MoM values for β-hCG, PAPP-A, and NT, the detection rate for trisomy 21 was estimated to be 89% at a fixed false-positive rate of 5%. At a fixed detection rate of 70%, the false-positive (amniocentesis) rate was estimated to be 1%. Detection is lower at younger maternal age (Table 14–12). In twins Spencer (2000) modeled an 80% detection, compared to 90% in singletons.

Following conclusions drawn from small data sets or exclusively based on statistical modeling (Biagiotti et al., 1998; De Biasio et al., 1999), Krantz and colleagues (2000) published the first large-scale prospective study. A total of 10,251 U.S. women of all ages were screened with PAPP-A and hCG using a dried blood spot method; 5809 also had NT measurement, using the Fetal Medicine Foundation criteria (Snijders et al., 1998). The sample contained 50 Down syndrome cases and 20 trisomy 18 cases. Using both ultrasound and serum analytes, detection rate for trisomy 21 was 87.5% (7/8) in women under age 35 years; in women over age 35 the detection rate was 92% (23/25), although with a higher false-positive (invasive procedure) rate. For trisomy 18, detection rates were 100% in both groups (n = 4 and n = 9). These impressive results indicate that first-trimester screening could be initiated if resources exist to perform assays and to handle problems. Schuchter et al. (2002) detected 12 of 14 Down syndrome cases among 4939 women tested. Spencer (2002) found that predicted risk (quantitatively) correlated quite well (r = 0.9995) with actual prevalence of Down syndrome. A NICHD sponsored multi-center cohort study reported highly favorable results in a cohort of 8514 women who completed screening between 74 and 97 days gestation (Wapner for the BUN Study Group, 2001; Wapner et al., 2002). The mean maternal age was 34.5 years. Using a mid-trimester screen positive cutoff of 1:270 identified 85.2% of the

▼ **Table 14–11.** SCREENING TO ACHIEVE AN 85% DETECTION RATE FOR DIFFERENT METHODS
• SHOWING THE FALSE-POSITIVE RATE, ODDS OF HAVING AN AFFECTED PREGNANCY GIVEN A
POSITIVE RESULT

Method of Screening (All include Maternal Age)	Risk Cutoff Level	False-Positive Rate (%)	Odds of Being Affected Given a Positive Result
First Trimester			
Combined test	1 in 540	4.9	1:45
Second Trimester			
Quadruple test	1 in 630	9.8	1:88
Triple test	1 in 830	14.5	1:131
Double test	1 in 1040	22.1	1:200
First and Second Trimester			
Integrated test:			
PAPP-A, NT + Quadruple	1 in 120	0.9	1:9
Integrated test variants:			
PAPP-A, NT + Triple	1 in 190	1:5	1:13
PAPP-A + Quadruple	1 in 410	5.2	1:47
PAPP-A + Triple	1 in 560	7.7	1:70

NT = nuchal translucency measurement; PAPP-A, pregnancy associated plasma protein A.
Double test: AFP, hCG; triple test: AFP, hCG, uE_3; quadruple test: AFP, hCG, uE_3, inhibin A.
From Wald NJ, Watt HC, Hackshaw AK: Integrated screening in Down's syndrome based on tests performed during the first and second trimesters. N Engl J Med 341:461, 1999.

61 trisomy 21 pregnancies at a false-positive rate (FPR) of 9.4% (predictably higher given maternal age of sample). At a false-positive rate of 5%, sensitivity would be 78.7%, and at a false rate of 1%, 63.9%. Of trisomy 18 cases, 90.9% were detected. Detection rate for trisomy 21 was 66.7% under age 35 years (at a 3.7% FPR) and 89.8% over age 35 years (15.2% FPR). Modeled for the age of the U.S. population and at 5% FPR yield 78.8% detection.

Concern exists that some trisomies detected in the first trimester represent pregnancies destined to be lost spontaneously if medical intervention had not been pursued; however, adjustment to take this into account would actually decrease the detection rate of potential liveborns relatively

▼ **Table 14–12.** DOWN SYNDROME DETECTION RATES AND FALSE-POSITIVE RATES ACCORDING
• TO MATERNAL AGE AND METHOD OF SCREENING*†

Age (years)	Double Test DR (%)	Double Test FPR (%)	Triple Test DR (%)	Triple Test FPR (%)	Quadruple Test DR (%)	Quadruple Test FPR (%)	Full Integrated Test DR (%)	Full Integrated Test FPR (%)
15–19	35	2.2	50	2.4	63	3.0	78	0.5
20–24	38	2.7	52	2.7	63	3.1	78	0.5
25–29	43	3.7	56	3.4	67	3.9	80	0.7
30–34	57	7.4	66	6.2	75	6.5	84	1.1
15–34	46	4.0	58	3.7	69	4.1	81	0.7
35–39	79	20	82	15	87	15	89	2.6
40 +	96	48	96	38	97	33	96	7.5
35 +	86	24	88	19	91	17	92	3.3
All	61	5.6	69	4.9	77	5.2	85	0.9

DR, detection rates; FPR, false positive rates.
* All tests include maternal age with gestational age estimated using ultrasound.
† Women are screen positive if the risk exceeds 1 in 250 for the double and triple tests, 1 in 300 for the quadruple test, and 1 in 120 for the integrated test.
From Wald NJ, Watt HC, Hackshaw AK: Integrated screening in Down's syndrome based on tests performed during the first and second trimesters. N Engl J Med 341:461, 1999.

little. A 3% decrease was estimated by Krantz and coworkers (2000). Wapner et al. (2002) estimated their 78.7% detection rate (given 5% FPR) in the first trimester would be equivalent to a 75% detection in the second trimester.

Is first-trimester screening, with its attraction of privacy and safer termination, preferable to second-trimester screening? Malone and colleagues (2000) editorialized that only large-scale trials allow a meaningful comparison of Down syndrome detection rates between various screening protocols. Trials are underway. Malone and associates (2000) believe that until the results of these trials are available, first-trimester methods for screening should be considered investigational and not an alternative to second-trimester screening. Not all agree, for the data of Krantz and colleagues (2000), Schuchter (2002), and Wapner et al. (2002) are convincing. Thus, we offer either first- or second-trimester noninvasive screening, depending upon patient preference. Patients desiring first-trimester screening who do not have access to sonographers specifically trained for NT measurements should be screened only using maternal serum analytes (PAPP-A and hCG).

INTEGRATED FIRST- AND SECOND-TRIMESTER SCREENING

Wald and coworkers (1997) first proposed first-trimester screening (ultrasound or maternal serum) followed by second-trimester serum screening. They called this approach "integrated," although "sequential" might be more descriptive. Detection rate was modeled to be at 91% given a 5% false-positive rate, or 71% at a 1% false-positive rate. One problem for U.S. application is that with integrated screening current algorithms require withholding first-trimester results until second-trimester values are obtained. If information is not withheld, sensitivity is said to decrease.

This model is now being tested in two cohort studies. In the United Kingdom, the SURUSS (Serum URine and Ultrasound Screening Study) trial is being conducted, and in the United States, the FASTER (First and Second Trimester Evaluation of Risk for Aneuploidy) trial is ongoing.

Some data are available from the SURUSS trial (Wald, 2002), which is performing in accordance with expectations (Tables 14–11 and 14–12). This 25 center (24 UK, 1 Austria) trial performed first trimester NT, PAPP-A, hCG and without disclosure second trimester inhibin A, free and total

hCG, uE$_3$, and AFP. Detection rates for trisomy 21 continued to improve as both first and second trimester analytes were added; however, urine ITA (invasive trophoblastic antigen) and total hCG were not useful. Assuming a constant Down syndrome detection rate of 85% the FPR rate progressively decreased in SURUSS as more tests were taken into account. The FPR was 5.6% at a 85% detection rate using only first trimester markers (PAPP-A, hCG, NT), 9.9% using only three second trimester markers (AFP, hCG, uE$_3$, but not inhibin A), and 5.6% using all four second trimester serum markers (inhibin A, AFP, hCG, uE$_3$). The FPR fell further to 2.4% using both first trimester PAPP-A plus the four second trimester analytes (hCG, AFP, uE$_3$, inhibin A), or 1.3% using NT plus first trimester serum analytes PAPP-A and hCG. With NT plus both first trimester PAPP-A and the four second trimester serum analytes, FPR was 0.9%.

In summary, there appears to be an incremental, albeit small benefit, of sequential first and second trimester screening. However, we would not favor combining first- and second-trimester screening (Wald et al., 1997) if this requires withholding information from first-trimester results merely to improve overall detection rates. Figure 14–3 provides rates of detection of Down syndrome and false-positives for various screening tests.

PROMISING NEW MARKERS: NASAL BONE; CELL-FREE FETAL DNA

New markers continue to be proposed as useful in noninvasive screening for Down syndrome. Most do not prove helpful after detailed testing. However, at least two appear exceptionally promising.

Cicero et al. (2001) reported that ultrasonographic absence of the nasal bone (NB) (10–12 weeks) correlated with fetal Down syndrome, yielding 82% detection with a FPR of 8.3%. Otaño et al. (2002) similarly found such a correlation. Cicero et al. (2001) further reported that NB and NT (nuchal translucency) could be combined to result in 92% detection for a FPR of 3.5% in the first trimester.

Intact fetal cells exists in the maternal blood, and if identified are definitive with a low false-positive rate (Chapter 17). Techniques are still too inconsistent to apply clinically but the attraction of performing serum or ultrasound screening followed by an invasive procedure only if fetal cells are also positive is appealing. Alternatively, cell-free fetal DNA is even more

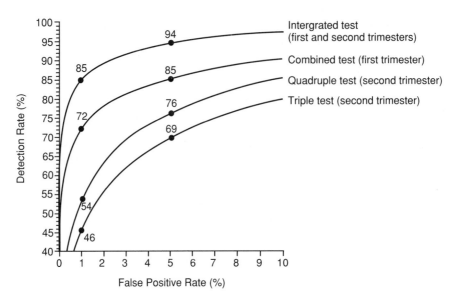

FIGURE 14–3 • Rates of detection of Down syndrome and false-positive rates for various noninvasive screening tests. Triple test: AFP, hCG, uE_3; quadruple test: AFP, hCG, uE_3, inhibin A; combined test: NT plus first-trimester serum analysis (PAPP-A, hCG); integrated test: combined test (first-followed by second-trimester tests). (From Wald NJ, Watt HC, Hackshaw AK: Integrated screening for Down's syndrome on the basis of tests performed during the first and second trimesters. N Engl J Med 341:461, 1999.)

abundant in maternal blood than intact fetal cells. Bianchi (2002) and Lee et al. (2001) showed cell-free fetal DNA is 1.7 × greater in Down syndrome pregnancies than in controls. Cell-free fetal DNA is as good a noninvasive marker as NT and likely independent. Adding DNA to second trimester maternal serum analyte testing (AFP, hCG, uE_3, inhibin A) would increase detection rate for Down syndrome from 73% to 87% albeit with slight increase in FPR (4% to 7%) (Bianchi, 2002).

Less Common Indications for Prenatal Cytogenetic Diagnosis

PARENTAL ANEUPLOIDY

If a parent has a numerical chromosomal abnormality (aneuploidy), the risk to offspring is increased. Empirically, approximately one third of reported offspring of females with 47,XX,+21 (Down syndrome) are aneuploid (Simpson, 1981; Bovicelli et al., 1982); therefore, antenatal chromosomal studies are indicated in the rare pregnant female with Down syndrome. This topic was discussed in Chapter 1, in which we explored reasons for the empirical risk's being lower than the theoretical 50% risk. Males with Down syndrome are almost always sterile; however, there are at least two well-documented

reports of an affected male fathering an unaffected child (Zühlke et al., 1994).

If a parent has sex chromosome aneuploidy, risks to offspring are increased. However, available risk figures are biased by the method of ascertainment. Approximately 20% of reported offspring of fertile 45,X/46,XY, 45,X/46,XX, and 45,X/46,XX/47,XXX subjects show chromosome abnormalities, but biases of ascertainment and reporting probably markedly influence the figure in the direction of overestimation (Simpson, 1981) (see Chapter 1). As evidence, women known to be 47,XXX or 46,XX/ 47,XXX only rarely have been shown to produce children with chromosome abnormalities. 47,XYY Men are at increased risk for chromosomally abnormal offspring, but few have been reported.

The most topical issue and the most informative data involve men with 47,XXY Klinefelter syndrome. Traditionally such men have been sterile, although those with mosaicism (46,XY/ 47,XXY) have long been recognized as potentially fertile. Pregnancy may now be achieved with intracytoplasmic sperm injection (ICSI).

Theoretical expectations would dictate that 50% of sperm should be hyperhaploid disomic, but as discussed in Chapters 1 and 12, the frequency of sex chromosomal polysomy in sperm (XY or XX disomy) or embryos (47,XXY or 47,XXX) is much less. The frequency of sex chro-

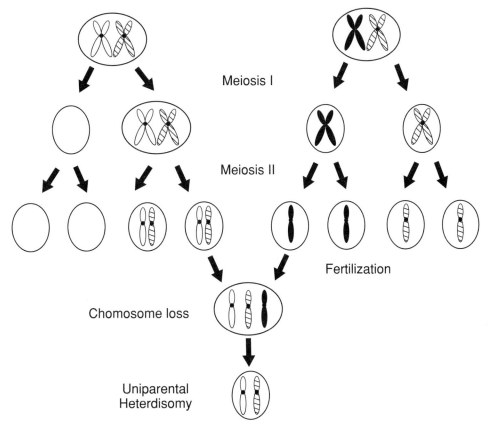

Meiosis I

Meiosis II

Fertilization

Chomosome loss

Uniparental
Heterodisomy

FIGURE 14–5 • Uniparental heterodisomy resulting from a disomic gamete arising from nondisjunction in meiosis I fertilizing a monosomic gamete with loss of the chromosome from the parent giving the single homolog.

hand, if an ostensibly balanced translocation is present in the fetus but in neither parent (a *de novo* translocation), the likelihood is 6.7% for reciprocal translocations and 3.7% for robertsonian translocations (Warburton, 1984). Presumably, the rearrangement is not actually balanced. In robertsonian translocation the phenotypical abnormality could reflect uniparental disomy, as already discussed (Berend et al., 2000; McGowan et al., 2002). Risks are not chromosome-specific but represent pooled data involving many chromosomes. Also recall that risks refer only to structurally anatomic abnormalities and cannot take into account risks of developmental delay (mental retardation) that may not be evident at birth. The risk for the fetus' being phenotypically abnormal is estimated at 9.4% for *de novo* inversions (Warburton, 1991) (Table 14–15).

MARKER CHROMOSOMES

Marker chromosomes, also called supernumerary chromosomes, are defined as chromosomes that cannot be fully characterized on the basis of standard cytogenetic analyses. They possess a paucity of banding landmarks. These small chromosomes usually contain a centromere, and a high percentage are derived from the short arm regions of the acrocentric chromosomes 13, 14, 15, 21, and 22. Marker chromosomes are observed in approximately 0.06% of the population (Sachs et al., 1987). Risks for phenotypical abnormalities are significant, 14.7% for a nonsatellited marker and 10.9% for a satellited marker (Warburton, 1991) (Table 14–16).

With the advent of FISH and other molecular cytogenetic techniques, the chromosomal origin of marker chromosomes can be established more readily. Chromosome-specific pericentric alphoid satellite probes that specifically hybridized to individual centromeres were first used in the mid 1990s (Blennow et al., 1995; Valerio et al., 1996b). Correlation between phenotype and chromosomal origin of markers is now being undertaken, and results may permit us to distinguish between those markers conferring a high risk for phenotypical abnormality and those conferring a low risk. Graf and colleagues (2000) analyzed 275 markers with PCR (microsatellite)

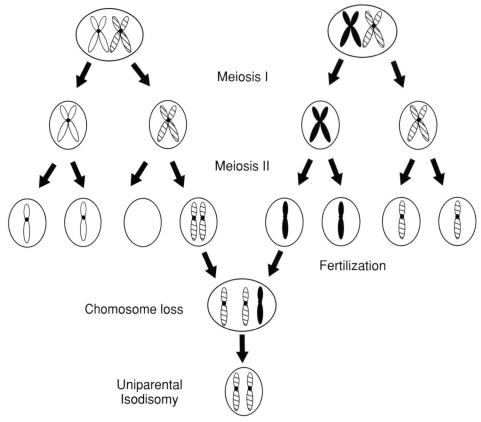

FIGURE 14–6 • Uniparental isodisomy occurring through a disomic gamete resulting from nondisjunction in meiosis II fertilizing a monosomic gamete with loss of the chromosome from the parent giving the single homolog.

and FISH (using yeast artificial chromosomes [YAC], bacterial artificial chromosomes [BAC], and cosmid probes). In over 40% the phenotype could be predicted on the basis of the presence or absence of specific genes. Whether the long established empirical risk data cited above should be altered as a result of FISH studies is not yet clear.

As with other structural chromosomal rearrangements, the risk for phenotypical abnormality should be correlated with whether the marker is *de novo* or familial. Risks are higher for *de novo* markers. In follow-up of 15 cases of marker chromosomes identified among 12,699 prenatal samples (11,055 amniotic fluids, 1644 chorionic villus samples), Brondum-Nielsen (1995) found five familial cases derived from acrocentric chromosomes 13, 14, 15, 21, and 22; all five pregnancies resulted in phenotypically normal offspring. Nine other markers represented *de novo* abnormalities.

▼ **Table 14–15.** PHENOTYPICAL OUTCOME OF DE NOVO BALANCED REARRANGEMENTS
• DIAGNOSED AT AMNIOCENTESIS

	Total Number	Percent with Abnormal Outcome	Live Birth		Elective Abortion		Fetal Death	
			Normal	Abnormal	Normal	Abnormal	Normal	Abnormal
Reciprocal translocation	144	5.5	118	6	15	2	3	0
Robertsonian translocation	51	3.9	48	2	1	0	0	0
Inversion	31	9.7	27	1	1	1	0	1
Total	226	5.75	193	9	17	3	3	1

Data from Warburton D, 1991.

▼ **Table 14–16.** INCIDENCE OF SUPERNUMERARY MARKER CHROMOSOMES

Source of Data	Number Studied	Incidence (per 1000)			Reference
		Overall	De Novo	Inherited	
Amniocentesis	52,965	0.60	–	–	Ferguson-Smith and Yates, 1984
	76,952	0.65	0.4	0.25	Warburton, 1984
	75,000	0.64	0.32	0.23	Hook et al., 1987
			–0.40	–0.32	
	10,000	1.5	0.9	0.6	Sachs et al., 1987
	377,357	–	0.4	–	Warburton, 1991
	42,000	0.88	0.52	0.21	LYF Hsu (unpublished data, Prenatal Diagnosis Laboratory)
Amniocentesis and CVS (combined)	39,105 (amniocentesis, 34,908; CVS, 4,197)	0.8	0.4 –0.5	0.3 0.4	Blennow et al., 1995
	12,699 (amniocentesis, 11,055; CVS, 1,644)	1.1	0.70	0.39	Brondum-Nielson and Mikkelsen, 1995
Newborns	59,452	0.18	0.05	0.10	Jacobs, 1981
	34,919	0.72	–	–	Nielsen and Wohlert, 1991

Tabulation by Hsu L: Chromosomal disorders. *In* Reece EA, Hobbins JC (eds): Medicine of the Fetus and Mother, 2nd ed. Philadelphia: Lippincott-Raven, 1999.

In two (one with a marker derived from chromosomes 14 or 17, the other with a ringlike marker derived from chromosome 17), pregnancies resulted in phenotypically normal infants delivered at term; however, the child with the derivative 17 showed minimal psychomotor retardation at age 2. All other pregnancies with *de novo* markers were terminated; three showed significant abnormalities at autopsy.

In reviewing 15,522 prenatal diagnostic procedures, Hume and colleagues (1995) identified 19 marker chromosomes: 5 (26%) from CVS specimens and 14 (74%) from amniotic fluid samples. In monitoring these pregnancies with high-resolution ultrasonography, the coexistence of a *de novo* marker chromosome with ultrasound evidence for anomalies was found to confer a poor prognosis. When ultrasound examination was normal, the likelihood of a phenotypically normal offspring was high.

Fluorescence in Situ Hybridization in Prenatal Diagnosis as an Alternative to Metaphase Analysis

FISH merges molecular genetics with cytogenetics, an exciting prospect. Using DNA sequences present only on the chromosome in question, chromosome-specific probes (e.g., nos. 13, 18, 21, the X, or the Y) can be created (Fig. 14–7). The probe is then labeled with a fluorochrome and hybridized with unknown DNA. Disomic cells (metaphase or interphase) usually (80 to 90%) show two separate signals; trisomic cells

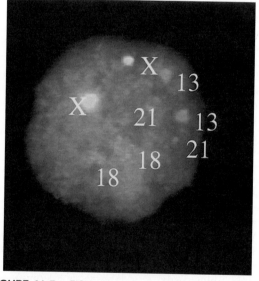

FIGURE 14–7 • FISH of interphase nucleus with a probe specific for chromosomes X, Y, 13, 18, and 21. Each chromosome would under microscopy be readily distinguished by virtue of chromosome-specific probes being different in color (fluorochrome). (Prepared by Dr. Farideh Bischoff, Baylor College of Medicine.) *See Color Plate*

show three signals. Because of geometric vicissitudes, not every trisomic cell shows three signals; however, the modal count is evident. Probes permit simultaneous assessment of multiple chromosomes (Bischoff et al., 1998). When several different fluores are used, computer-digitalized imaging is often employed to assess the number of signals. The attraction for diagnostic purposes is that FISH is applicable to interphase cells, permitting very rapid results.

In one early study, amniotic fluid cells were analyzed with five probes (21, 18, 13, X, and Y) by Klinger and coworkers (1992), who were able to diagnose accurately corresponding trisomies. Ward and colleagues (1993) reported a sensitivity of 88%; the 12% usually represented not errors but uninformative (no result) cases. No false-positive trisomies were diagnosed, but a false-negative sex chromosome abnormality was reported by Benn and coworkers (1992). CVS and placental samples (2709) hybridized with five probes (21, 18, 13, X, and Y; Bryndorf et al., 1996) showed that 93% of cases would be informative and that the detection rate for the numerical abnormalities of the tested chromosomes would be 82%.

When there is insufficient time to perform cultures for cytogenetic studies, very rapid (same day) diagnosis of aneuploidy is even possible by FISH. Usually laboratories prefer 24 or 48 hours. Unequivocal indications for using FISH include management involving a high-risk fetus (e.g., ultrasound findings of multiple anomalies), in which questions exist concerning appropriateness of performing cesarean section or necessity of neonatal surgery (Lapidot-Lifson et al., 1996). In the study of Witters et al. (2002) all trisomy 21 cases (n = 70) were detected by FISH within 48 hours. Rapid FISH analysis is also possible for translocations, using subtelomeric probes (Pettenati et al., 2002).

Whether FISH studies should be offered routinely to women undergoing amniocentesis or CVS is more controversial. Pergament and coworkers (2000) suggest that rapid FISH analysis for chromosomes X, Y, 13, 18, and 21 provides "anxiety relief" while patients await final cytogenetic results of amniocentesis or CVS. Although we would not dissuade couples from the option of FISH analysis while awaiting metaphase results, we prefer not to perform FISH obligatorily. If a laboratory recommends that no action be taken on abnormal FISH results pending cytogenetic studies, the FISH will have proved unnecessary and cost-inefficient. If FISH results were to show no abnormalities but the full cytogenetic result proved abnormal, the reassurance would have been unwarranted.

REFERENCES

Abushoufa RA, Talbot JA, Brownbill K, et al.: The development of a sialic acid specific lectin-immunoassay for the measurement of human chorionic gonadotropin gylcoforms in serum and its application in normal and Down's syndrome pregnancies. Clin Endocrinol 52:499, 2000.

ACOG Committee Opinion: Down syndrome screening. Publication No. 141, August 1994. Washington DC: American College of Obstetricians and Gynecologists, 1994.

ACOG Practice Bulletin: Prenatal diagnosis of fetal chromosomal abnormalities. Clinical Management for Obstetricians-Gynecologists Obstetrics and Gynecology Number 27. Obstet Gynecol 97:1, 2001.

Alberman ED: The abortus as a predictor of future trisomy. *In* De la Cruz FF, Gerald PS (eds): Trisomy 21 (Down Syndrome). Baltimore: University Park Press, 1981, p 69.

Antonarakis SE: The Down Syndrome Collaborative Group: Parental origin of the extra chromosome in trisomy 21 as indicated by analysis of DNA polymorphisms. N Engl J Med 324:872, 1991.

Bahado-Singh R, Oz U, Shahabi S, et al.: Urine hyperglycosylated hCG plus ultrasound biometry for detection of Down syndrome in the second trimester in a high-risk population. Obstet Gynecol 95:889, 2000.

Bar-Hava I, Yitzhak M, Krissi H, et al.: Triple-test screening in *in vitro* fertilization pregnancies. J Assist Reprod Genet 18:226, 2001.

Benn P, Ciarleglio L, Lettieri L, et al.: A rapid (but wrong) prenatal diagnosis. N Engl J Med 326:1638, 1992.

Benn PA, Leo MV, Rodis JF, et al.: Maternal serum screening for fetal trisomy 18: A comparison of fixed cutoff and patient-specific risk protocols. Obstet Gynecol 93:707, 1999.

Berend SA, Horwitz J, McCaskill C, et al.: Identification of uniparental disomy following prenatal detection of robertsonian translocations and isochromosomes. Am J Hum Genet 66:1787, 2000.

Berry E, Aitken DA, Crossley JA, et al.: Screening for Down's syndrome: Changes in marker levels and detection rates between first and second trimester. Br J Obstet Gynaecol 104:811, 1997.

Biagiotti R, Brizzi L, Periti E, et al.: First trimester screening for Down's syndrome using maternal serum PAPP-A and free beta hCG in combination with fetal nuchal translucency thickness. Br J Obstet Gynaecol 105:917, 1998.

Bianchi DW: Prenatal exclusion of recessively inherited disorders: should maternal plasma analysis precede invasive techniques? Clin Chem 48:689, 2002.

Bianchi DW: Fetomaternal cellular and DNA trafficking: the yin and the yang. 11th International Conference on Prenatal Diagnosis and Therapy, Buenos Aires, June 3–5, 2002, Presentation.

Bielanska M, Tan SL, Ao A: Fluorescence in-situ hybridization of sex chromosomes in spermatozoa and spare preimplantation embryos of a Klinefelter 46,XY/47,XXY male. Hum Reprod 15:440, 2000.

Bischoff FZ, Nguyen DD, Burt KJ, et al.: Estimates of aneuploidy using multicolor fluorescence in situ hybridization on human sperm. Cytogenet Cell Genet 66:237, 1994.

Bischoff FZ, Lewis DE, Nguyen DD, et al.: Prenatal diagnosis with use of fetal cells isolated from maternal blood: Five-color fluorescent in situ hybridization analysis on flow-sorted cells for chromosomes X, Y, 13, 18 and 21. Am J Obstet Gynecol 179:203, 1998.

Blennow E, Nielson KB, Telenius H, et al.: Fifty probands with extra structurally abnormal chromosomes characterized by fluorescence in situ hybridization. Am J Med Genet 55:85, 1995.

Bogart MH, Pandian MR, Jones OW: Abnormal maternal serum gonadotropin levels in pregnancies with fetal chromosome abnormalities. Prenat Diagn 7:623, 1987.

Bonduelle M, Wilikens A, Buysse A, et al.: A follow-up study of children born after intracytoplasmic sperm injection (ICSI) with epididymal and testicular spermatozoa and after replacement of cryopreserved embryos obtained after ICSI. Hum Reprod 1:196, 1998.

Boué A, Gallano P: A collaborative study of the segregation of inherited chromosome structural rearrangements in 1356 prenatal diagnoses. Prenat Diagn 4:45, 1984.

Bovicelli L, Orsini LF, Rizzo N, et al.: Reproduction in Down syndrome. Obstet Gynecol 59:13s, 1982.

Brambati B: Chorionic villus sampling. Curr Opin Obstet Gynecol 7:109, 1995.

Bricker L, Garcia J, Henderson J, et al.: Ultrasound screening in pregnancy: A systematic review of clinical effectiveness and women's views. Health Technol Assess 4:1, 2000.

Brondum-Nielsen K, Mikkelson M: A 10-year survey, 1980–1990, of prenatally diagnosed small supernumerary marker chromosomes identified by FISH analysis. Outcome and follow-up of 14 cases diagnosed in a serious of 12,699 prenatal samples. Prenat Diagn 15:615, 1995.

Brumfield CG, Wenstrom KD, Owen J, et al.: Ultrasound findings and multiple marker screening in trisomy 18. Obstet Gynecol 95:51, 2000.

Bryndorf T, Christensen B, Vad M, et al.: Prenatal detection of chromosome aneuploidies in uncultured chorionic villus sampling by FISH. Am J Hum Genet 59:918, 1996.

Bui TH, Iselius L, Lindsten J: European collaborative study on prenatal diagnosis: Mosaicism, pseudomosaicism and single abnormal cells in amniotic fluid cell cultures. Prenat Diagn (Special Issue) 4:145, 1984.

Canadian Collaborative CVS—Amniocentesis Clinical Trial Group. Multicentre randomised clinical trial of chorion villus sampling and amniocentesis. Lancet 1:1, 1989.

Canick JA, Knight GJ, Palomaki GE, et al.: Low second trimester maternal serum unconjugated oestriol in pregnancies with Down's syndrome. Br J Obstet Gynaecol 95:330, 1988.

Canick JA, Kellner LH, Saller DN, et al.: Second-trimester levels of maternal urinary gonadotropin peptide in Down syndrome pregnancy. Prenat Diagn 15:739, 1995.

Casati A, Giorgi R, Lanza A, et al.: Trisomy 21 mosaicism in two subjects from two generations. Ann Genet 35:245, 1992.

Chao AS, Chung CL, Wu CD, et al.: Second trimester maternal serum screening using alpha fetoprotein, free beta human chorionic gonadotropin and maternal age specific risk: Result of chromosomal abnormalities detected in screen positive for Down syndrome in an Asian population. Acta Obstet Gynecol Scand 78:393, 1999.

Christiansen M, Oxvig C, Wagner JM, et al.: The proform of eosinophil major basic protein: A new maternal serum marker for Down syndrome. Prenat Diagn 19:905, 1999.

Cicero S, Curcio P, Papageorghiou A, et al.: Absence of nasal bone in fetuses with trisomy 21 at 11–14 weeks of gestation: an observational study. Lancet 358:1665, 2001.

Claussen U, Schäfer H, Trampisch HJ: Exclusion of chromosomal mosaicism in prenatal diagnosis. Hum Genet 67:23, 1984.

Cuckle HS, Wald NJ, Thompson SG: Estimating a woman's risk of having a pregnancy associated with Down's syndrome using her age and serum alpha-fetoprotein level. Br J Obstet Gynaecol 94:387, 1987.

Cuckle HS, Iles RK, Chard T: Urinary beta-core human chorionic gonadotrophin: A new approach to Down's syndrome screening. Prenat Diagn 14:953, 1994.

Cuckle HS, Iles RK, Sehmi IK, et al.: Urinary multiple marker screening for Down's syndrome. Prenat Diagn 15:745, 1995.

Cuckle HS, Schmi I, Jones R, et al.: Maternal serum activin A and follistatin levels in pregnancies with Down syndrome. Prenat Diagn 19:513, 1999.

Daniel A, Hook EB, Wulf G: Risks of unbalanced progeny at amniocentesis to carrier of chromosome rearrangements: Data from United States and Canadian laboratories. Am J Med Genet 33:14, 1989.

De Biasio P, Siccardi M, Volpe G, et al.: First trimester screening for Down syndrome using nuchal translucency meas-urement with free beta-hCG and PAPP-A between 10 and 13 weeks of pregnancy—the combined test. Prenat Diagn 19:360, 1999.

de Michelena MI, Burstein E, Lama JR, et al.: Paternal age as a risk factor for Down syndrome. Am J Med Genet 45:679, 1993.

Extermann P, Bischof P, Marguerat P, et al.: Second trimester maternal serum screening for Down's syndrome: Free beta-human chorionic gonadotrophin (hCG) and alpha-fetoprotein, with or without unconjugated oestriol, compared with total hCG, alpha-fetoprotein and unconjugated oestriol. Hum Reprod 13:220, 1998.

Farra C, Giudicelli B, Pellissier MC, et al.: Fetoplacental chromosomal discrepancy. Prenat Diagn 20:190, 2000.

Featherstone T, Cheung SW, Spitznagel E, et al.: Exclusion of chromosomal mosaicism in amniotic fluid cultures: Determination of number of colonies needed for accurate analysis. Prenat Diagn 14:1009, 1994.

Ferguson-Smith MA, Yates JR: Maternal age specific rates for chromosome aberrations and factors influencing them: Report of a collaborative European study in 52,965 amniocentesis. Prenat Diagn 4:44, 1984.

Friedman JM: Genetic disease in the offspring of older fathers. Obstet Gynecol 57:745, 1981.

Frishman GN, Canick JA, Hogan JW, et al.: Serum triple-marker screening in in vitro fertilization and naturally conceived pregnancies. Obstet Gynecol 90:98, 1997.

Graf MD, Mowrey PN, Van Dyke DL, et al.: Molecular and cytogenetic delineation of marker chromosomes: Implications for phenotypic effects. Am J Hum Genet 67 (Suppl 2):60, 2000.

Guidelines for Women's Health: The American College of Obstetricians and Gynecologists, Washington, DC 20024, 1996.

Guttenbach M, Michelmann HW, Hinney B, et al.: Segregation of sex chromosomes into sperm nuclei in a man with 47,XXY Klinefelter's karyotype: A FISH analysis. Hum Genet 99:474, 1997.

Hackshaw AK, Densem J, Wald NJ: Repeat maternal serum testing for Down's syndrome screening using multiple markers with special reference to free alpha and free beta-hCG. Prenat Diagn 15:1125, 1995.

Haddow JE, Palomaki GE, Knight GJ, et al.: Prenatal screening for Down's syndrome with use of maternal serum markers. N Engl J Med 327:588, 1992.

Haddow JE, Palomaki GE: Prenatal screening for Down syndrome. In Simpson JL, Elias S (eds): Essentials of Prenatal Diagnosis. New York: Churchill Livingstone, 1993, p 185.

Haddow JE, Palomaki GE, Knight GJ, et al.: Second trimester screening for Down's syndrome using maternal dimeric inhibin A. J Med Screen 5:115, 1998a.

Haddow JE, Palomaki GE, Knight GJ, et al.: Screening of maternal serum for fetal Down's syndrome in the first trimester. N Engl J Med 338:955, 1998b.

Hall JG: Genomic imprinting: Review and relevance to human diseases. Am J Hum Genet 46:857, 1990.

Heinonen S, Ryynanen M, Kirkinen P, et al.: Effect of in vitro fertilization on human chorionic gonadotropin serum concentrations and Down's syndrome screening. Fertil Steril 66:398, 1996.

Hook EB: Rates of chromosomal abnormalities of different maternal ages. Obstet Gynecol 58:282, 1981.

Hook EB: Evaluation and projections of rates of chromosome abnormality in chorionic villus studies (CVS). Am J Hum Genet 43:A108, 1988.

Hook EB: Chromosome abnormalities: Prevalence, risks and recurrences. In Brock DH, Rodeck CH, Ferguson-Smith MA (eds): Prenatal Diagnosis and Screening. Edinburgh: Churchill Livingstone, 1992, p 351.

Hook EB, Cross PK, Schreinemachers DM, et al.: Chromosomal abnormality rates at amniocentesis and in liveborn infants. JAMA 249:2034, 1983.

Hook, EB, Cross PK, Jackson L, et al.: Rates of 47, +21 and other cytogenetic abnormalities diagnosed in 1st trimester chorionic villus sampling (CVS): Comparison with rates from 2nd trimester amniocentesis. Am J Hum Genet 41:A276, 1987.

Hook EB, Cross PK, Jackson LG, et al.: Maternal age-specific rates of 47, +21 and other cytogenetic abnormalities diagnosed in the first trimester of pregnancy in chorionic villus biopsy samples. Comparison with rates expected from observations at amniocentesis. Am J Hum Genet 42:797, 1988.

Howe D, Gornall R, Wellesley D, et al.: Six year survey of screening for Down's syndrome by maternal age and mid-trimester ultrasound scans. BMJ 320:606, 2000.

Hsu L: Prenatal diagnosis of chromosome abnormalities through amniocentesis. In Milunsky A (ed): Genetic Disorders and the Fetus, 4th ed. Baltimore: Johns Hopkins Press, 1998, p 155.

Hsu LYF: Chromosomal disorders. In Reece EA, Hobbins JC, Mahoney MJ, et al. (eds): Medicine of the Fetus and Mother. Philadelphia: JB Lippincott, 1992, p 447.

Hsu L, Kaffe S, Jenkins EC, et al.: Proposed guidelines for diagnosis of chromosome mosaicism in amniocytes based on data derived from chromosome mosaicism and pseudo-mosaicism. Prenat Diagn 12:555, 1992.

Hsu LY, Perlis TE: United States survey on chromosome mosaicism and pseudomosaicism in prenatal diagnosis. Prenat Diagn 4:97, 1984.

Hume RF Jr, Drugan A, Ebrahim SA, et al.: Role of ultra-sonography in pregnancies with marker chromosome aneuploidy. Fetal Diagn Ther 10:182, 1995.

Jacobs PA: Mutation rates of structural chromosome rearrangements in man. Am J Hum Genet 33:44, 1981.

Jorgensen FS, Valentin L, Salvesen KA, et al.: Multiscan—A Scandinavian multicenter second trimester obstetric ultrasound and serum screening study. Acta Obstet Gynecol Scand 78:501, 1999.

Jou HJ, Shyu MK, Chen SM, et al.: Maternal serum screening for Down syndrome by using alpha-fetoprotein and human chorionic gonadotropin in an Asian population. A prospective study. Fetal Diagn Ther 15:108, 2000.

Kalousek DK, Dill FJ, Pantzar T, et al.: Confined chorionic mosaicism in prenatal diagnosis. Hum Genet 77:163, 1987.

Kalousek DK, Howard-Peebles PN, Olson SB, et al.: Confirmation of CVS mosaicism in term placentae and high frequency of intrauterine growth retardation association with confined placental mosaicism. Prenat Diagn 11:743, 1991.

Kleijer WJ, Thompson EJ, Niermeijer MF: Prenatal diagnosis of the Hurler syndrome: report on 40 pregnancies at risk. Prenat Diagn 3:179, 1983.

Klinger K, Landes G, Shook D, et al.: Rapid detection of chromosome aneuploidies in uncultured amniocytes by using fluorescence in situ hybridization (FISH). Am J Hum Genet 51:55, 1992.

Knight GJ, Palomaki GE, Neveux LM, et al.: hCG and the free beta-subunit as screening tests for Down syndrome Prenat Diagn 18:235, 1998.

Krantz DA, Larson JW, Buchanan PD, et al.: First trimester Down syndrome screening; Free beta human chorionic gonadotropin and pregnancy-associated plasma protein A. Am J Obstet Gynecol 174:612, 1996.

Krantz DA, Hallahan TW, Orlandi F, et al.: First-trimester Down syndrome screening using dried blood biochemistry and nuchal translucency. Obstet Gynecol 96:207, 2000.

Lam YH, Tang MH: Second-trimester maternal serum inhibin-A screening for fetal Down syndrome in Asian women. Prenat Diagn 19:463, 1999.

Lapidot-Lifson Y, Lebo RV, Flandermeyer RR, et al.: Rapid aneuploid diagnosis of high-risk fetuses by fluorescence in situ hybridization. Am J Obstet Gynecol 174:886, 1996.

Ledbetter DH, Martin AO, Verlinsky Y, et al.: Cytogenetic results of chorionic villus sampling: High success rate and diagnostic accuracy in the U.S. Collaborative Study. Am J Obstet Gynecol 162:495, 1990.

Ledbetter DH, Zachary JM, Simpson JL, et al.: Cytogenetic results from the U.S. Collaborative Study on CVS. Prenat Diagn 12:317, 1992.

Liao AW, Heath V, Kametas N, et al.: First-trimester screening for trisomy 21 in singleton pregnancies achieved by assisted reproduction. Hum Reprod 16:1501, 2001.

Lorber BJ, Grantham M, Peters J, et al.: Nondisjunction of chromosome 21: Comparisons of cytogenetic and molecular studies of the meiotic stage and parent of origin. Am J Hum Genet 51:1265, 1992.

Malone FD, Berkowitz RL, Canick JA, et al.: First trimester screening for aneuploidy: Research or standard of care? Am J Obstet Gynecol 182:490, 2000.

Maymon R, Dreazen E, Weinraub Z, et al.: Antenatal screening for Down's syndrome in assisted reproductive pregnancies. Hum Reprod Update 5:530, 1999a.

Maymon R, Dreazen E, Tovbin Y, et al.: The feasibility of nuchal translucency measurement in higher order multiple gestations achieved by assisted reproduction. Hum Reprod 14:2102, 1999b.

McGowen KD, Weiser JJ, Horwitz J, et al.: The importance of investigating for uniparental disomy in prenatally identified balanced acrocentric rearrangements. Prenat Diagn 22:141, 2002.

Merkatz IR, Nitowsky HM, Macri JN, et al.: An association between low maternal serum α-fetoprotein and fetal chromosomal abnormalities. Am J Obstet Gynecol 148:886, 1984.

Mikkelsen M, Stene J: Previous child with Down's syndrome and other chromosome aberrations. In Murken JD, Stengel-Rutkowski S, Schwinger E (eds): Prenatal diagnosis: Proceedings of the Third European Conference on Prenatal Diagnosis of Genetic Disorders. Stuttgart, Germany: F Enke, 1979, p 22.

Moore GE, Ali Z, Khan RU, et al.: The incidence of uniparental disomy associated with intrauterine growth retardation in a cohort of thirty-five severely affected babies. Am J Obstet Gynecol 176:294, 1997.

Moosani N, Pattinson HA, Carter MD, et al.: Chromosomal analysis of sperm from men with idiopathic infertility using sperm karyotyping and fluorescence in situ hybridization. Fertil Steril 64:811, 1995.

MRC Working Party on the Evaluation of Chorion Villus Sampling. Medical Research Council European Trial of chorion villus sampling. Lancet 337:1491, 1991.

Neveux LM, Palomaki GE, Knight GJ, et al.: Multiple marker screening for Down syndrome in twin pregnancies. Prenat Diagn 16:29, 1996.

New England Regional Genetics Group Prenatal Collaborative Study of Down syndrome Screening: Combining maternal serum α-fetoprotein measurements and age to screen for Down syndrome in pregnant women under age 35. Am J Obstet Gynecol 160:575, 1989.

Nielsen J, Wohlert M: Chromosome abnormalities found among 34,910 newborn children: results from a 13-year incidence study in Arhus, Denmark. Hum Genet 87:81, 1991.

O'Brien JE, Dvorin E, Drugan A, et al.: Race-ethnicity-specific variation in multiple-marker biochemical screening: alpha-fetoprotein, hCG, and estriol. Obstet Gynecol 89:355, 1997a.

O'Brien JE, Dvorin E, Yaron Y, et al.: Differential increases in AFP, hCG, and uE$_3$ in twin pregnancies: Impact on attempts to quantify Down syndrome screening calculations. Am J Med Genet 73:109, 1997b.

Ognibene A, Ciuti R, Tozzi P, et al.: Maternal serum superoxide dismutase (SOD): A possible marker for screening Down syndrome affected pregnancies. Prenat Diagn 19:1058, 1999.

Okada H, Fujioka H, Tatsumi N, et al.: Klinefelter's syndrome in the male infertility clinic. Hum Reprod 14:946, 1999.

Otaño K, Aiello H, Igarzábal L, et al: First trimester absence of fetal nasal bone on ultrasound and Down syndrome. Prenat Diagn in press, 2002.

Palomaki GE, Haddow JE, Knight GJ, et al.: Risk-based prenatal screening for trisomy 18 using alpha-fetoprotein, unconjugated oestriol and human chorionic gonadotropin. Prenat Diagn 15:713, 1995.

Palomaki GE, Knight GJ, Haddow JE, et al.: Prospective intervention trial of a screening protocol to identify fetal trisomy 18 using maternal serum alpha-fetoprotein, unconjugated oestriol, and human chorionic gonadotropin. Prenat Diagn 12:925, 1992.

Palomaki GE, Knight GJ, Haddow JE, et al.: Cigarette smoking and levels of maternal serum alpha-fetoprotein, unconjugated estriol, and hCG: Impact of Down syndrome screening. Obstet Gynceol 81:675, 1993.

Pergament E, Chen PX, Thangavelu M, et al.: The clinical application of interphase FISH in prenatal diagnosis. Prenat Diagn 20:215, 2000.

Pettenati MJ, Von Kap-Herr C, Jackle B, et al.: Rapid interphase analysis for prenatal diagnosis of translocation carriers using subtelomeric probes. Prenat Diagn 22:193, 2002.

Perona M, Mancini G, Dall'Amico D, et al.: Influence of smoking habits on Down's syndrome risk evaluation at mid-trimester through biochemical screening. Int J Clin Lab Res 28:179, 1998.

Petersen MB, Adelsberger PA, Schinzel AA, et al.: Down syndrome due to de novo robertsonian translocation t(14q;21q): DNA polymorphism analysis suggests that the origin of the extra 21q is maternal. Am J Hum Genet 49:529, 1991.

Peterson MB, Frantzen M, Antonarakis SE, et al.: Comparative study of microsatellite and cytogenetic markers for detecting the origin of the nondisjoined chromosome 21 in Down syndrome. Am J Hum Genet 51:516, 1992.

Petrocik E, Wassman ER, Kelly JC: Prenatal screening for Down syndrome with maternal serum human chorionic gonadotropin levels. Am J Obstet Gynecol 161:1168, 1989.

Phillips OP, Elias S, Shulman LP, et al.: Maternal serum screening for fetal Down syndrome in women less than 35 years of age using alpha-fetoprotein, hCG, and unconjugated estriol: A prospective 2-year study. Obstet Gynecol 80:353, 1992.

Reubinoff BE, Abeliovich D, Werner M, et al.: A birth in non-mosaic Klinefelter's syndrome after testicular fine needle aspiration, intracytoplasmic sperm injection and preimplantation genetic diagnosis. Hum Reprod 13:1887, 1998.

Ribbert LS, Kornman LH, De Wolf BT, et al.: Maternal serum screening for fetal Down syndrome in IVF pregnancies. Prenat Diagn 16:35, 1996.

Richkind KE, Risch NJ: Sensitivity of chromosomal mosaicism detection by different tissue culture methods. Prenat Diagn 10:519, 1990.

Rodis JF, Vintzileos AM, Fleming AD, et al.: Comparison of humerus length with femur length in fetuses with Down syndrome. Am J Obstet Gynecol 165:1051, 1991.

Ron-El R, Strassburger D, Gelman-Kohan S, et al.: A 47,XXY fetus conceived after ICSI of spermatozoa from a patient with non-mosaic Klinefelter's syndrome: Case report. Hum Reprod 15:1804, 2000.

Sachs ES, Jahoda MG, Los FJ, et al.: Trisomy 21 mosaicisms in gonads with unexpectedly high recurrence risks. Am J Med Genet 7:186, 1990.

Sachs ES, Van Hemel JO, Den Hollander JC, et al.: Marker chromosomes in a series of 10,000 prenatal diagnoses: Cytogenetic and follow-up studies. Prenat Diagn 7:81, 1987.

Schreinemachers DM, Cross PK, Hook EB, et al.: Rates of trisomies 21, 18, 13 and other chromosome abnormalities of about 20,000 prenatal studies compared with estimated rates in live births. Hum Genet 61:318, 1982.

Schuchter K, Hafner E, Stangl G, et al.: The first trimester "combined test" for the detection of Down syndrome pregnancies in 4939 unselected pregnancies. Prenat Diagn 22:211, 2002.

Sebire NJ, Snijders RJM, Hughes K, et al.: Screening for trisomy 21 in twin pregnancies by maternal age and fetal nuchal translucency thickness at 10–14 weeks of gestation. BJOG 103:999, 1996.

Shaffer LG, Jackson-Cook CK, Stasiowski BA, et al.: Parental origin determination in 30 de novo robertsonian translocations. Am J Med Genet 43:957, 1992.

Sherman SL, Takaesu N, Freeman SB, et al.: Trisomy 21: Association between reduced recombination and nondisjunction. Am J Hum Genet 49:608, 1991.

Sikkema-Raddatz B, Castedo S, Te Meerman GJ: Probability tables for exclusion of mosaicism in prenatal diagnosis. Prenat Diagn 17:115, 1997.

Simoni G, Fraccaro M, Arslanian A, et al.: Cytogenetic findings in 4952 prenatal diagnoses: An Italian collaborative study. Hum Genet 60:63, 1982.

Simpson JL: Pregnancies in women with chromosomal abnormalities. *In* Schulman JD, Simpson JL (ed): Genetic Diseases in Pregnancy. New York: Academic Press, 1981, p 439.

Simpson, JL, Martin AO, Verp MS, et al.: Hypermodal cells in amniotic fluid cultures: Frequency interpretation and clinical significance. Am J Obstet Gynecol 143:250, 1982.

Simpson JL, Elias S, Morgan CD, et al.: Second trimester maternal serum human chorionic gonadotropin and unconjugated oestriol levels in blacks and whites. Lancet 16:1459, 1990.

Simpson JL, Elias S, Morgan CD, et al.: Does unexplained second trimester (15–20 weeks gestation) MSAFP evaluation presage adverse perinatal outcome? Pitfalls and preliminary studies with late second and third-trimester maternal serum alpha-fetoprotein. Am J Obstet Gynecol 164:829, 1991.

Simpson JL: Maternal serum screening in the United States: Current perspective. *In* Grudzinskas JG, Ward RHT (eds): Screening for Down Syndrome in the First Trimester Proceedings, Conference on First Trimester Screening, Royal College Ob/Gyn, London, 1997, p 95.

Simpson NE, Dallaire L, Miller JR, et al.: Prenatal diagnosis of genetic disease in Canada: Report of a collaborative study. Can Med Assoc J 115:739, 1976.

Smith-Bindman R, Hosmer W, Feldstein VA, et al.: Second-trimester ultrasound to detect fetuses with Down syndrome: A meta-analysis. JAMA 285:1044, 2001.

Snijders RJ, Noble P, Sebire N, et al.: UK multicenter project on assessment of risk of trisomy 21 by maternal age and fetal nuchal-translucency thickness at 10–14 weeks of gestation. Fetal Medicine Foundation First Trimester Screening Group. Lancet 352:343, 1998.

Snijders RJM, Sundberg K, Holzgreve W, et al.: Maternal age and gestation-specific risk for trisomy 21: Effect of previous affected pregnancy. Ultrasound Obstet Gynecol 13:167, 1999.

Spencer K: Is the measurement of unconjugated oestriol of value in screening for Down's syndrome? *In* Grudzinskas JG, Chard T, Chapman M, et al. (eds): Screening for

Down's syndrome. New York: Cambridge University Press, 1994, p 141.

Spencer K: Second trimester prenatal screening for Down's syndrome using alpha-fetoprotein and free beta-hCG: A seven year review. Br J Obstet Gynecol 106:1287, 1999.

Spencer K: Screening for trisomy 21 in twin pregnancies in the first trimester using free beta-hCG and PAPP-A, combined with fetal nuchal translucency thickness. Prenat Diagn 20:91, 2000.

Spencer K: Accuracy of Down syndrome risks produced in a first-trimester screening programme incorporating fetal nuchal translucency thickness and maternal serum biochemistry. Prenat Diagn 22:244, 2002.

Spencer K, Salonen R, Muller F: Down's syndrome screening in multiple pregnancies using alpha-fetoprotein and free beta hCG. Prenat Diagn 14:537, 1994.

Spencer K, Souter V, Tul N, et al.: A screening program for trisomy 21 at 10–14 weeks using fetal nuchal translucency, maternal serum free beta-human chorionic gonadotropin and pregnancy-associated plasma protein-A. Ultrasound Obstet Gynecol 13:231, 1999.

Staessen C: Fertility and assisted reproduction in XXY—ICSI and ART. In Simpson JL, et al.: Klinefelter Syndrome Conference "Expanding the Phenotype and Identifying New Research Directions." In preparation, 2002.

Stene J, Stene E, Mikkelsen M: Risk for chromosome abnormality at amniocentesis following a child with a non-inherited chromosome aberration. A European Collaborative Study on Prenatal Diagnosis 1981. Prenat Diagn 4:81, 1984.

The NICHD National Registry for Amniocentesis Study Group. Midtrimester amniocentesis for prenatal diagnosis: Safety and accuracy. JAMA 115:739, 1976.

Tournaye H, Camus M, Vandervorst M, et al.: Surgical sperm retrieval for intracytoplasmic sperm injection. Int J Androl 3:69, 1997.

Valerio D, Aiello R, Altieri V, et al.: Maternal serum screening of fetal chromosomal abnormalities by AFP, uE$_3$, hCG, and free-beta hCG. Prospective and retrospective results. Minerva Ginecol 48:169, 1996a.

Valerio D, Aiello R, Alteri V, et al.: Cytogenetic characterization of chromosome markers detected at amniocentesis: Implications for karyotype-phenotype correlations. Minerva Ginecologica 48:365, 1996b.

Vejerslev LO, Mikkelsen M: The European collaborative study on mosaicism in chorionic villus sampling: Data from 1986 to 1987. Prenat Diagn 9:575, 1989.

Wald NJ, Densem JW, Cheng R, et al.: Maternal serum free alpha- and free beta-human chorionic gonadotropin in pregnancies with insulin-dependent diabetes mellitus: Implications for screening for Down's syndrome. Prenat Diagn 14:835, 1994a.

Wald NJ, Densem JW: Maternal serum free α-human chorionic gonadotrophin levels in twin pregnancies: Implications for screening for Down syndrome. Prenat Diagn 14:717, 1994b.

Wald NJ, Kennard A, Hackshaw AK, et al.: First trimester serum screening for Down's syndrome. Prenat Diagn 15:1227, 1995.

Wald NJ, Densem JW, George L, et al.: Prenatal screening for Down's syndrome using inhibin-A as a serum marker. Prenat Diagn 16:143, 1996a.

Wald NJ, George L, Smith D, et al.: Serum screening for Down's syndrome between 8 and 14 weeks of pregnancy. International Prenatal Screening Research Group. Br J Obstet Gynaecol 103:407, 1996b.

Wald NJ, Kennard A, Hackshaw S, et al.: Antenatal screening for Down's syndrome. J Med Screen 4:181, 1997.

Wald NJ, Hackshaw AK, Diamandis EP, et al.: Maternal serum prostate-specific antigen and Down syndrome in the first and second trimesters of pregnancy. International Prenatal Screening Research Group. Prenat Diagn 19:674, 1999a.

Wald NJ, White N, Morris JK, et al.: Serum markers for Down's syndrome in women who have had in vitro fertilisation: Implications for antenatal screening. Br J Obstet Gynaecol 106:1304, 1999b.

Wald NJ, Watt HC, Hackshaw AK: Intergrated screening for Down's syndrome on the basis of tests performed during the first and second trimesters. N Engl J Med 341:461, 1999.

Wald N, Rodeck C: Antenatal screening for Down's syndrome: where are we now? 11th International Conference on Prenatal Diagnosis and Therapy, Buenos Aires, June 3–5, 2002, Presentation.

Waller KD, Mills JL, Simpson JL, et al.: Are obese women at higher risk for producing malformed offspring? Am J Obstet Gynecol 170:541, 1994.

Wapner RJ: Chorionic villus sampling. Obstet Gynecol Clin North Am 24:83, 1997.

Wapner RJ, Simpson JL, Golbus MS, et al.: Chorionic mosaicism: Association with fetal loss but not with adverse perinatal outcome. Prenat Diagn 12:347, 1992.

Wapner RJ for the BUN Study Group: First trimester aneuploid screening: results of the NICHD multicenter study. Am J Obstet Gynecol 185:(Suppl):S70, 2001.

Wapner RJ, Thom EA, Simpson JL, et al.: Feasibility and performance of first trimester aneuploidy screening at multiple North American centers. In Press 2002.

Wapner R, et al.: First trimester aneuploid screening: results of the NICHD multicenter study. In Preparation, 2002. **AU: OK?**

Warburton D: Outcome of cases of de novo structural rearrangements diagnosed at amniocentesis. Prenat Diagn 4:69, 1984.

Warburton D: De novo balanced chromosome rearrangements and extra marker chromosomes identified at prenatal diagnosis: Clinical significance and distribution of breakpoints. Am J Hum Genet 49:995, 1991.

Warburton D, Kline J, Stein Z, et al.: Does the karyotype of a spontaneous abortion predict the karyotype of a subsequent abortion? Evidence from 273 women with two karyotyped spontaneous abortions. Am J Hum Genet 41:465, 1987.

Ward BE, Gersen SL, Carelli MP, et al.: Rapid prenatal diagnosis of chromosomal aneuploides by fluorescence in situ hybridization: Clinical experience with 4,500 specimens. Am J Hum Genet 52:854, 1993.

Warren AC, Chakravarti A, Wong C, et al.: Evidence for reduced recombination on the nondisjoined chromosome 21 in Down syndrome. Science 237:652, 1987.

Wenstrom KD, Owen J, Chu DC, et al.: Free beta-hCG subunit versus intact hCG in Down syndrome screening. Obstet Gynecol 90:370, 1997.

Wenstrom KD, Owen J, Chu D, et al.: Prospective evaluation of free beta-subunit of human chorionic gonadotropin and dimeric inhibin A for aneuploidy detection. Am J Obstet Gynecol 181:887, 1999.

Weremowicz S, Sandstrom DJ, Thomas A, et al.: Chromosome analysis on fetal tissues: A revised protocol employing interphase FISH improves the success rate. Am J Hum Genet A835, 2000. **AU: Volum**

Witters I, Devriendt K, Legius E, et al.: Rapid prenatal diagnosis of trisomy 21 in 5049 consecutive uncultured amniotic fluid samples by fluorescence in situ hybridisation (FISH). Prenat Diagn 22:29, 2002.

Wolstenholme J: Confined placental mosaicism for trisomies 2, 3, 7, 8, 9, 16 and 22. Their incidence, likely origins, and mechanisms for cell lineage compartmentalization. Prenat Diagn 16:511, 1996.

Worton RG, Stern R: A Canadian collaborative study of mosaicism in amniotic fluid cell cultures. Prenat Diagn 4:131, 1984.

Zühlke C, Thies U, Braulke I, et al.: Down syndrome and male fertility: PCR-derived fingerprinting, serological and andrological investigations. Clin Genet 46:324, 1994.

Prenatal Diagnosis of Mendelian Disorders and Neural Tube Defects

The most common indication for prenatal genetic diagnosis is risk for chromosomal abnormalities. At age 35 years, the risk for Down syndrome is 1 in 365, whereas the risk for all chromosomal abnormalities is 1 in 200 (see Chapter 14). However, the risk may be much greater for either polygenic-multifactorial traits (2 to 5%) or mendelian disorders (25 to 50%). Principles underlying these genetic etiologies were discussed in Chapters 2 and 3. In this chapter we discuss general approaches to detection of polygenic-multifactorial or mendelian disorders *in utero*.

Mendelian Disorders

With localization of genes to specific chromosomes, increasing numbers of mendelian disorders are now detectable *in utero*. In the 1960s and 1970s, emphasis was on rare metabolic disorders, detectable on the basis of the presence or absence of a given enzyme (gene product). Antenatal diagnoses of the hemoglobinopathies and hemophilia were later accomplished by examining fetal blood, originally obtainable only by fetoscopic sampling (see Chapter 13).

DNA analysis now permits diagnosis of many more disorders using any available nucleated cell (e.g., chorionic villi, amniotic fluid cells). The nature of the mutant or absent gene product need not necessarily be known. Until recently it was almost never known. Now, we can predict confidently that in the foreseeable future almost all common mendelian disorders will be detectable as the location of the causative gene becomes known. The rapid progress and increasing complexity required to diagnose mendelian traits dictate a close liaison between the obstetrician/gynecologist and the geneticist. For this reason we will eschew offering the traditional list of detectable disorders, which by the time of publication would almost certainly be out of date.

INBORN ERRORS OF METABOLISM

Antenatal diagnoses are readily possible for approximately 100 inborn errors of metabolism. Most are transmitted in autosomal recessive fashion, although a few display X-linked recessive or autosomal dominant inheritance. Couples at increased risk are usually identified because they previously had an affected child. Occasionally genetic screening (see Chapter 4) can identify an at risk couple before birth of an affected child. Screening for disorders that fall outside the standard is not required, nor is it reasonable to expect obstetricians who are not geneticists to be fully cognizant of diagnostic possibilities for all these disorders. Ongoing communication with a reproductive geneticist is essential.

Detection of a metabolic disorder by enzymatic assay requires that the enzyme be expressed in amniotic fluid cells or chorionic villi. This requirement is fulfilled by most metabolic disorders, but a prominent exception is phenylketonuria (PKU). Fortunately, PKU can now be detected by molecular techniques. All metabolic disorders detectable in amniotic fluid have proved detectable as well in chorionic villi.

Cultured villi or amniotic fluid cells are usually necessary for diagnosis, although occasionally a diagnosis can be arrived at on the basis of analysis of amniotic fluid liquor. One prominent example is 17α-hydroxyprogesterone, an elevated value of which indicates adrenal 21-hydroxylase deficiency (congenital adrenal hyperplasia). This disorder is also detectable in villi or amniotic fluid cells, either by direct molecular analysis of known mutations (see Chapter 11) or by analysis of linked HLA markers. Another example is Smith-Lemli-Opitz syndrome, detectable on the basis of the presence of dehydroestriol and dehydropregnanetriol in maternal urine or blood. These compounds are undetectable in normal pregnancies (Shackleton et al., 2001).

DISORDERS DETECTABLE SOLELY BY TISSUE SAMPLING

If a gene causing a given disorder is not expressed in amniotic fluid or chorionic villi, enzymatic analysis of such tissues will not provide information concerning the presence or absence of the disorder. However, the gene might still be expressed in other tissues—blood, skin, muscle, or liver. Initially skin was obtained through fetoscopically directed biopsy, under direct vision; currently ultrasound-directed sampling permits use of even smaller instruments. Procedure-related losses following skin biopsy or other invasive procedures are presumably greater than those following CVS or amniocentesis; however, the severity of some disorders justifies tissue sampling if no other diagnostic method is available. Counseling a procedure-related loss of about 2 to 3% seems appropriate (see Chapter 13).

Molecular advances have made tissue sampling nearly obsolete, but sampling fetal skin may still be the only available method for diagnosing certain dermatologic abnormalities, such as variants of epidermolysis bullosa or congenital ichthyosis in which the chromosomal location of the gene is not known. This would preclude linkage analysis or direct DNA analysis. Linked polymorphic markers may also be uninformative in a given family. The proband could be the initial case who also represents a new mutation. In all these scenarios, tissue sampling may be the only diagnostic option. Histologic and electron microscopic analyses of fetal skin would be necessary.

Using the same reasoning, muscle biopsy for dystrophin (histochemistry) may be the only way to detect Duchenne muscular dystrophy in certain families.

DIAGNOSIS OF MENDELIAN DISORDERS BY MOLECULAR METHODS

The power of molecular prenatal diagnosis is that any available nucleated cell can be utilized for diagnosis. All diploid cells contain the same DNA; thus, the gene need not be expressed, unlike the situation in which a gene product (enzyme, a protein) must be analyzed. Through molecular techniques developed within the last decade, phenylketonuria, Duchenne muscular dystrophy, cystic fibrosis, adult-onset polycystic kidney disease, Huntington chorea, and a host of other heretofore undetectable or difficult to detect disorders are now detectable *in utero*.

To take advantage of these advances, the obstetrician/gynecologist must be aware of the analytic techniques that make possible diagnosis by molecular methods. These include polymerase chain reaction (PCR), Southern blotting, use of restriction endonucleases, and use of linkage analysis (see Chapter 2). More detailed reviews are available in standard genetic texts. For our discussion here it is convenient to divide mendelian disorders into (1) those in which the precise nucleotide abnormality is known, and (2) those in which the gene is localized to a given chromosomal region but in which the molecular basis is not known or for which diagnosis is not practical.

Approach with Known Molecular Etiology

Traditional Approaches. The major molecular categories of mendelian disorders include absence of the gene or point mutations leading to missense (single amino acid change) or nonsense (stop codon) mutations. The simplest situation conceptually arises with absence of DNA. One can determine whether a probe does or does not hybridize with the relevant sequence of DNA from an individual of unknown genotype. Duchenne muscular dystrophy is an example; 80% of cases are caused by a gene deletion. If the unknown DNA fails to show hybridization, the specimen presumably lacks the DNA sequence; thus, a gene deletion must exist, and the diagnosis is made.

If the sequence of a typical mutation were known, a restriction enzyme could be selected that acts at the altered site. For example, sickle cell anemia, codon 6 (the triplet signifying the sixth amino acid) has undergone a missense mutation from adenine to thymine ($6A \rightarrow T$). This results in the amino acid's being valine rather than glutamic acid (Glu6Val) (see Table 2–1 for nomenclature). Certain restriction enzymes (see Chapter 2) can be applied diagnostically because of their capacity to recognize the normal nucleotide sequence but not the mutant sequence. Mst II is such a restriction enzyme, acting on the normal nucleotide sequence at

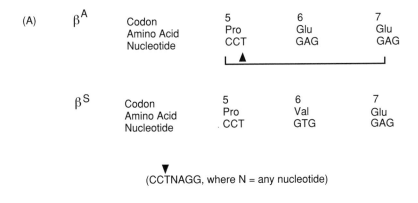

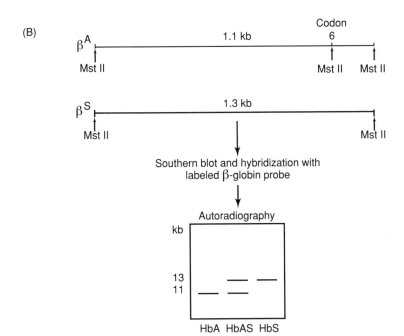

FIGURE 15–1 • Use of a radioactively labeled gene probe for β-globin for diagnosis of sickle cell anemia. The approach uses the choice of a specific restriction enzyme (A) followed by Southern blotting (B) to elicit differences in DNA lengths. A mutation from adenine (A) to thymine (T) results in loss of an Mst II restriction recognition site (CCTNAGG, when N = any nucleotide). (From Simpson JL: *In* Gabbe SA, Niebyl JL, Simpson JL (eds): Obstetrics: Normal and Problem Pregnancies, 3rd ed. New York: Churchill-Livingstone, 1996.)

codon 6 but not at the Mst II recognition site (Fig. 15–1). After exposure to Mst II, one can use a probe for β-globin to differentiate the longer DNA fragment connoting a sickle cell mutation.

Another diagnostic approach involves use of oligonucleotide or allele-specific probes. One can construct DNA probes for sequences of any desired number of nucleotides, usually 15–40 mer. Under conditions of high stringency (high temperature, low salt concentration, polar solvent), probes will hybridize only to sequences complementary for every single nucleotide. If even a single nucleotide is absent (or altered), the oligonucleotide probe will fail to hybridize. Hybridization indicates presence of the known or mutant sequence; failure of hybridization

indicates absence. One allele specific oligonucleotide (ASO) is used to detect the normal sequence, whereas another ASO is used to detect the mutant sequence. Figure 15–2 illustrates this approach for detection of sickle cell disease.

Several practical variations exist in ASO screening. One is to place the specimen containing unknown DNA on a filter and then add the probe, a technique called dot blot or slot blot (depending on shape of the blot). The converse is possible, placing probe(s) on the filter and then adding the unknown specimen DNA. This is called a reverse dot blot. If a single patient must be screened for a panel of mutations, called multiplex analysis, reverse dot blot is preferable (Fig. 15–3).

FIGURE 15–2 • Dot blood analysis. Oligonucleotides are constructed for sequences complementary to normal DNA (β^A) and mutant DNA (β^S). DNA challenged by the oligonucleotide probe will be hybridized if and only if the DNA contains all nucleotides connoted by the probe. Thus, AS individuals will respond to both (β^A and β^S, respectively). Homozygous individuals respond with a stronger (darker) signal than heterozygous individuals. (From Simpson JL: *In* Gabbe SA, Niebyl JF, Simpson JL (eds): Obstetrics: Normal and Problem Pregnancies, 4th ed. New York: Churchill-Livingstone, 2001.)

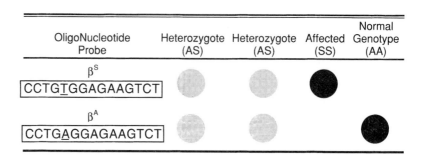

OligoNucleotide Probe	Heterozygote (AS)	Heterozygote (AS)	Affected (SS)	Normal Genotype (AA)
β^S CCTG<u>T</u>GGAGAAGTCT			●	
β^A CCTG<u>A</u>GGAGAAGTCT				●

Newer Approaches. Many other diagnostic modifications exist, all reflecting the underlying principles of PCR and hybridization. These were once used less for diagnosis than for detecting heretofore unknown mutations in a candidate gene believed responsible for a given disorder. However, this is now less true. Even techniques like comparative genome hybridization or microarrays are diagnostically applied.

Increasingly, the preferred alternative is to sequence directly the relevant portion of the target gene known to contain most mutations. Sequenc-

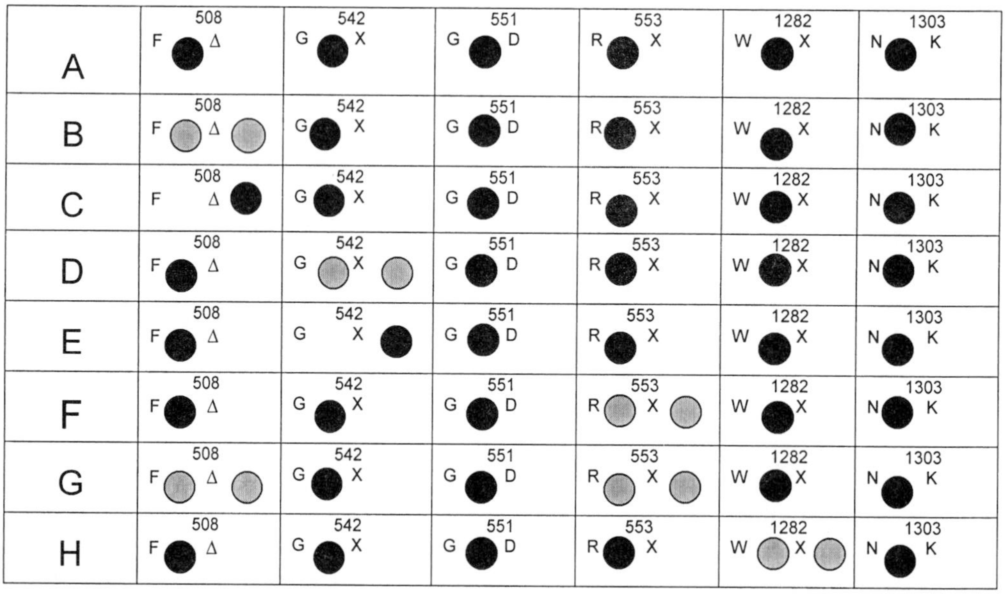

	508	542	551	553	1282	1303
A	F ● Δ	G ● X	G ● D	R ● X	W ● X	N ● K
B	F ◐ Δ ◐	G ● X	G ● D	R ● X	W ● X	N ● K
C	F Δ ●	G ● X	G ● D	R ● X	W ● X	N ● K
D	F ● Δ	G ◐ X ◐	G ● D	R ● X	W ● X	N ● K
E	F ● Δ	G X ●	G ● D	R ● X	W ● X	N ● K
F	F ● Δ	G ● X	G ● D	R ◐ X ◐	W ● X	N ● K
G	F ◐ Δ ◐	G ● X	G ● D	R ◐ X ◐	W ● X	N ● K
H	F ● Δ	G ● X	G ● D	R ● X	W ◐ X ◐	N ● K

FIGURE 15–3 • Allele-specific oligonucleotide probes are bound to the test strip to detect six common CF mutations; in this figure, each individual strip runs horizontally. DNA samples from individuals of unknown CF status are PCR-amplified and hybridized to separate test strips. Here, test strips for eight different individuals are shown (rows A through H). Following hybridization and colorimetric analysis, the patterns of dots on the strips are revealed—hence the CF status of the individuals. For each mutation on the strip (ΔF508, G542X, G551D, R553X, W1282X, and N1303K) the left dot, if present, indicates the person has a normal DNA sequence at that part of the CF gene. The right dot, if present, indicates the person has a CF mutation at that site. Individual A, then, has no CF mutations at the loci tested, as demonstrated by single dots on the left side of all mutations. In contrast, individuals B, D, F, and H are carriers, as demonstrated by the presence of two dots for one of the CF mutations. Individual C has CF, as demonstrated by a single dot on the right side of the ΔF508 panel; individual E has CF, as demonstrated by the single dot on the right side of the G542X panel. Individual G also has CF, but this person's CF arises from two different mutations—ΔF508 and R553X—as indicated by the pairs of dots in each of these panels. This is called compound heterozygosity.

ing may also obviate the inherent problem of decreased specificity in dot blot analysis compared to Southern blotting. As might be imagined, many approaches are under active evaluation in large laboratories. The exact choices that will prove applicable for widespread diagnosis are yet to be determined.

Other molecular techniques utilize FISH. Obstetricians tend to think of using FISH to detect numerical chromosomal abnormalities (aneuploidy) in interphase cells (see Chapters 1 and 14). However, the same principle can be applied to detect the presence of a gene. An SRY probe can detect presence of the gene differentiating testes (see Chapter 10). The microdeletion syndrome listed in Table 1–7 can be detected by FISH. These tests can be applied to amniotic fluid cells of a fetus having an uncharacterized marker chromosome (see Chapter 10) to determine probable phenotype. Two FISH signals can detect gene duplications, as in Charcot-Marie-Tooth disease.

Molecular Hetereogeneity. A major diagnostic problem in most mendelian disorders is their molecular hetereogeneity. Usually many different molecular mutations are responsible for a single clinical disorder. This was illustrated in Chapter 4 for cystic fibrosis. Hemophilia A and B, adult polycystic kidney disease, PKU, β-thalassemia, and almost all mendelian disorders not confined to a specific ethnic group fit into this category. Given molecular heterogeneity, it may be necessary to amplify the unknown DNA (PCR) and test with multiple ASOs (multiplex PCR). The mutation present may still not involve an allele corresponding to one of the mutations tested. Strategies may be different in different ethnic groups. Table 15–1 compares sensitivity of

▼ **Table 15–1.** LIKELIHOOD OF A GIVEN
• MUTATION FOR TAY-SACHS DISEASE BEING DETECTED IN JEWISH AND NON-JEWISH INDIVIDUALS KNOWN TO HAVE THE MUTATION

Mutation	Jewish	Non-Jewish
+ TATC 1278	.80	0.08
+ 1 IVS 12	.09	0.00
Gly269Ser	.03	0.05
Arg247Trp	.02	0.32
Arg249Trp	.00	0.04
+1 IVS 9	.00	0.10
Other	.01	0.02
Unknown	.05	0.39
	100	100

Data from Kaback M, Lim-Stule J, Dabhoekan D, et al., 1993.

detecting Tay-Sachs disease using molecular testing in the Ashkenazi Jewish and in the general (non-Ashkenazi) population. In the latter, molecular screening is unrealistic because detection rate is too low (40%) (Kaback et al., 1993; Gravel et al., 2001). The same would hold true for most mendelian traits in the general population. By contrast, within a given ethnic group almost all cases show the same mutation or a limited number of mutations; thus, molecular screening is easier. One can take advantage of this by screening for a limited panel of mutations likely to detect heterozygosity for several different disorders.

The clinical consequence is that despite molecular advances, a place still exists for prenatal genetic diagnosis using the gene product (protein or enzyme). Diagnostic use of microarray (chips) may eventually allow for analysis of most mutations. High thoughput sequencing is another possibility.

Approach When the Precise Molecular Basis is Not Known or Molecular Testing is Impractical

The molecular approaches described above are applicable when the precise molecular basis of a disorder is known. Unfortunately, this requirement is not fulfilled as often as one would desire. Certain genes may not yet be cloned and isolated. Or, their chromosomal location may be known but the sequence and common perturbations may not have been determined. We have also alluded to the limitation posed by heterogeneity at the molecular level in the previous section. Thus, even if the causative gene is known, searching for the mutation operative in a given family may (at present) not be practical. That is, sequencing the entire gene for every diagnostic situation is not practical, and even then the mutation might not be detected if it were located in a promoter region or involved in translation.

One way to address the dilemma is linkage analysis, taking advantage of the ostensibly innocuous differences in DNA that exist among individuals in the general population. These differences are called *polymorphisms* and are analogous to such well-known polymorphisims as the ABO blood group locus (A, B, O alleles). Despite being clinically insignificant, these differences in DNA yield variations in DNA fragment lengths following exposure to a given restriction endonuclease.

As discussed in Chapter 2, the molecular polymorphisms initially used were *restriction fragment length polymorphisms* (RFLPs). Irrespective of type of polymorphism used in linkage analysis, diagnosis is made not on the basis of the mutant gene or its product per se but rather on the basis of the presence or absence of a nearby marker in a given family. In RFLPs the marker is a DNA variant capable of being recognized or not recognized following exposure to a given endonuclease.

RFLPs are still used diagnostically, but increasingly the polymorphic marker used is a dinucleotide or trinucleotide tandem repeat polymorphism. Throughout the genome there exist polymorphisms in which the number of nucleotide repeats, e.g., the dinucleotides cytosine and adenine (CA) or guanine thymine (GT) vary among individuals at a given locus. Some individuals may show 6 CA repeats at a given locus, others 8, others 10. The almost innumer-

able polymorphisms are the scientific basis for use of DNA analysis in forensic pathology, i.e., DNA "fingerprinting." Major efforts are underway in industry and academic circles to provide more dense polymorphic markers throughout the genome, either dinucleotide repeats or single nucleotide polymorphisms.

Figure 15–4 illustrates linkage analysis, using a RFLP polymorphism. Assume that a given RFLP nucleotide repeat is known to lie close to or preferably within the mutant gene of interest. One next must deduce the *cis-trans* relationship between the mutant allele and the marker. Starting with an individual of known genotype, usually an affected fetus or child, one can then determine on which parental chromosome a given RFLP site or DNA marker is located. Is the marker located on the chromosome carrying the

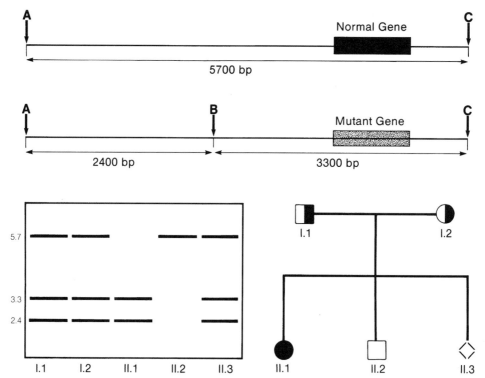

FIGURE 15–4 • Restriction fragment length polymorphisms (RFLPs), which are invaluable for certain prenatal diagnoses. Suppose one mutant gene is linked to another gene (B) that governs whether or not a restriction site (B) is present. If the restriction site is present, DNA is cut by a certain restriction enzyme *(arrow)* to produce 3300 and 2400 bp long fragments. If the segment conferring the restriction site is not present, the total fragment is 5700 bp long. The different lengths can serve as markers to allow genotypes to be deduced. If two obligate heterozygotes 1.1 and 1.2 have one affected child, and a probe for the gene hybridizes to the region A to C, the probe can identify three fragments (2400, 3300, and 5700 bp). If the affected child shows only the 2400 and 3300 bp fragments, it can be deduced that the mutant allele is in association (i.e., on the same chromosome) with the gene-conferring restriction site B and thus is producing both 2400 and 3300 bp fragments. The normal allele must be in association with the allele not conferring restriction B and thus is designated by the 5700 bp fragment. Genotypes can thus be predicted from DNA analysis of chorionic villi and amniotic fluid cells. Fetus 11.3 can be assumed to be heterozygous because all three fragments (2400, 3300, and 5700) are present. (From Simpson JL: *In* Gabbe SA, Niebyl JF, Simpson JL (eds): Obstetrics: Normal and Problem Pregnancies, 4th ed. New York: Churchill-Livingstone, 2001.)

mutant gene, or is it located on the chromosome carrying the normal gene?

Pitfalls in linkage analysis using polymorphic DNA are the same as those arising in any type of linkage analysis. First, the marker may or may not be informative in a given family. If all family members show identical DNA fragment patterns at a given locus, that locus is useless because affected and unaffected individuals cannot be distinguished from one another. If a given marker is uninformative, another marker must be sought that could prove informative. Theoretically, this should be successful, as the number of DNA markers is almost limitless. Second, the distance between the mutant gene and the marker is crucial because the likelihood of meiotic recombination is inversely related to the distance. As discussed in Chapters 1 and 2, recombination occurs during meiosis I between homologous chromosomes. Recombination can occur even between closely linked loci; thus, prenatal diagnosis based on linkage analysis is never 100% accurate. Using polymorphic markers on both sides of the mutant can minimize but never exclude a recombinational event.

Despite these caveats, linkage analysis permits prenatal diagnosis in many situations in which diagnosis is not otherwise possible. Linkage analysis is especially applicable to single-gene (mendelian) disorders characterized by molecular heterogeneity.

Polygenic-Multifactorial Disorders

DISORDERS DETECTABLE ONLY BY ULTRASOUND

Anomalies inherited in polygenic-multifactorial fashion (see Chapter 3) usually carry recurrence risks of 1 to 5% for first-degree relatives (siblings, offspring, parents). The risk is sufficiently high to justify invasive prenatal diagnosis for many couples. The number of genes responsible for these defects is unknown, but presumably there is more than one; thus, diagnosis on the basis of enzyme assays or DNA cannot be entertained seriously at present. Except for the few conditions amenable to amniotic fluid AFP analysis, the principal method of assessment involves visualization of fetal anatomy by ultrasound.

The typical couple at risk already has had a child with the anomaly in question, thus having a 1 to 5% risk for another affected child. To preserve all reproductive options, diagnosis should be made by 20 to 24 weeks' gestation. This is sufficiently early in gestation to weigh the alternatives of termination, fetal surgery, or preterm delivery followed by neonatal surgery. With PUBS, amniocentesis, or second-trimester transabdominal CVS, one can exclude chromosomal abnormalities if late second trimester interventions are contemplated. A careful search for other defects is necessary before selecting any option. For some conditions (e.g., hydrocephaly) an isolated anomaly is rare, but for others (e.g., posterior urethral) values, only a single malformation may be present.

Many volumes provide detailed information on ultrasound technique and accuracy. We merely note here that antenatal ultrasonography for anomaly detection should be performed only by highly experienced ultrasonographer. The problem is uncertainty concerning sensitivity, which can vary by operator, equipment, gestational age, and patient habitus (e.g., obesity). Physicians who routinely scan their obstetric patients only for fetal viability, multiple gestations, and placental location should explicitly inform their patients that anomaly assessment is not being attempted. Casual reassurance of fetal normalcy should be eschewed. It should further be realized that few physicians have sufficient experience to allow calculation of their own specificities or sensitivities. Sensitivity of detection is never 100%, even in the best of hands.

NEURAL TUBE DEFECTS

The sole group of polygenic-multifactorial disorders that we will specifically discuss are the neural tube defects (NTDs). This group is chosen because existing standards dictate that the obstetrician offer screening for these conditions.

Types of NTDs

NTDs result from failure of closure of the fetal neural tube. Anencephaly is the most severe form of NTD, arising at or before 3 weeks' gestation and resulting from failed closure of the anterior neural tube and overlying cranial bones, with subsequent underdevelopment of brain tissue. Fetuses with anencephaly either spontaneously abort or result in stillborns or neonatal deaths. Spina bifida arises later in embryonic development, at approximately 4 weeks' gestation, as a result of failure of closure of the middle or caudal region of the fetal neural tube. Patients with spina bifida have about an 80 to 90% 5-year survival, but almost all have at least some neurologic deficit. Perhaps 15 to 20% of patients with spina bifida have other malformations, such as cardiovascular abnormalities or abdominal wall defects. Few of these are part of an identifiable syndrome. However, NTDs have been reported in many different syndromes. Table 15–2 shows the spectrum of NTDs.

Open neural tubes are either not covered with skin or are covered only by a thin membrane over the brain, spinal cord, or nerves. Almost all cases of anencephaly (99%) and most cases of spina bifida (85 to 90%) are open defects. About 50% of encephaloceles are open. Closed defects are usually not detected by MSAFP screening (see below) because AFP does not leak into the surrounding amniotic fluid and secondarily into the maternal serum. Nonetheless, 70% of closed NTDs are associated with moderate or severe handicaps.

Incidence and Recurrence Risks

Incidence of NTDs varies with geography and ethnicity. An incidence of up to 1% of all live births was reported at one time in Northern Ireland, Scotland, and Wales (Elwood and Elwood, 1980). However, this incidence has decreased in recent years, even before prenatal screening (Wald and Cuckle, 1984; Eurocrat Working Group, 1991). The incidence is much lower in Japan. In the United States the incidence was once 1 to 2 in every 1000 live births, with the highest incidence rates in the Appalachian

▼ **Table 15–2.** SPECTRUM OF NEURAL TUBE
• DEFECTS

Polygenic-multifactorial isolated inheritance (90–95%)
Mendelian disorders
   Autosomal recessive (claims)
   X-linked recessive (claims)
   Meckel syndrome (most common)
   Robert syndrome
   Jarcho-Levin syndrome
   Median facial cleft syndrome
   HARDE (Walker-Warburg) syndrome
   Oculoauriculovertebral (Goldenhar) syndrome
   Other
Chromosomal aneuploidy and polyploidy
   Trisomy 18
   Trisomy 13
   Trisomy 21
   Triploidy
   Other
Teratogens
   Valproic acid
   Carbamazepine
   Aminopterin
   Thalidomide
Amniotic band sequence
Cloacal extrophy
Sacrococcygeal teratoma

region (8 per 10,000 livebirths) (Jorde et al., 1984). More recently Stevenson and colleagues (2000) reported that prevalence of NTDs decreased from 1.89 to 0.95 per 1000 live births in a surveillance program in South Carolina, a region of relatively high NTD incidence. Incidence is high in the Rio Grande Valley, especially on the Mexican side of the border. In general NTDs are more common in people of Irish, Scottish, and Egyptian ancestry and least common in people of African, Ashkenazi Jewish, and Asian ancestry. When a member of a low incidence ethnic group migrates to a new locale, the incidence rates for NTD reflect a middle ground between the ancestral homeland and the new location rates.

Both chromosomal and single-gene disorders may be associated with NTDs. NTDs have been documented as showing ostensible X-linked recessive or autosomal dominant inheritance patterns. Anencephaly in particular and NTDs in general are more common in female offspring and abortuses, a finding of still uncertain significance. Teratogens, for example valproic acid, can be associated with NTDs (Table 15–2).

The above data notwithstanding, most NTDs are isolated and presumably polygenic-multifactorial in etiology (Milunsky, 1998). Recurrence risks for these NTDs reflect the population incidence, number of affected persons in a family, ancestry, and geographical location (Table 15–3). In the United Kingdom (with its high incidence of NTDs), a woman who has had a child with an NTD has a 5% recurrence risk.

In the United States, couples who have had a child with an NTD have approximately a 2% risk of recurrence—1% for any subsequent offspring having spina bifida and 1% for any subsequent offspring having anencephaly (2% for any NTD). This holds true irrespective of the type of NTD present or the sex of the index case (proband). If a prospective parent has an NTD (i.e., spina bifida), the risk is also about 2%. These risks are predictable on the basis of polygenic-multifactorial etiology (see Chapter 3). Second-degree relatives (nieces, nephews, grandchildren) and third-degree relatives (first cousins) are less likely to be affected. A woman whose sister or brother had a child with an NTD carries a lower (0.5 to 1.0%) risk for NTD offspring. For reasons that remain unclear, the risk is even lower if the father's sibling had an NTD.

Amniotic Fluid AFP

Antenatal diagnosis of an NTD is best accomplished by determining levels of amniotic fluid

▼ **Table 15–3.** RECURRENCE RISK FOR NEURAL TUBE DEFECTS, REFLECTING RESULTS OF
• MULTIPLE STUDIES

	Risk of NTDs (%)		
Family History	United States	United Kingdom	Canada
One previous child with NTDs	1.4–3.2	4.6–5.2	2.4–6.0
Two previous children with NTDs	6.4	10–20	4.8
Three previous children with NTDs		21–25	
Affected parent and one sibling with NTDs		3	4.5
Affected parent and one sibling with NTDs		13	
All first cousins	0.26	0.4–0.6	
All maternal first cousins			0.9
All paternal first cousins			0.5
Affected maternal nephew/niece	0.99		0.6–1.3
One child with multiple vertebral anomalies		3–7	
One child with spinal dystrophism		4	
One sibling and a second-degree relative affected		9	
One sibling and a third-degree relative affected		7	

Modified from Milunsky A: Genetic Disorders of the Fetus, 4th ed. Baltimore: Johns Hopkins University Press, 1998, where references are found.

alpha-fetoprotein (AFP). Levels higher than 2.5 MoM are generally considered abnormal. AFP is a glycoprotein with a structure similar to that of albumin; its function is unknown. Genes for both albumin and AFP are located in tandem on chromosome 4q (Gibbs et al., 1987). AFP is initially produced by the yolk sac and liver. As gestation progresses, liver production of AFP increases, and by the end of the first trimester almost all AFP is produced by the fetal liver. A small amount of AFP is produced by the gastrointestinal tract. AFP is secreted into fetal serum, peaking around 3 mg/mL at 13 weeks after conception (Gitlin et al., 1966) (Fig. 15–5). Maternal serum AFP (MSAFP) continues to increase until approximately 30 weeks, when the concentration plateaus or slightly decreases.

Pregnant women having a previous affected child with NTD or themselves having NTD (e.g., spina bifida) should be offered amniocentesis to determine amniotic fluid AFP and acetylcholinesterase levels (see below). Diagnosis of NTD is possible in all cases of anencephaly and in all cases of open spina bifida. Diagnosis is not always possible in fetuses with closed spina bifida or in the 50% of fetal encephaloceles that are closed.

Can ultrasound replace amniotic fluid AFP analysis? Indeed, ultrasonography by experienced physicians should readily exclude anencephaly, and spina bifida theoretically can be excluded through serial views of the vertebral column and shape of the cranium, ventricles, cerebellum, and cisternal magna. However, it is rarely possible for individual ultrsonographers to state their sensitivity or specificity for detecting NTDs. Amniotic fluid AFP analysis should

be considered the standard method for detecting an NTD despite statements to the contrary. This statement is made despite the authors' awareness that some excellent obstetric ultrasonographers recommend avoiding invasive procedures if ultrasound examination reveals no anomalies.

Acetylcholinesterase (AChE) is produced from neuronal axons. AChE is present in the amniotic fluid of fetuses with open NTDs but absent in normal amniotic fluid. Acetylcholinesterase is thus an invaluable ancillary diagnostic method. Its presence or absence can be interpreted independent of gestational age. AChE can be used to exclude amniotic fluid AFP that is spuriously elevated because amniotic fluid contains fetal blood. If AChE is absent but fetal hemoglobin is present, elevated amniotic fluid AFP can be assumed to be due to fetal blood.

Elevated amniotic fluid AFP and maternal serum amniotic fluid AFP are associated with other polygenic-multifactorial anomalies (e.g., omphalocele, gastroschisis, cystic hygroma) (Table 15–4). In these disorders, AChE may or may not be elevated. MSAFP (see below) may or may not be elevated. With certain mendelian traits (e.g., congenital nephrosis) MSAFP is elevated but AChE is not. Ultrasonographic studies should be undertaken to corroborate elevated amniotic fluid AFP and to determine the nature of any defect present; however, again, failure to detect an anomaly by ultrasound does not necessarily indicate that elevated amniotic fluid AFP level was spurious. If amniotic fluid AFP is elevated and AChE is present, at our centers we counsel that the fetus is likely to be abnormal irrespective of ultrasound findings.

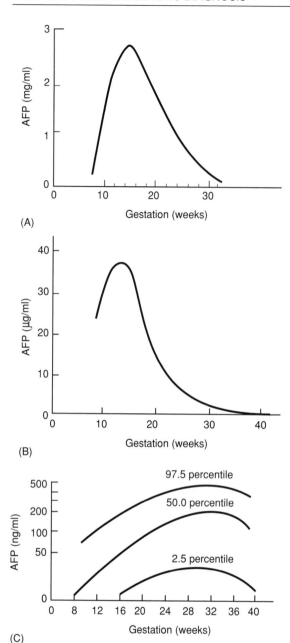

FIGURE 15–5 • Approximate relationship between AFP values in fetal serum (*A*), amniotic fluid (*B*), and maternal serum (*C*). Note varying laboratory units for each graph. (From Habib ZA: Maternal serum alpha-fetoprotein: Its value in antenatal diagnosis of genetic disease and obstetrical-gynaecological care. Acta Obstet Gynecol Scand 61:14, 1977. Copyright, 1977, Munksgaard International Publishers Ltd, Copenhagen, Denmark.)

MSAFP Screening

In adults, serum AFP levels are normally below 10 ng/mL. The level increases greatly during pregnancy until approximately 30 weeks' gestation, plateauing until 35 to 36 weeks, and finally

▼ **Table 15–4.** FETAL DISORDERS IDENTIFIED
• BY AMNIOTIC FLUID AFP TESTING OR
  MSAFP SCREENING

Fetal demise
Neural tube defects
    Anencephaly
    Spina bifida
    Encephalocele
Ventral wall defects
    Omphalocele
    Gastroschisis
Chromosomal abnormalities
Triploidy
Trisomies: 18, 13, 21
Amniotic band sequence
Pentalogy of Cantrell: omphalocele, lower sternal defect,
    deficiency of diaphragmatic pericardium, intracardiac
    abnormality, anterior diaphragm defect
Renal agenesis
Multiple gestation (elevated MSAFP)
Congenital nephrosis (Finnish type)
Sacrococcygeal teratoma
Determatologic disorders
    Epidermolysis bullosa
    Congenital icthyosiform erythroderma
Rh(D) or Kell isoimmunization

falling. The sharp rise reflects the very high concentration in fetal plasma, peaking at 3000 ug/mL (3 mg/mL) at 10 to 13 weeks before falling sharply (Habib, 1977) (see Fig. 15–5). Amniotic fluid AFP parallels this pattern. That AFP is so concentrated in the fetus probably indicates a key osmotic or immunoregulatory function. As discussed, amniotic fluid AFP is increased, often greatly so, with open NTDs. Paralleling this, maternal serum MSAFP is elevated (>2.5 MoM) in pregnancies characterized by open neural tube defects. Performing amniocentesis when MSAFP is >2.5 MoM leads to detection of fetal NTDs in 85 to 90% of open NTD cases. Because 95% of infants with NTDs are born without a family history of NTDs, MSAFP screening is the only practical way to decrease the incidence of NTDs in the general population.

If MSAFP is >2.5 MoM, women should be offered amniocentesis to determine amniotic fluid AFP and acetylcholinesterase levels. The same holds if amniocentesis is undertaken for another indication (e.g., maternal age). All women considered at low risk should be offered maternal serum marker screening between 15 and 20 weeks' gestation.

Several variables affect MSAFP levels. Definitive treatsies have explored this topic in detail (Milunsky, 1998; Wald and Leck, 2000), and we need mention here only those few variables for which adjustments are usually made.

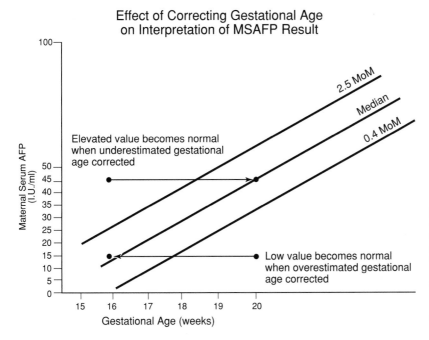

Effect of Correcting Gestational Age on Interpretation of MSAFP Result

Elevated value becomes normal when underestimated gestational age corrected

Low value becomes normal when overestimated gestational age corrected

Maternal Serum AFP (I.U./ml)

Gestational Age (weeks)

FIGURE 15–6 • Median MSAFP throughout gestation. Increasing values with increasing gestational age require accurate dating to interpret low or high levels of MSAFP. (From Simpson JL: *In* Gabbe SA, Niebyl JF, Simpson JL (eds): Obstetrics: Normal and Problem Pregnancies, 3rd ed. New York: Churchill-Livingstone, 1996.)

The most obvious is gestational age, the clinical effect of which is illustrated in Figure 15–6. A second variable is weight. Heavier women have lower MSAFP levels because of a vascular dilutional effect. Ethnicity is important because MSAFP is 10% higher in black women than in white women. Hispanic women in the U.S. have slightly lower values (Byrne et al., 1997), but standard curves used for the white population can be used for Hispanics. The same holds true for Asian women. Insulin-dependent diabetic patients have a 40% lower MSAFP than do non-diabetic women, probably reflecting weight but possibly also inadequate glycemic control. Recently, Sancken and Bartels (2001) reopened this question and concluded that MSAFP in diabetic women did not differ significantly from that in the general pregnancy population. Thus, taking into account diabetic status may no longer be necessary. However, offspring of at least poorly controlled diabetic women are at an increased risk for having a fetus with an NTD. Thus, a lower threshold for amniocentesis might still be appropriate. Finally, 30 to 60% of twin pregnancies have MSAFP values at or above 2.5 MoM.

A pregnant woman should explicitly be counseled that a normal MSAFP cannot completely exclude a fetal NTD. About 10 to 15% of open NTDs and anecephaly may fail to be detected with MSAFP screening, and closed NTDs generally are not detected.

Management of Elevated MSAFP Levels

Approximately 5% of women who undergo MSAFP screening have elevated MSAFP levels. Most prove to have normal fetuses. Elevated MSAFP, like elevated amniotic fluid AFP, may be associated with several different circumstances (Table 15–5), encompassing normal pregnancy, fetal NTD or other anomalies, maternal disease, or other adverse perinatal complications. If MSAFP is elevated, high quality ultrasonography should confirm gestational age and exclude multiple gestation, fetal demise, and overt anomalies. If gestational age is 18 weeks or less and MSAFP is between 2.5 and 2.99 MoM, repeating

▼ **Table 15–5.** EXPLANATIONS FOR ELEVATED
• MSAFP OTHER THAN FETAL ANOMALIES

Fetal demise
Multiple gestation (50% of twins and almost all triplets have MSAFP values that are elevated compared to singleton values)
Underestimation of gestational age
Maternal disorders
    Tumor of liver or yolk sac or ovarian teratomas
    Acute viral hepatitis
    Blood group sensitization [Rh(D) and Kell]
    Lupus autoantibody
Placental anomalies
    Hemangiomas of placenta, umbilical cord
    Placental lakes
    Retroplacental bleed

▼ **Table 15–6.** ODDS OF A GIVEN MSAFP VALUE AT 16 TO 18
• WEEKS' GESTATION BEING ASSOCIATED WITH OPEN SPINA
  BIFIDA, STRATIFIED BY POPULATION INCIDENCE

MSAFP (MoM)	Odds of NTDs	
	Incidence of 1 per 1000	Incidence of 2 per 1000
2.0	1:800	1:400
2.5	1:290	1:140
3.0	1:120	1:59
3.5	1:53	1:27
4.0	1:26	1:13
4.5	1:14	1:7
5.0	1:7	1:4

Data from Fourth Report of the U.K. Collaborative Study on Alpha-Fetoprotein in Relation to
Neural Tube Defects 1982. From Wald N, Leck I: Antenatal and Neonatal Screening, 2nd ed.
New York: Oxford University Press, 2000.
Multiple gestations are excluded. Odds assume no prenatal genetic diagnosis and no selective
abortion.

the MSAFP may be worthwhile. Finding a value
< 2.5 MoM avoids amniocentesis, reducing the
false-positive result rate (amniocentesis) by
about 40%, without decrease in detection rate.
MSAFP > 3.0 MoM is unlikely to fall below 2.5
MoM upon repeating.

If ultrasound fails to provide an explanation for
the elevated MSAFP and no structural anomalies
are visualized, amniocentesis should be offered.
Table 15–6 shows the likelihood that a given
MSAFP will prove abnormal, stratified by population incidence. Amniotic fluid should be analyzed for amniotic fluid AFP, AChE, and
chromosomes. AChE testing allows high sensitivity and specificity for NTD detection and is independent of gestational age between 15 and 22
weeks. AChE is sometimes observed with fetal
cystic hygroma, upper gastrointestinal obstruction, hydrops, and other rare anomalies. AChE is
usually negative in congenital nephrosis, an
uncommon explanation for markedly elevated
MSAFP. Table 15–7 lists common explanations
for false-positive and false-negative MSAFP levels.

Using ultrasonography in lieu of amniocentesis
in the evaluation of an elevated MSAFP remains
controversial and in our opinion is not recommended. Many cases of open spina bifida can
be detected by ultrasound examination, either
before or after learning the MSAFP results
(Richards et al., 1988). When patients were
referred in the 1980s for an elevated MSAFP
value to a center in the California prenatal screening program, 8.1% of NTDs were not detected
by ultrasound examination (Platt et al., 1992).
However, the false negative rate for NTD detection is undoubtedly much lower with more
modern ultrasound equipment. Detection is
highest with associated cranial features (i.e.,
"lemon" and "banana" signs). In open NTDs,

when present, ultrasound evaluation provides
perhaps 90 to 95% sensitivity for detecting fetal
NTDs. However, few can creditably claim the
near 100% detection rate that exists when amniotic fluid AFP and AChE are used to detect open
NTDs (Milunsky, 1998).

Perinatal Complications and Elevated MSAFP

Unexplained elevated MSAFP levels (i.e., normal
ultrasound and normal amniotic fluid AFP) may
be associated with adverse perinatal outcome
unrelated to NTDs. In a sentinel case-control
study from California, Waller and coworkers
(1991) reported that women with elevated levels
of serum AFP in the second trimester of pregnancy had an increased risk of fetal death, a risk
manifested as increased throughout pregnancy.
MSAFP levels 2.0 to 2.9 times the median were
associated with an elevated risk of fetal death
(odds ratio 2.4; 95% CI 1.7–3.4). Women with
higher MSAFP levels (≥ 3.0 MoM) have a higher
risk for fetal death (odds ratio, 10.4; 95% CI,

▼ **Table 15–7.** COMMON EXPLANATIONS FOR
• FALSE-POSITIVE AND FALSE-NEGATIVE
  MSAFP LEVELS

False-Positive
Gestation more advanced than estimated
Multiple gestations
Ethnicity (African-Americans have higher levels)
Low maternal weight (less than 90 lb)
Fetal bleeding (into maternal circulation)
Fetal demise (recent)

False-Negative
Gestation less advanced than estimated
Maternal insulin-dependent diabetes mellitus
Obesity

4.9–220). Fetal deaths were especially likely to be associated with maternal hypertension or placental infarction. There was a 2.4 relative risk for preterm deliveries, a 2.7 relative risk for small-for-gestational-age (SGA) fetuses, and a 4 to 5 relative risk for extremely SGA fetuses (Morssink et al., 1995). Adverse perinatal outcomes associated to elevated MSAFP could be secondary to a defective maternal-fetal placental barrier.

The clinical dilemma is that no consensus exists on the optimal method of surveillance of these pregnancies. The effectiveness of expensive monitoring (e.g., serial ultrasound examinations and/or biophysical profiles) in such cases has not been demonstrated (Elias et al., 1990). Follow up third-trimester MSAFP values surprisingly proved less predictive than second-trimester values (Simpson et al., 1995).

Folic Acid Supplementation to Prevent Neural Tube Defects

Folic acid can decrease the incidence of NTDs. Smithells and coworkers (1980) first championed this hypothesis, showing lower than expected recurrence risk when folic acid was administered to women having a prior NTD. In 1991 the Medical Research Council (MRC) Vitamin Study Group reported a prospective, randomized study finding that folic acid supplementation decreased the recurrence rate of NTDs by 71% in women who had a previous child with an NTD (Medical Research Council, 1991). This recurrence study was followed by a small but conclusive *occurrence* (no previously affected NTD offspring) study that showed efficacy (Czeizel and Dudas, 1992), and one U.S. case control study similarly showed benefit (Milunsky et al., 1989). One other U.S. study in Illinois and California failed to show a positive association between NTDs and folates (vitamins and diet) (Mills et al., 1989).

The Centers for Disease Control (CDC, 1993) and The American College of Medical Genetics now recommend daily supplemental folic acid (0.4 mg) for women throughout their reproductive years. The Centers for Disease Control favors food fortification to accomplish this (Centers for Disease Control and Prevention and Prevention Working Group on Folic Acid, 1993). In women who have had a child with a prior NTD, the American College of Obstetricians and Gynecologists recommends daily folate (4 mg), beginning at least 1 month prior to conception (ACOG, 1996).

In a case-control study comparing 203 children with spina bifida to 583 controls, de Franchis and co-workers (2002) found homozygosity for the 677C-T allele of 5, 10-methylenetetrahydrofolate reductase was associated with an odds ratio for spina bifida of 1.57 (95% CI, 1.02–2.38). For the 844ins68 allele of cystathionine-β-synthase, the odds ratio was 0.83 (95% CI, 0.39–1.64). For the joint genotype, the odds ratio was 3.69 (95% CI, 1.04–13.50). They concluded that interactions between common alleles of folate genes might contribute to susceptibility for spina bifida.

Obesity

An association between pregnancy weight and NTDs has been reported. A reported two- to four-fold increase risk of NTDs was reported in obese women, defined as body mass index >29 kg/m^2 or body weight > 80 kg. This risk appears independent of folic acid supplementation (Waller et al., 1994; Shaw et al., 1996). Obese patients should be counseled concerning the benefits of weight reduction prior to pregnancy.

REFERENCES

ACOG: Educational Bulletin: Nutrition and Women. American College of Medicine, October 1996.

Byrne JL, Waller DK, Rose E, et al.: Effect of Hispanic ethnicity on interpretation of maternal serum screening. Fetal Diagn Ther 12:102, 1997.

Centers for Disease Control and Prevention: Recommendations for the use of folic acid to reduce number of cases of spina bifida and other neural tube defects. JAMA 269:1233, 1993.

Centers for Disease Control and Prevention and Prevention Working Group on Folic Acid. Position paper on folic acid food fortification and the prevention of spina bifida and anencephaly (SBA). Atlanta: Centers for Disease Control and Prevention, 1993.

Czeizel AE, Dudas I: Prevention of the first occurrence of neural-tube defects by periconceptional vitamin supplementation. N Engl J Med 327:1832, 1992.

de Franchis R, Botto LD, Sebastio G, et al.: Spina bifida and folate-related genes: A study of gene-gene interactions. Genet Med 4:126, 2002.

Elias S, Simpson JL, Golbus MS: Re: Update on MSAFP policy statement from the ASHG. Am J Hum Genet 46:847, 1990.

Elwood JM, Elwood JH: Epidemiology of anencephalus and spina bifida. New York: Oxford University Press, 1980.

Eurocrat Working Group: Prevention of neural tube defects in twenty regions of Europe and impact of prenatal diagnosis, 1980-1986. J Epidemiol Community Health 45:52, 1991.

Gibbs PE, Zielinski R, Boyd C, et al.: Structure, polymorphism, and novel repeated DNA elements revealed by a complete sequence of the human alpha-fetoprotein gene. Biochemistry 26:1332, 1987.

Gitlin D, Boesman M: Serum alpha-fetoprotein, albumin, and gamma-G-globulin in the human conceptus. J Clin Invest 45:1826, 1966.

Gravel RA, Kaback MM, Proia RL, et al.: The GM2 gangliosi-doses. *In* Scriver CR, Beaudet AL, Sly WS, et al. (eds): The Metabolic and Molecular Bases of Inherited Disease. New York: McGraw Hill Medical Publishing, 2001, p 3827.

Habib ZA: Maternal serum alpha-fetoprotein: Its value in antenatal diagnosis of genetic disease and in obstetrical-gynecological care. Acta Obstet Gynecol Scand 61:1, 1977.

Jorde LB, Fineman RM, Martin RA: Epidemiology of neural tube defects in Utah, 1940-1979. Am J Epidemiol 119:487, 1984.

Kaback M, Lim-Steele J, Dabholkar D, et al.: Tay-Sachs disease—Carrier screening, prenatal diagnosis, and the molecular era. An international perspective, 1970 to 1993. The International TSD Data Collection Network. JAMA 270:2307, 1993.

Mills JL, Rhoads GG, Simpson JL, et al.: National Institute of Child Health and Human Developmental and Neural Tube Defects Study Group: The absence of a relation between the periconceptional use of vitamins and neural-tube defects. N Engl J Med 321:430, 1989.

Milunsky A: Genetic Disorders of the Fetus, 4th ed. Baltimore: Johns Hopkins University Press, 1998.

Milunsky A, Jick H, Jick SS, et al.: Multivitamin/folic acid supplementation in early pregnancy reduces the prevalence of neural tube defects. JAMA 262:2847, 1989.

Morssink LP, Kornman LH, Beekhuis JR, et al.: Abnormal levels of maternal serum human chorionic gonadotropin and alpha-fetoprotein in the second trimester: Relation to fetal weight and preterm delivery. Prenat Diagn 15:1041, 1995.

MRC Vitamin Study Research Group: Prevention of neural tube defects: Results of the Medical Research Council Vitamin Study. Lancet 228:131, 1991.

Platt LD, Feuchtbaum L, Filly R, et al.: The California mater-nal serum α-fetoprotein screening program: The role of ultrasonography in the detection of spina bifida. Am J Obstet Gynecol 166:1328, 1992.

Richards DS, Seeds JW, Katz VL, et al.: Elevated MSAFP with normal ultrasound: Is amniocentesis always appro-priate? A review of 26,069 screened patients. Obstet Gynecol 7:203, 1988.

Sancken U, Bartels I: Biochemical screening for chromosomal disorders and neural tube defects (NTD): Is adjustment of maternal alpha-fetoprotein (AFP) still appropriate in insulin-dependent diabetes mellitus (IDDM)? Prenat Diagn 21:383, 2001.

Shackleton CH, Roitman E, Kratz L, et al.: Dehydro-oestriol and dehydropregnanetriol are candidate analytes for pre-natal diagnosis of Smith-Lemli-Opitz syndrome. Prenat Diagn 21:207, 2001.

Shaw GM, Velie EM, Schaffer D: Risk of neural tube defect-affected pregnancies among obese women. JAMA 275:1093, 1996.

Simpson JL, Palomaki GE, Mercer B, et al.: Associations between adverse perinatal outcome and serially obtained second- and third-trimester maternal serum α-fetoprotein measurements. Am J Obstet Gynecol 173:1742 1995.

Smithells RW, Sheppard S, Schorah CJ, et al.: Possible pre-vention of neural-tube defects by periconceptional vitamin supplementation. Lancet 1:339, 1980.

Stevenson RE, Allen WP, Pai GS, et al.: Decline in prevalence of neural tube defects in a high-risk region of the United States. Pediatrics 106:677, 2000.

Wald NJ, Cuckle HS: Open neural tube defects. *In* Wald NJ (ed): Antenatal and neonatal screening. Oxford: Oxford University Press, 1984, p 25.

Wald N, Leck I: Antenatal and Neonatal Screening, 2nd ed. New York: Oxford University Press, 2000.

Waller DK, Lustig LS, Cunningham GC, et al.: Second-trimester maternal serum alpha-fetoprotein levels and the risk of subsequent fetal death. N Engl J Med 325:6, 1991.

Waller KD, Mills JL, Simpson JL, et al.: Are obese women at higher risk for producing malformed offspring? Am J Obstet Gynecol 170:541, 1994.

CHAPTER 16

Preimplantation Genetic Diagnosis

Preimplantation genetic diagnosis (PGD) is an attractive newer addition to the prenatal diagnostic armamentarium. Many couples choose PGD rather than traditional prenatal genetic diagnostic approaches for assessing mendelian disorders, aneuploidy, or chromosomal imbalance. Unlike early amniocentesis, CVS, and other invasive techniques discussed in Chapter 13, PGD is not just an earlier option for prenatal diagnosis. It allows genetic diagnosis prior to establishing a pregnancy, a preconceptional approach that has unique advantages. Moreover, potential application of PGD extends beyond traditional prenatal genetic diagnosis to improved pregnancy rates in assisted reproductive technology (ART) (Simpson, 2001a).

Yet PGD is a method of prenatal genetic diagnosis considerably more complicated than traditional approaches using amniocentesis or CVS (see Chapter 13). A successful preimplantation genetics diagnostic program requires (1) high quality ART, (2) micromanipulation skills sufficient to obtain a specimen (polar body or blastomere) for analysis, and (3) molecular technology more sophisticated than that required for traditional prenatal diagnosis. Close collaboration among clinical geneticists, laboratory investigators, and *in vitro* fertilization providers is necessary (Geraedts et al., 2002).

In this chapter we consider the current status of PGD as a method of prenatal genetic diagnosis. We begin by considering indications specific for PGD as opposed to being applicable to prenatal genetic diagnosis as well (see Chapters 14 and 15).

Unique Indications for Preimplantation Genetic Diagnosis

In addition to traditional indications for prenatal genetic diagnosis, couples may choose PGD for reasons different from those of couples selecting CVS or amniocentesis. In some circumstances no other option appears applicable to them.

AVOIDING CLINICAL PREGNANCY TERMINATION

Despite well-meaning efforts, proponents of prenatal genetic diagnosis almost unavoidably underestimate the anguish and psychological trauma incurred by couples who undergo pregnancy termination because of a genetically abnormal fetus. Physicians and geneticists may assume that couples who avail themselves of this reproductive option have resolved their ethical ambiguities. However, this is rarely true. A couple's angst is amplified in those unfortunate circumstances requiring repeated pregnancy terminations because of consecutively affected offspring. In the ESHRE PGD Consortium data (ESHRE PGD Consortium Steering Committee, 2002), 36.2% of 1561 couples stated that their reason for undergoing PGD was objection to pregnancy termination; another 21.1% had a previous termination after traditional prenatal genetic diagnosis.

PGD permits intervention before clinical recognition of pregnancy, thus avoiding this quandary. Couples who insist on avoiding a pregnancy termination for religious reasons may find PGD an acceptable alternative. Specifically, many Orthodox Jewish and Islamic authorities consider abortion acceptable prior to 40 days' embryonic age.

EXCEPTIONAL GENETIC RISK

Independent of the previous indication, PGD may be preferable to CVS or amniocentesis for couples at exceptionally high risk for genetic disorders. An example might involve a couple in which one partner is homozygous for an autosomal recessive disease whereas the other is heterozygous for the same condition. In this situation (pseudoautosomal dominant inheritance), 50% of offspring will be affected. Similar risks hold for autosomal dominant traits of high penetrance, such as Huntington disease or myotonic dystrophy.

PRENATAL DIAGNOSIS WITHOUT DISCLOSING PARENTAL GENOTYPE

An unusual indication for PGD arises when a couple desires to undergo prenatal genetic diagnosis without finding out their own genotype. The prototype may be Huntington disease, a severe adult onset neurologic disorder in which mean age of onset is not until the fifth decade. If a patient's parent has Huntington disease, the patient (male or female) would have a 50% risk of being affected even if he or she is clinically normal at the present time. The risk for his or her fetus is 25%. Prenatal genetic diagnosis is possible through molecular methods and traditionally would be performed by first determining if the parent had the mutant gene. Only then would prenatal diagnosis of the fetus be pursued. Unfortunately, there are enormous implications for an asymptomatic individual who learns that he or she has the Huntington disease gene. Yet the patient may still wish to avoid transmitting a mutant gene to his or her offspring. Through PGD, it is possible to perform prenatal genetic diagnosis without learning the parental genotype. All embryos could be screened, and only those that are unaffected could be transferred. A negative factor is that this scenario would need to be repeated in all subsequent cycles, or otherwise a patient could deduce his or her genotype.

PGD IN COUPLES ALREADY REQUIRING ART

PGD may be logically desired by couples already requiring ART to achieve pregnancy. This would hold for women aged 35 years or older. If ART is medically necessary in younger women and only a limited number of embryos can be transferred, it is logical to transfer only those embryos known to be genetically normal. It might also be acceptable to transfer embryos only of a given sex, provided that embryos of the opposite sex are donated to infertile couples.

PRESELECTION AND TRANSFER OF HLA-ANTIGEN IDENTICAL EMBRYOS

Although it is theoretically possible with traditional prenatal genetic diagnosis, PGD has made identification of embryos of specific HLA-type for transfer practical. The approach was illustrated by Verlinsky and colleagues (2001a), who performed PGD on a couple whose older daughter had Fanconi anemia, an autosomal recessive disorder in which bone marrow failure requires transplantation to restore hematopoiesis. Transplantation with cord blood is an attractive option, and success is likely if the cord blood is HLA-compatible. Given that prenatal genetic diagnosis was desirable in any pregnancy by the couple and given that only a few embryos are transferred per in vitro fertilization (IVF) cycle, it was reasonable to test the embryos not only for Fanconi anemia but also for HLA status. This would identify the 25% embryos who should be HLA-compatible with the older, moribund, sib. Of 30 embryos tested in four cycles, six were affected with Fanconi anemia. Of 24 unaffected embryos, five were HLA-identical with the older affected, sib. Only HLA-compatible, unaffected embryos were transferred. Pregnancy was achieved, and at birth cord blood was collected and transplanted successfully in the older sib without harm to the newborn.

By 2002 Rechitsky et al. (2002) reported 18 PGD cycles for indication of HLA matching 5 β-thalassemia, 6 Fanconi anemia, 1 Wiskott-Aldrich syndrome, 6 leukemia. This approach is applicable for a variety of hematopoietic disorders.

Obtaining Preimplantation Cells for PGD

PGD requires access to gametes (oocytes) or embryos before 6 days postconception, the time when implantation occurs. There are three potential approaches: (1) polar body biopsy, (2) blastomere biopsy or aspiration of 1 to 2 blastomeres from the six- to eight-celled embryos (2 to 3 days), and (3) trophectoderm biopsy from the 5- to 6-day blastocyst.

BLASTOMERE (SIX TO EIGHT CELLS) BIOPSY

Biopsy at this stage was the first technique developed. The approach is to aspirate one to two of the six to eight cells contained within the zona pellucida. This can be accomplished by mechanical

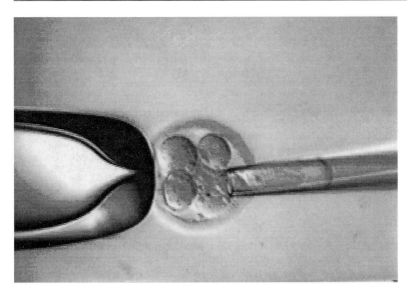

FIGURE 16-1 • Aspiration technique starts with stabilization of the embryo by suction on a holding pipette, penetration of the zona pellucida with a beveled pipette, and removal of blastomeres. (Courtesy of Dr. Pauline Cisneros and Dr. Sandra Carson, Baylor College of Medicine.)

(razor) or chemical (pronase, ethylenediamine-tetra-acetic acid [EDTA]) dissociation of the zona pellucida, followed by aspiration with a second pipette (Fig. 16–1). Sentinel work in this area was performed by Handyside and colleagues over a decade ago (Handyside et al., 1989, 1990, 1992).

Micromanipulation is now commonplace in ART units worldwide, specifically for intracytoplasmic sperm injection (ICSI). Embryo biopsy and assisted hatching techniques are less widely available. In the initial work of Handyside and colleagues (1989), a single cell was removed through a hole made in the zona pellucida by a drilling pipette (diameter 10–20 mm) containing acid Tyrode solution. A newer alternative to acid Tyrode is the laser (Boada et al., 1998). Even non-contact laser methods are available (Clement-Sengewald et al., 2002). Irrespective of technique, some biopsied embryos are naturally lost; however, with increasing technical prowess, this is becoming less of a problem. Removal of one or two cells does not affect glucose or pyruvate uptake or delay spontaneous hatching of blastocysts, the traditional markers of normal embryonic development (Hardy et al., 1990; Handyside et al., 1992). Most units only remove a single blastomere, but the center in Brussels (Van de Velde et al., 2000) routinely removes two cells to enhance accuracy. This group reports no decrease in pregnancy rate or implantation rate.

POLAR BODY BIOPSY

A second general approach is to remove either the first or second polar biopsy, or both. Literally this constitutes preconceptional diagnosis as opposed to preimplantation diagnosis *per se*. Suppose a woman and her mate were both heterozygous for the same autosomal recessive disorder. A polar body having the mutant allele should be complemented by a primary oocyte presumed to have the normal allele. The normal oocyte could thus be allowed to fertilize *in vitro* and then be transferred for potential implantation (Fig. 16–2). Conversely, if the polar body were normal, fertilization would not be allowed to proceed because the oocyte would contain the mutant allele. The same reasoning would apply to detecting aneuploidy. A polar body containing only one chromosome 21 (as determined by FISH with a chromosome-specific probe) should be complemented by a primary oocyte also containing a single No. 21. If the first polar body failed to show a 21, the oocyte can be presumed to have two No. 21, which would lead to a trisomic zygote.

Polar body biopsy (PBB) is technically similar to blastomere biopsy, but the embryo is not entered *per se*. Thus, PBB has theoretical advantages as well as certain disadvantages (Table 16–1). An advantage is no reduction in cell number following biopsy. Contamination with sperm is less likely. Disadvantages include inability to assess the paternal genotype, precluding its application if a father has an autosomal dominant disorder. Lacking information about paternal transmission also results in reproductive inefficiencies. The presence of a mutant autosomal recessive allele in a polar body precludes allowing that oocyte to be fertilized, whereas in reality the embryo resulting from fertilization of

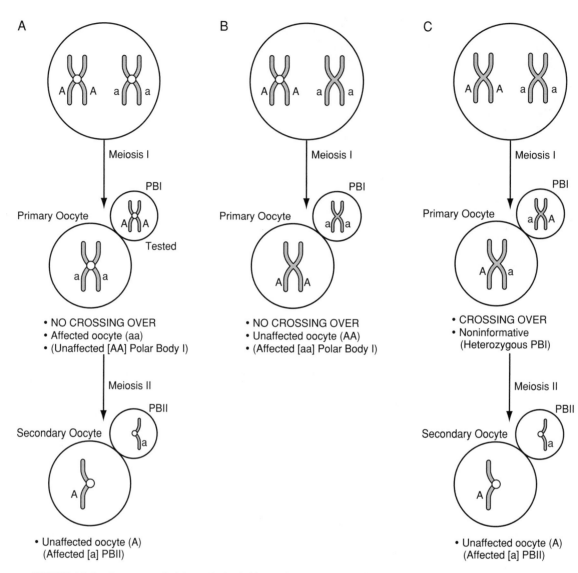

FIGURE 16–2 • Strategy underlying polar body biopsy. In the absence of crossing-over, analysis of the first polar body (PB 1) enables one to deduce the genetic status of the oocyte and, hence, whether the zygote could be affected. If PB 1 is heterozygous, crossing-over has occurred between homologous chromosomes and PB 1 analysis is noninformative. However, PB 2 analysis enables deduction of the maternal contribution to the zygote. Polar body analysis provides no information about paternal genotype and has the theoretical disadvantage of inefficiency in autosomal recessive disorders. If segregation of a mutant paternal autosomal dominant gene is sought, blastomere analysis rather than polar body analysis is necessary. A, normal allele; a, mutant allele.

that oocyte would be affected only if the sperm also contained the father's mutant allele. If it were known that the father's normal allele were transmitted, the embryo would be heterozygous and clinically normal.

Another disadvantage of PBB is recombination, the meiotic phenomenon that occurs routinely between homologous chromosomes (see Chapter 1). If crossing-over involves the region containing the gene in question, the single chromosome in the primary oocyte would not contain DNA sequences encoding both alleles. That is, the two chromatids of the single chromosome would differ in genotype (heterozygosity). The genotype of the secondary oocyte could then not be predicted without biopsy of not only the first but also the second polar body, or biopsy of the embryos *per se* (blastomere or blastocyst biopsy). Diagnostic hazards resulting from recombination are a greater problem for genes located nearer the telomeres because these genes display recombination frequencies approximating 50%. (Recombination is suppressed near the centromere.) Recombination can be addressed by biopsying both the first and second polar body (Verlinsky et al., 1997). The "problem" of

▼ **Table 16–1.** ADVANTAGES AND
• DISADVANTAGES OF POLAR BODY BIOPSY
COMPARED WITH BLASTOMERE BIOPSY

Advantages
- More time for analysis
- No reduction in mass of embryonic tissue
- No sperm contamination (polar body 1)
- ? Operator contamination would not lead to transfer of affected embryos
- ? Ethically more acceptable (literally preconceptional)

Disadvantages
- Greater technical difficulty
- Inefficient because fewer embryos to transfer (*paternal genotype not known*)
- Unable to determine sex
- Not applicable if father has dominant disorder
- Recombination may necessitate sequential polar body 1 and polar body 2 biopsies

recombination actually can then be beneficial; the presence of two alleles at the first polar body excludes allele drop out and one can be confident of the accuracy of a second polar body biopsy showing only one allele. The topic is revisited in more detail below.

BLASTOCYST (TROPHECTODERM) BIOPSY

An underlying difficulty when aspirating either the polar body or a blastomere from the six- to eight-celled embryo is that diagnosis must depend upon only a single cell, or occasionally two. Many more cells would be available if one biopsied the 5- to 6-day blastocyst, which contains hundreds of cells. The strategy is to biopsy the trophectoderm overlying the anembryonic pole. The safest approach appears to involve slitting the zona pellucida to allow extrusion of 10 to 30 cells, followed by excision and analysis of the herniated cells. This technique proved to be the least disruptive of four techniques evaluated by Carson and colleagues (1993) in the mouse and by Dokras and coworkers (1990) in the human. Laser drilling is a new alternative (Veiga et al., 1997).

One major problem is that blastocysts are less readily obtainable as six- to eight-celled embryos. Blastocysts can be obtained by culture *in vitro*, but this process has traditionally proved very inefficient. After 3 to 4 days *in vitro*, embryonic development is not sustained efficiently to the blastocyst stage. With media now being developed specifically for 4- to 6-day embryos, there has been greater recent success. Some argue that culturing to the blastocyst stage selects out abnormal embryos and improves pregnancy success; however, many chromosomal abnormalities are still present at this stage. Coonen and coworkers (2000) studied 299 blastocysts and found the mean percent of (normal) diploid cells in ostensibly normal embryos to be only 72 ± 17%; of all blastocysts studied, 11% were chaotic and 5% monosomic. Among 50 blastocysts, Sandalinas and coworkers (2000) found 17 aneuploides (34%) using FISH probes for X, Y, 13, 15, 16, 18, 21, and 22. The 17 included 14 trisomies, 2 monosomies 21, and 1 monosomy X. Thus, culture of blastocysts does not eliminate chromosomally abnormal embryos, even though the proportion of chromosomal abnormalities could decrease from the cleavage embryo stage. Finally, an increased rate of monozygotic twinning has been reported following transfer of nonbiopsied blastocysts (Veiga et al., 1997). Transferring blastocysts stripped of their zona pellucida has been said to minimize monozygotic (MZ) twinning (Trounson et al., 1998).

An attractive but still unrealized clinical alternative involves recovery of blastocysts by uterine lavage, a technique developed initially by Buster and colleagues for use in infertile couples (Bustillo et al., 1984; Buster et al., 1985). In order to be practical for PGD, uterine lavage to recover blastocysts probably requires superovulation to yield multiple embryos, the strategy employed routinely by IVF programs. Lavage has proved surprisingly difficult. Carson and coworkers (1991) superovulated 15 fertile women in 29 cycles, using four different ovulation induction regimens coupled with either natural intercourse or intracervical donor insemination. In 29 cycles only two morulas, one blastocyst, and four unfertilized ova were recovered. Formigli and colleagues (1990) had similarly disappointing results. The poor experience with superovulated donors has led to approaches utilizing natural ovulation. A single success was reported by Carson and coworkers (1991), but PGD by lavage remains unavailable clinically. If perfected, however, lavage would provide a far less expensive method of PGD than polar body or blastomere biopsy.

Technical Considerations in Diagnosing Chromosomal Abnormalities

Cytogenetic analysis in preimplantation genetic diagnosis would clearly be useful for a variety of reasons. Sex determination (XX or XY) may be desirable for couples at risk for X-linked recessive disorders in which an exact diagnosis is not possible. Aneuploidy, translocations, or other chromosomal rearrangement could be excluded. Cytogenetic methodologies are well established in traditional prenatal genetic diagnosis (CVS, amniocentesis); however, accuracy is more an issue in PGD because of the inherent limitations of analyzing only one or two cells.

METAPHASE ANALYSIS

When prenatal genetic diagnosis involves chorionic villi or amniotic fluid cells, cytogenetic analysis typically involves a relatively large number of cells. Only certain cells are informative, namely, those either spontaneously entering metaphase or those arrested in metaphase after addition of the mitotic spindle inhibitor colcemid. Morphologically suitable metaphases are selected for analysis. Usually about 20 cells are counted, and a few are karyotyped chromosome by chromosome. Of the 20, perhaps 18 or 19 cells typically show the modal number of chromosomes (2n = 46). Perhaps one or two cells prove hypomodal, presumably representing a broken cell. Unless the same hypomodal or hypermodal count is found in the other cells, the nonmodal is generally assumed to be artifactual, i.e., pseudomosaicism.

In PGD, diagnosis may depend upon information from a single cell. There is little margin for error. Metaphase analysis is possible for only a single cell, but this is not optimal. In animal studies an interpretable metaphase can be obtained in perhaps 80% of cases from a single blastomere (Dyband, 1991; Kola and Wilton, 1991; Gimenez et al., 1993). Given that an 80% information rate is not acceptable clinically, new techniques are being developed. One approach involves fusing the second polar body with a one-celled mouse embryo (Verlinsky et al., 1994). Another method is to inject the second polar body into an enucleated oocyte, following which the haploid pronucleus can be treated with okadaic acid to induce premature chromosome condensation (Verlinsky and Evsikov, 1999). Metaphase preparations can also be produced by inserting the polar body or a single blastomere into an activated enucleated bovine egg (Willadsen et al., 1999) or an activated enucleated mouse zygote (Verlinsky et al., 2000a). This investigational technique yields heterokaryons that could be arrested in metaphase of the first cleavage division, thus suitable for whole chromosome painting or hybridization with telomeric or centromeric

probes using enucleated mouse zygotes. Approximately 80% of either blastomeres or oocytes were informative (Verlinsky et al., 2000a). The most recent update by the same group reported fall karyotyping in 89% of 412 blastomeres (Cieslak et al., 2002).

Other approaches to determine chromosomal status include comparative genome hybridization (Wells and Delhanty, 2000; Wilton et al., 2001), microarray chips (Weier et al., 2001) and chromosome painting. All these techniques are applicable for single-cell analysis, but in none can an individual result be guaranteed clinically. The most salutary results to date utilize comparative genome hybridization. Wilton et al. (2002) performed CGH on embryos from 20 patients with implantation failure. Biopsied embryos were cryopreserved while analysis proceeded; pregnancy rate was 20% per cycle or 15% per embryo.

FISH WITH CHROMOSOME-SPECIFIC PROBES

Given the limitations cited above, the current approach for chromosomal analysis in PGD involves FISH with chromosome-specific probes. FISH is a molecular genetic technique based on analysis of DNA sequences that are chromosome-specific. Chromosome-specific probes can hybridize to denatured DNA, either metaphase or interphase. In interphase cells, the number of FISH signals should equal the number of a given chromosome. Using a chromosome 21-specific probe would detect trisomy 21 if three signals were visualized in the nucleus. Simultaneous use of probes for more than one chromosome is possible using different colored fluorochromes. This approach is also well suited for sex determination, X and Y probes being the first used concurrently (Grifo et al., 1992).

Pitfalls include geometric vicissitudes that preclude every trisomic cell showing three signals. Sometimes one chromosome (signals) is superimposed on another, a pitfall difficult to recognize using only two-dimensional analysis (see Chapter 1 and Fig. 1–7). In amniotic fluid cells two signals in about 90% of normal disomic cells are typically seen (Klinger et al., 1992); the percentage of trisomic cells with three signals is stochastically lower, approximately 80%. Conversely, in about 1% of normal disomic cells three signals will be observed (false-positive). These cells are presumably undergoing cell division, their chromatids already having separated. FISH accuracy in blastomeres seems at least as high as and probably

failure to transfer an embryo that is phenotypically normal but actually only heterozygous (not homozygously affected). If the abnormal allele has "dropped out," the embryo would type as homozygously normal rather than the actual heterozygous genotype. In any case, the embryo would be clinically normal.

PCR failure is a greater problem if one depends on absence of a mutant autosomal dominant allele to connote normalcy. Transferring only embryos known to have the normal allele addresses this problem. This approach is used in myotonic dystrophy (Sermon et al., 1997).

FLUORESCENT PCR FOR GREATER ACCURACY

ADO might merely be a quantitative phenomenon rather than the qualitative phenomenon it ostensibly seems to be. One allele might simply be amplified to a much greater extent than the other. If so, the less well amplified allele could still prove detectable by a method more sensitive than traditional approaches (ethidium bromide staining). Such a technique could be fluorescent PCR, which relies on qualitative identification of all potential alleles (Findlay et al., 1995, 1998). Fluorescent PCR usually detects alleles by recording qualitatively distinct peaks. Even if the heights of the peaks differ (see Fig. 16–3), they can still be distinguished. With fluorescent PCR rather than use of traditional ethidium bromide stained gels, several groups are reporting diagnosis of compound heterozygosity (Findlay et al., 1998; Santaló et al., 1999). Multiplex fluorescent PCR for diagnosis of both aneuploidy and a mendelian disorder is possible (Findlay et al., 2001).

ADO IN NUCLEOTIDE REPEAT DISORDERS

A special problem arises in single cell PCR when the disorder is characterized by triplet nucleotide repeats. Fragile-X (FMR-1), myotonic dystrophy, and Huntington disease are the relevant examples. Amplification across repeat nucleotide sequences proves to be less reliable than for unique sequences for point mutations; PCR amplification "skips" across portions of the gene to yield a shorter product than would be expected. In myotonic dystrophy ADO is 20 to 30%, for which reason Sermon and coworkers (1997) offer PGD only by studying linked polymorphic markers. Only embryos whose biopsied blastomeres show the normal allele are transferred.

SEQUENTIAL ANALYSIS IN FIRST AND SECOND POLAR BODY BIOPSY TO EXCLUDE ADO

Various approaches have been utilized for decreasing errors caused by allele dropout. As mentioned, it is possible to resolve the recombination dilemma inherent in polar body analysis (Verlinsky and Kuliev, 1992; Verlinsky et al., 1997). This strategy paradoxically relies on benefiting from recombination occurring at the first meiotic division. If both mutant and normal alleles can be shown to be amplified from the first polar body, it can be deduced whether ADO did or did not occur. Although the first polar body alone may have been uninformative, the second polar body can be analyzed with the confidence of having excluded ADO. One now expects only one type of DNA, mutant or normal, and an accurate diagnosis can be offered. If the second polar body biopsy reveals the mutant allele, the complementary secondary oocyte can confidently be assumed to be genetically normal. Figure 16–6 shows the strategy.

CONCURRENT ANALYSIS FOR THE MUTANT GENE AND A LINKED POLYMORPHIC MARKER TO EXCLUDE ADO

ADO presumably occurs in part as result of the chromosomal region that is in question being lost

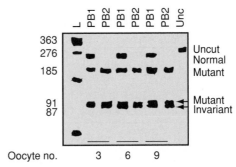

FIGURE 16–6 • Triplet pregnancy resulting from PGD for thalassemia mutation IVS 1–6 using sequential first (PB 1) and second (PB 2) polar body multiplex PCR. Polyacrylamide gel analysis of *sfan1* restriction digestion of PCR product from PB 1 and PB 2 in three oocytes. Restriction digestion gave rise to a 276-bp fragment (normal allele), a 185-bp fragment (mutant allele), a 91-bp fragment (mutant allele) and an 87-bp invariant fragment. All three oocytes (3, 6, and 9) were predicted to be normal based on a heterozygous PB 1 and a hemizygous mutant PB 2. They were transferred, resulting in triplet pregnancy and the birth of three unaffected children. (From Verlinsky Y, Kuliev A: An Illustration Textbook and Reference for Clinicians: An Atlas of Preimplantation Genetics Diagnosis. New York: Parthenon Publishing, 2000.)

or failing to be available physically for PCR primer annealing. This phenomenon could be recognized if a closely linked DNA sequence were simultaneously analyzed (see Fig. 16–4). If both the mutant and the expected linked polymorphic variant (in *cis)* are present, ADO would be excluded. Conversely, ADO would be suspected if one analysis revealed mutant gene but there were two alleles at the locus-linked polymorphic locus; ADO involving only the mutant allele must have occurred. Thus, transfer of an affected embryo would be avoided. Using this approach to exclude diagnostic errors, accuracy for single gene PGD is very high (Verlinsky et al., 2001e). Rechitsky (2001) summarized their experience with sequential analysis of 1047 oocytes using polar body biopsy. ADO occurred in 8.5%, but in less than 1% it was not appreciated clinically through concomitant analysis of linked polymorphic markers.

CONTAMINATION AS A DIAGNOSTIC PROBLEM

Another problem is contamination from ambient DNA. Actually this can be even more castastrophic than PCR failure in autosomal recessive traits (Simpson et al., 1994). Table 16–4 shows the consequences of contamination from ambient cells, namely, transfer of a genetically abnormal embryos assumed erroneously to be genetically normal. By contrast, PCR failure is only inefficient in that it decreases the number of embryos transferable; however, in contrast to what occurs with contamination, no false-negative results would occur for autosomal recessive traits (see Table 16–4).

Mendelian Indications for PGD

SEX DETERMINATION FOR X-LINKED RECESSIVE DISORDERS

Sex determination requires analysis of blastomeres or blastocysts. Polar body analysis provides no information concerning transmission of paternal genes and is not helpful. The first PGD cases were performed on couples at risk for X-linked recessive disorders (Handyside et al., 1989). The strategy was to transfer only female (XX) embryos, which whether they were heterozygous or homozygously normal would nonetheless be clinically normal. Initially, the diagnosis was made on the basis of the presence or absence of a Y-specific DNA signal, such as SRY.

Current molecular strategy for determining embryonic sex is to amplify using primers that anneal to sequences common to both the X and Y. X and Y sequences internal to the common primer annealing sites are selected on the basis of differing in some minor but recognizable fashion, for example, number of intervening nucleotides or presence or absence of a restriction endonuclease site. Sex determination is then possible by analysis of gels or by fluorescent PCR (Findlay et al., 1998). The amelogenin or ZXY/ZXX systems are commonly used.

For the last several years sex determination has been preferentially based on FISH with chromosome-specific probes. FISH analysis also addresses the possibility that PCR "failure" has occurred because the analyzed cell is monosomic or haploid. Simultaneous FISH can be used for the X, Y, and one or more autosomes used as controls to verify that an intact nucleus is being analyzed.

▼ **Table 16–4.** CONSEQUENCES OF DNA CONTAMINATION TO PGD

True Embryonic Genotype	Contaminant DNA Speciously Amplified	"Diagnosis" after Spurious Amplification	Interpretation and Clinical Action
BB	b	Bb	Amplification of both actual and contaminant DNA. Transfer performed. (Acceptable error because heterozygote clinically normal)
BB	b	bb	Amplification of only contaminant DNA. No transfer despite normal genotype. (Tolerable error despite loss of opportunity for pregnancy)
bb	B	BB	Amplification only of contaminant DNA with transfer of embryo of incorrect (affected) genotype. (Unacceptable error)
bb	B	Bb	Amplification of both actual DNA and ambient DNA. Transfer of embryo of incorrect (affected) genotype. (Unacceptable error)

Performing PGD for sex determination in couples at risk for X-linked recessive disorders carries the obvious pitfall that the 50% of male embryos inheriting the normal maternal X and, hence, being clinically normal cannot be transferred (or in polar body analysis allowed to fertilize). Detecting the specific mutation would obviously be preferable to sex determination alone because unaffected male embryos could be transferred as well as female embryos. However, sometimes the specific mutation is not known, and at other times it is not practical to analyze for an X-linked mutation unique to a single family. Linkage analysis using polymorphic loci should be possible, as described above, but laborious and expensive. Indications for using PGD to determine sex thus extend to X-linked disorders not amenable to direct mutational analysis, either because the gene has not been sequenced or because no mutation-specific assay has been validated.

COMMON MENDELIAN DISORDERS: INDICATIONS AND EXPERIENCE

Table 16–5 list the most common mendelian disorders for which PGD is currently offered. These include cystic fibrosis (ΔF508 homozygosity) (ESHRE PGD Consortium Steering Committee, 2002; Verlinsky et al., 2002), Tay-Sachs disease, Rh (D), sickle cell anemia (Kuliev et al., 2001), certain β-thalassemias (Kuliev et al., 1998; Kanavakis et al., 1999; Chamayou et al., 2002; Kalakoutis et al., 2002), phenylketonuria (Verlinsky et al., 2001c), spinal muscular atrophy, and myotonic dystrophy (Sermon et al., 1997, 2002), and many more (Verlinsky and Kuliev, 2000). Several autosomal dominant disorders are amenable to diagnosis, including adenosis polyposis coli (Ao et al., 1998) and Li-Fraumeni syndrome (Simpson, 2001b; Verlinsky et al., 2001b). A more detailed list of disorders for which PGD has been performed is provided by the ESHRE PGD Consortium Steering Committee (1999, 2002) and by Verlinsky and Kuliev (2000). However, any mendelian disorder whose gene is localized or whose molecular basis is known is potentially detectable by linkage analysis if not otherwise.

Worldwide, the number of PGD cycles for mendelian traits has been increasing steadily. Approximately 500 had been tabulated in a 1999 publication (Verlinsky and Kuliev, 1999). The September 1999 meeting of the 9th International Working Group on PGD estimated 600 mendelian cycles worldwide, with 100 pregnancies (Verlinsky et al., 2000b). By June 2000 the estimate had

▼ **Table 16–5.** SELECTED DISORDERS FOR
• WHICH PGD IS OFFERED*

Autosomal-Dominant
Adenomatous polyposis coli
Marfan syndrome
Huntington disease
Li-Fraumeni syndrome (p53)
Myotonic dystrophy
Charcot-Marie-Tooth disease

Autosomal-Recessive
Cystic fibrosis
Fanconi Anemia
Tay-Sachs disease
β-thalassemia
Sickle cell disease
Gaucher disease
Spinal muscular dystrophy
Phenylketonuria
Epidermolysis bullosa
Rh(D)
PLA-1 isoimmunization

X-linked
Identification of sex
Lesch-Nyhan syndrome
Duchenne muscular dystrophy
Hemophilia A and B
Fragile X syndrome
Retinitis pigmentosa
Ornithine transcarbamoylase deficiency
Severe combined immunodeficiency
Ocular albinism 1

Chromosomal
Aneuploidy (13,16,18,21,22,X, Y) by chromosome-specific probes
Balanced translocations

---

* For most disorders, not all mutations are detectable directly for a given disorder. Linkage analysis may be the applicable approach. PLA-1, platelet antibody A.

increased to 750, with at least 150 pregnancies and more than 100 children (Verlinsky et al., 2001e). The largest number was performed by polar body biopsy, by which 23 different disorders were tested in 66 cycles. This led to 23 pregnancies and 17 normal offspring. Half these cases were for sex determination (X-linked disorders). Cystic fibrosis was the next major indication and the largest single mendelian diagnosis.

In the most recent report (Verlinsky et al., 2002) by the group with greatest experience, 15% of 1643 PGD cycles were for Mendelian indications, 6% for translocations and 79% for aneuploidy. The approximately 25% pregnancy rate for all mendelian PGD cases worldwide parallels that for IVF in general, judged by national registries (ASRM/SART, 2000). However, it could be argued that only the most successful ART centers attempt PGD; in these centers pregnancy rates are higher than registry averages, and thus PGD pregnancies perhaps should be higher. Of note is that PGD is not a technology restricted to highly developed countries. An example is availability of PGD in 6 centers in China (Zhang, 2002). Indeed, PGD has now taken its place as part of pre-pregnancy genetic screening and traditional prenatal genetic diagnosis (Simpson, 2002).

PGD FOR ADDITIONAL MENDELIAN DISORDERS

In theory all mendelian disorders should be detectable by preimplantation genetic diagnosis. However, obstacles exist. One major impediment is expense. Assisted reproduction costs 6000 to 12,000 U.S. dollars per cycle, and is not always reimbursed by third-party carriers in North America. Second, not all centers with genetic expertise have a highly successful ART program, and the converse. Third, the requisite molecular assay may not be facile. A specific molecular strategy must be devised for each situation, and experience must be gained in single cell molecular analysis. PGD diagnosis of a given disorder can confidently be offered to a patient only if most individuals affected with a mendelian disorder have the same mutant DNA sequence. If molecular heterogeneity exists, PGD may be unavailable simply because of the impracticality of devising a strategy for only a single case.

Examples of common disorders characterized by molecular heterogeneity and for which all genotypes are not necessarily applicable for PGD include β-thalassemia (Kuliev et al., 1998), hemophilia A, polycystic kidney disease, Marfan syndrome (Blaszczyk et al., 1998), Duchenne and muscular dystrophy, and hemophilia A. In these and other conditions, diagnosis is still possible on the basis of linkage analysis using polymorphic DNA markers. Rechitsky and coworkers (1999, 2001), Verlinsky and coworkers (1999a) and Verlinsky and Kuliev (2000) illustrate this approach, particularly as applied to polar body biopsy.

Of special note is the adult onset autosomal dominant disorders for which PGD has been accomplished, including Huntington disease, Marfan syndrome, and Li-Fraumeni syndrome (Verlinsky et al., 2001b). Although some have difficulty with pursuing diagnosis for adult-onset disorders, the consensus is to the contrary (Simpson, 2001b).

Conceptionally simple but more technically daunting is the alternative of high throughput molecular technology, sequencing an entire gene or selected exons. Readily feasible from genomic DNA, this is not currently possible from a single cell. However, the trajectory of molecular advances suggests that it will be available in the foreseeable future. Microarray technology is another possibility.

NUCLEOTIDE REPEAT DISORDERS: FRAGILE X SYNDROME (FMR-1), MYOTONIC DYSTROPHY, HUNTINGTON DISEASE

Distinct diagnostic problems arise in mendelian disorders whose pathogenesis involves nucleotide repeats: FMR-1, Huntington disease (HD), and myotonic dystrophy (DM). These disorders are attractive indications for PGD, but as noted above amplification across triplet repeats is unpredictable. The number of triplet repeats may be underestimated by PCR, leading to false-negative conclusions. While ADO is a manageable 5% for unique sequence DNA, the rate is an unacceptable (30%) for nucleotide repeat sequences.

Perhaps the preferred strategy at present is to bypass molecular analysis of the expansion *per se* in favor of analysis of linked polymorphic markers. This approach has already been described. Briefly, transmission of a marker *cis* to the normal allele (i.e., on the same chromosome and shown not to have undergone recombination) indicates a normal embryo. Sermon and coworkers (1997, 1998) thus determined whether the embryo had or had not inherited the normal allele from the parent affected with myotonic dystrophy. Only if the normal allele is present is embryo transfer performed; information concerning presence or absence of the mutant *per se* is not taken into account. The same approach is applicable to FMR-1 (Sermon et al., 1999; Apessos et al., 2001). More recently, strategies are being developed to allow direct exclusion of the mutation, thus avoiding the pitfall of diagnostic error due to recombination. With experience success appeared to be increasing. Sermon et al. (2002) analyzed 94 PGD cycles for DM within 19 pregnancies: 6 of 39 in Huntington disease, 3 of 18 for FRAXA.

A confounding factor in pursuing PGD for triplet nucleotide repeat disorders is that women heterozygous for FMR-1 and perhaps also DM have ovarian dysfunction. They respond poorly to ovulation stimulation, producing fewer oocytes and, hence, fewer embryos. Pregnancy rates are lower than for PGD in other mendelian traits.

Cytogenetic Indications for PGD

ANEUPLOIDY DETECTION FOR ADVANCED MATERNAL AGE OR PRIOR TRISOMY

Using FISH with chromosome-specific probes to confirm euploidy is the indication for two thirds of all PGD cases performed worldwide (Verlinsky et al., 2000, 2001e). The most common cytogenetic indication is maternal age older than 35 years in women already requiring ART to achieve pregnancy. The attraction of PGD in this context is that women who must undergo ART to become pregnant are naturally reticent to undergo invasive procedures such as CVS because a valued pregnancy could be jeopardized. Experience is increasing rapidly. Using polar body biopsy, Verlinsky and coworkers (1999b) reported 614 cycles transferring aneuploidy-free embryos (13, 18, 21); 131 clinical pregnancies resulted, producing 88 healthy children. By 2000, 917 cycles by that group yielded 182 clinical pregnancies and 140 children (Verlinsky et al., 2001d). Decreased abortion rates and increased implantation rates have also been reported by Gianaroli and colleagues (1997, 1999) and by Munné and colleagues (1998a, 1999).

By 2000 worldwide estimates totaled 1500 cycles for chromosomal diagnosis yielding 400 clinical pregnancies (Verlinsky et al., 2001e). Cytogenetic indications are now the most common category for PGD, constituting 79% of indications in the most experienced center (Verlinsky et al., 2002). The potential is even greater. Over half of the ART cycles in the U.S. are performed in women 35 years or older. This totaled 56.4% (17,250) of all 30,598 cycles (Table 16–6). Thus, the potential for chromosomal diagnosis is even greater than currently practiced.

Aneuploidy detection by PGD is also applicable to couples having prior aneuploid offspring,

▼ **Table 16–6.** MATERNAL AGES IN ASRM/SART
• REGISTRY DATA (1998 CYCLES)

Maternal Age (Yrs)	Indication		
	Female Factor Infertility (n)	Male Factor Infertility (n)	Percent Maternal Age
< 35	16,648	7,546	47.6%
35–37	8,524	3,147	22.9%
38–40	7,063	2,366	18.5%
> 40	4,348	1,129	10.7%
	36,583	14,188	100%

constituting some of the indications in the series cited above. As reviewed in Chapter 14, the recurrent risk is about 1%.

STRUCTURAL CHROMOSOMAL ABNORMALITIES

A parental chromosomal rearrangement (e.g., balanced translocation) places offspring at increased risk (see Chapters 1, 5, and 14) and increases the risk of spontaneous abortion. Prenatal genetic diagnosis has long been offered for this indication, and with amniocentesis or CVS full karyotypic analysis is performed. With PGD, unbalanced translocations can be detected in a single cell using FISH with chromosome-specific probes. A few cases have been analyzed using nuclear transfer techniques to generate a metaphase (Verlinsky et al., 2001c), and comparative genome hybridization is possible (Wilton et al., 2000, 2001).

Strategy depends on analyzing numbers of FISH signals and their geometric proximity. Presence or absence of a translocation chromosome can be identified during interphase using fluores of different colors, each connoting a specific and different chromosome-specific DNA sequence. If signals are closer together than expected in normal diploid cells, the translocation chromosome is present. An unbalanced state can be deduced by tallying the total numbers of signals or their relative proximities (Verlinsky and Kuliev, 2000).

Initially break point specific probes had to be designed expressly for a particular reciprocal translocation (Weier et al., 1999). This was highly accurate but very expensive. Using telomeric and centromeric probes diagnostic of the translocation in question (Scriven et al., 1998; Munné et al., 2000) became possible after development of telomeric probes for every chromosome (Ning et al., 1996). Telomeric probes can also be used to detect cryptic translocations (McKenzie et al., 2002). Offering PGD to translocation heterozygotes not only excludes chromosomally abnormal liveborns but decreases spontaneous abortion rates (Conn et al., 1999; Munné et al., 2000; Munné, 2001). In 38 cases studied by Munné and coworkers (2000), the spontaneous rate was 90% (35/38) prior to PGD and 10% (12/116) after PGD transfer of only balanced embryos. A consistent finding is that surprisingly few embryos prove normal. The frequency of abnormal segregants is greater in reciprocal than in robertsonian translocations (Gianaroli et al., 2002; Van Assche et al., 2002); however, interchromosomal effects (monosomy and trisomy for other chromosomes) seem perhaps higher in robertsonian (Gianaroli et al., 2002).

Implantation rate was 38.5% in the Gianaroli et al. (2002) series of 42 cycles; pregnancy rates in another series of 24 cycles was 21.4% for reciprocal and 28.6% for robertsonian translocations (Van Assche et al., 2002). A drawback to using telomeric rather than break point specific probes is that with the former it is not possible to distinguish translocation heterozygotes from chromosomally abnormal embryos; identifying unbalanced blastomeres is not a problem. Figures 16–7 and 16–8 show the strategy employed at our institution.

Inversions can be detected using the same strategy (Iwarsson et al., 1998). As in translocation, it is not possible to distinguish genetically balanced inversion carriers from genetically normal ones without the inversion.

Evolving Indications for PGD

PGD SOLELY FOR REPEAT SPONTANEOUS ABORTIONS OR IVF FAILURE

In Chapter 5 we showed that recurrent aneuploidy exists in repetitive clinical abortions. There is a tendency for otherwise normal women to have numerical abnormal (aneuploid) offspring in successive pregnancies. Presumably the pathogenesis involves perturbation of meiotic or mitotic processes. The phenomenon of recurrent aneuploidy appears to extend to preimplantation embryos as well. In 14 couples with repeated abortions, PGD revealed 10-fold higher aneu-

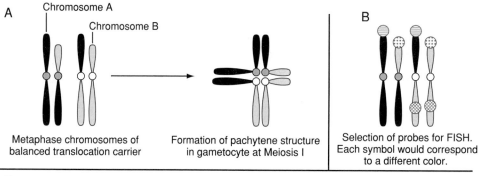

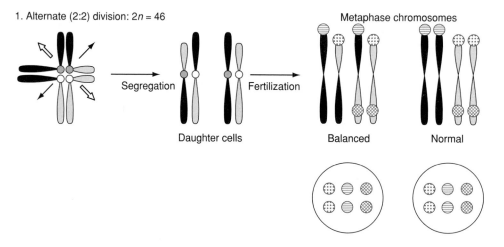

FIGURE 16–7 • Schematic diagram illustrating the use of two telomeric and a locus-specific probe to distinguish genetically balanced from genetically unbalanced embryos. Each symbol would correspond to a probe characterized by distinct fluorochromes differing in color. A reciprocal translocation between chromosomes A and B leads to the pachytene configuration (see Chapter 1) shown in Panel A. Panel B shows selection of requisite probes. Panel C shows consequences of alternate, adjacent 1, and adjacent 2 segregation. Only the former (C, 1) produces daughter cells (gametes) that are genetically normal and, hence, lead to genetically balanced or genetically normal (no translocation) embryos. In both cases interphase nuclei would show two signals for each of the three probes. Distinguishing genetically normal from balanced heterozygosity is not possible. In Panel C, 2 and C, 3, adjacent 1 and adjacent 2 segregates are shown. All products are unbalanced as shown by other than two signals existing per cell. (Courtesy of Dr. Farideh Bischoff, Baylor College of Medicine.) *Illustration continued on opposite page*

2. Adjacent 1(2:2) Division: 2n = 46

3. Adjacent 2 (2:2) Division: 2n = 46

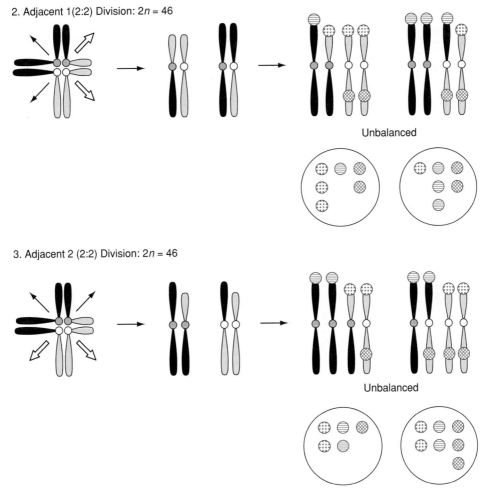

FIGURE 16–7 • *Continued.*

ploidy rates for chromosome 13 and three to four-fold higher for chromosomes 16, 18, 21, and 22 compared with PGD embryos from controls with normal reproductive histories (Rubio et al., 2000). For the latter four chromosomes, background rates were 4 to 8% versus 11 to 25% in repetitive aborters. Percentages of aneuploid PGD embryos tend to be similar in successive IVF cycles (Ferraretti et al., 2000). Not surprisingly, some couples experience repeated IVF failures because of recurrent aneuploidy.

Couples experiencing either repeated abortion or inexplicable IVF failure could benefit from PGD for aneuploidy detection and transfer of euploid embryos. For several years applying these indications has been known to increase the implantation rate and lower the abortion rate (Gianaroli et al., 1997, 2001; Munné et al., 1998a, 1999, 2000). It seems likely that the liveborn rate will be improved as well (Ferraretti et al., 1999).

The relationship between recurrent aneuploidy and chromosomally chaotic embryos, also discussed in Chapter 5, is less clear. Of significance here is that chromosomally chaotic embryos are also nonrandomly distributed. Among eight women undergoing PGD in successive cycles and who contributed embryos that could be disaggregated and subjected to FISH, all 24 chaotic embryos were found in a subset of only four women; in the four other women studied no chaotic embryos were found, even when sought in successive cycles (Delhanty et al., 1997). If certain women were predisposed to chaotic embryos, it could be worthwhile to analyze six- to eight-celled embryos and transfer only the (few) euploid embryos (Conn et al., 1999). Ferraretti and colleagues (2000) found that the percentage of abnormal embryos remained high in successive unsuccessful IVF cycles (64%, 66%, and 61%). Two thirds were aneuploid,

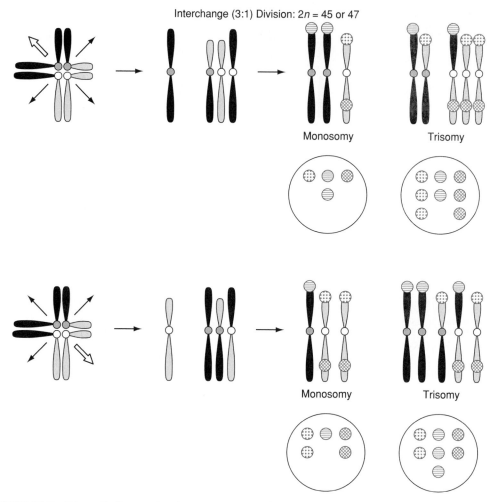

Interchange (3:1) Division: 2n = 45 or 47

Monosomy   Trisomy

Monosomy   Trisomy

FIGURE 16–8 • Schematic diagram showing consequences of 3:1 segregation of the translocation shown in Figure 16–7. Two different divisions can occur, tertiary (3:1) and interchange (3:1). All products of either division are abnormal. (Courtesy of Dr. Farideh Bischoff, Baylor College of Medicine.) *Illustration continued on opposite page*

lending support to the use of PGD in women experiencing repeated IVF failure.

PGD SOLELY FOR IMPROVING THE ART PREGNANCY RATE

If PGD for transferring aneuploid-free embryos improves outcome in couples experiencing repeated IVF failures or repeated abortions, it follows that PGD could improve pregnancy rates in IVF in general. Although chromosomal abnormalities are increased in morphologically abnormal embryos and in slowly growing embryos, many morphologically normal embryos are nonetheless aneuploid and could be chosen for transfer. Aneuploidy further increases with advancing maternal age, regardless of whether embryos are morphologically normal or abnor-

mal (Munné et al., 1995). Transferring morphologically normal, euploid, embryos should improve the pregnancy rate in routine couples undergoing ART because aneuploid embryos not able to yield a clinical pregnancy would be given no opportunity to implant. Thus, the potential for the remaining (euploid) embryos to produce a pregnancy should be increased.

If this approach were pursued, it would seem obligatory to detect those trisomies compatible with life: 13, 18, and 21. Screening for X and Y is usually performed as well, and screening for chromosomes 14, 16, and 22 could be useful. Detection of trisomies that are lethal but not uncommon in abortuses (e.g., 16) is especially appealing (Verlinsky et al., 1998). Bahçe et al. (1999) wonder if the trisomies for which one should screen to improve ART should be the lethal trisomies 1, 15, 16, 17, and 22. The strat-

Tertiary (3:1) Division: $2n = 45$ or 47

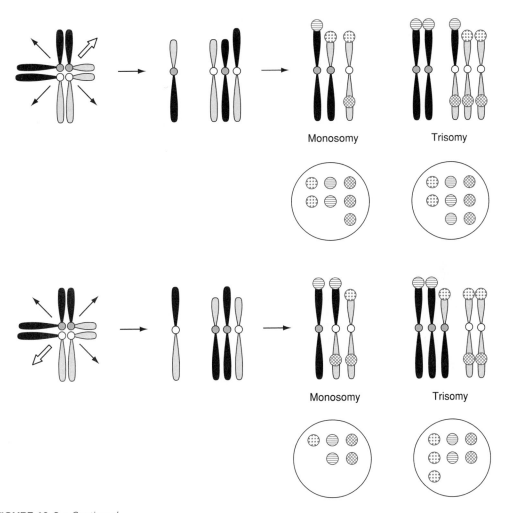

FIGURE 16–8 • *Continued.*

egy of the several groups is to perform two rounds of hybridization. Locus-specific probes (e.g., 13, 21, 22) might be used in the first round, perhaps in conjunction with some centromeric alphoid repeats (e.g., 16, 18); in the second round of hybridization only alphoid repeat probes (e.g., X, Y, 1, 15) are applied.

Transferring only embryos euploid for selected chromosomes has for several years been shown to increase implantation rates and decrease clinical pregnancy losses in older women (≥38 years usually) (Gianaroli, 1999, 2001; Munné et al., 1998a, 1999). Worldwide experience already cited (Verlinsky et al., 2000, 2001e, 2002) for aneuploidy detection has largely been generated by this indication. Disappointingly, the expected increase in liveborns was initially not observed. One possible explanation is unappreciated

damage following embryo biopsy, effects of which should be mitigated against by experience. In 1999, Ferraretti and coworkers compared outcome in 38- to 43-year-old IVF subjects in Bologna. Their study compared 109 cycles in which PGD was performed (patient choice) to 182 cycles in which PGD was not performed. Testing involved chromosomes 13, 14, 15, 16, 18, 21, 22, X, and Y. Sample size was small, and logistic regressions had not yet been performed to take into account potential confounding variables, but impressive differences were observed: increased implantation rate (26.6% PGD versus 15.6% non-PGD), decreased abortions (4.3% versus 14%), and increased livebirths as assessed by cumulative rates over three cycles (90% versus 50%). In 2000 the same group reported further progress of an ongoing randomized trial in which

PGD was or was not performed in women ≥38 years old (Feliciani et al., 2000). Using PGD and transferring only two embryos, the pregnancy rate per embryo transfer was 31% compared with that of younger women; without PGD, the pregnancy rate was only 10%. More recently, reasons for some studies failing to show salutary results have become clear. Those women of advanced maternal age who respond well to ovulation stimulation show significantly improved pregnancy rates, for example 44.1 versus 23.5% in controls in one series (Munné et al., 2002). In women who failed to respond favorably (e.g., < 7 embryos), even PGD does not yield sufficient numbers of normal embryos to improve the dismal prognosis.

"OBLIGATORY" PGD SHOULD MANDATED RESTRICTION BE PLACED ON EMBRYO TRANSFERS

If regulatory bodies were to restrict the number of embryos that could be transferred, routine PGD for aneuploidy detection would become relatively more attractive. In fact, it would seem irresistible to transfer only euploid embryos. This follows from 50% of embryos appearing morphologically normal at the eight-cell stage but actually being chromosomally abnormal (aneuploid, mosaic, or chaotic) (see also Chapter 5).

NONANEUPLOID MARKERS FOR ART SUCCESS

Nongenetic indications for PGD could be envisioned if a specific marker were shown to predict implantation success. Potential markers might include presence of a particular cell cycle gene, demonstration that embryonic rather than maternal protein synthesis (or mRNA) had been initiated, or physiologic evidence of differentiation through nanomolar technology. The obvious strategy would then involve transferring only those embryos having the positive predictive marker. One example might be presence or absence of a gene like Oct, a gene that if not expressed confers lethality.

PGD FOR GENE THERAPY

When gene therapy becomes available, two general approaches can be envisioned. *First*, gene therapy could be directed toward cells or organs of a given type, such as liver or bone marrow. If so, transfer of cells having a normal gene inserted (or an abnormal disrupted) would ordinarily be deferred until after organogenesis, either while still *in utero* or postnatally. *Second*, and more relevant here, gene correction might be applicable nonspecifically. It might suffice to insert that gene into a cell destined to become distributed anywhere in the body. The early embryo would then be the logical target, especially if genetically corrected cells were to have a selective advantage that could facilitate repopulating an erstwhile abnormal embryo. One would make a diagnosis, insert a normal gene into one or more cells of the early (abnormal) embryo, and transfer freshly corrected embryos.

Strategies pursued in animal models already seem promising and applicable to human PGD. For example, chimeras can be created by inserting genetically normal donor blastomeres into an affected embryo. Feasibility of success is predicated on only a few donor cells needing to be incorporated into the desired organ for proper function and, hence, a clinically normal offspring. These techniques have not yet been applied for human gene therapy, but their application can be anticipated.

Safety of Assisted Reproductive Technologies: ART, ICSI, PGD

Like any prenatal invasive technique, blastomere and polar body biopsy must prove relatively safe if PGD is to prove a viable option for conventional prenatal genetic diagnostic procedure (see Chapter 14). Data are still limited, but there is every reason to believe PGD be able to serve as an alternative to CVS and amniocentesis.

In this section our consideration of PGD safety begins by reviewing the safety of ART in general, the more general technology of which PGD is a small subset and for which considerable data exist.

SPONTANEOUS ABORTIONS IN ART

After ART not involving PGD, the spontaneous abortion rate is almost 20%. The clinical loss rate in the 1997 United States cycles was 18.1% (ASRM/SART, 2000). In 1998 U.S. cycles, the latest published data, the loss rate in all U.S. (n = 58,937) IVF cycles nationwide was 17.6% (SART/ASRM, 2002). This is generally considered higher than that of the general population (see Chapter 5). Although not large, the increase is of potential concern because we have observed that 50 to 60% of clinically recognized spontaneous abortions show chromosomal abnormalities. If the etiology of the increased spontaneous abortions in ART were cytogenetic, liveborns could be at increased risk for cytogenetic abnormalities.

Is the spontaneous abortion rate, in fact, really increased over background? One difficulty in analysis is that the interval of observation is longer in women undergoing ART than in pregnant women in the general population. In ART pregnancies, surveillance during the cycle of conception is more rigorous than in spontaneously conceived pregnancies. An ideal comparison would involve a life table analysis taking into account the differing number of weeks of observation. Even if the increase is real, it has long been assumed to reflect hormonal perturbations secondary to ovulation indication.

Another problem is that the ART population is not necessarily comparable to the general population. The underlying infertility that necessitated ART may be associated with factors that increase the rate of pregnancy loss or pregnancy complications. Women undergoing ART are usually older (mean age > 35 years) than women conceiving naturally (mean age 27 or 28 years). Advanced maternal age is associated with increased risk of pregnancy loss and chromosomal abnormalities, whereas advanced paternal age is associated with fresh mendelian mutations. Potential confounding variables not often taken into account include maternal disease, maternal toxin exposure, and advanced paternal age. Direction of bias when failing to take into account potential confounding variables is not even certain. Despite certain unfavorable correlates in the ART population, the older maternal age in women undergoing ART is probably associated with fewer exposures to toxins such as alcohol and cigarettes. These should confer a more favorable outcome, which could counterbalance negative correlates like age and prior reproductive failure.

ANOMALIES IN ART

Anomalies may plausibly be increased in ART (and, hence, PGD) for several reasons. (1) *In vivo* selective mechanisms against morphologically abnormal sperm might not be comparable to *in vitro* mechanisms. Given the increased likelihood of polyspermic fertilization, an increase in triploidy is especially possible. (2) Altered hormonal milieu *in vitro* may predispose to perturbations of meiosis or mitosis, leading to chromosomal aneuploidy. (3) Point mutations could result from various chemical and environmental exposures during *in vitro* fertilization.

In addition to problems cited in the previous section, other pitfalls exist in assessing anomalies after ART (Simpson, 1998). One is the differing rigor of evaluation. Neonatal examination following ART pregnancies could be more extensive than that following conventional pregnancies. Absolute anomaly rates might thus spuriously appear increased in ART compared with the less rigorously assessed general population. A variant of this problem arises when ART outcome is assessed over a protracted time interval after birth. In the birth defects registries utilized to derive the 2 to 3% anomaly rates cited in the general population, ascertainment is restricted to anomalies detected during the brief interval of hospitalization following delivery (1 to 3 days). Assessment carried out over a longer interval naturally results in more anomalies being recorded in ART than in population-based birth defects registries. Minor anomalies may also be recorded in ART surveys but not in birth defect surveillance programs: small umbilical hernias, nonpigmented skin, "hip clicks" that may or may not indicate congenital hip dislocations and an extra digit. If ultrasound is routinely performed, internal anomalies may be detected and included even if not associated with externally evident symptoms. Overall, ART anomaly rates have the real potential of being spuriously overestimated if not assessed using standards comparable to those of population-based birth defects registries.

The above pitfalls notwithstanding, ART surveillance registries have generally failed to show increased rates of anomalies (Simpson, 1998; Simpson and Lamb, 2001). The U.S. registry has never shown an increase in anomalies after ART. In the 1990 AFS/SART cohort, for example, 38 congenital anomalies were observed in 28 pregnancy outcomes derived from 3110 infants (Medical Research Intl, 1992). This report recorded total anomalies per total infants rather than more conventionally recording the number of infants with anomalies per number of children. The latter rate would seem to have been 28/3110, or 0.9%. Certain anomalies recorded in registries would surely not have been detected on neonatal examination. Examples from the 1990 AFS/SART cohort (Medical Research Intl, 1992) included periventricular cyst, hydronephrosis, pyloric stenosis, retinopathy, and pulmonary hypoplasia. In addition, anomalies detected in pregnancy termination cases were sometimes pooled with anomalies detected among liveborns. This well-meaning attempt at completeness is hazardous because some of the pregnancies that were terminated might have been lost spontaneously if iatrogenic intervention had not occurred. Despite the above, the malformation rate in early U.S. ART registries only reached 1%, lower than the expected 2 to 3%. Higher anomaly rates were reported in the 1993 cohort of 6321 clinical pregnancies that resulted into 5103 deliveries and 6870 infants (Society for Assisted Reproduction Technology, 1995). In that cohort there were 2.3 "birth defects per 100 neonates delivered"; however, not all these anomalies were major. In the U.S. report of 1997 cycles, the anomaly rate was 1.6% in 7353 deliveries (ASRM/SART, 2000).

Registry data from other countries are not dissimilar to the U.S. experience. An early report from ART units in Australia and New Zealand tabulated the incidence of major congenital anomalies as 2.2% (37/1697 infants) (Saunders et al., 1989). Because 6 of the 37 infants had spina bifida, Lancaster (1987) claimed a relationship between neural tube defects (NTDs) and ovulation-indication agents. However, case control data collected in the U.S. failed to confirm this concern (Mills et al., 1990), nor have other registries. The latest data from Australia continue to show an increase in NTDs in ART offspring, despite no overall increase in anomalies in the population (Lancaster et al., 2000). In another well-publicized Australian study (Hansen et al., 2002) the risk of a major malformation was twice as high in IVF offspring as in the normal population. Again, the proper control group is an infertile and not a normal population. On the positive side, an Australian cohort of 314 cases matched with controls provided reassuring information concerning growth and neurologic development; the offspring were 22 to 25 months old (Lancaster, 1996; Saunders et al., 1989).

A population-based data set in Sweden was used to compare anomalies in the general population (control) of 1,690,577 births with those of 9111 IVF pregnancies (Ericson and Kallen, 2001). Like the Australian data, the overall anomaly rate was not different (OR 0.89) in the IVF group once appropriate adjustments were made. However, again a three-fold increase in NTDs was observed. Alimentary atresia and omphalocele were also increased three-fold. This study expanded earlier analyses of Bergh and colleagues (1999) and Wennerholm and coworkers (2000). More recently, Koivurova et al. (2002) reported a four-fold increase in cardiac malformations in IVF offspring compared to the general population in northern Finland, even while no increase was found in other anomalies.

In the U.K., the Medical Research Council Working Party on Children Conceived through IVF surveyed 1267 pregnancies resulting from IVF or gamate intra fallopian tube (GIFT) transfer (Beral and Doyle, 1990). The 1978–1987 data set covered all U.K. clinics registering with a voluntary licensing authority. One or more congenital anomalies were detected in the first week of life in 35 of 1581 infants (2.2%). A slight increase in central nervous system anomalies did not reach statistical significance. The 2.2% of individuals with one or more malformations is comparable to that for the general U.K. population. A more thorough analysis was later conducted on a subset of the U.K. survey described above, namely, cases from the Bourne-Hallam unit founded by Robert Edwards. Of 961 Bourne-Hallam infants born between 1978 and 1987, 763 still resided in the U.K. In this group the malformation rate was 2.7% in multiple births and 2.4% in singletons (Rizk et al., 1991). Congenital anomalies following ART seemed comparable to those detected in the first week of life in the general population. Rates of individual anomalies were comparable to those expected on the basis of maternal age-adjusted rates in a Liverpool Congenital Malformations Register.

An excellent data set is compiled by the French National INF registry (FIVNAT). A 1993 report of 1986 to 1990 data revealed rates of anomalies of about 2% (FIVNAT, 1993), which remained essentially unchanged by the time of a later report (FIVNAT, 1995). Follow-up of 375 French cases at 6 to 13 years revealed that height, weight, and scholastic performance were no different than expected (Oliveness et al., 1997).

ANOMALIES FOLLOWING INTRACYTOPLASMIC SPERM INJECTION (ICSI)

More analogous to PGD than conventional IVF are outcomes following ICSI. ICSI is frequently performed for oligospermia and azoospermia and is the mainstay of male infertility treatment.

Recent U.S. data reported the malformation rate to be 1.7% in 4949 ICSI/IVF pregnancies (62.9% singletons) (ASRM/SART, 2000). In Australia the frequency of malformation in 4260 ICSI births or terminations was 2.5%, similar to that following IVF without ICSI (Lancaster et al., 2000). In the Swedish IVF Registry ICSI infants showed an anomaly rate of 47/1,139 or 4% (Ericson and Kallen, 2001). Hypospadias was increased in ICSI offspring, seven detected cases yielding a relative risk of 2.9 (95%, CI 1.4, 5.4). Hypospadias could have reflected inheritance of mutant paternal genes that were the cause for the spermatogenic abnormalities necessitating ICSI. Wennerholm and coworkers (2000) favor this explanation. Teratogenic effect of exogenously administered progesterone in humans is another possibility (Silver et al., 1999), although critical analysis by one of us led to the conclusion that administration of progesterone was not associated with fetal hypospadias (Simpson and Kaufman, 1998). Of interest, NTDs were not increased after ICSI in the Swedish cohort.

Outstanding surveillance is being conducted in Brussels by Bonduelle and coworkers (1994, 1995, 1996a, b, 1997, 1998, 1999, 2001, 2002). In the 1994 report, these investigators studied 163 couples undergoing subzonal insemination, ICSI, or both. Couples were followed in cohort fashion, including a systematic neonatal examination by a geneticist. Follow–up was performed at 12 months and again at 2 years of age. In the cohort, 21 children were born after subzonal insemination, 24 after ICSI, and 10 after a combination of the two techniques. Only 2 of the 55 infants showed major malformations. One case involved bilateral inguinal hernia. The second case involved cheilopalatoschisis and duplication of the pyelus; psychomotor development was normal at 1 year of age. None of the 55 infants had chromosomal abnormalities.

Bonduelle and coworkers (1995) initially matched 130 children born after ICSI to 130 children born after IVF. Surveillance consisted of prenatal chromosomal studies, prenatal ultrasound examination, and physical examinations at birth, 2 months, and 1 year of age. Five major anomalies were detected in the ICSI group compared with six in a matched group. In 1999, the major malformation rate in the Brussels sample of 1987 ICSI/IVF offspring was reported to be 2.3% (Bonduelle et al., 1999). This is not increased over background considering rigorous surveillance. There was also no evidence that any particular malformation was increased following ICSI. In the most recent reports, Bonduelle and colleagues (2001, 2002) reported a malformation rate of 3.4% following ICSI (n = 2840); the rate was 3.8% following standard IVF (n = 2955). Taking into account malformations in stillborns, terminations, and liveborns, total major malformation rates were 4.2% in ICSI and 4.6% in IVF. (Note that these rates are ascertained differently from traditional birth defects registry data, which are restricted by liveborn neonates.) Using the same criteria for hypospadias as Wennerholm and coworkers (2000b), Bonduelle and associates (2002) found 0.28% hypospadias in ICSI (8/2840) versus 0.47% in

IVF (14/2955) infants. No differences were found for ICSI using ejaculated epididymal and testicular sperm.

The genetic abnormality for which greatest concern has been raised in ICSI is chromosomal. Prenatal cytogenetic studies have been performed in many ICSI pregnancies (Bonduelle et al., 1997, 1999, 2002); cytogenetic outcome of ICSI pregnancies in 1987 are shown in Table 16–7. The sex chromosomal abnormality rate of 0.8% was increased over population expectations (see Chapter 1) but was much lower than the alarming rate reported by In't Veld and coworkers (1995) in a small sample. The frequency of de novo structural aberrations was also increased. The most recent tabulation of Bonduelle and coworkers (2002) continued to find increased de novo chromosomal aberrations (1.56%). Aboulghar and colleagues (2001) reported 3.5% chromosomal abnormalities in 430 ICSI babies (15/430); six had sex chromosomal abnormalities, eight autosomal, and one both. A French study found a higher malformation rate using testicular rather than epididymal spermatozoa (Bajirova et al., 2001).

The explanation for this low but ostensibly increased rate of de novo and sex chromosomal abnormalities is unclear. Several explanations seem worth considering (Simpson and Lamb, 2001). (1) The site of needle insertion could interfere with the meiotic spindle (Terada et al., 2000), a possible mechanism being preferential localization of the X and Y in the sub-acrosomal region (Sbracia et al., 2002). Atypical decondensation of the sperm nucleus and delayed DNA replication may occur after ICSI (Terada et al., 2000). (2) Oligospermic men who require ICSI could in fact be low grade 47,XXY mosaics. (3) A nonspecific interchromosomal effect could exist, supported by 2% of women and 4% of men in ICSI

▼ **Table 16–7.** FREQUENCY OF CHROMOSOMAL
• ABNORMALITIES IN ICSI PREGNANCIES

Chromosomal Abnormalities	N	Percentage
De Novo		
Sex chromosomal	9	0.83
Autosomal		
Aneuploidy	4	0.36
Structural	5	(0.46)
Subtotal	9	(0.83)
Inherited		
Balanced	9	(0.83)
Unbalanced	1	(0.09)
Subtotal	10	(0.92)
Grand Total	28	(2.57)

Based on 1082 prenatal genetic diagnosis from 1987 ICSI pregnancies. Data from Bonduelle M, Wilikens A, Buysse A, et al., 1998; and Bonduelle M, Camus M, De Vos A, et al., 1999.

cycles having somatic (blood) chromosomal rearrangements (Simpson and Lamb, 2001). In 2002 the American Society for Reproductive Medicine Male Infertility Best Practice Policy Committee (Sharlip et al., 2002) recommended that karyotyping "should be offered to men with nonobstructive azoospermia or severe oligospermia." (4) A generalized meiotic or mitotic perturbation could reflect a mutant gene, perhaps with pleiotropic effect. Meiotic abnormality could predispose gametes to aneuploidy. Palermo et al. (2002) reported aneuploidy in 11.4% of sperm with nonobstructive azoospermia, compared to only 1.8% in epididymal sperm in obstructive azoospermia and 1.5% in ejaculated sperm. That sex chromosomal and not autosomal aneuploidy is observed could merely reflect greater lethality in the latter. (5) A nonspecific, nongenetic effect could exist secondary to an inhospitable cellular millieu. Simpson and Lamb (2001) discuss these explanations in more detail elsewhere.

Obstetric outcomes (birth weight, prematurity) in 424 ICSI pregnancies are similar to those observed after conventional IVF (Wisanto et al., 1995; Bonduelle et al., 1999, 2002).

ANOMALIES AFTER PGD

Experience is more limited in PGD, but neither anomaly rates nor spontaneous abortion rates seem increased after PGD compared with conventional ART without embryo biopsy. A confounding factor is that the population of women undergoing PGD for mendelian diagnosis is young compared with those undergoing ART for infertility or PGD for cytogenetic indications.

In a 1999 report of 500 PGD cycles for mendelian/sex determination, the pregnancy rate was 20% (Verlinsky and Kuliev, 1999). The anomaly rates were not increased. No increase in anomalies was found in the 79 neonates born in the ESHRE Preimplantation Genetic Diagnosis Consortium (ESHRE PGD Consortium Steering Group, 1999); the majority of PGD cases were studied for chromosomal indications. The 10th (2000) International Working Group on PGD (Verlinsky et al., 2001e) tabulated an anomaly rate of 4.7% in 136 newborns in two registries, a figure seemingly not increased over background given rigorous surveillance of these infants. The incidence of monozygotic twinning is increased after assisted hatching (Hershlag et al., 1999), and this bears surveillance in PGD as well.

More detailed information concerning outcome in PGD liveborns in one center was reported by Strom and coworkers (2000). A follow-up of 97 pregnancies after polar body biopsy yielded 109 livebirths. PGD had been performed for cytogenetic indications in 91 and for mendelian indications in 18. Six infants had either some major or minor birth defects, a number well within expected numbers. The six included two with definite major anomalies (unilateral transverse limb reduction due to amniotic band syndrome; neonatal seizures with cerebral infarcts). One infant had asymptomatic thickening of the tricuspid valve, which did not require surgery and may or may not be major. Three other infants unequivocally had minor anomalies: strawberry hemangiomas on both arms; minor hemangioma; and bilateral syndactyly toes. Only 1 of 44 infants followed up to 6 months had developmental delay. Mean birth weight in singletons was normal. A later follow-up of 202 liveborn PGD offspring from the same center (138 singleton pregnancies, 46 twin gestations, 18 triplet pregnancies) found only 3 with major defects (amniotic bands, ventricular septal defect, cardiomegaly) (Ginsberg et al., 2002). Fisher et al. (2002) reported outcome of 39 PGD infants (19 singleton, 7 twins, 2 triplets). Only 3 had malformations, and one of these had the autosomal dominant disorder lymphoedema-distichiasis, clearly not related to PGD.

Two ongoing international registries continue to collect data: (1) International Preimplantation Genetic Diagnosis (PGD) Consortium (Y. Verlinsky, Chicago; *e-mail:rgi@flash.net),* and (2) European Society of Human Reproduction and Embryology (www.eshre.com) PGD Consortium.

Pregnancy rates have traditionally been considered essentially zero after cryopreservation of a biopsied embryo, presumably because ice crystals form in the embryo that lacks an intact zona pellucida (Joris et al., 1998; Magli et al., 1999). Indeed, survival rate after thawing biopsied embryos is significantly lower after including thawing of nonbiopsied embryos. However, successful pregnancies after thawing cryopreserved biopsied embryos were recently reported (Lalic et al., 2001; Wilton et al. 2001, 2002).

RECOMMENDED SURVEILLANCE FOR CONGENITAL ANOMALIES FOLLOWING ART OR PGD

Verifying PGD safety ideally necessitates a cohort approach, recording data systematically in standard fashion. Prospective evaluation should begin as soon as possible after pregnancy is recognized and recorded on standard forms. One approach was suggested by Simpson and

▼ **Table 16–8.** RECOMMENDED SYSTEMATIC ANOMALY ASSESSMENT

Instrument	Time	Purpose
Intake information	Recognition of pregnancy	Sociodemographic history; ethnic origin; occupation; family history, obstetric and medical history; current drug exposure; exposure to tobacco, alcohol, and other toxins
Surveillance during pregnancy	End of first trimester	Exposure to infections or drug/toxins since completing intake form (A): interim changes in medical status; results of interim prenatal exams and ultrasound exams
Fetal loss	Recognition of fetal loss	Determine timing of fetal loss; potential explanation.
Neonatal assessment	Defined time (e.g., 1 week) after delivery	Pregnancy complications and exposures not previously recorded; infant weight, length, head circumference, systematic search for major anatomic abnormalities

From Simpson JL, Liebaers I: Assessing congenital anomalies after preimplantation genetic diagnosis. J Assist Reprod Genet 13:170, 1996.

Liebaers (1996) (Table 16–8). Background data should include family history, obstetric history, number of prior spontaneous abortions, medical illnesses, drug ingestion, and exposures to smoking and alcohol. Shortly after the end of the teratogenic period (e.g., 12 weeks), surveillance is recommended again to record intervening changes in health status that might affect pregnancy outcome. Such events might include exposure to infections or ingestion of medications.

A standard definition of major anomaly must be utilized. We recommend three: death, serious handicaps, or necessity for surgery. All three outcomes are readily measurable. A hemangioma requiring surgery is defined as a major anomaly, whereas one not requiring surgery is considered minor by definition. Geneticists should confirm abnormal findings and verify the presence or absence of mendelian disorders or known malformation syndromes; however, geneticists should not perform surveillance examinations routinely because their diagnostic acumen should be greater than that of pediatricians who lack genetic training. Rigorous examinations by specialists in dysmorphology could yield a spurious increase in anomaly rates if a control group were not comparably scrutinized.

It is crucial to record and analyze separately internal anomalies detected only by ultrasound. If an anomaly rate in a PGD or ART cohort includes internal anomalies recognized in asymptomatic fetuses or neonates, the calculated rate will spuriously be higher because surveillance would be more vigorous than in the general population; the latter would be far less likely to undergo routine, comprehensive, ultrasound surveys during pregnancy. If, on the other hand, ultrasound was performed as a result of a clinically abnormal situation (e.g., polyhydramnios), it would be appropriate to include it as an anomaly. Major anomalies identified in abortuses, spontaneous or induced, should also be assessed separately, again the rationale being that birth defects registries do not record anomalies in abortuses.

A final requirement is that neonatal anomaly assessment be restricted to a specified time interval, such as within 1 week after delivery or the 2 to 3 days coinciding with routine postpartum stay. Detection rate for anomalies increases as the length of surveillance after delivery increases. Restricting anomaly assessment to perhaps 1 week after delivery allows surveillance comparable to that of the birth defects registry data, which typically ascertain cases only while neonates are hospitalized.

REFERENCES

Aboulghar H, Aboulghar M, Mansour R, et al.: A prospective controlled study of karyotyping for 430 consecutive babies conceived through intracytoplasmic sperm injection. Fertil Steril 76:249, 2001.

Ao A, Wells D, Handyside AH, et al.: Preimplantation genetic diagnosis of inherited cancer: Familial adenomatous polyposis coli. J Assist Reprod Genet 15:140, 1998.

Apessos A, Abou-Sleiman PM, Harper JC, et al.: Preimplantation genetic diagnosis of the fragile X syndrome by use of linked polymorphic markers. Prenat Diagn 21:504, 2001.

ASRM/SART: Assisted reproductive technology in the United States: 1997 results generated from the American Society for Reproductive Medicine/Society for Assisted Reproductive Technology Registry. Fertil Steril 74:641, 2000.

Bahçe M, Cohen J, Munné S: Preimplantation genetic diagnosis of aneuploidy: Were we looking at the wrong chromosome? J Assist Reprod Genet 16:176, 1999.

Bajirova M, Francannet C, Pouly JL, et al.: FIVNAT final report on the malformation risk after ICSI using epididymal or testicular spermatozoids. Hum Reprod 16:40(Abstract O–100), 2001.

Beral V, Doyle P: Births in Great Britain resulting from assisted conception, 1978–87, MRC Working Party on Children Conceived in In vitro Fertilization. Br J Med 300:1229, 1990.

Bergh T, Ericson A, Hillensjö T, et al.: Delivery and children born after in-vitro fertilization in Sweden 1982–1995; a retrospective cohort study. Lancet 354:1579, 1999.

Blaszczyk A, Tang YX, Dietz HC, et al.: Preimplantation genetic diagnosis of human embryos for Marfan's syndrome. J Assist Reprod Genet 15:281, 1998.

Boada M, Carrera M, De La Iglesia C, et al.: Successful use of a laser for human embryo biopsy in preimplantation genetic diagnosis: Report of two cases. J Assist Reprod Genet 15:302, 1998.

Bonduelle M, Desmyttere S, Buysse A, et al.: Prospective follow-up study of 55 children born after subzonal insemination and intracytoplasmic sperm injection. Hum Reprod 9:1765, 1994.

Bonduelle M, Legein J, Derde MP, et al.: Comparative follow-up study of 130 children born after intracytoplasmic sperm injection and 130 children born after *in vitro* fertilization. Hum Reprod 10:3327, 1995.

Bonduelle M, Legein J, Buysse A, et al.: Prospective follow-up study of 423 children born after intracytoplasmic sperm injection. Hum Reprod 11:1558, 1996a.

Bonduelle M, Wilikens J, Buysse A, et al.: Prospective study of 877 children born after intracytoplasmic sperm injection, with ejaculated epididymal and testicular spermatozoa and after replacement of cryopreserved embryos obtained after ICSI. Hum Reprod 11:131, 1996b.

Bonduelle M, Devroey P, Liebaers I, et al.: Commentary: Major defects are overestimated. BMJ 7118:1265, 1997.

Bonduelle M, Wilikens A, Buysse A, et al.: A follow-up study of children born after intracytoplasmic sperm injection (ICSI) with epididymal and testicular spermatozoa and after replacement of cryopreserved embryos obtained after ICSI. Hum Reprod 13:196, 1998.

Bonduelle M, Camus M, De Vos A, et al.: Seven years of intracytoplasmic sperm injection and follow-up of 1987 subsequent children. Hum Reprod 14(Suppl):243, 1999.

Bonduelle M, Deketelaere V, Liebaers L, et al.: Pregnancy outcome after ICSI: A cohort study of 2995 IVF children and 2899 ICSI children. Hum Reprod 16:40(Abstract O–99), 2001.

Bonduelle M, Liebaers I, Deketelaere V, et al.: Neonatal data on a cohort of 2889 infants born after intracytoplasmic sperm injection (ICSI) (1991–1999) and of 2995 infants born after *in vitro* fertilisation (IVF) (1983–1999), in press, 2002.

Buster JE, Bustillo M, Rodi IA, et al.: Biologic and morphologic development of donated human ova recovered by nonsurgical uterine lavage. Am J Obstet Gynecol 153:211, 1985.

Bustillo M, Buster JE, Cohen SW, et al.: Nonsurgical ovum transfer as a treatment in infertile women. Preliminary experience. JAMA 251:1171, 1984.

Carson SA, Gentry WL, Smith AL, et al.: Trophectoderm microbiopsy in murine blastocysts: comparison of four methods. J Assist Reprod Genet 10:427, 1993.

Carson SA, Smith AL, Scoggan JL, et al.: Superovulation fails to increase human blastocyst yield after uterine lavage. Prenat Diagn 11:513, 1991.

Chamayou S, Alecci C, Ragolia C, et al.: Successful application of preimplantation genetic diagnosis for β-thalassaemia and sickle cell anaemia in Italy. Hum Reprod 17:1158, 2002.

Cieslak J, Evsikov S, Galat V, et al.: Nuclear transfer for full karyotyping and PGD for chromosomal translocations. Reprod BioMed Online 4:Suppl 2:23(Abstract O-30), 2002.

Clement-Sengewald A, Buchholz T, Schütze K, et al.: Noncontact, laser-mediated extraction of polar bodies for prefertilization genetic diagnosis. J Asst Reprod Genet 19:183, 2002.

Conn CM, Cozzi J, Harper JC, et al.: Preimplantation genetic diagnosis for couples at high risk of Down syndrome pregnancy owing to parental translocation or mosaicism. J Med Genet 36:45, 1999.

Coonen E, Dumoulin JCM, Derhaag JG, et al.: Genetic make-up of human embryos grown *in vitro* until the blastocysts stage. Hum Reprod 15:182(Abstract P–212), 2000.

Delhanty JD, Harper JC, Ao A: Multicolour FISH detects frequent chromosomal mosaicism and chaotic division in normal preimplantation embryos from fertile patients. Hum Genet 99:755, 1997.

Desnick RJ, Schuette JL, Golbus MS, et al.: First-trimester biochemical and molecular diagnoses using chorionic villi: High accuracy in the U.S. Collaborative Study. Prenat Diagn 12:357, 1992.

Dokras A, Sargent IL, Ross C, et al.: Trophectoderm biopsy in human blastocysts. Hum Reprod 5:821, 1990.

Dyband AP: Reliable technique for chromosomal preparations from mammalian oocytes, preimplantation embryos and isolated blastomeres. *In* Verlinsky Y, Kuliev A (eds): Preimplantation Genetics. New York: Plenum Press, 1991, p 293.

ESHRE PGD Consortium Steering Committee: Preimplantation Genetic Diagnosis (PGD) Consortium: Preliminary assessment of data from January 1997 to September 1998. Hum Reprod 14:3138, 1999.

ESHRE PGD Consortium Steering Committee: ESHRE preimplantation genetic diagnosis consortium: data collection III (May 2001). Hum Reprod 17:233, 2002.

Ericson A, Kallen B: Congenital malformations in infants born after IVF: A population-based study. Hum Reprod 16:504, 2001.

Feliciani E, Ferraretti AP, Gerin F, et al.: PGD for aneuploidy as a tool to avoid the need of transferring more than two embryos. Hum Reprod 15:182(Abstract P–219), 2000.

Ferraretti AP, Gianaroli L, Fortini D, et al.: Clinical outcome in repeated cycles with preimplantation genetic diagnosis for aneuploidy according to the patient's age. Hum Reprod 15:182(Abstract P-220), 2000.

Ferraretti AP, Gianaroli L, Magli MC, et al.: The impact of preimplantation genetic diagnosis for aneuploidy on the implantation and abortion rates in patients over 37 years old. Hum Reprod 14:99, 1999.

Findlay I, Corby N, Rutherford A, et al.: Comparison of FISH PRINS, and conventional and fluorescent PCR for single-cell sexing: Suitability for preimplantation genetic diagnosis. J Assist Reprod Genet 15:258, 1998.

Findlay I, Matthews PL, Mulcahy BK, et al.: Using MF-PCR to diagnose multiple defects from single cells: Implications for PGD. Mol Cell Endocrinol 183:Suppl 1:S5, 2001.

Findlay I, Ray P, Quirke P, et al.: Allele drop-out and preferential amplification in single cells and human blastomeres: Implications for preimplantation diagnosis of sex and cystic fibrosis. Hum Reprod 10:1609, 1995.

Fischer J, Escudero T, Chen S, et al: Obstetric outcome of 100 cycles of PGD of translocations and other structural abnormalities. Reprod BioMed Online 4:Suppl 2:26(Abstract O-37), 2002.

FIVNAT: Pregnancies and birth resulting from *in vitro* fertilization; French National Registry: Analysis of data 1986 to 1992. Contracept Fertil Sex 23:S141, 1995.

FIVNAT: French National IVF Registry: Analysis of 1986 to 1990 data. Fertil Steril 59:587, 1993.

Formigli L, Roccio C, Belotti G, et al.: Non-surgical flushing of the uterus for pre-embryo recovery: Possible clinical applications. Hum Reprod 58:329, 1990.

Geraedts JPM, Harper J, Braude P, et al.: Preimplantation genetic diagnosis (PGD), a collaborative activity of clinical genetic departments and IVF centres. Prenat Diagn, in press, 2002.

Gianaroli L, Magli MC, Ferraretti AP: The *in vivo* and *in vitro* efficiency and efficacy of PGD for aneuploidy. Mol Cell Endocrinol 183:Suppl 1:S13, 2001.

Gianaroli L, Magli MC, Ferraretti AP, et al.: Robertsonian and reciprocal translocations. Reprod BioMed Online 4:Suppl 2:26(Abstract O-38), 2002.

Gianaroli L, Magli MC, Ferraretti AP, et al.: Preimplantation diagnosis for aneuploidies in patients undergoing *in vitro* fertilization with a poor prognosis: Identification of the categories for which it should be proposed. Fertil Steril 72:837, 1999.

Gianaroli L, Magli MC, Ferraretti AP, et al.: Preimplantation genetic diagnosis increases the implantation rate in human *in vitro* fertilization by avoiding the transfer of chromosomally abnormal embryos. Fertil Steril 68:1128, 1997.

Gimenez C, Egozcue J, Vidal F: Cytogenetic sexing of mouse embryos. Hum Reprod 8:470, 1993.

Ginsberg N, Cieslak J, Rechitsky S, et al.: Clinical outcome following PGD in one large center. Reprod BioMed Online 4:Suppl 2:31(Abstract O-47), 2002.

Grifo JA, Boyle A, Tang Y-X, et al.: Preimplantation genetic diagnosis. In situ hybridization as a tool for analysis. Arch Pathol Lab Med 116:393, 1992.

Handyside AH, Delhanty JD: Preimplantation genetic diagnosis: Strategies and surprises. Trends Genet 13:270, 1997.

Handyside AH, Kontogianni EH, Hardy K, et al.: Pregnancies from biopsied human preimplantation embryos sexed by Y-specific DNA amplification. Nature 344:768, 1990.

Handyside AH, Lesko JG, Tarin JJ, et al.: Birth of a normal girl after *in vitro* fertilization and preimplantation diagnostic testing for cystic fibrosis. N Engl J Med 327:905, 1992.

Handyside AH, Pattinson JK, Penketh RJ, et al.: Biopsy of human preimplantation embryos and sexing by DNA amplification. Lancet 1:347, 1989.

Hardy JK, Martin KL, Leese HJ, et al.: Human preimplantation development *in vitro* is not adversely affected by biopsy at 8–cell stage. Hum Reprod 5:708, 1990.

Hansen M, Kurinczuk JJ, Bower C, et al.: The risk of major birth defects after intracytoplasmic sperm injection and *in vitro* fertilization. N Engl J Med 346:725, 2002.

Hershlag A, Paine T, Cooper G, et al.: Monozygotic twinning associated with mechanical assisted hatching. Fertil Steril 71:144, 1999.

In't Veld P, Brandenburg H, Verhoeff A, et al.: Sex chromosomal abnormalities and intracytoplasmic sperm injection. Lancet 346:773, 1995.

Iwarsson E, Ahrlund-Richter L, Inzunza J, et al.: Preimplantation genetic diagnosis of a large pericentric inversion of chromosome 5. Mol Hum Reprod 4:719, 1998.

Joris H, Vitrier S, De Vos A, et al.: Reduced survival after embryo biopsy and cryopreservation of human embryos obtained after abnormal fertilization. Hum Reprod 13 (Suppl. 1):61, 1998.

Kanavakis E, Vrettou C, Palmer G, et al.: Preimplantation genetic diagnosis in 10 couples at risk for transmitting beta-thalassemia major: Clinical experience including the initiation of six singleton pregnancies. Prenat Diagn 19:1217, 1999.

Klinger K, Landes G, Shook D, et al.: Rapid detection of chromosome aneuploides in uncultured amniocytes by using fluorescence in situ hybridization (FISH). Am J Hum Genet 51:55, 1992.

Koivurova S, Hartikainen A-L, Gissler M, et al.: Neonatal outcome and congenital malformations in children born after *in vitro* fertilization. Hum Reprod 17:1391, 2002.

Kola I, Wilton L: Preimplantation embryo biopsy: Detection of trisomy in a single cell biopsied from a four-cell mouse embryo. Mol Reprod Dev 29:16, 1991.

Kuliev A, Rechitsky S, Verlinsky O, et al.: Preembryonic diagnosis for sickle cell disease. Mol Cell Endocrinol 183:Suppl 1:S19, 2001.

Kuliev A, Rechitsky S, Verlinsky O, et al.: Preimplantation diagnosis of thalassemia. J Assist Reprod Genet 15:219, 1998.

Lalic I, Catt J, McArthur S: Pregnancies after cryopreservation of embryos biopsied for PGD. Hum Reprod 16: 32(Abstract 76), 2001.

Lancaster PA: Congenital malformations after *in vitro* fertilization. Lancet 2:1392, 1987.

Lancaster PA, Hurst T, Shafir E: Congenital malformations and other pregnancy outcome after microinsemination. Reprod Toxicol 14:74(Abstract), 2000.

Lancaster PA, Shafir E: High incidence of neural tube defects after assisted conception. Hum Reprod 11:39(Abstract 83), 1996.

Ledbetter DH, Zachery JM, Simpson JL, et al.: Cytogenetic results from the US Collaborative Study on CVS: High diagnostic accuracy in over 11, 000 cases. Prenat Diagn 12:317, 1992.

Magli MC, Gianaroli L, Fortini D, et al.: Impact of blastomere biopsy and cryopreservation techniques on human embryo viability. Hum Reprod 14:770, 1999.

Medical Research International Society for Assisted Reproductive Technology (SART): The American Fertility Society: *In vitro* fertilization-embryo transfer (IVF-ET) in the United States: 1990 results from IVF-ET Registry. Fertil Steril 57:15, 1992.

McKenzie LJ, Cisneros PL, Torsky S, et al.: PGD of a cryptic translocation: implications for segregation products. Reprod BioMed Online 4:Suppl 2:30(Abstract O-45), 2002.

Mills JL, Simpson JL, Rhoads GG, et al.: Risk of neural tube defects in relation to maternal fertility and fertility drug use. Lancet 336:103, 1990.

Munné S, Sadowy S, Walmsley R, et al.: PGD of aneuploidy for good responder IVF patients. Reprod BioMed Online 4:Suppl 2:25(Abstract O-35), 2002.

Munné S: Preimplantation genetic diagnosis of structural abnormalities. Mol Cell Endocrinol 183:Suppl 1:S55, 2001.

Munné S, Alikani M, Tomkin G, et al.: Embryo morphology, developmental rates and maternal age are correlated with chromosome abnormalities. Fertil Steril 64:382, 1995.

Munné S, Cohen J: Chromosome abnormalities in human embryos. Hum Reprod Update 4:842, 1998.

Munné S, Magli C, Bahçe M, et al.: Preimplantation diagnosis of the aneuploidies most commonly found in spontaneous abortions and livebirths: XY, 13, 14, 15, 16, 18, 21, 22. Prenat Diagn 18:1459, 1998a.

Munné S, Magli C, Cohen J, et al.: Positive outcome after preimplantation diagnosis of aneuploidy in human embryos. Hum Reprod 14:2191, 1999.

Munné S, Marquez C, Magli C, et al.: Scoring criteria for preimplantation genetic diagnosis of numerical abnormalities for chromosome X, Y, 13, 16, 18 and 21. Mol Hum Reprod 4:863, 1998b.

Munné S, Sandalinas M, Escudero T, et al.: Outcome of preimplantation genetic diagnosis of translocations. Fertil Steril 73:1209, 2000.

Ning Y, Roschke A, Smith ACM, et al.: A complete set of human telomeric probes and their clinical application. National Institutes of Health and Institute of Molecular Medicine Collaboration. Nat Genet 14:86, 1996.

Olivennes F, Kerbrat V, Rufat P, et al.: Follow-up of a cohort of 422 children aged 6 to 13 years conceived by *in vitro* fertilization. Fertil Steril 67:284, 1997.

Palermo GD, Colombero LT, Hariprashad JJ, et al.: Chromosome analysis of epididymal and testicular sperm in azoospermic patients undergoing ICSI. Hum Reprod 17:570, 2002.

Rechitsky S, Strom C, Verlinsky O, et al.: Accuracy of preimplantation diagnosis of single-gene disorders by polar body analysis of oocytes. J Assist Reprod Genet 16:192, 1999.

Rechitsky S, Strom C, Verlinsky O, et al.: Allele dropout in polar bodies and blastomeres. J Assist Reprod Genet 15:253, 1998.

Rechitsky S, Verlinsky O, Kuliev A, et al.: Preimplantation non-disease testing. Reprod BioMed Online 4:Suppl 2:23(Abstract O-32), 2002.

Rechitsky S, Verlinsky O, Rechitsky AM, et al.: Reliability of preimplantation diagnosis for single gene disorders. Mol Cell Endocrinol 183:Suppl 1:S65, 2001.

Rizk B, Doyle P, Tan SL, et al.: Perinatal outcome and congenital malformations in *in vitro* fertilization babies from the Bourn-Hallam group. Hum Reprod 6:1259, 1991.

Rubio C, Vidal F, Minguez Y, et al.: High incidence of chromosomal abnormalities in preimplantation embryos from recurrent spontaneous abortion patient. Hum Reprod 15:O–203, 2000.

Sandalinas M, Sadowy S, Calderon F, et al.: Survival of chromosome abnormalities to blastocyst stage. Hum Reprod 15:P–027, 2000.

Santaló J, Pérez N, Egozcue J, et al.: First case of preimplantation genetic diagnosis in a couple carrying the 1609delCA mutation for cystic fibrosis. Hum Reprod 14:42(Suppl 1), 1999.

SART/ASRM: Assisted reproductive technology in the United States: 1998 results generated from the American Society for Reproductive Medicine/Society for Assisted Reproductive Technology Registry. Fertil Steril 77:18, 2002.

Saunders DM, Lancaster P: The wider perinatal significance of the Australian *in vitro* fertilization data collection program. Am J Perinatol 6:252, 1989.

Sbracia M, Baldi M, Cao D, et al.: Preferential location of sex chromosomes, their aneuploidy in human sperm, and their role in determining sex chromosome aneuploidy in embryos after ICSI. Hum Reprod 17:320, 2002.

Scriven PN, Handyside AH, Ogilvie CM: Chromosome translocations: Segregation modes and strategies for preimplantation genetic diagnosis. Prenat Diagn 18:1437, 1998.

Sermon K, De Vos A, Van de Velde, et al.: Fluorescent PCR and automated fragment analysis for the clinical application of preimplantation genetic diagnosis of myotonic dystrophy (Steinert's disease). Mol Hum Reprod 4:791, 1998.

Sermon K, Lissens W, Joris H, et al.: Clinical application of preimplantation diagnosis for myotonic dystrophy. Prenat Diagn 17:925, 1997.

Sermon K, Seneca S, Venderfaeillie A, et al.: Preimplantation diagnosis for fragile X syndrome based on the detection of the non-expanded paternal and maternal CGG. Prenat Diagn 19:1223, 1999.

Sermon K: PGD for dynamic mutations. Reprod BioMed Online 4:Suppl 2:24(Abstract O-33), 2002.

Sharlip ID, Jarow JP, Belker AM, et al.: Best practice policies of male infertility. Fertil Steril 77:873, 2002.

Silver RI, Rodriguez R, Chang TS, Gearhart JP: *In vitro* fertilization is associated with an increased risk of hypospadias. J Urol 161:1954, 1999.

Simpson JL: PGD as part of pre-pregnancy genetic screening. Reprod BioMed Online 4:Suppl 2:10(Abstract O-2), 2002.

Simpson JL: Celebrating preimplantation genetic diagnosis of p53 mutations in Li-Fraumeni syndrome. Reprod BioMed Online 3:2, 2001b.

Simpson JL: Changing indications for preimplantation genetic diagnosis (PGD). Mol Cell Endocrinol 183:Suppl 1:S69, 2001a.

Simpson JL: Are anomalies increased after ART and ICSI? *In* Kempers RD, Cohen J, Haney AF, et al. (eds): Fertility and Reproductive Medicine (Preceedings of the XVI World Congress on Fertility and Sterility, San Francisco). Amsterdam, San Francisco: Elsevier Science, 1998, p 199.

Simpson JL, Carson SA, Buster JE, et al.: Preimplantation genetic diagnosis: Indications and Pitfalls. *In* Mori T, Aono T, Tominago T, et al. (eds): Frontiers in Endocrinology: Perspectives on Assisted Reproduction. Rome: Ares-Serono Symposia Publications, 1994, p 689.

Simpson JL, Kaufman R: Fetal effects of progestogens and diethylstilbestrol. *In* Fraser IS, Jansen RPS, Lobo RA, et al. (eds): Estrogens and Progestogens in Clinical Practice. London: Churchill Livingstone, 1998, p 533.

Simpson JL, Lamb D: Genetic effects of intracytoplasmic sperm injection. Semin Reprod Med 19:239, 2001.

Simpson JL, Liebaers I: Assessing congenital anomalies after preimplantation genetic diagnosis. J Assist Reprod Genet 13:170, 1996.

Society for Assisted Reproductive Technology and The American Society for Reproductive Medicine: Assisted Reproductive Technology in the United States and Canada: 1993 results generated from the American Society for Reproductive Medicine/Society for Assisted Reproductive Technology. Fertil Steril 64:13, 1995.

Strom CM: Preimplantation genetic diagnosis of mendelian disorders. *In* Sciarra J (ed): Gynecology and Obstetrics. vol. 5, ch 109. Philadelphia: Lippincott Williams and Wilkins, 2001.

Strom CM, Levin R, Strom S, et al.: Neonatal outcome of preimplantation genetic diagnosis by polar body removal: The first 109 infants. Pediatrics 106:650, 2000.

Terada Y, Luetjens CM, Sutovsky P, et al.: Atypical decondensation of the sperm nucleus, delayed replication of the male genome, and sex chromosome positioning following intracytoplasmic human sperm injection (ICSI) into golden hamster eggs: Does ICSI itself introduce chromosomal anomalies? Fertil Steril 74:454, 2000.

Trounson A, Anderiesz C, Jones GM, et al.: Oocyte maturation. Hum Reprod 13:Suppl 3:52, 1998.

Van Assche E, Staessen C, Ogur G, et al.: PGD for reciprocal and Robertsonian translocations in 41 treatment cycles. Reprod BioMed Online 4:Suppl 2:27(Abstract O-39), 2002.

Van de Velde H, Van Ranst H, Sermon K, et al.: Implantation after biopsy of one or two cells for preimplantation genetic diagnosis. Hum Reprod 15:82(Abstract O–205), 2000.

Veiga A, Sandalinas M, Benkhalifa M, et al.: Laser blastocyst biopsy for preimplantation diagnosis in the human. Zygote 5:351, 1997.

Verlinsky Y, Kuliev A: Micromanipulation of gametes and embryos in preimplantation genetic diagnosis and assisted fertilization. Curr Opin Obstet Gynecol 4:720, 1992.

Verlinsky Y, Dozortsev D, Evsikov S: Visualization and cytogenetic analysis of second polar body chromosomes following fusion with one-cell mouse embryo. J Assist Reprod Genet 11:123, 1994.

Verlinsky Y, Rechitsky S, Cieslak J, et al.: Preimplantation diagnosis of single gene disorders by two-step oocyte genetic analysis using first and second polar body. Biochem Mol Med 62:182, 1997.

Verlinsky Y, Cieslak J, Ivakhnenko V, et al.: Preimplantation diagnosis of common aneuploidies by the first and second polar body FISH analysis. J Assist Reprod Genet 15:285, 1998.

Verlinsky Y, Rechitsky S, Verlinsky O, et al.: Prepregnancy testing for single-gene disorders by polar body analysis. Genet Test 3:185, 1999a.

Verlinsky Y, Cieslak J, Ivakhnenko V, et al.: Prevention of age-related aneuploidies by polar body testing of oocytes. J Assist Reprod Genet 16:165, 1999b.

Verlinsky Y, Evsikov S: Karyotyping of human oocytes by chromosomal analysis of the second polar bodies. Mol Hum Reprod 5:89, 1999.

Verlinsky Y, Cieslak J, Evsikov S, et al.: Preimplantation genetic diagnosis (PGD) for translocations using nuclear transfer techniques to convert single blastomeres and polar bodies into metaphase chromosomes. Am J Hum Genet 67:421, 2000a.

Verlinsky Y, Munné S, Gianaroli L, et al.: Preimplantation genetic diagnosis — an integral part of assisted reproduction. J Assist Reprod Genet 17:75, 2000b.

Verlinsky Y, Kuliev A: An Illustration Textbook and Reference for Clinicians: An Atlas of Preimplantation Genetics Diagnosis. New York: Parthenon Publishing, 2000.

Verlinsky Y, Rechitsky S, Schoolcraft W, et al.: Preimplantation diagnosis for Fanconi anemia combined with HLA matching. JAMA 285:3130, 2001a.

Verlinsky Y, Rechitsky S, Verlinsky O, et al.: Preimplantation diagnosis for P53 tumour suppressor gene mutations. Reprod BioMed Online 2:102, 2001b.

Verlinsky Y, Rechitsky S, Verlinsky O, et al.: Preimplantation testing for phenylketonuria. Fertil Steril 76:346, 2001c.

Verlinsky Y, Cieslak J, Ivakhnenko V, et al.: Chromosomal abnormalities in the first and second polar body. Mol Cell Endocrinol 183:S47, 2001d.

Verlinsky Y, Munne S, Gianaroli, et al.: Tenth anniversary of preimplantation genetic diagnosis. J Assist Reprod Genet 18:64, 2001e.

Verlinsky Y, Cieslak J, Rechitsky S, et al.: Present status and impact of PGD: experience in one large center. Reprod BioMed Online 4:Suppl 2:10(Abstract O-3), 2002.

Weier HU, Munné S, Fung J: Patient-specific probes for preimplantation genetic diagnosis of structural and numerical aberrations in interphase cells. J Assist Reprod Genet 16:182, 1999.

Weier HG, Munné S, Lersch RA, et al.: Towards a full karyotype screening of interphase cells: "FISH and chip" technology. Mol Cell Endocrinol 183:Suppl 1:S41, 2001.

Wells D, Delhanty JD: Comprehensive chromosomal analysis of human preimplantation embryos using whole genome amplification and single cell comparative genomic hybridization. Mol Hum Reprod 6:1055, 2000.

Wennerholm UB, Bergh C, Hamberger L, et al.: Incidence of congenital malformations in children born after ICSI. Hum Reprod 15:944, 2000a.

Wennerholm UB, Bergh C, Hamberger L, et al.: Obstetric outcome of pregnancies following ICSI, classified according to sperm origin and quality. Hum Reprod 15:1189, 2000b.

Willadsen S, Levron J, Munné S, et al.: Rapid visualization of metaphase chromosomes in single human blastomeres after fusion with in-vitro matured bovine eggs. Hum Reprod 14:470, 1999.

Wilton L, Williamson R, McBain J, et al.: Preimplantation diagnosis of aneuploidy using comparative genomic hybridization. Reprod BioMed Online 4:Suppl 2:13(Abstract O-10), 2002.

Wilton L, Williamson R, McBain J, et al.: Use of comparative genomic hybridization in karyotype embryos prior to implantation: The achievement of a successful pregnancy. Hum Reprod 16:33(Abstract 78), 2001.

Wilton L, Williamson R, Slater H, et al.: Determination of aneuploidy in human embryos using comparative genomic hybridization. Hum Reprod 15:13(Abstract 32), 2000.

Wisanto A, Magnus M, Bonduelle M, et al.: Obstetric outcome of 424 pregnancies after intracytoplasmic sperm injection. Hum Reprod 10:2713, 1995.

Zhuang GL: PGD: China's experience. Reprod BioMed Online 4:Suppl 2:39(Abstract O-63), 2002.

▼

CHAPTER 17

Prenatal Diagnosis by Intact Fetal Cells or Cell-free DNA in Maternal Blood

Fetal cells circulate in the maternal blood during pregnancy, and their analysis represents a new approach to prenatal genetic diagnosis. Although it is not yet a standard approach, fetal cell recovery promises to be an attractive addition to noninvasive prenatal diagnosis. Use of cell-free DNA is yet another, more recent, approach. Consensus exists that detection is possible for fetal aneuploidy and for selected mendelian disorders. Already useful is the ability to detect the existence of Rh(D) fetuses in a sensitized Rh-negative mother through the study of maternal blood. Investigation now is focusing on the consistency with which fetal cells can be recovered, the reliability with which diagnosis can be made, and the sensitivity of detecting various disorders. The question now is whether fetal cell analysis can become competitive in sensitivity and specificity to other types of noninvasive screening (Chapter 14). Alternatively, intact fetal cells or cell-free fetal DNA may prove complementary to multiple maternal analyte or ultrasound to increase sensitivity and specificity or noninvasive aneuploidy detection.

Historical Overview (1969–1989)

Walknowska and coworkers (1969) first reported XY metaphases in maternal blood of pregnant women carrying male fetuses. De Grouchy and Trubuchet (1971) confirmed this finding, as did other groups (Schindler and Martin-du-Pan, 1972; Takahara et al., 1972; Whang-Peng et al., 1973). The fact that not all women carrying male fetuses showed 46,XY

metaphases was explained by fetal cells being rare findings in maternal blood. That XY metaphases were also present in some women carrying female fetuses was explained by assuming that clones of fetal cells were established in the mother's bone marrow during prior pregnancies. When others were unable to confirm these results on a consistent basis, however, the lower quality XY metaphases available during this era were thought by many to have represented cytogenetic misclassifications (Sargent et al., 1994). Y-chromatin-positive cells were also claimed to exist in maternal blood by several groups (Schroder and de la Chapelle, 1972; Grosset et al., 1974; Schroder et al., 1974; Zilliacus et al., 1975). Again, results were considered by some to reflect confusion in areas of autosomal fluorescence, which can mimic Y-chromatin.

In 1979, Herzenberg and colleagues were the first to report use of flow cytometry to enrich fetal cells (Herzenberg et al., 1979; Iverson et al., 1981). The strategy was to study HLA-A2 negative women who conceived with an HLA-A2 positive male. HLA-A2 antigen cells present in maternal blood can only result from having been present on a fetal cell containing the allele inherited from the father. Y-chromatin was used as an independent marker in pregnancies in which the fetus was male. Maternal blood samples indeed showed HLA-A2 positive cells that were also Y-chromatin positive. Again, however, results could not be universally confirmed.

Existence of fetal cells in maternal blood was not definitively confirmed to the satisfaction of the scientific community until molecular methods were applied in the later 1980s. Using nested primer PCR to amplify for Y-sequences, Lo and coworkers (1989, 1990) verified fetal cells in unsorted nucleated cells, and many others confirmed these results using various separation schemes (Bianchi et al., 1990; Müeller et al., 1990; Wachtel et al., 1991; Kao et al., 1992).

Time of Appearance of Fetal Cells

Using nested primer PCR for Y-specific DNA, signals can be detected early in pregnancy in the peripheral blood of pregnant women carrying male fetuses. Y-specific signals were detected at between 33 and 40 days' gestation by Thomas and colleagues (1994). By 6 weeks' gestation, 18 of 18 pregnancies having a male fetus showed a Y-specific signal in maternal blood. Liou and coworkers (1993, 1994) found Y sequences indicative of male fetal cells in 19 of 19 pregnancies by 10 to 11 weeks.

Fetal Cell Type

Diagnosis of chromosomal abnormalities initially required analysis of intact fetal interphase cell analysis by FISH with chromosome-specific probes. To be pragmatic, one must enrich the rare intact fetal cells by targeting a specific cell type. Candidate fetal cell types are trophoblasts, lymphocytes, granulocytes, nucleated red blood cells, and endothelial cells.

TROPHOBLASTS

Trophoblasts are attractive candidate cells because of their distinctive morphology, which readily permits definitive microscopic identification. Commonly shed into the maternal circulation extensively during the first trimester, trophoblasts in normal pregnancies are cleared rapidly by the pulmonary circulation. In addition to this difficulty, there are a lack of trophoblast-specific monoclonal antibodies (Covone et al., 1984, 1988; Bertero et al., 1988). Many claims of fetal-specific trophoblast antibodies have not been verified. Perhaps better results can be obtained by HASH-2, human placental lactogen, or HLA-G (Moreau et al., 1994; Latham et al., 1996; van Wijk et al., 1996, 1998, 2001).

A further concern with trophoblasts is that as part of the placenta, these cells are known from CVS studies to show 1 to 2% chromosomal mosaicism. Thus, genetic analysis of a placental trophoblast might not be fully representative of the fetal karyotype. In addition, trophoblasts may be multinucleated and therefore pose difficulty in interphase FISH and DNA analyses. Despite these technical and biologic concerns, several groups have indeed isolated trophoblasts from the maternal circulation and performed morphologic and genetic diagnoses on them (Müeller et al., 1990; Hawes et al., 1994a, b). However, the detection rate per case has not been determined. Current workers seeking to isolate fetal trophoblasts favor depletion technologies, i.e., removing all cells except trophoblasts. Van Wijk et al. (2001) use HLA-G or HASH2 (van Wijk et al., 1998).

LYMPHOCYTES

In the initial studies in this field, Walknowska and colleagues (1969) appeared to demonstrate the presence of a Y chromosome in mitogen-stimulated cells that were widely presumed to be fetal lymphocytes. Studies in the early 1970s showing interphase analysis with the quinacrine-staining Y body were also presumed to involve fetal lymphocytes. Two papers demonstrated the presence of apparent male lymphocytes in the blood of pregnant women, 1 and 5 years after birth of a male infant, respectively (Schroder et al., 1974; Ciaranfi et al., 1977). These were taken to indicate that the fetal cells were not only lymphocytes but also could persist postpartum. Fetal lymphocytes or mononuclear cells were therefore logically used as targets for flow-sorting experiments by Herzenberg and colleagues (1979). As noted, this group successfully used monoclonal antibody to HLA-A2 and flow-sorted fetal HLA-A2 positive cells in pregnant women who did not have this antigen.

Recent studies of fetal lymphocytes in the maternal circulation have been limited. One reason is lack of monoclonal antibodies specific for uniquely fetal lymphocyte antigens. In addition, there is concern regarding whether a particular lymphocyte originates from a previous pregnancy. Finally, it would be necessary to perform HLA typing of both parents prior to enrichment. Few if any workers appear to be emphasizing this cell at present.

ERYTHROBLASTS

The fetal nucleated red cell (erythroblast) is an attractive candidate because nucleated red blood cells (NRBCs) constitute about 10% of red cells in the 11-week fetus and 0.5% in the 19-week fetus. Nucleated red blood cells do not persist longer than perhaps 5 days in the adult and are rare in peripheral adult blood.

Bianchi and coworkers (1990) were the first to focus on NRBCs, flow-sorting for transferrin receptor (CD71) expression and performing PCR for a Y sequence. After enrichment, Y sequences were found in six of eight pregnancies in which women were carrying male fetuses. Our group was later successful when sorting not only for CD71 but also for cell size, cell granularity, and glycophorin-A positivity (Price et al., 1991; Wachtel et al., 1991). Using nested primers for a Y-specific sequence, we correctly identified male fetuses in 12 of 12 flow-sorted samples (Wachtel et al., 1991). We identified female fetuses in five of six samples.

Our group later became the first to detect fetal aneuploidy by maternal blood analysis. Analyzing interphase cells by FISH with chromosome-specific probes, we detected trisomy 18 (Price et al., 1991) in 1992 and trisomy 21 (Elias et al., 1992) in 1992 (Fig. 17–1). Our initial experience with 69 maternal blood samples proved promising, with no false-positive results (Simpson and Elias, 1993, 1994). The premise of the U.S. NICHD multi-center that we and others are pursuing has been that fetal erythroblasts can be isolated from maternal blood. Current results will be discussed below (Bianchi et al., 2002).

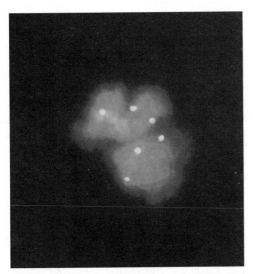

FIGURE 17–1 • The first detected case of trisomy 21 from analysis of maternal blood. In each of two cells there are three signals for the chromosome 21 specific probe (FISH) (From Elias S, Price J, Dockter M, et al.: First trimester prenatal diagnosis of trisomy 21 in fetal cells from maternal blood. Lancet 340:1033, 1992.) *See Color Plate*

Frequency of Fetal Cells in Maternal Blood

Relatively few fetal cells exist in maternal blood, the best estimates being perhaps 1 cell per mL of maternal blood. Using an avidin-biotin-based immunoaffinity system, Hall and Williams (1992) estimated that the ratio of fetal nucleated cells to maternal nucleated cells was 1:4.75 × 10^6 to 1.6 × 10^7. Hamada and associates (1993) estimated the ratio of fetal nucleated cells to maternal nucleated cells by performing FISH on unsorted maternal blood using a DNA probe specific for the repetitive Y-DNA sequence DYZ1. Frequencies in successive trimesters became higher—0.27, 3.52, and 8.56 × 10^5, respectively. We estimate frequency to be at 1:1 × 10^7 or 1 × 10^8 based on flow cytometry data. Using quantitative PCR, Bianchi and coworkers (1997) estimated that a 16-mL maternal blood sample contains perhaps 19 fetal cells ("DNA equivalents").

Exceptional results were obtained by Wachtel and colleagues, who believe that fetal cells in maternal blood are much more frequent. Their conclusions are derived from a technique called charged flow separation, whose principle is based on physical differences between fetal and maternal cells. In our opinion, most of the cells recovered by this group were not fetal. (They stated that 30% of NRBCs in maternal blood are fetal, Wachtel et al., 1998.) However, in very few samples was FISH with chromosome-specific probes the end point. Using charged flow separation, no relationship is seen between fetal cells and gestational age (Shulman et al., 1998).

Persistence of Fetal Cells After Pregnancy

A potential pitfall is that fetal cells from a prior pregnancy could persist in the maternal circulation and, hence, lead to diagnostic error. This would be especially troublesome if aneuploid cells were to persist after a chromosomally abnormal live born offspring or after a chromosomally abnormal spontaneous abortion.

Fortunately for diagnostic purposes, fetal cells disappear in large part after delivery. One week after gestation, 26 of 28 women delivering males showed XFY and SRY sequences in their blood (Hsieh et al., 1993). By 4 months, only 2 of 23 did. Others have had similar experiences, including our group (Elias et al., 1996). Lo and coworkers (1998a) followed eight women delivered of male fetuses postpartum, obtaining serial blood samples for analysis of Y sequences in maternal *plasma*. All eight women showed fetal DNA sequences, but amounts of fetal DNA fell rapidly postpartum. By 2 hours, levels were undetectable in most women.

Bianchi and colleagues (1996) clarified some of the ostensible contradiction by showing that the fetal cells persisting from prior pregnancies are indeed detectable, but not by using the same selection criteria employed to isolate cells for prenatal diagnosis. Positive selection for persisting clones is achieved not with CD71 (see below), but by CD38 and CD34. If appropriate selection criteria are chosen, clones of fetal cells established in prior pregnancies should not interfere with diagnosis.

Detecting Chromosome Abnormalities

ENRICHMENT TECHNIQUES FOR INTACT FETAL CELLS

Assuming the consensus of no more than 1 fetal cell per 100,000 maternal cells (1 mL blood) and probably closer to 1 per 1–10 million, FISH analysis for fetal chromosomal abnormalities requires enrichment. The general strategy underlying enrichment is not to achieve a pure sample of fetal cells but merely to generate a sample relatively more likely to contain fetal cells. Even after enrichment, most cells are still likely to be maternal, perhaps 100:1. However, even 1% frequency of fetal cells can still permit an efficient search for fetal aneuploidy using FISH with chromosome-specific probes.

Enrichment is approached initially by density gradient or protein separation techniques (Troeger et al., 1999; Samura et al., 2000). Some groups have long believed that fetal diagnosis is possible solely after the relatively minor enrichment achieved by single Ficoll density gradient (Oosterwijk et al., 1998), but until recently most groups believed more refined enrichment is necessary. The initial approaches used flow cytometry (Lewis et al., 1996) (Fig. 17–2). The alternative is magnetic-activated cell sorting (MACS) (Fig. 17–3) (Ganshirt-Ahlert et al., 1993). With either, the principle is that one selects against (negatively) those cells of the undesired type and selects for (positively) those cells of the desired type.

Flow cytometry once seemed most useful in our hands, but the technology is more expensive than MACS (Simpson and Elias, 1995a, b), and appears predisposed to loss of rare fetal cells. Other problems in flow sorting include physical stress on separated cells and the unavoidable inverse relationship between degree of cell fixation (for preservation) and success of FISH analysis (Lewis et al., 1996).

In the alternative of MACS (see Fig. 17–3) antibodies directed against the cells sought for enrichment are conjugated to magnetic beads; these beads (and, hence, the desired cell type) are retained under a magnetic field, when cells in solution pass through (positive selection). Cells that lack the antigen in question fail to attach to beads, are not retained in the magnetic field, and pass through unimpeded to be discarded. After releasing the magnet, cells attached to the beads can be collected for subsequent analysis. The converse can be performed, target cells being allowed to pass through and nontargeted cells being retained in the magnetic field. Rather than use of magnetic beads, ferro fluids can also be used. The advantage of MACS is its lower cost compared with fluorescence activated cell-sorting (FACS) and its ease of use. The disadvantage is its inability to select for more than one marker and lack of efficiency in the hands of some investigators. In the U.S. NICHD NIFTY trial recovery was better with MACS than FACS (Bianchi et al., 2002).

More recently the trend is toward even less obtrusive separation, perhaps selecting negatively for progenitor stem cells (Bischoff et al., 2002a).

ANTIGEN SELECTION

No single selection criterion is ideal, and none are universally utilized. Initially, Bianchi and colleagues (1990) used antibodies against CD71 (transferrin receptor), and our group (Price et al., 1991) utilized positive selection (antibodies) for both glycophorin-A and CD71 (transferrin). Later we abandoned glycophorin-A in FACS (Simpson et al., 1995b). Troeger and colleagues (1999) still find anti-glycophorin-A more useful than anti-CD36 and anti-CD71. Negative depletion may be utilized as well, for example anti-CD45 to remove lymphocytes. Unfortunately, all selection techniques are still relatively nonspecific, with negative selection inadvertently excluding many cells of interest. It has been estimated by quantitative PCR that a 16-mL blood sample contains approximately 19 fetal cells, although FISH analysis usually reveals no more than one to three fetal cells and often (40–50%) zero.

The theoretically attractive approach of using various embryonic fetal hemoglobins (ε- and

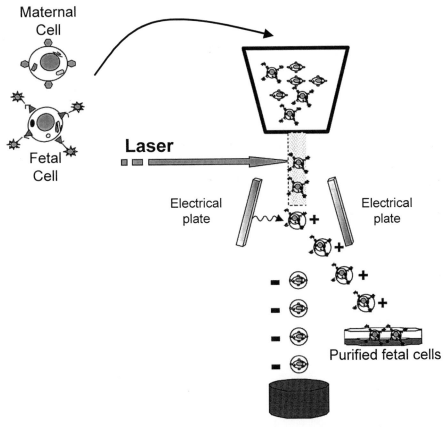

FIGURE 17–2 • Fluorescence activated cell sorting (FACS). Fetal cells are labeled with an antibody conjugated to a fluorochrome. Cells are passed through a liquid stream in single file and fluorescent-labeled antibodies are exited. Labeled fetal cells are deflected to a collection and unlabeled maternal cells are discarded.

ξ-globin), has not proved as useful as might be imagined, although Choolani et al. (2002) continue to pursue this strategy. Selection for γ-globin (fetal) and selection against β-globin (maternal) seems more efficacious in most hands. Ultimately a truly unique fetal specific antigen will be identified. Perhaps the gene product of a developmental gene will prove the talisman. The significance of such a marker would be enormous, for sensitivity of fetal cell analysis would jump to nearly 100%. Fetal cell analysis would then probably quickly supplement ultrasound or serum marker screening as the favored method of noninvasive screening.

FISH ANALYSIS (CHROMOSOME-SPECIFIC PROBES)

Initially sequential or selected use of probes for selected chromosome-specific probes was employed: X, Y, and usually 21 or 18. A genuine screening program requires, however, prospective analysis of all chromosomes that would be detected in at least maternal serum screening programs. Simultaneous analysis for numerical abnormalities of X and Y is thus required at a minimum; five-color FISH technology with the addition of 13 and 18 is preferable. Analysis of physically stressed flow-sorted fetal cells is difficult, but Bischoff and coworkers have shown the ability to analyze efficiently (98%) all five chromosomes simultaneously (Bischoff et al., 1998). Directly labeled probes that intercalate into DNA (Vysis Inc., Downers Grove, IL) are utilized. See Chapters 1 and 14 for discussions concerning FISH and its accuracy in detecting aneuploidy.

SENSITIVITY OF FETAL ANEUPLOIDY DETECTION

In determining the accuracy of detecting chromosomal abnormalities in fetal blood, the

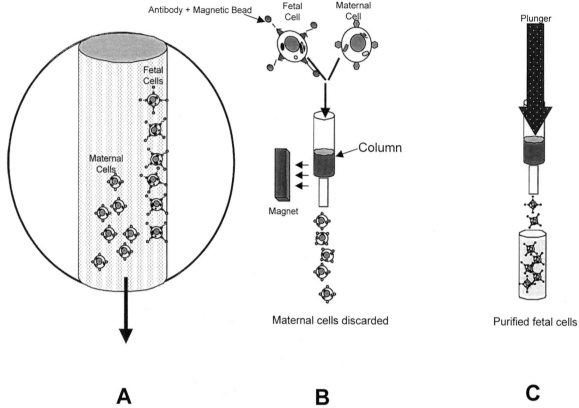

A   **B**   **C**

FIGURE 17-3 • Magnet activated cell sorting (MACS). *A,* Fetal cells are labeled with an antibody conjugated to a magnetic bead and are drawn to the side of the column. *B,* Unlabeled maternal cells pass through the column. *C,* Purified magnetically activated fetal cells are then flushed through the column for collection.

approach is usually to determine the number of pregnancies characterized by a male fetus in which male (XY cells) are detected. Actually, this may underestimate sensitivity because it seems likely from both clinical evaluation (Price et al., 1991; Simpson and Elias, 1993) and quantitative PCR studies (Bianchi et al., 1997) that several fold more fetal cells are present in the maternal blood in aneuploid pregnancies than in euploid pregnancies. Some do not agree with these statements, but offer support, predominantly based on morphologic criteria (NRBCs). However, maternal erythroblasts also increase during pregnancy; thus, we believe that studies should utilize FISH with chromosome-specific probes as an unequivocal fetal marker.

In the United States collaborative study, NIFTY (National Institute of Child Health and Human Development *Fetal Cell Study*) (Bianchi et al., 1999), outcome assessed is numbers of pregnancies in which fetal trisomies are detected per numbers of pregnancies in which fetal trisomies exist. In the initial analysis (1995–1999), 2 of the 4 sites used FACS and two MACS. If fetal trisomy

exists, usually one to three trisomic (and, hence, fetal cells) were detected (Bianchi et al., 2002) per 20 to 30 mL specimen. Over 3600 cases were studied prospectively. At least one aneuploid cell was found in 74.4% of 43 autosomal trisomies false-positive rates below the 5% observed in maternal serum analyte screening. MACS seemingly gave better results than FACS, but univariate analysis would be inappropriate because gestational age was lower in MACS than in FACS sorted specimens. One conclusion from the NIFTY trial is that cell loss must be minimized. Thus, efforts are being pursued to use minimally disruptive separation techniques such as whole blood progenitor cell enrichment (Bischoff et al., 2002a).

Very favorable results were also reported from Spain by Rodriguez de Alba and coworkers (1999). The group sequentially used a double-density gradient, MACS with positive selection for CD71, postseparation identification of NRBCs by Kleihauer staining, and FISH for 13, 18, 21, X, and Y. Among 66 samples, all six aneuplodies were detected: two trisomy 18 and four trisomy 21. In 46,XY fetuses usually one or two XY cells are found, but in the six trisomic fetuses there were far more fetal (aneuploid) cells: 15, 3, 50, 2 for the trisomy 21 cases; 20 and 5 for the trisomy 18.

Issues of potential concern include whether a woman's blood type or Rh status influences the detection of fetal cells in maternal blood. In 1052 women of mean maternal age of 36.2 years carrying a male fetus with a mean gestational age of 14.0 weeks, Elias and coworkers (2000) initially found no relationship between likelihood of having a Y signal by FISH maternal ABO or Rh status. Analysis of the complete NIFTY data (Bianchi et al., 2002) confirmed these preliminary findings. Similarly, maternal race appears to have no effect on fetal cell recovery (Evans et al., 2000). As determined by numbers of XY cells recovered, sensitivity is inversely related to gestational age, earlier than 14 weeks being favorable. That trisomic cells are very rare in nontrisomic pregnancies is key to the potential usefulness of fetal cell analysis. Combining intact fetal cell or cell free DNA analysis with nuchal translucency or maternal serum analyte screening (see Chapter 15) offers the additional promise of greater sensitivity at lower false positive rates.

In some cases, fetal cell analysis seems even more sensitive than chorionic villus analysis. Bischoff and coworkers (1995) detected seven 47,XXY cells in a maternal blood specimen enriched by CD71+ selection. All 15 metaphases in standard chorionic villus analysis were normal. Not until FISH studies of an additional 500 cells was performed was the aneuploid fetal cell line verified (47,XXY cells). The clinical significance of such low levels of mosaicism is unclear.

Cheung and coworkers (1996) enriched fetal cells by Ficoll separation and MACS, identified them after enrichment on the basis of zeta or epsilon hemoglobin staining, physically removed these cells, and subjected pooled cells to PCR to detect hemoglobinopathies. Using this approach, sickle cell anemia and β-thalassemia were excluded in couples at risk. This approach could be combined with Takabayashi's method of morphologically identifying cells (Takabayashi et al., 1995). However, despite promising initial work this method has not proved to be useful in most hands. Still, new antibodies continue to be utilized (Choolani et al., 2002).

Detecting Fetal Mendelian Disorders from Maternal Blood

Detection of fetal mendelian disorders by analysis of fetal cells does not necessarily require

enrichment. PCR-based technology alone may suffice, since the DNA may be derived from any type of fetal cell. Mendelian diagnosis thus does not necessarily necessitate targeting of any specific fetal cell type or enrichment.

DIAGNOSING FETAL SEX DETERMINATION BY PCR OF MATERNAL BLOOD

Determining fetal sex is obviously useful in couples at risk for X-linked recessive traits and can be performed easily. Nested primer analysis for Y-DNA sequences was used initially by Lo and coworkers (1989, 1990) to establish that fetal cells exist in maternal blood. As already noted, detection rates for fetal sex approach 100% by the end of the first trimester (Liou et al., 1993, 1994).

Primer extension *in situ* techniques can also be employed to detect fetal Y-DNA sequences (Orsetti et al., 1998).

DIAGNOSING OF FETAL AUTOSOMAL DOMINANT AND RECESSIVE DISORDERS BY PCR ALONE

The principle of detecting mendelian disorders by analysis of DNA of the fetal cells present in maternal blood was first shown by Camaschella and colleagues (1990). DNA was obtained from maternal blood of three pregnancies at risk for β-thalassemia/hemoglobin Lepore$_{Boston}$. Hemoglobin Lepore$_{Boston}$ is a hybrid δ-β-globin gene that results from unequal crossing-over between misaligned β- and δ-genes, leading to a 7-kb deletion. Camaschella and colleagues (1990) used PCR to amplify for hemoglobin Lepore$_{Boston}$-specific DNA in unsorted maternal blood of women whose male partners carried the Lepore$_{Boston}$ mutation. The mutation was correctly identified in two fetuses and excluded in a third.

Another circumstance permitting detection of a mendelian disorder through analysis of fetal cells in maternal blood arises when the father is heterozygous (Aa) and the mother homozygously abnormal (aa) for an autosomal recessive trait. The normal allele, which may or may not be transmitted by the heterozygous father, should be readily detectable. If blood from the homozygous mother reveals DNA of the normal paternal allele (A), the fetus could be deduced to be heterozygous (Fig. 17–4). An example of PCR in maternal blood to detect an autosomal recessive disorder is identifying pregnancies at risk for fetal Rh(D)

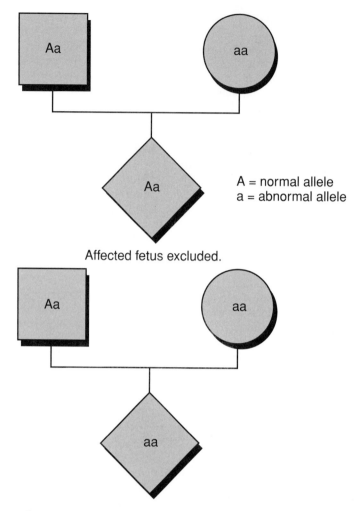

A = normal allele
a = abnormal allele

Affected fetus excluded.

Either affected fetus or no fetal cells present.
Results are therefore inconclusive.

FIGURE 17–4 • Exclusion of an autosomal recessive disorder by analysis of fetal cells isolated from maternal blood.

disease. The molecular basis for an individual's being Rh(D)-negative (dd) is usually a gene deletion, d representing lack of the DNA sequence that if present encodes D. If the mother is Rh-negative and the father is homozygous for Rh(D) (Rh-positive), all fetuses must be heterozygous: (Dd); every pregnancy would then be a risk for RhD-isoimmunization. If the father is heterozygous, however, the likelihood is 50% that the fetus would inherit his RhD gene and, hence, be affected; the other 50% of pregnancies would not be at risk for Rh-isoimmunization. Nested primers can be constructed such that the CE sequence is concurrently amplified, allowing an "internal control" that assures lack of D is not the result of primers failing to anneal or absence of cellular DNA in the sample tested. Several sets of primers are available (Geifman-Holtzman et al., 1996).

Lo and coworkers (1998b) studied 57 RhD-negative women throughout pregnancy. All RhD-positive fetuses in the second and third trimesters were correctly identified; 10 of 12 in the first trimester were also detected. This study actually analyzed fetal DNA in maternal plasma (see below).

FETAL DNA IN MATERNAL PLASMA

Until now the discussion has implied that fetal DNA that is to be analyzed is present in the

Thomas MR, Williamson R, Craft I, et al.: Y chromosome sequence DNA amplified from peripheral blood in women in early pregnancy. Lancet 343:413, 1994.

Troeger C, Holzgreve W, Hahn S: A comparison of different density gradients and antibodies for enrichment of fetal erythroblasts by MACS. Prenat Diagn 19:521, 1999.

Tyndall A, Gratwohl A: Microchimerism: Friend or foe? Nat Med 4:386, 1998.

Valerio D, Aiello R, Altieri V, et al.: Culture of fetal erythroid progenitor cells from maternal blood for non-invasive prenatal genetic diagnosis. Prenat Diagn 16:1073, 1996.

Valerio D, Aiello R, Altieri V: Isolation of fetal erythroid cells from maternal blood based on expression of erythropoietin receptor. Mol Hum Reprod 3:451, 1997a.

Valerio D, Altieri V, Antonucci FR, et al.: Characterization of fetal haematopoietic progenitors circulating in maternal blood of seven aneuploid pregnancies. Prenat Diagn 17:1159, 1997b.

Valerio D, Altieri V, Cavallo D, et al.: Detection of fetal trisomy 18 by short-term culture of maternal peripheral blood. Am J Obstet Gynecol 183:222, 2000.

van Wijk IJ, van Vugt JM, Mulders MA, et al.: Enrichment of fetal trophoblast cells from the maternal peripheral blood followed by detection of fetal deoxyribonucleic acid with a nested X/Y polymerase chain reaction. Am J Obstet Gynecol 174:871, 1996.

van Wijk IJ, van Vugt JM, Könst AA, et al.: Identification of HASH2 positive extravillus trophoblast cells in the peripheral blood of pregnant women. Trophoblast Res 11:23, 1998.

van Wijk IJ, Griffioen S, Tjoa ML, et al.: HLA-G expression in trophoblast cells circulating in maternal peripheral blood during early pregnancy. Am J Obstet Gynecol 184:991, 2001.

Wachtel SS, Sammons D, Twitty G, et al.: Charge flow separation: Quantification of nucleated red blood cells in maternal blood during pregnancy. Prenat Diagn 18:455, 1998.

Wachtel SS, Elias S, Price J, et al.: Fetal cells in the maternal circulation—isolation by multiparameter flow cytometry and confirmation by PCR. Hum Reprod 6:1466, 1991.

Walknowska J, Conte FA, Grumbach MM: Practical and theoretical implications of fetal/maternal lymphocyte transfer. Lancet 1:1119, 1969.

Whang-Peng J, Leikin S, Harris C, et al.: The transplacental passage of fetal leukocytes into the maternal blood. Proc Soc Exp Biol Med 142:50, 1973.

Zilliacus R, de la Chapelle A, Schroder J, et al.: Transplacental passage of fetal blood cells. Scan J Haemetol 15:333, 1975.

Zimmermann B, Holzgreve W, Zhong XY, et al.: Inability to clonally expand fetal progenitors from maternal blood. Fetal Diagn Ther 17:97, 2002.

Ethics and Legal Issues

Ethical and Legal Issues in Reproductive Genetics

On July 31, 1989, the cover of *Time* magazine showed a snake with fangs and forked tongue bared coiled around a staff, parodying a caduceus, the insignia symbolizing a physician. The cover story, entitled "Doctors and Patients: Image vs. Reality" discussed the "infected climate" of the physician-patient relationship that in recent years has led to a lack of trust due to cost containment, threats of malpractice suits, dehumanizing technologies, and uncertainties of diagnosis and treatment. The article concluded, "the practice of medicine, though it may become ever more precise, will never again be simple, never cheap and never magic" (*Time*, 1989). Indeed, it is no surprise that modern physicians face numerous ethical dilemmas with uncertainty and confusion while practicing in a climate in which medical malpractice suits can threaten even the most competent and conscientious practitioner. Nowhere are these concerns more apparent than in medical practices and technological innovations involving human genetics and reproduction.

Doctrine of Informed Consent

The entire purpose of the doctrine of informed consent is to permit individuals to decide for themselves on a course of action and to give the individual the objective, material information needed to make a decision in a reasonable

This chapter reflects previous works coauthored by one of us (Sherman Elias) with George J. Annas, J.D., M.P.H., Edward Utley Professor and Chair, Department of Health Law, Boston University Schools of Medicine and Public Health, Boston, MA.

manner. No matter how irrational the decision of a woman or couple to have a child may seem to the counselor, in the context of prenatal diagnosis it must be remembered that it is the individual's or couple's child, not the counselor's, and the individual's or couple's decision.

As two leading legal commentators have put it:

The very foundation of the doctrine of informed consent is every man's right to forego treatment or even cure if it entails what *for him* are intolerable consequences or risks, however warped or perverted his sense of values may be in the eyes of the medical profession, or even of the community, so long as any distortion falls short of what the law regards as incompetency. *Individual freedom here is guaranteed only if people are given the right to make choices which would generally be regarded as foolish* [emphasis added] (Harper and James, 1968).

Genetic Counseling and Prenatal Diagnosis

A woman seeking prenatal care can properly expect to be fully informed of any reason that her fetus might be handicapped and of the existence of diagnostic tests that might identify the precise genetic condition. The physician incurs this duty to disclose such information because it is this type of information that the pregnant woman who seeks prenatal care wishes to discover—to learn all she can to help her have a healthy child (Elias and Annas, 1987; Annas and Elias, 1996).

The term "malpractice" refers to professional misconduct that embodies a failure to exercise reasonable prudence in carrying out professional duties. The purpose of the medical-malpractice lawsuit is to afford recovery for damages sustained as a result of a physician's failure to exercise ordinary and reasonable care in the diagnosis and treatment of a patient and to deter such conduct. To prevail in a malpractice action, the plaintiff must prove four elements: duty, breach, damages, and causation (Annas, 1989a).

In prenatal diagnosis cases in which the physician fails to inform the parents of the existence of a test applicable to their situation, negligently performs the test, fails to refer to a specialist who could perform the test, or inaccurately informs the couple about their risks of having an affected child, the courts now almost universally permit the parents to sue their physician for depriving them of their right to make a decision about commencing or continuing a pregnancy. Such a lawsuit is sometimes termed a "wrongful birth" case. A wrongful birth suit must allege and prove not only that the physician was negligent in the care of the pregnant woman but also that had the negligent act not been committed, the child would not have been born (e.g., had the woman been properly informed that she was at risk to have a child with Down syndrome, she could have sought amniocentesis or chorionic villus sampling and had an abortion if her fetus were so affected).

The rationale for permitting parents to recover damages in such a case is set forth in typical language by a Texas court:

"It is impossible for us to justify a policy which at once deprives the parents of information by which they could elect to terminate the pregnancy likely to produce a child with a defective body, a policy which in effect requires that the deficient embryo be carried to full gestation until the deficient child is born, and which policy then denies recovery from the tortfeasor of costs of treating and caring for the defects of the child" (Jacobs v. Theimer, 1975).

In so-called "wrongful life" suits, the plaintiff is the child (through its parents or guardian) who seeks damages against the physician for being born. Until recently, most courts rejected lawsuits by the child because they thought it was impossible to put a monetary value on life in an impaired condition compared with nonexistence. The choice for these children is *never* to be healthy, but either to be born with a handicap (such as Down syndrome or Tay-Sachs disease) or not to be born at all. We believe that future courts are likely to limit such actions to *serious* handicaps, those in which fetuses, if they could speak to us (which, of course, they can

only do through their parents), would agree with an "objective societal consensus" that their own best interest would be served if they were aborted. Put another way, they would be better off *from their own perspective* if they never existed. Conditions like deafness and Down syndrome would not qualify, whereas conditions like Tay-Sachs would qualify. Measuring damages *is* problematic, but courts are likely to award at least the additional medical costs caused by the handicap itself. However, because medical costs can be recovered in a wrongful birth case directly, wrongful life cases are only likely to be brought in those rare instances in which for some reason (e.g., the child has been given up for adoption) the parents have lost the right to sue on their own behalf (Annas and Elias, 1990).

We have proposed the following guidelines concerning the ethical and legal responsibilities of the physician in relation to genetic counseling and prenatal diagnosis (Annas and Elias, 1993, 1996):

1. *Physicians must give accurate information to the parents and should not withhold vital information.* These principles are consistent with the doctrine of informed consent and the reasonable expectations of pregnant women under a physician's care (Annas, 1981). The physician does not guarantee a healthy child, but the reasonable expectation of the patient is that she will be apprised of any information the physician has that the child might be handicapped and of the alternative ways to proceed so that the patient can determine what action to take (Annas and Coyne, 1975).

2. *Physicians cannot be required to perform prenatal diagnostic procedures (e.g., chorionic villus sampling or genetic amniocentesis).* Indeed, many are not qualified to perform these procedures and for them to do so may itself be malpractice.

3. *Genetic counseling should be nondirective.* The counselor should remain impartial and objective in providing information that will allow competent counselees to make their own informed decision.

4. *To ensure the patient's interest in both autonomy and privacy, no information obtained in genetic counseling or screening should be disclosed to any third party, including insurers and employers, without the patient's informed consent* (Annas, 1976; President's Commissions, 1983). Such strict nondisclosure policies should be maintained unless and until specific legislation is enacted that would clearly delineate the circumstances in which

confidentiality must be breached, e.g., in relation to certain contagious diseases, gunshot wounds, or child abuse. On the other hand, counselors should be permitted to attempt to persuade patients to allow them to make disclosures of important information to potentially affected relatives if there is a high probability of serious harm and if the disclosure is limited to pertinent genetic information. We recommend that the genetic counselor make clear, both verbally and in writing, the policy that he or she follows so that the patient can refuse to be screened or counseled if he or she is not in agreement with the disclosure policy.

Genetic Screening

Today's screening tests usually focus on conditions that occur either in the family or in the racial or ethnic group of one or both prospective parents. As our ability to identify genes associated with particular diseases increases, a panel of screening tests to identify carriers of numerous genes will be offered more routinely. It will then become increasingly difficult—if not impossible—to inform those offered screening or testing for reproductive purposes about all the genetic information that can be obtained and the implications of that information.

Consent for Screening

Our current model for screening and testing requires pretest counseling (Elias and Annas, 1987). Such counseling is a method of obtaining informed consent, and the obligation to counsel can be seen as inherent in the fiduciary nature of the physician–patient relationship (Annas, 1989b; Andrews et al., 1994). For ordinary medical procedures, the physical risks and treatment alternatives are the chief items of information that must be disclosed. There are few physical risks in genetic screening. What must be conveyed in counseling regarding genetic screening is that the tests may yield new information that may ultimately force some unwelcome choices (such as whether to marry, abort, or adopt). Self-determination and rational decision making are the central values protected by informed consent (Annas, 1989b). In the setting of reproductive genetics, what is at stake is the right to decide whether or not to have a genetic test, with emphasis on the right to refuse if the potential harm (in terms of stigma or unacceptable choices) outweighs, for the individual person or family, the potential benefits.

Generic Consent for Genetic Screening*

As the Human Genome Project continues, tens if not hundreds of new genetic screening tests will compete for introduction into routine clinical practice. Already some researchers have suggested population-based screening to identify carriers of the genes for such conditions as the fragile X syndrome and myotonic dystrophy. Each new screening test presents the same questions: What information should be given to which patients, when should it be presented, who should present it, and how and by whom should the results by conveyed? It will soon be impossible to do meaningful prescreening counseling about all available carrier tests. Giving too much information ("information overload") can amount to misinformation and make the entire counseling process either misleading or meaningless (Rodwin, 1993). To prevent disclosure from being pointless or counterproductive, we believe that strategies based on general or "generic" consent should be developed for genetic screening. Their aim would be to provide sufficient information to permit patients to make informed decisions about carrier screening, yet avoid the information overload that could lead to "misinformed" consent (Annas and Elias, 1992).

Traditionally, goals of reproductive genetic counseling, including counseling about screening carrier status, involve helping the person or family:

1. Comprehend the medical facts, including the diagnosis, the probable course of the disorder, and the available management.
2. Appreciate the way heredity contributes to the disorder and the risk of recurrence in specified relatives.
3. Understand the options for dealing with the risk of recurrence.
4. Choose the course of action that seems appropriate to them in view of their risk and their family goals and act in accordance with that decision.
5. Make the best possible adjustment to the disorder in an affected family member and/or to the risk of recurrence of that disorder (Fraser, 1974).

For example, in the current context of counseling a couple, at least one of whom is of Italian ancestry, each of these issues would be discussed

*This section has been adapted from Elias and Annas (1994) with permission.

as it relates specifically to β-thalassemia, with explanation of the use of hemoglobin electrophoresis as a screening test to determine carrier status. If consideration of another prenatal test were appropriate—as in the case of screening of maternal serum for alpha-fetoprotein, human chorionic gonadotropin, or unconjugated estriol to detect fetal aneuploidy, open neural-tube defects, and other abnormalities—a separate discussion about these tests, including information on their sensitivity and specificity and of each of the possible associated fetal disorders, would also be required. Even knowledgeable couples could become confused, frustrated, and anxious if faced with scores of such options for genetic screening.

By contrast, an approach based on generic consent would emphasize broader concepts and common-denominator issues in genetic screening. We envision a situation in which patients would be told of the availability of a panel of screening tests that can be performed on a single blood sample. They would be told that these tests could determine whether they carry genes that put them at increased risk of having a child with a birth defect that could involve serious physical abnormalities, mental disabilities, or both. Several common examples could be given to indicate the frequency and spectrum of severity of each type or category of condition for which screening was being offered. For example, prenatal screening could include tests for fetal conditions, such as neural-tube defects, and chromosome abnormalities, such as cystic fibrosis and fragile X syndrome. In the future, a sample of fetal blood cells may be retrievable from maternal blood to be used not only for estimation of risks but also perhaps for definitive diagnosis (Elias et al., 1996) (see Chapter 17).

In the course of such counseling, important factors common to all genetic screening tests would be highlighted. Among these are the limitations of screening tests, especially the fact that negative results cannot guarantee a healthy infant; the possible need for additional invasive tests, such as chorionic villus sampling or amniocentesis, to establish a definitive diagnosis; the reproductive options that might have to be considered, such as prenatal diagnosis, adoption, gamete donation, abortion, or acceptance of risks; the costs of screening; issues of confidentiality, including potential disclosure to other family members; and the possibility of social stigmatization, including discrimination in health insurance and employment. If carrier status is detected in the woman, it must be emphasized that the partner should also be screened. Before prenatal testing was agreed to in such cases, the woman would need to be told that she would be advised to consider abortion if the fetus was found to be affected with a non-treatable condition (Andrews et al., 1994).

This type of generic consent to genetic screening can be compared to obtaining consent to perform a physical examination. Patients know that the purpose of the examination or test is to locate potential problems that are likely to require additional follow-up and that could present them with choices they would rather not have to make. The patient is not generally told, however, about all the possible abnormalities that can be detected by a routine physical examination or routine blood work, but only about the general purpose of each. On the other hand, tests that may produce especially sensitive and stigmatizing information, such as screening of blood for the human immunodeficiency virus, should not be performed without specific consent. Similarly, because of its reproductive implications, genetic testing has not traditionally been carried out without specific consent. Even in a generic model, tests for untreatable fatal diseases such as Huntington disease should not be combined with other tests or performed without specific consent (Andrews et al., 1994).

What is central in the concept of generic consent for genetic screening is not a waiver of the individual patient's right to information. Rather, it would reflect a decision by the genetics community that the most reasonable way to conduct a panel of screening tests to identify carriers of serious conditions is to provide basic, general information to obtain consent for the screening and much more detailed information on specific conditions only after they have been detected. Since, in the vast majority of cases, no such conditions will in fact be found, this method is also the most efficient and cost-effective.

Limits to Generic Consent

Some people require more specific and in-depth information on which to base their decision regarding screening. It is therefore essential to build into the screening program ample opportunity for patients to obtain all the additional information they need to help them make decisions. Clinicians, of course, must be open and responsive to the concerns and questions of patients. Counseling could be provided in person by a physician or other health professional. Alternatively, audiovisual aids could be used, which would help ensure consistency in the information provided, be more efficient, and respond to the shortage of genetic counselors.

Generic consent for genetic screening should help prevent information overload and avert the wasting of time on useless information. It would not, however, solve what is likely to be an even more central problem in genetic screening: Are there genetic conditions for which screening should not be offered to prospective parents? Examples might include genes that predispose a person to a particular disease late in life (such as Alzheimer disease, Parkinson disease, or breast cancer) (Biesecker et al., 1993; Andrews et al., 1994). From the perspective of the fetus, life with the possibility—or even the high probability—of developing these diseases in late adulthood is much to be preferred to no life at all. Thus, in this case, unlike that of the fetus with anencephaly, for example, no reasonable argument could be made that precluding abortion by denying this information could amount to forcing a "wrongful life" on the child (Elias and Annas, 1987). Because of a personal experience with a friend or family member who suffered from one of these diseases, however, the couple might see abortion as a reasonable choice under such circumstances.

We must address this question directly and publicly. Are there genetic diseases and predispositions for which screening of prospective parents and testing of fetuses should not be offered as a matter of good medical practice and public policy, regardless of the technical ability to screen and the wishes of the couple? Offering carrier screening to assist couples in making reproductive decisions is not a neutral activity but, rather, implies that some action should be taken on the basis of the results of the test. Thus, merely offering screening for a breast-cancer or colon-cancer gene could suggest to couples that artificial insemination, adoption, and abortion are all reasonable choices if they are found to be carriers of such a gene. To some this may prove especially troublesome, given adult-onset of the disorders. Even these autosomal dominant forms of high risk (50%) have not proved amenable to traditional prenatal genetic diagnosis (amniocentesis, chorionic villus sampling); however, with preimplantation genetic diagnosis (PGD) more options exist for severe conditions (Simpson, 2001; Verlinsky et al., 2001).

A standard of care for genetic screening and consent in the face of hundreds of available genetic tests will inevitably be set. We believe the medical profession should take the lead in setting such standards and that, with public input, the model of generic consent for genetic screening will ultimately be accepted.

Guidelines for Decision-Making

Medical decisions are usually made by individual patients with the advice and recommendations of their physicians. Often more than one course of action may be morally justifiable based on examination of basic principles. At times, no course of action will seem correct, yet a decision will have to be made and supported with ethical reasoning. The American College of Obstetricians has provided the following useful guidelines for ethical (and legal) analysis of the various factors when attempting to resolve such difficulties.*

1. *Identify the decision makers.* The first step in addressing any problem is to answer the question "Whose decision is it?" In general, the patient is presumed to have the capacity to choose among medically acceptable alternatives or to refuse treatment.
   a. At times the patient's ability to make a decision is not clear. A person's capacity to make a decision depends on that person's ability to understand information and appreciate the implications of that information for his or her own personal decision. In contrast, *competence and incompetence* are legal determinations that may or may not truly reflect functional capacity. Assessment of a patient's capacity to make decisions must at times be made by professionals with expertise in making such determinations. Decisions about competence can be made only in a court of law.
   b. If a patient is thought to be incapable of making a decision or has been found legally incompetent, a surrogate decision maker must be identified. In the absence of a durable power of attorney, family members have been called on to render proxy decisions. In some situations, the court may be called on to appoint a guardian. A surrogate decision maker should make the decision that the patient would have wanted or, if the patient's wishes are not known, that will promote the best interests of the patient. The physician has an obligation to assist those representing the patient in examining the issues and reaching a resolution.
   c. In the obstetric setting, a pregnant woman is generally considered the appropriate decision maker for the fetus that she is carrying.

---

*From American College of Obstetricians and Gynecologists. Ethics in Obstetrics and Gynecology. Washington, DC, © ACOG, 2002.

2. *Collect data, establish facts.*
   a. It is important to be aware that perceptions about what may or may not be relevant or important to a case are based on personal values. One should remain as objective as possible when collecting the information on which a decision will be based.
   b. Use consultants as needed to ensure that all available information about the diagnosis, treatment, and prognosis has been obtained.
3. *Identify all medically appropriate options.*
   a. Use consultation as necessary.
   b. Identify other options raised by the patient or other concerned parties.
4. *Evaluate options according to the values and principles involved.*
   a. Start by gathering information about the values of the involved parties, and try to get a sense of the perspective and values each is bringing to the discussion. The values of the decision maker will be the most important as decision making proceeds.
   b. Decide whether any of the options violates ethical principles that all agree are important. Eliminate those options that, after analysis, are found to be morally unacceptable by all parties.
   c. Reexamine the remaining options according to the interests and values of each party. Some alternatives may be successfully combined.
5. *Identify ethical conflicts and try to set priorities.*
   a. Try to define the problem in terms of the ethical principles involved (e.g., beneficence versus autonomy).
   b. Weigh the principles underlying each of the arguments made. Does one of the principles appear more important than others as the conflict is examined? Does one proposed course of action seem to have more merit than the others?
   c. Consider respected opinions about similar cases and decide to what extent they can be useful in addressing the current problem. Look for morally relevant differences and similarities between this and other cases. Usually, it will be found that the basic dilemma at hand is not a new one and that points considered by others in resolving past dilemmas can be useful.
6. *Select the option that can be best justified.* Try to arrive at a rational resolution to the problem, one that can be justified to others in terms of ethical principles with universal appeal.
7. *Reevaluate the decision after it is acted upon.* Repeat the evaluation of the major options in light of information gained during the implementation of the decision. Was the best possible decision made? What lessons can be learned from the discussion and resolution of the problem?

REFERENCES

Andrews LB, Fullarton JE, Holtsman NA, et al.: Assessing Genetic Risks: Implications for Health and Social Policy. Washington, DC: National Academy Press, 1994.

Annas GJ, Coyne B: "Fitness" for birth and reproduction: Legal implications of genetic screening. Family Law Q 9:463, 1975.

Annas GJ, Elias S: Legal and ethical implications of fetal diagnosis and gene therapy. Am J Med Genet 35:215, 1990.

Annas GJ, Elias S: Legal and ethical issues in genetic screening, prenatal diagnosis, and gene therapy. *In* Simpson JL, Elias D (eds): Essential of Prenatal Diagnosis. New York: Churchill-Livingstone, 1996, p 1281.

Annas GJ, Elias S: Legal and ethical issues in genetic screening, prenatal diagnosis, and gene therapy. *In* Simpson JL, Elias S (eds): Essential of Prenatal Diagnosis. New York: Churchill-Livingstone, 1993, p 393.

Annas GJ, Elias S: Legal and ethical issues in obstetric practice. *In* Gabbe SG, Niebyl JR, Simpson JL (eds): Obstetrics: Normal and Problem Pregnancies, 3rd ed. New York: Churchill-Livingstone, 1996, p 1281.

Annas GJ, Elias S: Social Policy Research Priorities for the Human Genome Project. *In* Annas GJ, Elias S (eds): Mapping Our Genes: Using Law and Ethics as Guides. New York: Oxford University Press, 1992, p 269.

Annas GJ: Righting the wrong of "wrongful life." Hastings Center Rep 11:8, 1981.

Annas GJ: Genetics and the Law. New York: Plenum Press, 1976.

Annas GJ: The Rights of Patients, 2nd ed. Carbondale: Southern Illinois University Press, 1989b.

Annas GJ: Who's afraid of the human genome? Hastings Cent Rep 19:19, 1989a.

Biesecker BB, Boehnke M, Calzone K, et al.: Genetic counseling for families with inherited susceptibility to breast and ovarian cancer. JAMA 269:1970, 1993.

Elias S, Annas GJ: Generic consent for genetic screening. N Engl J Med 330:1611, 1994.

Elias S, Annas GJ: Reproductive Genetics and the Law. Chicago: Yearbook 1987.

Elias S, Lewis DE, Bischoff FZ, et al.: Isolation and genetic analysis of fetal nucleated red blood cells from maternal blood: The Baylor College of Medicine experience. Early Hum Dev 47:S85, 1996.

Fraser FC: Genetic counseling. Am J Hum Genet 26:636, 1974.

Harper FV, James F: The Law of Torts (Supp) Sec 171.1,61, 1968.

Jacobs v Theimer, 519 SW 2d 846, 849 (Tex), 1975.

President's Commissions for the Study of Ethical Problems in Medicine and Biomedical and Behavioral Research: Screening and Counseling for Genetic Conditions, Feb. 1983. Library of Congress No. 83-600502, Washington, DC: U.S. Government Printing Office, 1983.

Rodwin M: Medicine, Money and Morals. New York, Oxford University Press, 1993.

Simpson JL: Celebrating preimplantation genetic diagnosis of p53 mutations in Li-Fraumeni syndrome. Reprod BioMed Online 3:2, 2001.

Time: Doctors and Patients: Image vs. Reality, July 31, 1989.

Verlinsky Y, Rechitsky S, Verlinsky O, et al.: Preimplantation diagnosis for p53 tumor suppressor gene mutations. Reprod BioMed Online 2:102, 2001.

Index

Note: Page numbers followed by f refer to illustrations; page numbers followed by t refer to tables.

Polycystic ovarian syndrome (*Continued*)
  frequency in female relatives, 196–198, 197t
  genetic mechanisms of, 199
  molecular basis of, 199–200
  pregnancy loss and, 115
Polydactyly
  as dominant inherited trait, 44f, 44–45
  short ribs with, 306t
Polygenic multifactorial inheritance, in polycystic ovarian
    syndrome, 199
Polygenic-multifactorial inheritance
  basis of, 75–77, 76f-77f, 76t
  concordance in twins, 78
  difference between polygenic and multifactorial, 77
  disorder characteristics in, 78–79
  disorders, prenatal diagnosis of, 405. *See also* Neural
      tube defects.
  heritability in, 79
  in discontinuous variation, 77–78, 78f
  incidence of, 78
  quantitative linkage analysis of, 77t, 79, 80f, 80t
  recurrence risk in, 79
  traits in, 75t
Polyglandular autoimmune syndrome, premature ovarian
    failure and, 272
Polymerase chain reaction (PCR)
  failure of, FISH simultaneous with, 424
  for diagnosis and sequencing, 61–62
  for DNA amplification, 60–61, 61f-62f
  in mendelian disorder diagnosis, 400
    failure of (allele dropout), 421f, 421–424, 422t
    fluorescent, 420f, 423
    nested, 62f, 416
    nucleotide repeat disorders and, 423
  of maternal blood
    fetal aneuploidy detection by, 451
    fetal autosomal dominant or recessive inheritance
        detected by, 449–450, 450f
    fetal sex determination by, 449
Polymorphism
  chromosomal, 26
  definition of, 403
  DNA, types of, 55–57
  in quantitative linkage analysis, 55–57
Polyploidy
  detection of, 18
  incidence of, 106, 108
  pregnancy loss and, 110
  recurrence of, 373t
Polysomy
  definition of, 16
  sex chromosomal, 21–22
    complements in, 110
    mental retardation from, 134
    spontaneous abortion incidence in, 106t
Polysomy X. *See also specific named polysomy e.g.,*
    47,XXY.
  in females, 332–333
  incidence of, 323
Polysomy Y, in males, 333–334.
Porphyria, acute intermittent, 163t
Position effect, 26
Prader-Willi syndrome, 27t, 137t, 143, 303t
  imprinting in, 51, 54f
Pre-eclampsia
  causes of, 163
  definition of, 162
  factor V Leiden mutation and, 155–156
  family studies of, 162, 163–164
  genes causing, 164–166

Pre-eclampsia (*Continued*)
  in autosomal dominant polycystic kidney disease, 162
  in twin pregnancies, 162
  incidence of, 162
  paternal imprinting and, 166
Pregnancy, effect of,
  aortic dissection in, 157
  breast cancer and, 222
  fetal cell persistence in maternal blood after, 445–446
  in autosomal dominant polycystic kidney disease, 162
  in cystic fibrosis, 92–93
    complications in, 148
    fetal and maternal death rate in, 148
    incidence of, 147
  in Ehlers-Danlos syndrome, 158–159
  in factor V Leiden mutation, 155–156, 164
  in idiopathic hypertrophic subaortic stenosis, 161
  in Marfan syndrome, 156–157
  in myotonic dystrophy, 159–160
  in phenylketonuria, 149–150, 150t
  in sickle cell disease, 151
  in thalassemias, 152–153
  in Turner syndrome, 252
  in von Willebrand disease, 154–155
  termination of. See Abortion, voluntary.
Pregnancy loss, 101–102. *See also* Abortion, spontaneous.
  alcohol intake and, 124
  alloimmune disease and, 121–123
  antifetal antibodies and, 121
  antiphospholipid and anticardiolipin antibodies and,
      119–120
  antisperm antibodies and, 120
  autosomal trisomy and, 108–110
  caffeine and, 123–124
  chemotherapy and, 123
  chromosomal abnormalities and, 108, 109t
    in first trimester, 106t
    in second trimester, 108
    in third trimester, 108
    IVF and, 107–108
    preimplantation, 103–107, 104f-105f, 106t
  chromosomal inversions and, 113
  chromosomal translocations and, 112
  cigarette smoking and, 124
  contraceptive agents and, 124
  diabetes mellitus and, 115
  embryotoxic antibodies and, 121
  environmental chemicals and, 123
  Factor V Leiden mutation, 120–121
  hypercoagulable conditions and, 120–121
  imprinting and, 111–112
  incidence of, 101–103
  incompetent cervix and, 116–117
  incomplete müllerian fusion and, 116
  infections and, 117–120
  intrauterine adhesions (synechiae) and, 115–116
  leiomyomas and, 116
  luteal phase defects and, 113–115, 114t
  maternal illness and, 125
  maternal subfertility and, 111
  Mendelian factors in, 125t, 125–126
  oligomenorrhea and, 115
  ovulation day conception and, 101
  polycystic ovary disease and, 115
  preimplantation, 101, 103–108
  psychological factors in, 124–125
  recurrent
    aneuploidy and, 109t, 110–111
    risks for, 102t, 102–103
  thyroid abnormalities and, 115

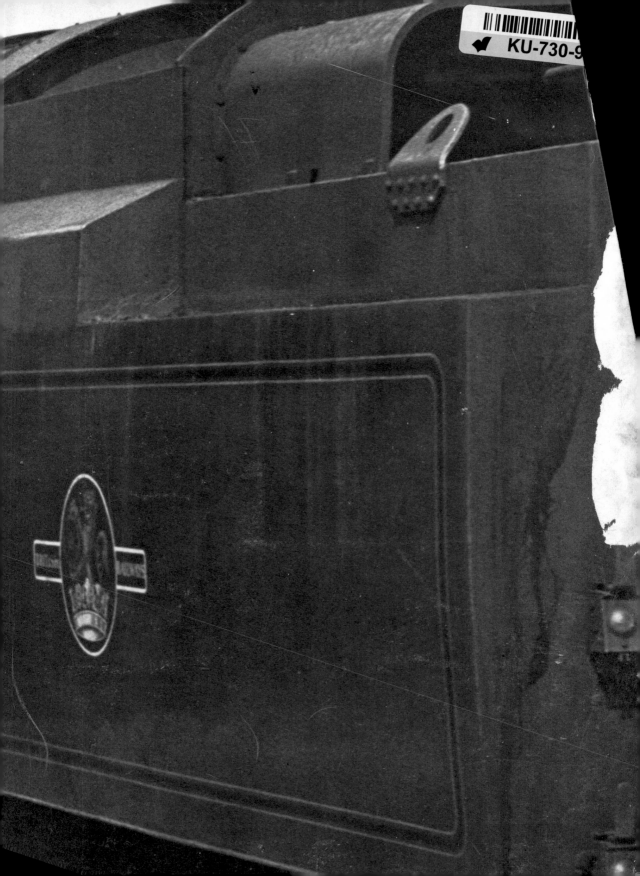
KU-730-9

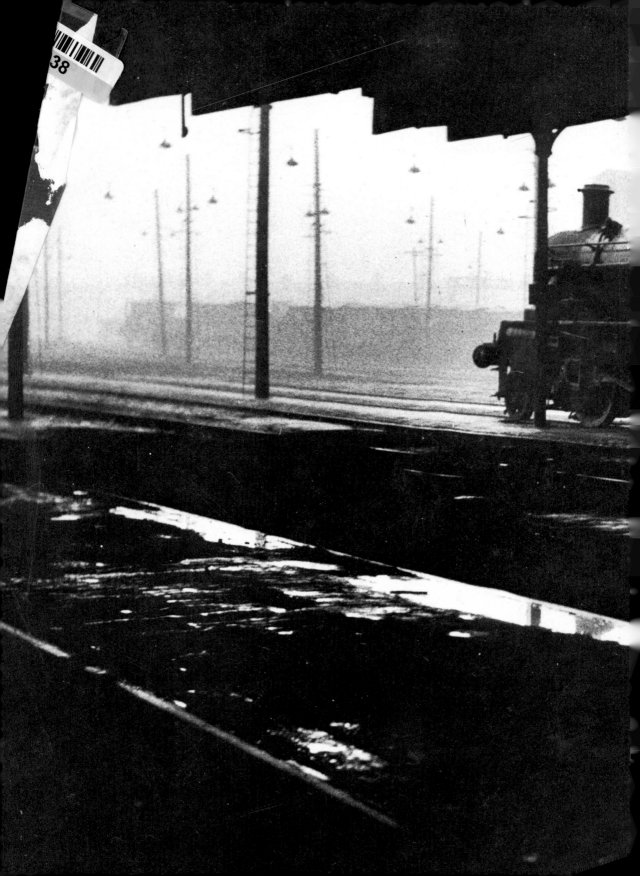

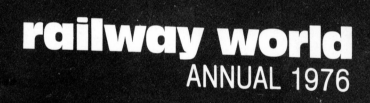

railway world
ANNUAL 1976

Edited by
ALAN WILLIAMS

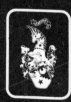

LONDON
IAN ALLAN LTD

Contents

STAFFORDSHIRE
COUNTY
LIBRARY

A 17. OCT. 1975

C 385.05

WITHDRAWN AND SOLD
STAFFORDSHIRE LIBRARY

First published 1975

ISBN 0 7110 0652 0 — 9/75

All rights reserved. No part of this book may be reproduced or transmitted in any form or by any means, electronic or mechanical, including photocopying, recording or by any information storage and retrieval system, without permission from the Publisher in writing.

© Ian Allan Ltd, 1975

Published by Ian Allan Ltd, Shepperton, Surrey, and printed in the United Kingdom by Ian Allan Printing Ltd.

Front cover: Preserved LNER Class V2 2-6-2 No 4771 swings round the curve at Borwick, near Carnforth with an enthusiasts' special on June 16 1974 *E. R. Osmotherley*

Title page: A decade ago, in 1965, a bleak November day at Willesden finds grubby BR Standard Mogul No 78033 resting in a half-empty shed, while in the mist beyond the overhead equipment for its electric successors is already taking shape. *Anthony Brown*

Experimental Section

H. A. V. Bulleid

The Midland Railway and, later, the LMS operated a small Experimental Section in the Locomotive Drawing Office at Derby. But I think Johnson, Deeley, Fowler, Hughes and Stanier would all have given different answers if asked "What is it for?"

Every new design of engine, or even every batch of a similar design, contains development items that could fairly be termed experimental, yet all that work went straight to the main design sections of the Drawing Office. In practice they (or their Chief Draughtsman) used the Experimental Section in three ways — for minor investigation of design queries, for overflow jobs when the main sections were hard pressed, and for exploring novel ideas. Besides these, the section was responsible for all dynamometer car trials.

When I was junior draughtsman on the Experimental Section between August and December 1935, most of its current jobs were influenced by the number of new Stanier engines then running, including six Pacifics, 100 three-cylinder 4-6-0s, 100 two-cylinder 4-6-0s, 40 2-6-0s and 60 2-6-4Ts and 2-6-2Ts.

The ghastly steaming of the three-cylinder 4-6-0s had just about been cured, thanks to some heroic work on the tubes and blastpipe by Riddles and Bond at Crewe, and all these engines were giving general satisfaction — which was just as well, since the total in traffic had reached 540 by the end of 1935. By mid-1935, the three-cylinder 4-6-0s around Derby were gradually ousting the over-taxed Compounds on the Sheffield-St. Pancras expresses, while their black sisters were doing excellently up and down the Manchester Bank.

My first three jobs involved problems not yet solved. They involved arrangements for vacuum tubes and pyrometers in the smokeboxes of the three-cylinder 4-6-0s for further blastpipe and superheater experiments, and a modification to the top-feed clack-boxes for all the taper-boiler engines. Then there was a sudden spate of trouble caused by well-intentioned busy fingers screwing down the protruding limit studs on the top feeds — thereby preventing feed! So we duly issued "Derby Drg. 2787: Sketch for Motive Power Depots showing why NOT to screw down studs protruding from top-feed clack-boxes."

The bogie side-check springs for the first Pacifics were, I seem to recall, first designed for an initial 2ton and a maximum 3ton compression. This was a typical designer's "first shot," to be modified according to the practical riding of the engine. In fact, it was decided that rather more centring force was needed, and we calculated and drew out springs to give the same maximum compression but with initial compression increased to $2\frac{1}{2}$ tons.

Brick arches somehow seemed to be on the agenda, the back end having quite an effect on steaming, the front end sometimes accumulating ash, and the whole affair causing panic when it collapsed into the fire! The compounds always had a tendency to clog the bottom row of tubes with ash, impairing steaming and making cleaning difficult. Several compounds, including Nos. 936, 1045, 1048/9 and 1061 accordingly had their brick arches rebuilt with four spaces in the front row of bricks, to let the ash drop back into the fire. The only one I ever examined was No. 936, on which I found the two centre spaces clogged solid but the two corner spaces free. We had expected it to be the other way about, and of course most bottom tubes were

3

still blocked. Some engines seemed to take a delight in baffling the experimenter!

About this time I also had to check the arch of a black 5 4-6-0, No. 5069, which had been indignantly reported as unsafe with a 3in gap at the centre. Measurement showed that the gap was 2½in, the firebox ½in over-width, and the bricks undersize. This was before full standardisation of the black 5s, and it was disconcerting to find that "bricks for the back six rows are F.264, engines 5020-5069 only." Standardisation was helped by our later drawing DRS 2772 from which the Pattern Shop mocked up a wooden "part firebox" and bricks to enable further study on brick arches.

It is always extremely tricky, with a new design, to sort out the serious from the trivial defect reports. One usually relies on repetition, watching more closely for a second complaint if the subject seems potentially serious. Sometimes the first complaint is merely a rogue case, virtually a false alarm.

Nevertheless, when it was reported that a motion arm had shaken loose on a black 5 we panicked slightly — bits of Walschaerts valve gear flying about loose are not healthy! By "motion arm" the shed meant "crosshead arm," the terminology still being novel at Derby. On other railways it was sometimes called the crosshead tail-piece. In this case, it was secured by studs and a large solid key fitted into a slot milled in the crosshead. After assembly it was not possible to see if the key and slot were a snug fit, which was of course essential to prevent rocking and ultimate loosening. We did not like blind fits at Derby and, based on this one report, we offered a version with a solid key on the crosshead and slot in the arm, so that the fit could be tested after assembly. When this sketch reached Coleman he responded with the view that there were plenty of existing problems about to tackle without inventing new ones! In the event, he proved to be right, for we had no more trouble.

The filing system in the Derby Loco Drawing Office was good and everyone was en-couraged to see what had been done in the past before dashing off a new design. So when complaints poured in about the cab front windows on the new engines, and it became clear that an improved window catch was necessary, we simply copied the old Midland Railway standard type!

There were no side windows on any Midland Railway engines, on the LMS Compounds built in 1926, or for that matter on the Claughtons, and there was only a fixed window at each side on the Scots. In contrast, all the Stanier engines had sliding side windows so that the rear half could be opened or closed at will. This involved a grooved sill upon which a driver or fireman naturally rested his forearm when seated at the open window. Soon complaints began to come in thick and fast about the agony to flesh and wreckage to clothes caused by these damned grooves. Worse still, bits of wood were being wedged in as protectors, looking ghastly and bending the frames, as well as rendering the windows totally inoperative.

So would the experimental section please design a folding armrest *instantly!* I only discovered later that the job had been delayed by being considered rather infra dig by the main part of the drawing office! It turned out to be as simple as it sounds and was very popular

Top right: Pre-war scene at Carlisle Upperby shed, with Stanier 'Black Five' 4-6-0s No 5139 and 5299 resting between turns, while on the left Fowler 2P 4-4-0 No 652 noses up alongside. *Eric Treacy*

Right: Looking much neater with a Stanier high-sided tender, unrebuilt Royal Scot 4-6-0 No 6166 *London Rifle Brigade* takes a drink from Tebay troughs as it hurries south with a Carlisle-Euston train in late LMS days. *M. W. Earley*

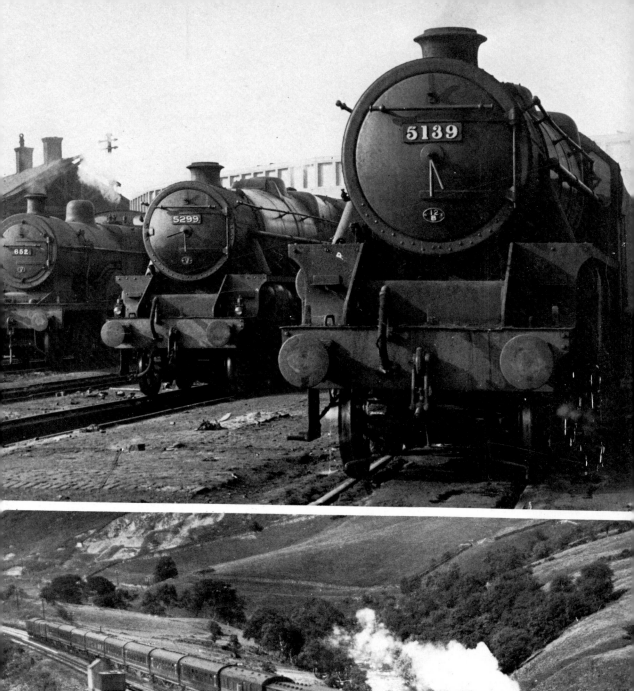
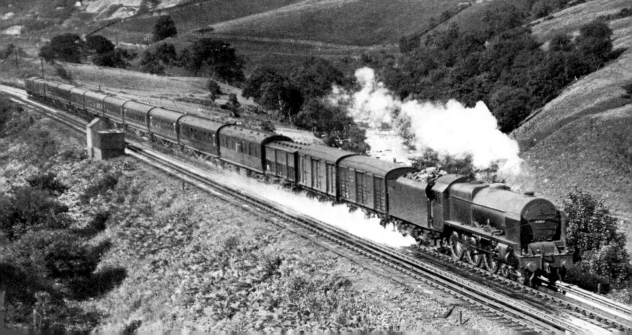

with the footplate staff; as a result I endured about a week of jocular fame!

Some jobs were aimed strictly at economy. I remember doing masses of calculations as a result of which a reduction was permitted in the minimum size before scrapping of crank axle bearings on the Class 4F 0-6-0s.

Shed Jobs were an interesting detraction from the normal work. In 1935 there was one of those periodic worries about stresses set up in boilers and fireboxes by heating up too fast from cold. Possibly Stanier had seen and disliked the practice at Crewe North Shed which, when pushed for an engine, got it going in an hour from cold by taking fire from the sand-drying furnace and using a separate steam supply for the blower. With this tough procedure the engine would be in steam while the lowest water spaces would still only be tepid. But, so the theory went, with a circulator fitted there would only be a few degrees difference between the hottest and coldest parts throughout heating-up.

Comparative experiments were carried out on Class 4F No. 3994 fitted with a circulator. Other apparatus needed included the portable blower occasionally used in 4 Shed, Derby and an adjacent Class 2P 4-4-0 to supply external steam at 160lb sq in. The portable blower, which fitted down the chimney and stood in for the engine's own blower, had a semi-official status; its use was reckoned to be officially taboo but unofficially tolerated in a genuine crisis. Experiments like this one on No. 3994 tacitly admitted its existence and therefore lent slight official support to its use!

Four tests were carried out, each starting from cold with the normal lighting-up process of firelighters, wood and coal, and subsequent firing as necessary. The results are shown below.

The total amount of coal used was not greatly affected, although of course there was an unmeasured contribution from the "external" steam. The notes on smoke were prompted by the Railway's genuine anxiety about excessive smoke emission, particularly from Sheds near residential areas. Smoke during early-morning lighting-up in cold weather always seemed particularly noisome and sulphurous, and people living nearby did not seem impressed when told that it was mildly disinfectant!

There was a tremendous economy drive in 1935 and as the case for fitting circulators was far from compelling, there the matter rested.

I was "borrowed" from the Works for the first two weeks of October 1934 for work with Dynamometer Car No. 2 (as the 1912 L&Y car was called) on the "Mid-day Scot," testing Royal Scot class 4-6-0 No. 6158 *Loyal Regiment,* with driver Garrett of Crewe North

test condition	time, cold to steam	coal used (cwt/qr)	smoke emission	circulation
normal.	$3\frac{1}{4}$ hrs	4·3	bad	poor
external steam to portable blower.	$1\frac{1}{4}$ hrs	4·1	negligible	very bad
external steam to circulator	$2\frac{1}{2}$ hrs	3·3	bad	excellent
external steam to portable blower and to circulator	$1\frac{1}{4}$ hrs	4·0	negligible	good

Shed. Each Monday and Wednesday we took over the 4.31pm Crewe-Glasgow, and each Tuesday and Thursday the 1.30pm out of Glasgow as far as Crewe, a distance of 243 miles. The trains normally loaded to 11 coaches plus the dynamometer car, about 400 tons in all. Normal timings were observed, and we were on time six out of the eight trips. On both occasions that we were late — and once we were very late! — the delays were due to permanent way and traffic delays rather than locomotive troubles. The weather was fine the first week, but colder and windy the second. Coal usage averaged 41lb per mile (minimum 39) the first week, 51lb per mile (maximum 60) the second.

There are some parallels between the petrol consumption of a car and coal consumption of a steam engine. The former is often boasted about on a "long journey" basis, with a minimum of acceleration and braking. The steam locomotive also dislikes short runs, yet these are in effect just what it gets if there are many signal checks and severe permanent way delays. They also involve fiercer accelerations in an attempt to regain lost time. On our worst run, when we were over half an hour late, the extra stopping and starting, the harder than usual working necessary to regain some of the lost time, and the simple fact of keeping the locomotive and train warm for the extra time all account for the somewhat startling jump from 40 to 60lb per mile, though some of the blame at least must also go down to adverse weather conditions.

My duties included keeping the coal records, a laborious chore in 1934 before the advent of auto coaling plants! The drill was to weigh a wagon of locomotive coal, load the tender, then re-weigh the wagon to calculate the amount loaded, usually around 7½ tons. At the end of the journey we weighed an empty wagon, slung the remaining coal on it, and then re-weighed it to calculate what you had got left. The least we ever had was 1¼ tons — and a "Scot" tender looked uncomfortably empty at that level!

The Sheds co-operated excellently in the coaling ritual, which involved four shunts each time, only occasionally giving a gentle reminder that they had other work to do, and sometimes grumbling at weighing empty trucks when the tare weight was already painted on. But it had to be done, because a combination of rain, residues, and the state of mechanical gear could affect the official tare weight by half a hundredweight.

Whilst the traffic people naturally took all steps to avoid delays to the "Mid-day Scot", the situation changed immediately we arrived at Glasgow Central — we slid to the bottom of the priority list for our road back to Polmadie Shed! When at last a path was found for us, *Loyal Regiment,* running tender first, would push the dynamometer car rather gingerly through the lights and the misty shine of the Glaswegian night south to Polmadie. Then, however late, the remaining coal had to to be weighed off, for one daren't delay this job for fear some of it might get "borrowed" to light up a nearby engine early the following morning!

The L&Y dynamometer car had an excellent kitchen, in which cooking, usually bacon and eggs, was almost a pleasure — except when coasting down Beattock at 80 mph! Switching to a cold meal for a change one day, I remember buying a home-grown cos lettuce in a shop near Crewe North Shed for 1d! Wages were low in those days but money went far. A craftsman on 30 per cent bonus but working the current economy drive "short" week (Saturday mornings were neither worked nor paid for) got about £3.50 per week, and a top-link driver a little more. As a junior draughtsman on a full week I got about £3.25 but expenses were very good at 80p for every complete 24 hours spent away from home, paid irrespective of claims, and we made the most of this by doing our own catering and cooking and where practicable, as at Polmadie, sleeping in the dynamometer car. It had luxuriously-cushioned long wide bench-type seats — thanks to the old L&Y!

But what about the engine, 6158 *Loyal Regiment?* It steamed very well and the fire responded to the dampers. It rode well and the cab was comfortable by 1930s standards. Despite the vast smokebox and deflectors, I thought the look-out ahead was reasonably good. The firing position was convenient and we had no injector troubles, live or exhaust. I found it an admirable engine, and so did driver Garrett and his fireman. At times we could have done with more steam, and have put it to good use, and this explains why the engines were so much improved when subsequently fitted with particularly free-steaming, good-circulation taper boilers by Stanier. The original boilers failed to incorporate all Churchward's findings, though they were as good as most of their contemporaries.

The 127 ton engine and tender, gleaming in polished maroon and black, made an impressive sight enjoyed by many as it set back with the dynamometer car onto the train at Crewe. With boiler nearly full and injector on we would just manage not to blow off steam before getting the right away. Driver Garrett would make one of his impeccable starts, knowing that slipping is exceptionally upsetting in a dynamometer car because it sends the chart pens flying, spoils the chart and usually wipes out all the important data on draw-bar pull during the initial acceleration.

The most exhilerating part of the run would be the approach to Shap in the gathering October twilight. The bank really starts with two miles at 1 in 110 just before Oxenholme, despite which we should, and did, take the easy curve of Oxenholme station at nearly 60mph. Then come seven miles at an average of 1 in 120 to Grayrigg which we did well (with a "Scot" and at least 400 tons) to pass at about 45mph on each occasion. From Grayrigg to Tebay is a six mile level stretch during which a driver aims to attain the maximum possible speed consistent with having a full head of steam at Tebay, the start of the five-mile climb to Shap proper at 1 in 75. Driver Garrett would get speed up to about 60mph at the start of the bank, but we would be down to around 25mph by the summit, with full regulator and about 35 per cent cut-off, and the beat of the engine down from a continuous roar to a nearly staccato 10 per second.

The heavy working of the engine, the last light over the Western hills, the white trail of steam in the dark sky and the bright lights of the train curving behind, all go to make the memory of the climb of Shap so dramatic. An open locomotive cab (unless running tender-first!) has always enough ambient heat to give what is now well-known as an "air curtain" effect, insulating the cab from the outside cold but allowing immediate access to the external conditions if you simply leaned out of the cab a few inches. By so doing, one was instantly translated from the typical cosy atmosphere and smell of the footplate into the keen — very keen — air of the fell country. But not always. Suddenly a fast goods would rattle by on the up line, leaving behind it a distinctly fishy aroma. On one trip, Garrett had just remarked that they often passed this particular fish special about the same place, and I had just expressed astonishment that you could smell it, on Shap, from another engine, when a tremendous tumult broke out. The engine started buck-jumping and even over the shindig you could hear the hail of cinders on the cab roof. Slipping! Garrett had the regulator closed in an instant and then eased it open again while winding back to a later cut-off. And it only seemed a few seconds before we were back to normal. Garrett attributed this sudden unladylike behaviour to a small drift of leaves on the track and said he was ready for such problems at that time of year. A few passengers may have noticed the slight snatch on the train at the time, but I am sure it was long forgotten by the time Garrett brought 6158 and his train to a halt in Glasgow Central, smoothly and on time.

Live Wires

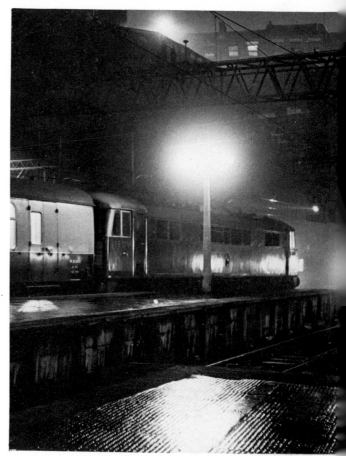

Right: The rapid spread of 25kV electrification during the past decade has brought overhead equipment and electric trains into the everyday life of London, the Midlands, the North West and Clydeside. Here, Class AL6 (now Class 86) No E3144 is ready to depart from Birmingham New Street with empty stock for Edge Hill on a wet night in January 1967. *P. Gerald*

Bottom: The first section of the West Coast main line to be electrified was that from Manchester Piccadilly to Crewe, and the early designs of overhead structure were on the heavy side, as this panorama of Stockport Edgeley in 1970 bears witness. An unidentified Class 86 is approaching on a passenger train, while on the left a mixed freight trundles by behind an English Electric Class 37 Co-Co *M. Dunnett*

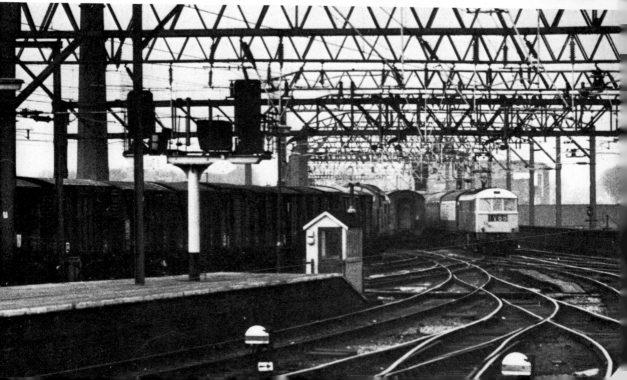

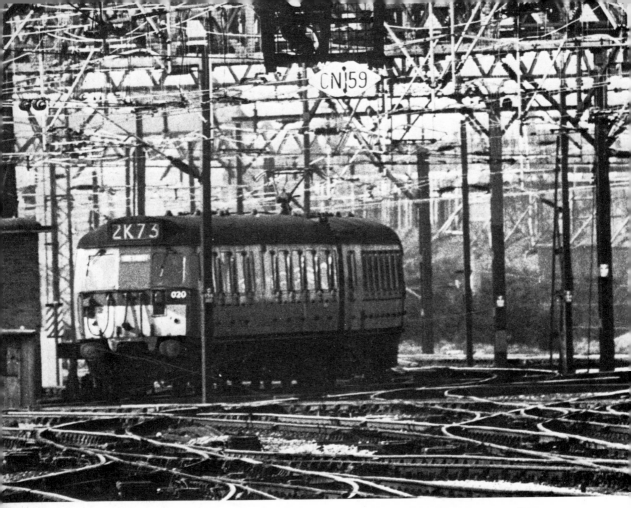

Above: But perhaps the greatest amount of suspended steel, copper and porcelain hangs above the complicated junction at the north end of Crewe Station, emphasised here by the telephoto lens as the camera catches Class 304/2 unit No 020 coming into the station off the Manchester line in April 1970. *M. Dunnett*

Top right: The LNER electrified both its Liverpool Street-Shenfield and Manchester-Sheffield routes on the 1500V dc overhead system and provided similar three-car suburban multiple units, with air-operated doors, for both schemes. But whereas the Shenfield units were rebuilt to 25kV standards when the remainder of the Great Eastern suburban lines were electrified on that system, the Manchester-based units remain 1500V dc, despite the fact that they share Manchester Piccadilly with West Coast 25kV electric trains, and that the neighbouring Altrincham line, also originally 1500V dc, was recently converted to 25kV standards. Here, two of the dc units make their way into Piccadilly alongside the ac lines on the 13·59 Hadfield-Manchester working on October 24 1973. *Philip Hawkins*

Centre right: Glasgow Central is now the Northern terminus of the electrified West Coast main line. But for a decade before the Electric Scots came, the station was already the terminus for the busy South Clydeside 25kV electric services, worked by handsome Class 303 and 311 three-car units. Here, a member of the class picks its way through the complicated approaches to the terminus and passes a two-car Cravens diesel unit on a suburban working. Electrification of the main line in May 1974 also included further stretches of the suburban system, including the branch to Lanark, thus enabling the further reduction of diesel workings into Glasgow and the better utilisation of the electric units. *British Rail*

Bottom right: Despite the demise of the steam engine, Liverpool Lime Street is evidently not pollution-free! A suburban diesel unit adds its exhaust to the haze as it shunts clear of the crossover prior to setting back into another platform while on the right a Class 86 waits quietly to depart with the 10·40 to Euston on April 12 1973 *D. Griffiths*

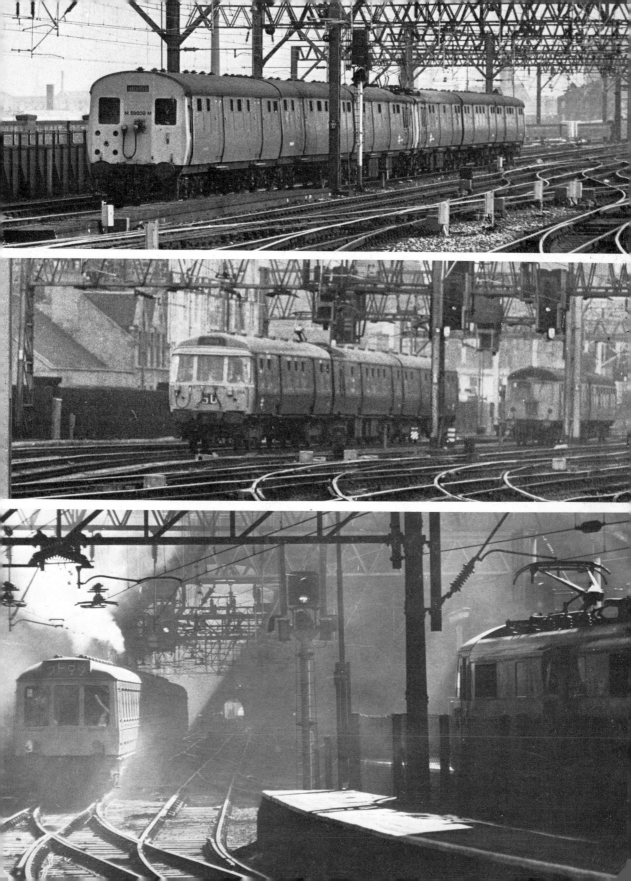

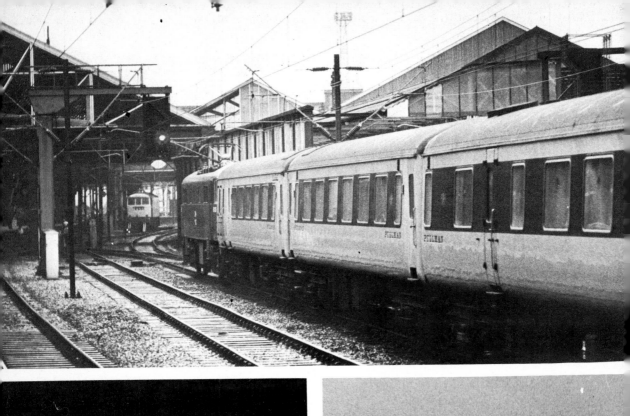

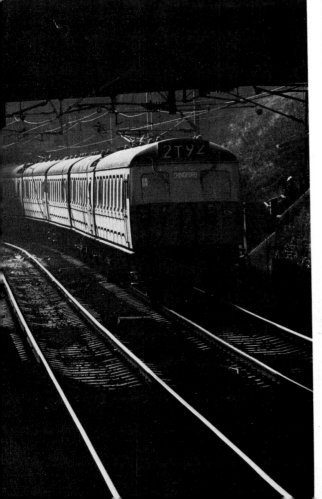

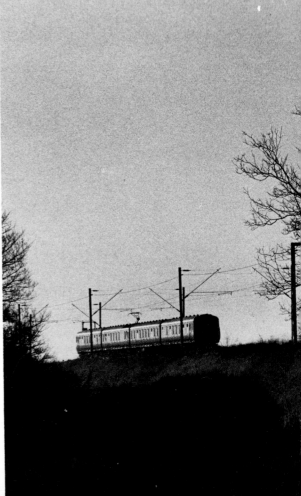

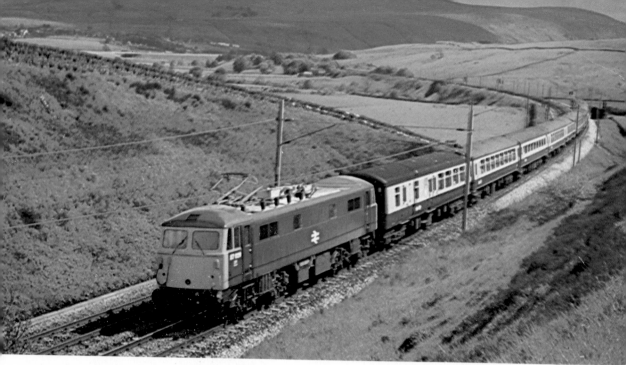

Above: Just a month after the inauguration of through electric services from England to Scotland, Class 87 Bo-Bo No 87029 hurries a Birmingham-Glasgow train past Greenholme on June 8 1974. *J. H. Cooper-Smith*

Right: Passenger services on the 1500V dc Manchester-Sheffield line via Woodhead have been withdrawn but freight traffic is still very heavy. Some of the Class 76 Bo-Bos have been fitted for multiple working, and two are seen here in tandem at Hazlehead with a Merry-go-round train for Fiddler's Ferry on June 28 1970. *P. N. Bradley*

Top left: Running 35 minutes late, the down morning Manchester Pullman picks its way carefully through Crewe on February 6 1974 in the charge of Class 86/2 Bo-Bo No 86230. *Philip Hawkins*

Far left: Underneath the arches of Clapton comes Class 305/1 unit No 417 at the head of a Liverpool Street-Chingford working on January 25 1972. *J. H. Cooper-Smith*

Left: Sunrise over Hampton-in-Arden on January 25, 1974 finds Class 310 unit No 074 hurrying towards the Midlands metropolis on the 08·32 Coventry-Birmingham New Street working. *Philip Hawkins*

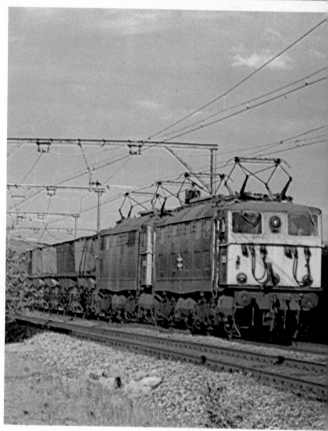

Last of the true narrow gauge?

Isle of Man Railway 2-4-0T No 11 *Maitland* is reflected in the waters of the Silver Burn as it draws gently away from Castletown with the 11·40 Douglas-Port Erin train on August 14 1972. *D. L. Percival*

For me, true narrow gauge railway operation in this country ceased in November 1965. For in that month the Isle of Man Railway announced the "temporary" withdrawal of services for urgent maintenance, and normal services were never resumed.

I should hasten to say that I have no wish to decry the valiant efforts of the narrow gauge railway preservationists — indeed I am one of them myself — but I fear the provision of viable year-round services on narrow gauge metals in the British Isles is now an impossible task.

But what made the old IMR so different from its Welsh counterparts? I can do no better than describe my first three visits to the Island, and in fact my first taste of the 3ft gauge.

I hate crowds and, having heard tales of how busy the IMR could be at the height of the holiday season, I chose the last but one week of the winter service for my visit. One train a day ran from the capital, Douglas, along the south coast of the island to Port Erin and another to the west coast town of Peel. The trains were conveniently timed so you could travel on both the same day. Winter services on the St. John's to Ramsey line, once owned by the Manx Northern Railway, had by then been withdrawn completely.

My request for a holiday runabout ticket so early in the year was treated by the Douglas

14

booking clerk as a whim of one of these mad enthusiasts, but by Tuesday lunchtime I had had my 12s 6d worth of travel.

Monday morning dawned foggy, as did most days that week. As I walked to Douglas station, the coastal fog siren booming out its warning to sailors, men on ladders were sticking up the new season's posters for the bus and train services, for both forms of transport shared the same management.

At the steam shed nothing stirred, but at 10am, with a roar and a cloud of exhaust, one of the ex-County Donegal railcars emerged, with its brother obediently in tow. But for more than an hour the other end of Douglas station had been a hive of activity. A never-ending stream of lorries was ferrying the inwards parcels and goods off the recently-arrived steamer from the mainland to the station.

A time-and-motion study man would have wept. Those parcels had been unloaded from the ship to a lorry, driven about half a mile to the station, then unloaded, booked in and loaded onto the train. On arrival at the destination station they would, as likely as not, be unloaded again to be put on yet another lorry for the final delivery! No wonder regular *commercial* services on the IMR had to stop!

Parcels for stations along the Peel line (Crosby, St. John's and Peel itself) were by now being loaded into one of the IMR grey "G" class vans standing at the stop blocks. The railcars backed gently onto it, coupled up and promptly at 10.25 we set out — the driver, the guard and yours truly, their solitary passenger.

Because it was a damp day, the driver had taken the precaution of walking along the platform, sprinkling sand on the rails, so we had little difficulty in starting. Our return from Peel was to prove this a wise move!

The outward journey was uneventful, though I wondered how much those crossing keepers along the line were paid for opening the gates twice daily in winter. Surely some

form of ungated level crossing could have been accepted by the island Parliament, Tynwald?

At St. John's, Station Master George Crellin, certainly the best-known character of the IMR (though now sadly deceased) came to meet our train as if it were a crack express, bustling from the booking office to the signal box, and on to the level crossing gates. At Peel, on the other hand, the huge station building seemed almost deserted.

The railcars backed out and into a siding to drop the van, and to shunt onto another already loaded and waiting in the goods shed. They could not run round in the normal way because the shunting neck was too short for two coaches! By the following year Douglas works had fitted a through brake pipe on one of the "G" vans and this was coupled permanently between the two railcars.

How pleased I was to be joined by a handful of passengers for my return to Douglas. Presumably they were taking advantage of the interchange arrangements whereby rail tickets could also be used for return on the bus, for there would be no train back to Peel that day.

By now the mist had turned to rain and as we climbed to St. John's the railcars slipped to a halt. The driver climbed down and gave the sandbox a hefty clout with a spanner. This evidently cleared the blockage and we were able to start off and crawl towards Douglas, where I was able to cast my eyes for the first time on one of those Beyer beauties — No 12 *Hutchinson*.

Fortunately the powers-that-be had decreed a solitary railcar was not powerful enough to pull its brother and a van over the gradients of the south line, and so they still steamed one of the 2-4-0Ts for the midday train to Port Erin and back.

Despite its inconvenient timing, a few passengers joined me in the two bogie coaches and we eventually set off, providing my first steam ride on the three foot gauge. I was amazed at the speeds attained at times — and

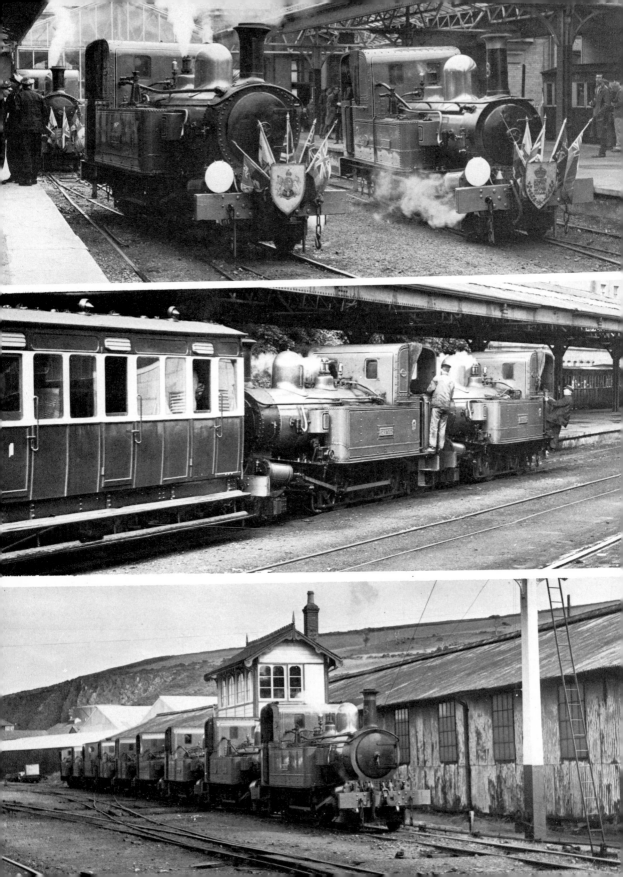

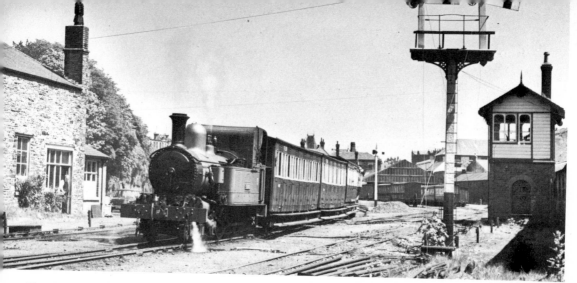

Top: Out of Douglas past a decidedly droopy junction signal comes IOMR No 11 *Maitland* with the 14·05 to Port Erin, in the south-west of the island, on June 14 1968. *G. D. King*

Top left: Three of the IOMR 2-4-0Ts, Nos 8 *Fenella*, 10 *G. M. Wood* and 12 *Hutchinson* were specially decorated for the 1967 re-opening of the Railway on Saturday June 3 and are seen here at the buffer stops at Douglas. *G. W. Morrison*

Centre left: As the 16·34 from Peel rolls into Douglas station on June 22 1968, the firemen of both No 10 *G. M. Wood* and No 11 *Maitland* swing out of their cabs ready to uncouple — an operation often completed before the train finally came to a stand. *G. D. King*

Bottom left: In recent years, spare locomotives have been exhibited at Douglas Station rather than simply left in the shed. Here, No 13 *Kissack* shunts a string of eight sister locomotives — including the solitary 0-6-0T *Caledonia* — back to the shed at the end of the day's operation on July 1 1971. *G. D. King*

at the rough ride. The diesels certainly had many advantages in that respect.

This journey passed uneventfully, except that on the return trip I was joined in my compartment by a Castletown teacher who, it transpired, used the train each day to go home to Douglas.

The rest of my holiday week was spent on the IMR, the Douglas horse trams and the Manx Electric line, where I bought a workman's contract ticket. This entitled me to seven trips from Douglas to Ramsey for 12s 6d and I found I could even fit in a trip

over much of the line after high tea. There was no fear of missing the last train back to Douglas, because the crew changed over wherever the two cars passed!

But fascinating as I found the MER, my heart lay with the steam railway and I vowed to return soon, as I did the following year, 1964, in July when they were operating the "early high season" timetable.

This provided a much busier scene. At St John's, where trains were divided and changed engines, one could see trains from Douglas, Peel and Ramsey arrive within a few minutes of each other — and leave together as well. Steam reigned almost supreme, with the diesel railcars relegated to a solitary return working along the Ramsey line to Kirk Michael (where the railway owned a pleasure park) during the afternoon. Even so, they were invariably packed with passengers and on one occasion a party of Irish nurses sang Irish airs at the top of their voices all the way back to Douglas, bringing back memories of the cars' early days on the County Donegal lines.

Sunday provided another spectacle on the IMR. The only trains of the day made the short run from Douglas along the Peel line to Kirk Braddan, where an open air church service is held.

By 1964 the IMR had this off to a fine art, using a solitary locomotive and the railcars. Two sets of coaches would be standing ready

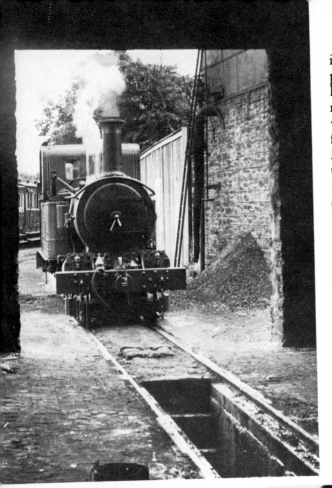

in the Port Erin platforms at Douglas; early passengers would be ushered into the first, the locomotive coupled up and an early start made for Braddan, where the passengers would alight at the ground-level cinder platform. Then the train continued to Union Mills, the next station along the line, where there was a passing loop. The locomotive would run round its train and propel the coaches further along the line towards Peel before returning light engine to Douglas to pick up the now well-filled second train and take the passengers to Braddan. When it reached Union Mills, and while it was running round these coaches, the staff would shut up Douglas station and set out on the railcars, with any late passengers.

At Braddan the railcars waited ahead of the locomotive, which uncoupled and stood a little forward of its coaches, in accordance with IMR Rules and Regulations. The Station Master from Douglas would unlock the little wooden booking hut and put up poster boards by the road inviting passengers to return to Douglas by train for the princely sum of 6d.

After the open air service the railcars filled first and returned to Douglas. Then came the

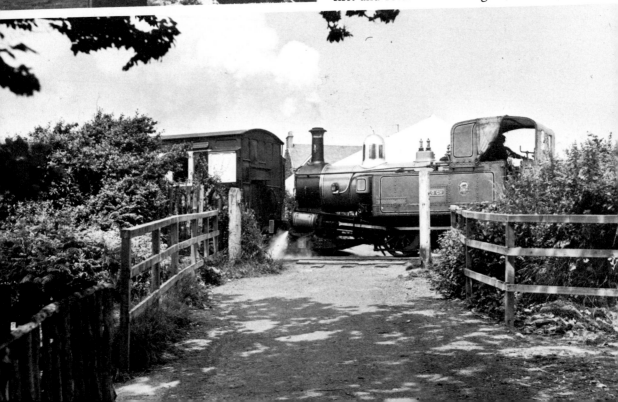

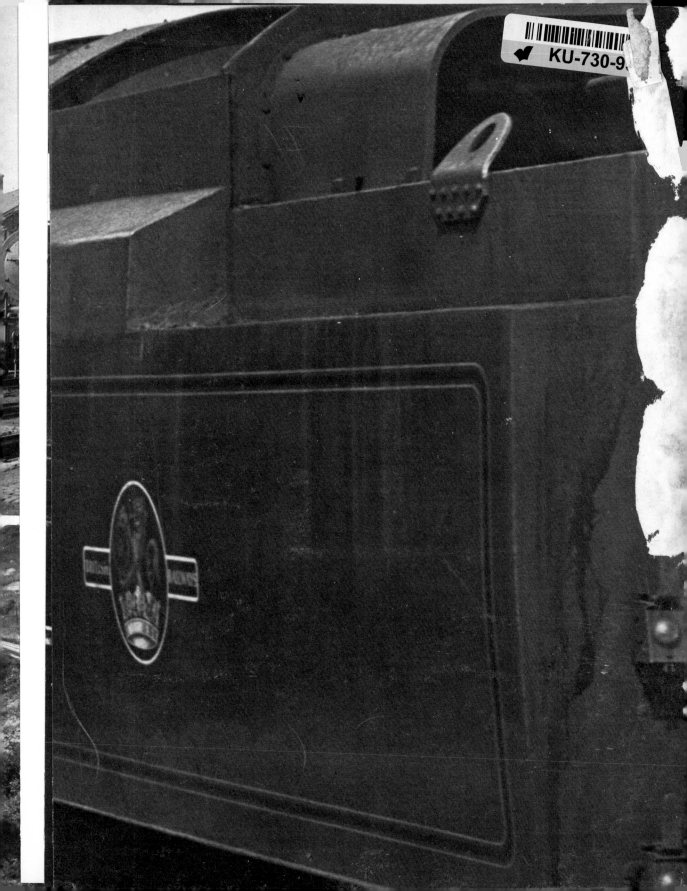

KU-730-9

with the footplate staff; as a result I endured about a week of jocular fame!

Some jobs were aimed strictly at economy. I remember doing masses of calculations as a result of which a reduction was permitted in the minimum size before scrapping of crank axle bearings on the Class 4F 0-6-0s.

Shed Jobs were an interesting detraction from the normal work. In 1935 there was one of those periodic worries about stresses set up in boilers and fireboxes by heating up too fast from cold. Possibly Stanier had seen and disliked the practice at Crewe North Shed which, when pushed for an engine, got it going in an hour from cold by taking fire from the sand-drying furnace and using a separate steam supply for the blower. With this tough procedure the engine would be in steam while the lowest water spaces would still only be tepid. But, so the theory went, with a circulator fitted there would only be a few degrees difference between the hottest and coldest parts throughout heating-up.

Comparative experiments were carried out on Class 4F No. 3994 fitted with a circulator. Other apparatus needed included the portable blower occasionally used in 4 Shed, Derby and an adjacent Class 2P 4-4-0 to supply external steam at 160lb sq in. The portable blower, which fitted down the chimney and stood in for the engine's own blower, had a semi-official status; its use was reckoned to be officially taboo but unofficially tolerated in a genuine crisis. Experiments like this one on No. 3994 tacitly admitted its existence and therefore lent slight official support to its use!

Four tests were carried out, each starting from cold with the normal lighting-up process of firelighters, wood and coal, and subsequent firing as necessary. The results are shown below.

The total amount of coal used was not greatly affected, although of course there was an unmeasured contribution from the "external" steam. The notes on smoke were prompted by the Railway's genuine anxiety about excessive smoke emission, particularly from Sheds near residential areas. Smoke during early-morning lighting-up in cold weather always seemed particularly noisome and sulphurous, and people living nearby did not seem impressed when told that it was mildly disinfectant!

There was a tremendous economy drive in 1935 and as the case for fitting circulators was far from compelling, there the matter rested.

I was "borrowed" from the Works for the first two weeks of October 1934 for work with Dynamometer Car No. 2 (as the 1912 L&Y car was called) on the "Mid-day Scot," testing Royal Scot class 4-6-0 No. 6158 *Loyal Regiment,* with driver Garrett of Crewe North

test condition	time, cold to steam	coal used (cwt/qr)	smoke emission	circulation
normal.	$3\frac{1}{4}$ hrs	4·3	bad	poor
external steam to portable blower.	$1\frac{1}{4}$ hrs	4·1	negligible	very bad
external steam to circulator	$2\frac{1}{2}$ hrs	3·3	bad	excellent
external steam to portable blower and to circulator	$1\frac{1}{4}$ hrs	4·0	negligible	good